Obstructive Sleep Apnea

Diagnosis and Treatment

SLEEP DISORDERS

Obstructive Sleep Apnea

Diagnosis and Treatment

Edited by
Clete A. Kushida
Stanford University
Stanford, California, USA

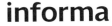
informa
healthcare

New York   London

Informa Healthcare USA, Inc.
52 Vanderbilt Avenue
New York, NY 10017

International Standard Book Number-10: 0-8493-9182-2 (Hardcover)
International Standard Book Number-13: 978-0-8493-9182-8 (Hardcover)

Library of Congress Cataloging-in-Publication Data

Obstructive sleep apnea: Diagnosis and treatment / edited
by Clete A. Kushida.
    p. ; cm. -- (Sleep disorders ; 4)
  Includes bibliographical references and index.
  ISBN-13: 978-0-8493-9182-8 (hb : alk. paper)
  ISBN-10: 0-8493-9182-2 (hb : alk. paper) 1. Sleep apnea syndromes. I. Kushida,
Clete Anthony, 1960- II. Title: Diagnosis and treatment.
III. Series: Sleep disorders (New York, N.Y.) ; 4.
  [DNLM: 1. Sleep Apnea, Obstructive--diagnosis. 2. Sleep Apnea,
Obstructive--therapy.   WF 143 O139 2007]

  RC737.5.O265 2007
  616.2'09--dc22   2007000617

Visit the Informa Web site at
www.informa.com

and the Informa Healthcare Web site at
www.informahealthcare.com

Preface

"When in doubt, pressurize the snout."

—attributal to Philip R. Westbrook

I often thought of this mantra during my on-call nights when, as a Stanford sleep medicine fellow, I was awakened from sleep by a technologist informing me that one of the clinic patients had repetitive obstructive apneas with significant oxygen desaturations. The technologist would typically ask, *"can I start the patient on CPAP?"* Invariably, I would mutter a drowsy "yes," often chiding myself that on the previous day I should have clearly written the respiratory thresholds for starting continuous positive airway pressure on the patient's sleep-study order sheet. This anecdote illustrates the fact that continuous positive airway pressure has become such an important and ubiquitous treatment for obstructive sleep apnea since its development over a quarter century ago. The modern sleep specialist has new diagnostic tools and other treatments, such as upper airway surgery and oral appliances, for patients with obstructive sleep apnea; nevertheless, our field is still in its adolescence with respect to the diagnosis and treatment of obstructive sleep apnea and other sleep disorders.

The reader might wonder why a neurologist is editing a two-volume set of books on obstructive sleep apnea, since it is a sleep-related breathing disorder and would therefore appear to be within the domain of pulmonary physicians. However, besides pulmonologists—neurologists, psychiatrists, internists, pediatricians, and otolaryngologists have entered the field of sleep medicine. Many clinicians now treat patients with sleep disorders on a full-time basis. Sleep medicine has truly become multidisciplinary, and a sleep clinician is expected to diagnose and treat a wide range of sleep disorders, from insomnia to restless legs syndrome, that were previously referred by internists to other specialists.

It is indeed a testament to the ever-increasing knowledge base on obstructive sleep apnea that there is a need for a two-volume set of books on this topic. The first volume, *Obstructive Sleep Apnea: Pathophysiology, Comorbidities, and Consequences* covers the pathophysiology, comorbidities, and consequences of obstructive sleep apnea, with sections exploring the features, factors, and characteristics of this disorder as well as its associations and consequences. This volume focuses on the diagnosis and treatment of obstructive sleep apnea, and includes a section on special conditions, disorders, and clinical issues. The authors and I have tried to conform the conditions and disorders described in this book to the second edition of the *International Classification of Sleep Disorders: Diagnostic & Coding Manual* published by the American Academy of Sleep Medicine in 2006, although some terms, such as obstructive sleep apnea syndrome and sleep-disordered breathing, have been retained in a few statements when appropriate. We have also tried to discuss new entities and findings such as complex sleep apnea, oxidative stress, cyclic alternating pattern, and adaptive servo-ventilation. However, given the rapidity with which the area of sleep medicine is advancing, it is highly conceivable that two volumes might not be sufficient to cover the topic of obstructive sleep apnea in just a few short years!

These books could not exist without the excellent contributions of a talented group of international authors; their detailed and comprehensive works are greatly appreciated. I am deeply indebted to the renowned and true pioneers of our field of sleep, William Dement, Christian Guilleminault, Sonia Ancoli-Israel, Chris Gillin, and Allan Rechtschaffen, who served as my mentors through various stages of my career. In all of my endeavors, I can always count on my parents, Samiko and Hiroshi Kushida, to assist me; these books were no exception. I have been very fortunate to serve, along with Dr. Dement, as Principal Investigator of the multicenter, randomized, double-blind, placebo-controlled Apnea Positive Pressure Long-Term Efficacy Study, sponsored by the National Heart, Lung, and Blood Institute of the National Institutes of Health. To date, this is the largest controlled trial funded by the National Institutes of Health in the field of sleep.

This book is dedicated not only to my parents but also to the marvelous core team of the Apnea Positive Pressure Long-Term Efficacy Study, consisting of William Dement, Pamela Hyde, Deborah Nichols, Eileen Leary, Tyson Holmes, Dan Bloch, as well as National Heart, Lung, and Blood Institute officials (Michael Twery and Gail Weinmann), site directors, coordinators, consultants, committee members, key Stanford site personnel (Chia-Yu Cardell, Rhonda Wong, Pete Silva, Jennifer Blair), Data and Safety Monitoring Board members, and other personnel without whom this project could not have functioned in such a meticulous and efficient manner.

It is my sincere hope that the reader will strive to become expert in the field of sleep. Although there is always room for improvement, awareness of sleep disorders by patients, physicians, and the general public is at an all-time high. However, available funding for sleep research and the number of young investigators interested in a career in basic or clinical sleep research are areas that need enhancement. The interested reader can directly contribute to this field in several ways: applying for membership in the American Academy of Sleep Medicine or Sleep Research Society, serving on committees in these organizations, becoming board certified in sleep medicine, submitting a sleep-related grant proposal to the National Institutes of Health, and/or just simply learning more about sleep and its disorders.

Lastly, etched forever in my memory is a sticker posted on the door of Mary Carskadon's former office at Stanford that contained words to live by: "Be alert. The world needs more lerts."

Clete A. Kushida

Contents

Contributors

Maha Alattar Department of Neurology, University of North Carolina, Chapel Hill, North Carolina, U.S.A.

Mark S. Aloia Butler Hospital, Providence, Rhode Island, U.S.A.

Sonia Ancoli-Israel Department of Psychiatry, University of California, San Diego and Veterans Affairs San Diego Healthcare System, San Diego, California, U.S.A.

Laurent Argaud Emergency and Intensive Care Department, Edouard Herriot Hospital, Lyon, France

Antoine Aschmann Medica Surgical Private Clinics, Mülheim, Germany

Najib T. Ayas Sleep Disorders Program and Respiratory Division, University of British Columbia, Vancouver, British Columbia, Canada

M. Safwan Badr Division of Pulmonary, Allergy, Critical Care, and Sleep Medicine, Wayne State University School of Medicine, Detroit, Michigan, U.S.A.

Robert D. Ballard Advanced Center for Sleep Medicine, Presbyterian/St. Luke's Medical Center, Denver, Colorado, U.S.A.

Richard B. Berry Division of Pulmonary, Critical Care, and Sleep Medicine, University of Florida, Gainesville, Florida, U.S.A.

Meeta H. Bhatt New York University School of Medicine and New York Sleep Institute, New York, New York, U.S.A.

Daniel B. Brown Greenberg Traurig, LLP, Atlanta, Georgia, U.S.A.

Peter R. Buchanan Royal Prince Alfred Hospital, Woolcock Institute of Medical Research and The University of Sydney, Sydney, Australia

Sudhansu Chokroverty Department of Neurology, NJ Neuroscience Institute at JFK Medical Center, Edison, New Jersey and Seton Hall University, South Orange, New Jersey, U.S.A.

Peter A. Cistulli Centre for Sleep Health & Research, Royal North Shore Hospital and The University of Sydney and Woolcock Institute of Medical Research, Sydney, Australia

Nancy A. Collop Division of Pulmonary/Critical Care Medicine, Johns Hopkins University, Baltimore, Maryland, U.S.A.

M. Ali Darendeliler Discipline of Orthodontics, Faculty of Dentistry, The University of Sydney and Department of Orthodontics, Sydney Dental Hospital, Sydney, Australia

William C. Dement Stanford Sleep Research Center, Palo Alto, California, U.S.A.

Julie A. Dopheide   Schools of Pharmacy and Medicine, University of Southern California, Los Angeles, California, U.S.A.

Francesco Fanfulla   Centro di Medicina del Sonno ad indirizzo cardio-respiratorio, Istituto Scientifico di Montescano IRCCS, Fondazione Salvatore Maugeri, Montescano (Pavia), Italy

Lavinia Fiorentino   Department of Psychiatry, University of California, San Diego and Veterans Affairs San Diego Healthcare System, San Diego, California, U.S.A.

Peter C. Gay   Pulmonary, Critical Care, and Sleep Medicine, Mayo Clinic College of Medicine, Rochester, Minnesota, U.S.A.

Charles F. P. George   University of Western Ontario, London Health Sciences Centre, London, Ontario, Canada

Ronald R. Grunstein   Royal Prince Alfred Hospital, Woolcock Institute of Medical Research and The University of Sydney, Sydney, Australia

Jerome E. Hester   Department of Otolaryngology/Head and Neck Surgery, Stanford University Medical Center, Palo Alto, California, U.S.A.

Max Hirshkowitz   Sleep Center, VA Medical Center and Departments of Medicine and Psychiatry, Baylor College of Medicine, Houston, Texas, U.S.A.

Amit Khanna   Department of Family Medicine, Case Western Reserve University, Cleveland, Ohio, U.S.A.

Vidya Krishnan   Division of Pulmonary/Critical Care Medicine, Johns Hopkins University, Baltimore, Maryland, U.S.A.

Scott M. Leibowitz   The Sleep Disorders Center of Cardiac Disease Specialists, Atlanta, Georgia, U.S.A.

Kasey K. Li   Sleep Apnea Surgery Center, East Palo Alto, California, U.S.A.

Michael R. Littner   VA Greater Los Angeles Healthcare System, Sulpulveda, California and David Geffen School of Medicine, University of California, Los Angeles, California, U.S.A.

Alan T. Mulgrew   Sleep Disorders Program and Respiratory Division, University of British Columbia, Vancouver, British Columbia, Canada

Nirav P. Patel   Division of Pulmonary, Critical Care, and Allergy, Center for Sleep & Respiratory Neurobiology, University of Pennsylvania Medical Center, Philadelphia, Pennsylvania, U.S.A.

Rafael Pelayo   Stanford University Center of Excellence for Sleep Disorders, Stanford, California, U.S.A.

Nelson B. Powell   Department of Otolaryngology/Head and Neck Surgery, Stanford University Medical Center and Division of Sleep Medicine, Department of Behavioral Sciences, Stanford School of Medicine, Palo Alto, California, U.S.A.

Rory Ramsey   Division of Pulmonary and Critical Care Medicine, Department of Medicine, Case Western Reserve University, Cleveland, Ohio, U.S.A.

Robert W. Riley   Department of Otolaryngology/Head and Neck Surgery, Stanford University Medical Center and Division of Sleep Medicine, Department of Behavioral Sciences, Stanford School of Medicine, Palo Alto, California, U.S.A.

Dominique Robert   University Claude Bernard and Edouard Herriot Hospital, Lyon, France

Richard J. Schwab   Division of Sleep Medicine, Pulmonary, Allergy, and Critical Care Division; University of Pennsylvania Medical Center, Philadelphia, Pennsylvania, U.S.A.

Donald M. Sesso   Department of Otolaryngology/Head and Neck Surgery, Stanford University Medical Center, Palo Alto, California, U.S.A.

Krista Sigurdson   Sleep Disorders Program and Respiratory Division, University of British Columbia, Vancouver, British Columbia, Canada

Riccardo A. Stoohs   Somnolab Sleep Disorders Centers—Dortmund, Essen, Dortmund, Germany

Kingman P. Strohl   Division of Pulmonary and Critical Care Medicine, Department of Medicine, Case Western Reserve University, Cleveland, Ohio, U.S.A.

Bradley V. Vaughn   Department of Neurology, University of North Carolina, Chapel Hill, North Carolina, U.S.A.

1   History and Physical Examination

Rory Ramsey
Division of Pulmonary and Critical Care Medicine, Department of Medicine,
Case Western Reserve University, Cleveland, Ohio, U.S.A.

Amit Khanna
Department of Family Medicine, Case Western Reserve University, Cleveland,
Ohio, U.S.A.

Kingman P. Strohl
Division of Pulmonary and Critical Care Medicine, Department of Medicine,
Case Western Reserve University, Cleveland, Ohio, U.S.A.

INTRODUCTION

The patient-physician encounter is an inquiry designed to disclose and test disease hypotheses. Physicians detect "cues" early in a patient interview and use them to generate predictions about a disease presence or state. They then ask questions to test the likelihood of hypothesized disease(s) and answers modify perceived probability. This process continues until a reasonable list of potential problems, a differential diagnosis, is shaped and decisions become more explicit. Physicians rely on their own experience, skill, and knowledge base to assign values to the presence or absence of key clinical features.

The purpose of this chapter is to identify those features in sleep history taking that are more likely to assign diagnostic value. The chapter will start by outlining some of the cues that physicians use to direct a general sleep history and then detail the contribution of other elements important in the consideration of obstructive sleep apnea (OSA). A sleep-specific physical examination will then be discussed. Adult and pediatric issues will be compared.

It is important to recognize that there are major limitations in the current literature. To a considerable extent, the recommendations in this chapter result from data from uncontrolled studies, case series, consensus guidelines, practice parameters, and other less rigorous forms of evidence like expert opinion; most of this literature is not focused on how a history and physical help in patient management or outcome. There is an enormous heterogeneity in study design, quality and in populations studied, so that a concordance among studies on the history and physical is difficult to discuss at more than a superficial level. Finally, clinical studies express associations in terms that are not always interchangeable, for example, relative risk (RR), odds ratio (OR), correlation coefficient (r), positive predictive value, likelihood ratio (LR), sensitivity, specificity, and so on. These features led to challenges in producing this review.

Yet, there is value still present in a general medical examination. No features or combination of features are ever fully sensitive and specific for sleep apnea or for sleep problems. A physician–patient encounter should do more than just capture a single suspected diagnosis. The process may involve not only a sleep outcome, but can disclose comorbid conditions and personal issues that could optimize testing and treatment.

MAIN CUES
Excessive Daytime Sleepiness

Excessive daytime sleepiness (EDS) is very common. Epidemiological studies estimate the prevalence to be 8% to 30% in the general population (1–3) depending on the definition of sleepiness and the population sampled. A primary care clinic-based study found that 38.8% experienced wake time tiredness or fatigue at least three to four times per week (4) and a study of sleep clinic patients found 50% complaining of excess sleepiness (5).

EDS is a challenging symptom because of a significant overlap with features of fatigue and the difficulty patients and physicians have in differentiating between the two symptoms. Sleepiness is the tendency to fall asleep, whereas fatigue involves a task context with musculoskeletal and/or neurasthenic qualities. For instance, one author has described fatigue as a drive for rest, and daytime sleepiness as a drive for sleep (6). Sleepiness may occur more often during "passive" conditions, such as watching television or sitting as a passenger in a car; but in its most severe form, sleepiness can intrude into "active" conditions, such as talking to someone or driving a car.

Several instruments have been developed to identify and measure symptoms of EDS (7). Currently, the most useful instrument may be the Epworth sleepiness scale (8). It is a list of eight questions that measure the propensity to sleep in familiar situations and has good test–retest reliability (9).

EDS is not particularly useful in directing one towards the consideration of any one disease. It is, however, very important in the quantification of the problem of sleepiness and should be described in regard to onset, situation, and chronicity. Specifics about functional sleepiness are probably the most useful. It is also important to note that people often underestimate their sleepiness (10). While the differential diagnosis of EDS is wide, sleep-related disorders should be considered early on.

Snoring (See Also Chapter 18)

Community-based studies have estimated that as many 30% to 40% of the general population (2,3,11) snores and others have shown that more than 50% of primary care populations snore (4). Studies from community, primary care, and sleep clinics have all shown a significant relationship between the presence of snoring and sleep apnea (2,4,12–15), and some have incorporated snoring into clinical prediction rules for sleep apnea (4,12–14). While snoring is clearly helpful in suggesting sleep apnea as a diagnostic possibility, its high prevalence in widespread populations impairs its ability to identify real disease. Nevertheless, this symptom should be described in regard to onset, severity, frequency, quality, and chronicity.

Witnessed Apneas/Bed Partner's Reports of Choking or Gasping

Polls have estimated that the prevalence of witnessed apneas in the general adult population ranges from 3.8% to 6% (2,11,16). A primary care population survey found that 11.1% of responders had observed breathing pauses at least one to two times per month (4). Community-, primary care-, and sleep clinic-based studies have all demonstrated a strong relationship between sleep apnea and witnessed apneas or nocturnal choking and several have incorporated these reports into multivariate prediction models for sleep apnea (12,14,17). One community-based study found that the report of apnea increased the odds of sleep apnea nine-fold (2) and another sleep clinic-based study found that it increased the odds 19-fold (18). In the Sleep Heart Health Study, witnessed apneas had the highest prevalence of all collected demographic and predictor variables in patients with an apnea–hypopnea index (AHI) ≥ 15 (15). However, the utility of this report is limited by a low sensitivity as only 9% of these sleep apnea subjects reported this symptom (15). Two additional limitations include the fact that not everyone has a bed partner and people may be poor reporters when it comes to describing respiratory events at night (19).

Insomnia
Insomnia is a repeated difficulty with sleep initiation, duration, consolidation, or quality that occurs despite adequate time and opportunity for sleep and results in some form of daytime impairment (20). Collectively, insomnia encompasses: adequate sleep opportunity, a persistent sleep difficulty, and associated daytime dysfunction. Among adults, insomnia typically manifests as difficulty initiating sleep, maintaining sleep, waking up too early, or sleep that is chronically nonrestorative or poor in quality. When considering adults who experience daytime sleepiness a few days a week versus those who do not, 73% complain of at least one symptom of insomnia, while only 25% carry a diagnosis of a sleep disorder (21). Detailed inquiry regarding the use of sleep aids is important when assessing patients for insomnia.

Sleep Hygiene
Addressing the sleep environment and associated behaviors that revolve around sleep onset are crucial pieces of history when trying to understand the etiology of one's sleep complaints and potential confounding or contributing factors. Understanding the location of one's sleep environment, the nature of temperature, light and sound exposure, and whether or not the bed is shared (i.e., number of persons, pets, etc.) can help address a patient's sleep complaints. Activities prior to bedtime must also be discussed. Ingestions (food, caffeine, alcohol, medications, tobacco, illicit substances) close to bedtime can have varied effects on one's sleep. Stimulating activities prior to bedtime, such as exercise (within 6 hours), television watching, reading, working, music listening, can all affect sleep quality. The location of where such activities are occurring must also be appreciated. Bedtime rituals (i.e., bathing, clothing worn to sleep, etc.) can also enhance one's insight to a patient's sleep complaints.

Sleep-Wake Schedule
Asking the patient for his/her Sleep-Wake schedule is important in demarcating a sleep complaint. Schedule abnormalities in wake and sleep times are clues to the more common sleep disorders (i.e., insomnia and circadian rhythm disorders) and can also be useful in suggesting the presence of other sleep disorders (i.e., narcolepsy and sleep apnea). It can be important to elicit prebedtime rituals, such as caffeinated/acidic foods, prescription/illicit/over-the-counter (OTC)/herbal pharmaceuticals, tobacco, and presleep physical, emotional, or cognitive stimulations. Nocturnal waking behaviors, especially nocturia, are proposed as a clue for sleep apnea (22).

An inquiry would include details on usual bedtime, time to falling asleep (sleep latency), awakenings from sleep (frequency, length, identifiable causes), final wake-up time (naturally; prompted by alarm, pet, or another person), and nap times and nap length. A formal sleep log over several days to weeks can be useful, since there can often be a discrepancy between remembrance reports on the first visit and prospectively recorded events.

Cataplexy

Cataplexy is specifically used in the diagnosis of narcolepsy. Cataplexy refers to a sudden loss of postural tone that is precipitated by the experience of strong emotion. Triggers include joy, sadness, anger, and hilarity. Laughter is the most common trigger (23,24). Cataplexy can manifest in many ways including head nodding, collapsing, dropping an item, and so on. The knees, face, and/or neck are the most common muscle groups involved; oculomotor involvement can also occur, affecting one's vision. Respiratory muscles are not affected by cataplexy. Loss of consciousness is rare (23). Cataplectic events are usually short, ranging from a few seconds to at most several minutes, and recovery is immediate and complete (23). People found to have narcolepsy, however, often carry a variety of other diagnoses such as periodic paralysis, absence seizures, and fugue states, often because the trigger events are not elicited or ignored. Other associated features of narcolepsy include sleep paralysis, hypnagogic hallucinations, and reports of poorly consolidated sleep (described below). These symptoms can however occur, albeit infrequently, in normal patients and isolated symptoms may be present in those with other sleep disorders.

A curious correlation is reported with one's month of birth and increased odds of manifesting narcolepsy. Retrospectively, when 800 birthdates were reviewed from confirmed narcoleptics with cataplexy in North America and Europe, the monthly distribution of birth yielded a peak in March with a maximal OR at 1.45 and a trough in September with a minimal OR at 0.63 (24,25).

Sleep Paralysis

Sleep paralysis is a transient, generalized inability to move or to speak during the transition between sleep and wakefulness. Such experiences can be frightening to the patient, as muscle control is regained within a few minutes. The sensation of being unable to breathe is sometimes perceived. Sleep paralysis is reported in 40% to 80% of narcoleptics, and may occur with sleep deprivation and can be familial (20).

Hypnagogic Hallucinations

Hypnagogic hallucinations are vivid perceptual (visual, tactile, auditory) experiences typically occurring at sleep onset. These experiences are often accompanied by feelings of fear. Recurring themes include being caught in a fire, being attacked, or flying through the air. Recurrent hypnagogic hallucinations are experienced by 40% to 80% of patients with narcolepsy and cataplexy (20).

Movements During Sleep

This class of symptoms can encompass a number of disparate but important entities including restless leg syndrome (RLS), periodic limb movement disorder (PLMD), and parasomnias. RLS is characterized by an irresistible urge to move the legs and is usually accompanied by uncomfortable and unpleasant sensations in the legs (dysesthesias). Spontaneous unpleasant sensations (e.g., "creepy-crawly," "ants marching up my legs") of the limbs occur at rest and are usually relieved by movement. This typical description is extremely suggestive if not diagnostic. RLS is estimated to occur in approximately 2.5% to 15% of the population, with a female predominance, occurring 1.5 to 2 times more commonly in women, and its prevalence increases with age (26–29). Other considerations include conditions such as muscle cramps and myotonic jerks, positional discomfort, hypotensive akathisias, sleep starts (hypnic jerks), neuroleptic-induced akathisias, sleep-related leg cramps, pain associated with arthritis, vascular conditions, injuries, and neuropathy can all mimic RLS to a certain degree.

A majority of patients with RLS also have concomitant periodic limb movements during sleep (PLMS). These PLMS primarily manifest by kicking or jerking leg movements at night, but they can also affect the arms. PLMS can be mistaken as leg kicks that occur around the time of arousal following an apnea or more rarely as a seizure. The individual leg movements that comprise PLMS need to meet specific polysomnographic criteria (i.e., 25% of baseline amplitude, 0.5–5 seconds duration, separated by 4–90 seconds, train of four individual leg movements equals one periodic leg movement) as well as resulting in a clinical sleep disturbance or daytime fatigue in order to meet the criteria for PLMD (20).

For the most part, parasomnias involve complex, seemingly purposeful, and goal-directed behaviors. There are 12 core categories of parasomnias, with only rapid eye movement (REM) sleep behavior disorder (RBD) requiring polysomnographic confirmation for diagnosis (20). Although the remaining 11 categories are clinical diagnoses, coexisting polysomnographic collaboration findings can be very helpful adjuncts at confirming or excluding certain diagnoses. OSA-induced arousals from REM or non-REM (NREM) sleep with complex or violent behaviors may trigger parasomnias, including: RBD, confusional arousals, sleepwalking, and sleep terrors, and sleep-related eating disorder. The differential diagnosis would include nocturnal complex seizures or nocturnal dissociative states. It is suggested that rebound slow-wave sleep with initiation of therapy for sleep apnea could trigger parasomnia phenomena.

SPECIFIC CUES FOR SLEEP APNEA WITH AN EMPHASIS ON ADULT PRESENTATIONS
Demographics
Sleep apnea is a very prevalent disorder in important populations. Epidemiological studies estimate the prevalence to be 2% to 4% in the general population (3,30,31), while other, more selected population studies achieved a prevalence range of 7% to 16% (2,32). Prevalence estimates (and therefore pretest probability) increase in clinical populations due to an enrichment of medical problems. Rates encountered in the primary care or hospital settings are particularly high: primary care (high risk 37.5%) (4), obese 40% to 60% (33), bariatric surgery evaluation 71% to 87% (34,35), hypertension 38% (36), stable outpatient congestive heart failure (CHF) > 50% (37,38), coronary artery disease (CAD) > 50% (39), acute stroke > 70% (40,41), and sleep clinic 67% (29).

In regards to the presentation of sleep apnea, studies show a strong relationship between age and sleep apnea (see also Chapter 16) (15,30,42,43). Duran (2) found that sleep apnea prevalence increased with age with an OR of 2.2 for each 10-year increase. The Sleep Heart Health Study noted that prevalence rose steadily with age up to 60 years at which point a plateau in prevalence occurs around 20% (15). It has also been shown that the severity of sleep apnea (42) and the effect of body mass index (BMI) seem to decrease with age (15,43) and that the magnitude of associations for sleep apnea, snoring, and breathing pauses also decreases with age (15).

Men have a higher prevalence of sleep apnea than women across all ages in epidemiological (3,31,44) and clinic-based studies (see also Chapter 14). This effect diminishes with time, however, and both sexes achieve a similar incidence by age 50 (43). A study of OSA incidence and its risk factors found the risk for sleep apnea in men increased only marginally with age, while it increased very significantly in women: the OR (confidence interval) for increased AHI per 10-year increase was 2.41 in women (1.78–3.26) and only 1.15 (0.78–1.68) in men (43). A study of Hong Kong women found a 12-fold rise in the prevalence of sleep apnea in women between the fourth and sixth decades (31). There is a large amount of literature to support the role of menopause in modulating this increased risk for sleep apnea in women around the age of 50 (44–46). In general, men and women are present with the same constellation of sleep-related symptoms and complications (47). Women with OSA may be slightly older, more obese, more likely to use sedatives, and complain of insomnia and depression (48).

It is not clear if race can be categorically used to confer risk, or if race difference is just a surrogate for a different risk profile. A study of sleep apnea risk factors in the Sleep Heart Health Study did not show a significantly higher prevalence in African-Americans (15) and another did not note any differences in respiratory disturbance index (RDI) when adjusted for known confounders (49). In contrast, a study of older community dwelling adults found that African-Americans had a 2.5 times greater odds of having an AHI > 30 (50), and the Cleveland Family Study found the prevalence of sleep apnea in young African-Americans was higher than that of Caucasians (51).

Studies in Asia estimate the prevalence of sleep apnea to be similar to that of the West (30,31). This is an intriguing finding given that obesity, the risk factor believed to modulate a large part of the risk for sleep apnea in the West, is less common in Asia. Other factors must therefore act in the expression of this disorder. Craniofacial morphology has been implicated as a modifier of risk in nonobese populations but could also interact with obesity as well (52–54).

History of Present Illness

General issues in the presentation would be the age of onset of symptoms as well as some consideration of the trajectory of illness severity. Some of these features are listed in Table 1, and includes features important in both adult and pediatric populations. The pediatric examination is also discussed in a separate section below.

Sleepiness is very common in sleep apnea patients: 38% to 51% in one epidemiological study (55) and 47% to 73% in a sleep clinic population (56). Despite this it is not associated with sleep apnea in clinical studies. This is in large part due to difficulty in differentiating sleep from fatigue. In a study of sleep apnea patients' perception of their problems, lack of energy, tiredness, and fatigue were more prevalent complaints than sleepiness (56).

Snoring is extremely common in sleep apnea patients and its absence should make OSA less likely (13). In one study only 6% of patients with OSA did not report snoring. Keep in mind however, that many patients have misperceptions about their snoring and tend to underestimate it (57). Some studies have shown that a report of "loud" habitual snoring strengthens by seven-fold the statistical association with sleep apnea and snoring (4,15,58). Witnessed apneas are relatively specific for sleep apnea, but have a low sensitivity (15).

Insomnia complaints are highly prevalent in OSA. Fifty-five percent of patients being referred for possible evaluation of OSA were noted to have complaints of insomnia, with difficulties maintaining sleep (38.8%) being more common than

TABLE 1 Features of Emphasis in the Adult and Pediatric Examination

Impact on daytime functioning	Irritability, mood swings, hyperactivity, automatic behaviors, work or academic performance, behavior of concern (inappropriate napping, inattentiveness), absences from work or school
Sleep/wake schedules	Usual bedtime, fall asleep time, wake time, napping habits, weekday/weekend variations
Customs surrounding sleep	Presleep routines and related transitional objects (television, pacifier, toy, etc.)
Sleep environment	Shared or private room, bed partners (including pets/toys/stuffed animals); electronics or other toys that may impede sleep routines; persistence or resolution of sleep complaints in other environments (hotels, sleepovers, etc.)
Body position(s) during sleep	Side sleeping and/or neck hyperextension to relieve obstruction
Exposures	Caffeinated beverages, tobacco products, recreational drugs
Other sleep behaviors	Snoring, witnessed apneas, paradoxical breathing, mouth breathing with dry mouth and throat, morning headaches, gastroesophageal reflux, sweating (may suggest increased work of breathing), stereotypic movements/complaints suggestive of seizure or movement disorders (including parasomnias and restless legs syndrome)

difficulties initiating sleep (33.4%) or early morning awakenings (31.4%). Despite the overall high prevalence of insomnia complaints in this study population, insomnia was more common in patients without rather than with significant sleep-disordered breathing (81.5% with AHI < 10 vs. 51.7% with AHI > 10) (59). The high prevalence of insomnia complaints may be attributable to the fact that the sleep disruption associated with OSA may be perceived as insomnia, or perhaps such patients with insomnia and OSA are more symptomatic, thus more likely to seek medical attention.

Weight gain increases the probability of sleep apnea. One large population-based study found a 10% weight gain and predicted a 32% increase in AHI. This translated to a six-fold increase in the odds of developing (moderate-to-severe) sleep apnea (32). Inversely, a decrease in weight leads to an improvement in sleep apnea. Studies in bariatric surgery patients show a dramatic improvement in RDI after weight loss (35,60).

Frequent awakening from sleep to urinate is common in sleep apnea patients. One retrospective study found a prevalence of 49% in sleep apnea patients (61) and others have noted frequent nocturia is related to sleep apnea severity (61–63).

Nocturnal angina may be related to apneas in some patients with ischemic heart disease and sleep-disordered breathing. Small series in patients with ischemic heart disease and relatively severe sleep apnea suggested a link between myocardial ischemia and apneas (64,65). However, these findings conflict with a larger study that included patients with less severe sleep apnea and failed to appreciate a significant association (66).

Past Medical History

OSA will coexist with other sleep disorders. A retrospective analysis of 643 OSA patients found that 31% had another sleep disorder: 14.5% had poor sleep hygiene and 8.1% had PLMD (67). In two other studies more than 50% of sleep apnea patients complained of insomnia (59,68).

Sleep apnea is not only associated with cardiovascular disease but may directly contribute to its pathogenesis. It was present in 38% of hypertensive subjects in one study (36). A dose–response relationship is present (69) and several trials found a small but significant improvement in hypertension with sleep apnea treatment (70–72). Others suggest that the prevalence of sleep apnea in patients with CAD, postmyo-cardial infarction, CHF, and poststroke to be > 50% (37–41). Results from the Sleep Heart Health Study show increasing odds of self-reported heart failure, stroke, and CAD in subjects with a high AHI (73). Additionally, a pathogenic role is suggested by observational studies that show fewer adverse cardiovascular outcomes in treated versus untreated patients (74–76).

Several studies have found that sleep apnea is independently associated with glucose intolerance and insulin resistance (33,77). The Sleep Heart Health Study found that patients with mild and moderate/severe OSA had increased adjusted ORs for fasting glucose intolerance: 1.27 (0.98, 1.64) and 1.46 (1.09, 1.97), respectively (77). At least one treatment study has found improvement in glucose control in patients treated for sleep apnea (78).

Depression is linked to sleep apnea in a number of correlation studies. Most are small, use different instruments to measure depression, and indicate that 24% to 58% of sleep apnea patients have some measure of depression (79,80). In a larger European telephonic survey, 17.6% with a Diagnostic and Statistical Manual of Mental Disorders (DSM-IV) breathing-related sleep disorder also had a diagnosis of a major depressive disorder (81).

Sleep apnea in the setting of pulmonary diseases is called the "overlap syndrome." Chronic obstructive pulmonary disease is the most common of these, but has a prevalence in the sleep apnea population similar to that of the general population (82). Pulmonary arterial hypertension is another disease but is much less common and the prevalence of sleep apnea in these patients is not well studied (83).

Hypothyroidism symptoms of fatigue can overlap with those of sleep apnea. Case series have reported improvement or resolution of sleep apnea in selected patients treated with thyroxine alone (84). Nonetheless, the limited evidence available suggests the prevalence of hypothyroidism in sleep apnea patients is no different than that seen in the general population (85) and routine screening in the absence of other signs of hypothyroidism is not cost-effective. Cases have also described lingual thyroids causing airways obstruction at night (86).

Glaucoma (87), end-stage renal disease (88,89), and gastroesophageal reflux disease (90,91) have been reported to occur with OSA, but the specificity of the asso-ciations are not established.

The occurrence of sleep disturbances during pregnancy is well documented, but the prevalence and incidence of specific sleep disorders is not confirmed in large-scale population studies. A spectrum of association between pregnancy and sleep disturbances ranges from an increased incidence of excessive sleepiness, insom-nia, nocturnal awakenings, and parasomnias (especially restless legs syndrome) to snoring, and both obstructive and central sleep apnea (92). Although specific sleep disorders tend to emerge during different stages of pregnancy, the third trimester appears to be the most vulnerable. Of special attention are those women who gain excessive weight during pregnancy. Thus, during routine perinatal obstetrical care, the sleep history should be periodically revisited.

Social History

Sleep apnea significantly worsens after heavy alcohol ingestion (93,94). The effect of more moderate levels of alcohol ingestion on sleep apnea are not as clear and results are conflicting (95,96). Some proposed mechanisms include increased nasal resistance due to edema, and reduced hypoglossus motor nerve activity.

Data from the Wisconsin Sleep Cohort Study found current smokers to have an increased risk of having moderate sleep apnea compared to nonsmokers (OR 4.44). Heavy smokers had the higher risk (OR 40.47) (97). One sleep clinic study found current smokers to have increased adjusted odds of sleep apnea [OR 2.5, confidence interval (CI) 1.3–4.7, $p = 0.0049$] (98).

Family History

The Cleveland Family Study found that there is a familial aggregation to sleep apnea. Families with an index case of sleep apnea had a higher prevalence of sleep apnea than in those without (21% vs. 9%, $p = 0.02$) and risk increased with additional affected members (99). Ongoing genetic studies are trying to find the relative role of different anatomical risk factors in mediating this increased risk. At the present time routine assessment and testing of family members is not advocated in the absence of clinical illness.

The sleepiness and lack of concentration that accompanies sleep apnea impair work performance, driving ability (100,101) and have deleterious effects on family relationships. Commercial drivers are a special group that is receiving an increasing amount of attention, as driving risk becomes a public safety issue. Moreno et al. (102) administered the Berlin questionnaire to a large group of truck drivers and found that 26% were at high risk for sleep apnea; however, the presence of inactivity and obesity were also strongly implicated in this pretest probability estimate.

Medication History

There is an accounting of medication use for sleep apnea in Chapter 17. In general, medications to note during the history and physical fall into three categories: (*i*) those that are associated with OSA, (*ii*) those that sedate and/or decrease respiratory drive, and (*iii*) those that impair sleep onset or maintenance (Table 2).

Drug-induced sleepiness is the most commonly reported side effect of central nervous system active pharmacological agents; the 1990 Drug Interactions and Side Effects Index of the Physicians' Desk Reference lists drowsiness as a side effect of 584 prescription or OTC preparations (103).

Allergies

Nasal obstruction contributes to the worsening of sleep-disordered breathing, but the extent to which this might be related to allergic rhinitis is not known. One case-control study did show that sleep apnea patients had a higher rate of perennial allergic rhinitis and atopy than controls (104).

THE PHYSICAL EXAMINATION FOR ADULT SLEEP APNEA

A sleep physical examination is directed at modifying the probability of sleep-disordered breathing based on the history, looking for evidence of associated or complicating disease, and excluding other potential causes for neurologic or cardio-vascular symptoms. A broader examination incorporating many of the other organ systems should be employed when considering other sleep disorders that may be caused by or confounded by other diagnoses.

TABLE 2 Medications as Clues to Predisposing Factors

Medications associated with OSA	Medications that sedate and/or reduce respiratory drive	Medications that impair sleep onset or maintenance
Barbiturates	Alpha-blockers	Adrenocorticotropin and
Benzodiazepines	Anticonvulsants	corticosteroids
Ethanol, illicit narcotics	Antidiarrheal agents	Alpha-agonists
Hypertensive and diabetic	Antiemtics	Anticholesterol agents
treatments	Antihistamines	Anticonvulsants
	Antimuscarinic	Antineoplastic agents
	Antipsychotics	Appetite suppressants
	Antispasmotics	Atypical antidepressants
	Antitussives	Benzodiazepines
	Anxiolytics	Beta-blockers
	Atypical antidepressants	Caffeine, nicotine, ethanol,
	Barbituates	illicit narcotics
	Benzodiazepines	Decongestants
	Beta-blockers	Diuretics
	Dopaminergics	Dopaminergics
	Diphenhydramine, phenylhydramine	Monoamine oxidase inhibitors
	Ethanol, illicit narcotics	NSAIDs
	Genitourinary smooth muscle	Opiates
	relaxants	Oral contraceptives
	Hydantoins	Pemoline, dextroampheta-
	Melatonin receptor agonists	mines, methylphenidates
	Monoamine oxidase inhibitors	Progesterone
	Muscle relaxants	Pseudoephedrine, ephedrine,
	Nonbenzodiazepine hypnotics	phenylpropanolamine
	Opiate agonists	Quinidine
	Selective serotonin reuptake	Quinolone antibiotics
	inhibitors	Theophylline, albuterol,
	Succinimides	ipratropium, terbutaline,
	Tricyclic antidepressants	salmeterol, metaproterenol,
	Valerian root, kava kava, melatonin,	xanthine derivatives
	chamomile, passiflora	Thyroid supplements
		Tranquilizers

Abbreviations: NSAIDs, nonsteroidal anti-inflammatory drugs; OSA, obstructive sleep apnea.

Blood Pressure

Many population-based studies have shown that hypertension is independently associated with sleep-disordered breathing studies (105–110). Blood pressure has been integrated into several clinical prediction rules for sleep apnea (4,12,17,18). One study found hypertension to have an adjusted OR of 11.9 for an AHI ≥ 30 (17). More recently, a causal relationship has been suggested by a number of studies that have shown an improvement in hypertension with sleep apnea treatment (70–72).

Obesity

Although a number of different measures of obesity have been used in clinical studies the BMI is probably the best and certainly the most practical. It has been found to be strongly associated with the presence of sleep apnea (4,12–15,18,108,111–115) and has been incorporated into a number of clinical prediction rules (4,13,14,18) for this disorder (see also Chapter 2).

Neck Circumference

Neck circumference is, in part, a surrogate for obesity but clinical studies have also found an independent association with sleep apnea (12,15,113,114), and one study has incorporated it into a multivariate clinical prediction rule for sleep apnea (12). One epidemiological study found the OR for an AHI $\geq$ 15 with an increment of one standard deviation (SD) in neck circumference to be 1.5 (15).

Nasal Function

Nasal obstruction has been implicated as a potential cause of sleep apnea. It can lead to higher inspiratory upper airway pressures and increased collapsibility of pharyngeal walls (116). Also, it appears to predispose to mouth breathing and the downward and backward displacement of the mandible (111), which may worsen airway obstruction at the level of the base of the tongue. Nasal resistance, as measured by posterior rhinometry, was significantly higher in patients with sleep apnea (115). A combination of nasal obstruction and a high Mallampati score (3 or 4; see below) are associated with an increased risk for the diagnosis of sleep apnea (RR 2.45, CI 1.23–4.84) (113). In this latter study, obstruction was measured by having the patient gently block one nostril, breathe through the other and having the physician listen for evidence of obstruction.

The external nasal valve comprises the columella, the nasal floor, and the nasal rim [inferior border of the lower lateral alae nasi (nasal cartilage)], which normally is dilated by the nasalis muscle during inspiration. Collapse of the nasal rim upon inspiration through the nose alone, is also often a sign of OSA-associated nasal resistance (Fig. 1).

Pharyngeal and Craniofacial Features

Pharyngeal and craniofacial morphology play an important role in the etiology of sleep apnea. Some anatomical variants result in a crowded oropharyngeal space

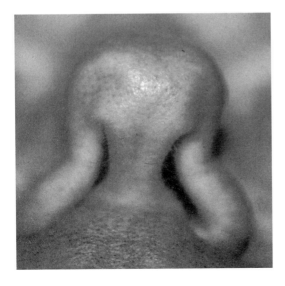

FIGURE 1 (*See color insert.*) Bilateral collapse of the nasal rim that is frequently observed during inspiration in patients with obstructive sleep apnea-associated nasal resistance. *Source*: Photograph courtesy of Kannan Ramar, M.D.

Class 1   Class 2   Class 3   Class 4

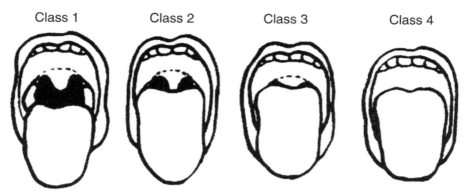

FIGURE 2 Mallampati classification system based on visualization of posterior oropharyngeal structures. *Class 1*, soft palate, fauces, uvula, anterior and posterior pillars visible; *Class 2*, soft palate, fauces and uvula visible; *Class 3*, soft palate and base of uvula visible; *Class 4*, soft palate not visible.

and predispose to obstruction during sleep. Many clinical studies have taken different measures of pharyngeal and craniofacial morphology and found associations between them and the presence of sleep apnea. Their utility however, has been notably impaired by their lack of simplicity and practicality at the bedside.

One measure used in the assessment is the Mallampati score (Fig. 2). Designed originally by anesthetists to grade intubation difficulty, the Mallampati grade correlated well with the severity of RDI: $r = 0.34$, $p < 0.001$ (117). In another study comparing apneic versus nonapneic patients, sleep apnea patients more often had a Mallampati score of 3 or 4 (78.8% vs. 46%, $p < 0.001$) (112).

Two other pharyngeal measurements that were independently associated with sleep apnea: tonsillar enlargement (OR 2.6) and lateral narrowing of the pharyngeal wall (OR 2.0) (Fig. 3) (118). Other potentially useful pharyngeal measures include tongue size (118), uvula size (118,119), and palatal height (112,114). "Scalloping" or dental impressions at the edge of the tongue may indicate the presence of an enlarged tongue that habitually presses against the teeth.

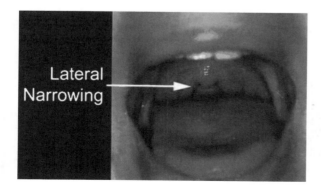

FIGURE 3 (*See color insert.*) Lateral narrowing of the pharyngeal wall. *Source*: Photograph courtesy of Kannan Ramar, M.D.

Retrognathia, micrognathia, and overbite (120) are craniofacial features that capture jaw factors that are associated with a restricted posterior pharynx. These are recognized qualitatively by noting the relative size of the jaw to the maxilla, forward protrusion of the upper teeth over the lower teeth, and absent lower teeth that were surgically removed due to crowding. Quantitative measures of these features are typically obtained by cephalometric radiographs and may be useful in modifying disease probability.

Other Features in the Examination

There is no intention of ignoring other features of the physical examination, as no one feature or collection of findings is ever fully sensitive and specific for sleep apnea and since the physician-patient encounter is designed to do more than just capture a suspected diagnosis. A respiratory, cardiovascular, and neurologic examination can contribute to the sleep workup. A normal neurological examination is particularly important in a patient suspected of having restless legs syndrome and/or PLMD with an emphasis on spinal cord and peripheral nerve function. Similarly, a normal peripheral vascular examination would exclude pathology that might be mistaken for restless legs syndrome.

THE EXAMINATION OF THE PEDIATRIC PATIENT

Sleep complaints or disorders occur in 1% to 28% of the pediatric population (121–123) (More information on the examination of the pediatric patient can be found in Chapter 15.). The incidence of OSA in children can range from 1% to 10%, while snoring can occur in 3% to 12% (123–126). These studies often emphasize the idea that the presentation of sleep disorders in children is different from those in adults. While this literature is interesting, for the purposes of this chapter, the basic elements of the history and physical have limitations in regard to common measures and approaches from which to make firm evidence-based conclusions.

One issue is relatively clear however. Children, with the possible exception of those who are obese, less commonly present with EDS (127). Rather, they present with a failure to thrive, attention and behavior problems, and show impaired academic performance. Thus, the approach and the thresholds for clinical suspicion of sleep disorders differ somewhat in the pediatric population.

History Taking

It is crucial that an appropriate historian (parent, guardian or other adult caregiver) is involved in the diagnostic process. A substantial proportion of pediatric sleep disorders involve psychosocial issues that can only be assessed by talking with the primary caregiver, and the value of teacher input is emphasized in this literature as well. The parent-child interaction should be observed closely for clues to extrinsic problems, such as sleep-onset association, limit setting disorder, or child maltreatment syndrome (126).

An age-appropriate history should be obtained. Certain elements stressed or elaborated on during a pediatric sleep-related history are similar to adults, while others are not (Table 1). As with the adult patient, features of the age of onset, degree of severity/stability, and frequency of the patient's sleep complaint, as well as responses to any attempts at treating the problem can give clues. Any new daytime or nocturnal symptoms or signs can also provide information; for instance, new-onset enuresis in a child can indicate a sleep disorder like sleep apnea. Occasionally, a child is recognized with a sleep disorder during a family vacation when there is greater opportunity for parents to observe children while sharing hotel rooms. Home-video footage both of waking and sleep behaviors can also provide invaluable information, if available.

Physical Examination

Routine key vital statistics include blood pressure, respiratory rate, heart rate, height, weight, age-appropriate BMI (for children with OSA can be either too thin or too heavy), and their position (relative population-based percentile standing) on age-appropriate growth charts.

A thorough examination would include mention of the child's general appearance and craniofacial characteristics such as midface hypoplasia, micrognathia, and occlusal relationships. In infants, septal deviation, choanal atresia, nasolacrimal cysts, and nasal aperture stenosis must be excluded, while in older children, nasal polyps and turbinate hypertrophy must be considered as a cause for upper airway obstruction (128).

Adenotonsillar hypertrophy is a common finding not only in the general pediatric population but in pediatric OSA patients as well. Oral assessment includes screening for signs of mouth breathing, tissue redundancy, and cleft lip/palate, as well as evaluation of tongue size, dentition, and tonsillar grading, including Mallampati staging (Fig. 2). Consideration for adenoid assessment with lateral neck radiography or nasopharyngoscopic examination can also be helpful.

Neuromuscular disorders, such as myotonic dystrophy, can be associated with chronic obstructive hypoventilation from a combination of oropharyngeal muscle weakness that leads to airway collapse and hypoventilation from diminished respiratory muscle excursion (126). Hoarseness of the voice, decreased gag reflex, and abnormal tendon reflexes could be clues to brainstem abnormalities, such as Chiari malformation (129).

Congenital craniofacial syndromes are associated with OSA. Children who have syndromes with craniosynostosis, such as Apert's syndrome, Crouzon's disease, Pfeiffer's syndrome, and Saethre-Chotzen syndrome; abnormalities of the skull base; and accompanying maxillary hypoplasia may have nasopharyngeal obstruction (126). Children with syndromes that involve micrognathia, such as Treacher Collins syndrome, Pierre Robin syndrome, and Goldenhar's syndrome, become obstructed at the hypopharyngeal level; and children with trisomy 21 often have a narrow upper airway combined with macroglossia and hypotonic musculature predisposing them to OSA (126).

CONCLUSIONS

The clinical evaluation for a patient being evaluated for presumed OSA represents an essential first step in the diagnosis of this common sleep disorder. The primary care physician or sleep specialist needs to inquire about the key symptoms of sleep apnea, such as EDS, snoring, and witnessed sleep-disordered breathing symptoms; other important symptoms or practices that affect the patient's sleep such as insomnia, sleep hygiene, and the patient's Sleep-Wake schedule also need to be assessed. Symptoms of other sleep disorders, such as those associated with narcolepsy, restless legs syndrome, PLMD, and parasomnias should be ruled out as possible contributors to the patient's sleep complaints. The experienced clinician should be aware of the high prevalence of sleep apnea; the relationships between this disorder and age, gender, and ethnicity; and the more complex associations including those between OSA and cardiovascular disease, glucose intolerance and insulin resistance, depression, pulmonary disease, and hypothyroidism. A careful evaluation of the patient's social, family, medication, and allergy history is critical for identifying or discounting possible risk factors for sleep apnea. The physical examination for adult patients with suspected OSA should be comprehensive, and should include assessment of blood pressure, indicators of obesity (e.g., BMI, neck circumference), nasal function, pharyngeal, and craniofacial features. Lastly, the examinations of pediatric versus adult patients with suspected OSA are not identical, since the presentation, symptoms, and physical signs associated with childhood OSA are markedly distinct from those associated with adult OSA.

REFERENCES

1. Bixler EO, Vgontzas AN, Lim HM, et al. Excessive daytime sleepiness in a general population sample: the role of sleep apnea, age, obesity, diabetes, and depression. J Clin Endocrinol Metab 2005; 90(8):4510–4515.
2. Duran J, Esnaola S, Rubio R, et al. Obstructive sleep apnea-hypopnea and related clinical features in a population-based sample of subjects aged 30 to 70 yr. Am J Respir Crit Care Med 2001; 163(3 Pt 1):685–689.
3. Young T, Palta M, Dempsey J, et al. The occurrence of sleep-disordered breathing among middle-aged adults. N Engl J Med 1993; 328(17):1230–1235.
4. Netzer NC, Stoohs RA, Netzer CM, et al. Using the Berlin questionnaire to identify patients at risk for the sleep apnea syndrome. Ann Intern Med 1999; 131(7):485–491.
5. Seneviratne U, Puvanendran K. Excessive daytime sleepiness in obstructive sleep apnea: prevalence, severity, and predictors. Sleep Med 2004; 5(4):339–343.
6. Roth T. Excessive sleepiness: What it means for us all. Consultant 2006; February (suppl):2–4.
7. Pigeon WR, Sateia MJ, Ferguson RJ. Distinguishing between excessive daytime sleepiness and fatigue: toward improved detection and treatment. J Psychosom Res 2003; 54(1):61–69.
8. Johns MW. A new method for measuring daytime sleepiness: the Epworth sleepiness scale. Sleep 1991; 14(6):540–545.
9. Sleep-related breathing disorders in adults: recommendations for syndrome definition and measurement techniques in clinical research. The Report of an American Academy of Sleep Medicine Task Force. Sleep 1999; 22(5):667–689.
10. Engleman HM, Hirst WS, Douglas NJ. Under reporting of sleepiness and driving impairment in patients with sleep apnoea/hypopnoea syndrome. J Sleep Res 1997; 6(4):272–275.
11. Ohayon MM, Guilleminault C, Priest RG, et al. Snoring and breathing pauses during sleep: telephone interview survey of a United Kingdom population sample. BMJ 1997; 314(7084):860–863.
12. Flemons WW, Whitelaw WA, Brant R, et al. Likelihood ratios for a sleep apnea clinical prediction rule. Am J Respir Crit Care Med 1994; 150(5 Pt 1):1279–1285.
13. Viner S, Szalai JP, Hoffstein V. Are history and physical examination a good screening test for sleep apnea? Ann Intern Med 1991 115(5):356–359.
14. Maislin G, Pack AI, Kribbs NB, et al. A survey screen for prediction of apnea. Sleep 1995; 18(3):158–166.
15. Young T, Shahar E, Nieto FJ, et al. Predictors of sleep-disordered breathing in community-dwelling adults: the Sleep Heart Health Study. Arch Intern Med 2002; 162(8):893–900.
16. Teculescu DB, Hannhart B, Benamghar L, et al. Witnessed breathing pauses during sleep: a study in middle-aged French males. Respir Med 2005; 99(10):1268–1274.

17. Martinez Garcia MA, Soler Cataluna JJ, Roman Sanchez P, et al. Clinical predictors of sleep apnea-hypopnea syndrome susceptible to treatment with continuous positive airway pressure. Arch Bronconeumol 2003; 39(10):449–454.
18. Crocker BD, Olson LG, Saunders NA, et al. Estimation of the probability of disturbed breathing during sleep before a sleep study. Am Rev Respir Dis 1990; 142(1):14–18.
19. Haponik EF, Smith PL, Meyers DA, et al. Evaluation of sleep-disordered breathing. Is polysomnography necessary? Am J Med 1984; 77(4):671–677.
20. The International Classification of Sleep Disorders: Diagnostic and Coding Manual. 2nd ed. Westchester, IL: American Academy of Sleep Medicine, 2005.
21. Foley D, Ancoli-Israel S, Britz P, et al. Sleep disturbances and chronic disease in older adults: results of the 2003 National Sleep Foundation Sleep in America Survey. J Psychosom Res 2004; 56(5):497–502.
22. Chasens ER, Umlauf MG. Nocturia: a problem that disrupts sleep and predicts obstructive sleep apnea. Geriatr Nurs 2003; 24(2):76–81,105.
23. Gelb M, Guilleminault C, Kraemer H, et al. Stability of cataplexy over several months—information for the design of therapeutic trials. Sleep 1994; 17(3):265–273.
24. Okun ML, Lin L, Pelin Z, et al. Clinical aspects of narcolepsy–cataplexy across ethnic groups. Sleep 2002; 25(1):27–35.
25. Dauvilliers Y, Carlander B, Molinari N, et al. Month of birth as a risk factor for narcolepsy. Sleep 2003; 26(6):663–665.
26. Phillips B, Hening W, Britz P, et al. Prevalence and correlates of restless legs syndrome: results from the 2005 national sleep foundation poll. Chest 2006; 129(1):76–80.
27. Allen RP, Walters AS, Montplaisir J, et al. Restless legs syndrome prevalence and impact: REST general population study. Arch Intern Med 2005; 165(11):1286–1292.
28. Allen RP, Earley CJ. Restless legs syndrome: a review of clinical and pathophysiologic features. J Clin Neurophysiol 2001; 18(2):128–147.
29. Punjabi NM, Welch D, Strohl K. Sleep disorders in regional sleep centers: a national cooperative study. Coleman II Study Investigators. Sleep 2000; 23(4):471–480.
30. Ip MS, Lam B, Lauder IJ, et al. A community study of sleep-disordered breathing in middle-aged Chinese men in Hong Kong. Chest 2001; 119(1):62–69.
31. Ip MS, Lam B, Tang LC, et al. A community study of sleep-disordered breathing in middle-aged Chinese women in Hong Kong: prevalence and gender differences. Chest 2004; 125(1):127–134.
32. Peppard PE, Young T, Palta M, et al. Longitudinal study of moderate weight change and sleep-disordered breathing. JAMA 2000; 284(23):3015–3021.
33. Punjabi NM, Sorkin JD, Katzel LI, et al. Sleep-disordered breathing and insulin resistance in middle-aged and overweight men. Am J Respir Crit Care Med 2002; 165(5):677–682.
34. Frey WC, Pilcher J. Obstructive sleep-related breathing disorders in patients evaluated for bariatric surgery. Obes Surg 2003; 13(5):676–683.
35. Rasheid S, Banasiak M, Gallagher SF, et al. Gastric bypass is an effective treatment for obstructive sleep apnea in patients with clinically significant obesity. Obes Surg 2003; 13(1):58–61.
36. Worsnop CJ, Naughton MT, Barter CE, et al. The prevalence of obstructive sleep apnea in hypertensives. Am J Respir Crit Care Med 1998; 157(1):111–115.
37. Javaheri S, Parker TJ, Liming SD, et al. Sleep apnea in 81 ambulatory male patients with stable heart failure. Types and their prevalences, consequences, and presentations. Circulation 1998; 97(21):2154–2159.
38. Javaheri S, Parker TJ, Wexler L, et al. Occult sleep-disordered breathing in stable congestive heart failure. Ann Intern Med 1995; 122(7):487–492.
39. Andreas S, Schulz R, Werner GS, et al. Prevalence of obstructive sleep apnoea in patients with coronary artery disease. Coron Artery Dis 1996; 7(7):541–545.
40. Dyken ME, Somers VK, Yamada T, et al. Investigating the relationship between stroke and obstructive sleep apnea. Stroke 1996; 27(3):401–407.
41. Turkington PM, Bamford J, Wanklyn P, et al. Prevalence and predictors of upper airway obstruction in the first 24 hours after acute stroke. Stroke 2002; 33(8):2037–2042.
42. Bixler EO, Vgontzas AN, Ten Have T, et al. Effects of age on sleep apnea in men: I. Prevalence and severity. Am J Respir Crit Care Med 1998; 157(1):144–148.

43. Tishler PV, Larkin EK, Schluchter MD, et al. Incidence of sleep-disordered breathing in an urban adult population: the relative importance of risk factors in the development of sleep-disordered breathing. JAMA 2003; 289(17):2230–2237.
44. Bixler EO, Vgontzas AN, Lim HM, et al. Prevalence of sleep-disordered breathing in women: effects of gender. Am J Respir Crit Care Med 2001; 163(3 Pt 1):608–613.
45. Young T, Finn L, Austin D, et al. Menopausal status and sleep-disordered breathing in the Wisconsin Sleep Cohort Study. Am J Respir Crit Care Med 2003; 167(9):1181–1185.
46. Resta O, Bonfitto P, Sabato R, et al. Prevalence of obstructive sleep apnoea in a sample of obese women: effect of menopause. Diabetes Nutr Metab 2004; 17(5):296–303.
47. Young T, Hutton R, Finn L, et al. The gender bias in sleep apnea diagnosis. Are women missed because they have different symptoms? Arch Intern Med 1996; 156(21):2445–2451.
48. Quintana-Gallego E, Carmona-Bernal C, Capote F, et al. Gender differences in obstructive sleep apnea syndrome: a clinical study of 1166 patients. Respir Med 2004; 98(10):984–989.
49. Scharf SM, Seiden L, Demore J, et al. Racial differences in clinical presentation of patients with sleep-disordered breathing. Sleep Breath 2004; 8(4):173–183.
50. Ancoli-Israel S, Klauber MR, Stepanowsky C, et al. Sleep-disordered breathing in African-American elderly. Am J Respir Crit Care Med 1995; 152(6 Pt 1):1946–1949.
51. Redline S. Epidemiology of sleep-disordered breathing. Semin Respir Crit Care Med 1998; 19:113–122.
52. Kubota Y, Nakayama H, Takada T, et al. Facial axis angle as a risk factor for obstructive sleep apnea. Intern Med 2005; 44(8):805–810.
53. Ito D, Akashiba T, Yamamoto H, et al. Craniofacial abnormalities in Japanese patients with severe obstructive sleep apnoea syndrome. Respirology 2001; 6(2):157–161.
54. Li KK, Powell NB, Kushida C, et al. A comparison of Asian and white patients with obstructive sleep apnea syndrome. Laryngoscope 1999; 109(12):1937–1940.
55. Kapur VK, Baldwin CM, Resnick HE, et al. Sleepiness in patients with moderate to severe sleep-disordered breathing. Sleep 2005; 28(4):472–477.
56. Chervin RD. Sleepiness, fatigue, tiredness, and lack of energy in obstructive sleep apnea. Chest 2000; 118(2):372–379.
57. Hoffstein V, Mateika S, Anderson D. Snoring: is it in the ear of the beholder? Sleep 1994; 17(6):522–526.
58. Kripke DF, Ancoli-Israel S, Klauber MR, et al. Prevalence of sleep-disordered breathing in ages 40–64 years: a population-based survey. Sleep 1997; 20(1):65–76.
59. Krell SB, Kapur VK. Insomnia complaints in patients evaluated for obstructive sleep apnea. Sleep Breath 2005; 9(3):104–110.
60. Buchwald H, Avidor Y, Braunwald E, et al. Bariatric surgery: a systematic review and meta-analysis. JAMA 2004; 292(14):1724–1737.
61. Hajduk IA, Strollo PJ Jr, Jasani RR, et al. Prevalence and predictors of nocturia in obstructive sleep apnea-hypopnea syndrome—a retrospective study. Sleep 2003; 26(1):61–64.
62. Umlauf MG, Chasens ER, Greevy RA, et al. Obstructive sleep apnea, nocturia and polyuria in older adults. Sleep 2004; 27(1):139–144.
63. Fitzgerald MP, Mulligan M, Parthasarathy S. Nocturic frequency is related to severity of obstructive sleep apnea, improves with continuous positive airways treatment. Am J Obstet Gynecol 2006; 194(5):1399–1403.
64. Schafer H, Koehler U, Ploch T, et al. Sleep-related myocardial ischemia and sleep structure in patients with obstructive sleep apnea and coronary heart disease. Chest 1997; 111(2):387–393.
65. Franklin KA, Nilsson JB, Sahlin C, et al. Sleep apnoea and nocturnal angina. Lancet 1995; 345(8957):1085–1087.
66. Mooe T, Franklin KA, Wiklund U, et al. Sleep-disordered breathing and myocardial ischemia in patients with coronary artery disease. Chest 2000; 117(6):1597–1602.
67. Scharf SM, Tubman A, Smale P. Prevalence of concomitant sleep disorders in patients with obstructive sleep apnea. Sleep Breath 2005; 9(2):50–56.
68. Krakow B, Melendrez D, Ferreira E, et al. Prevalence of insomnia symptoms in patients with sleep-disordered breathing. Chest 2001; 120(6):1923–1929.

69. Peppard PE, Young T, Palta M, et al. Prospective study of the association between sleep-disordered breathing and hypertension. N Engl J Med 2000; 342(19):1378–1384.
70. Pepperell JC, Ramdassingh-Dow S, Crosthwaite N, et al. Ambulatory blood pressure after therapeutic and subtherapeutic nasal continuous positive airway pressure for obstructive sleep apnoea: a randomised parallel trial. Lancet 2002; 359(9302):204–210.
71. Faccenda JF, Mackay TW, Boon NA, et al. Randomized placebo-controlled trial of continuous positive airway pressure on blood pressure in the sleep apnea-hypopnea syndrome. Am J Respir Crit Care Med 2001; 163(2):344–348.
72. Becker HF, Jerrentrup A, Ploch T, et al. Effect of nasal continuous positive airway pressure treatment on blood pressure in patients with obstructive sleep apnea. Circulation 2003; 107(1):68–73.
73. Shahar E, Whitney CW, Redline S, et al. Sleep-disordered breathing and cardiovascular disease: cross-sectional results of the Sleep Heart Health Study. Am J Respir Crit Care Med 2001; 163(1):19–25.
74. Peker Y, Hedner J, Norum J, et al. Increased incidence of cardiovascular disease in middle-aged men with obstructive sleep apnea: a 7-year follow-up. Am J Respir Crit Care Med 2002; 166(2):159–165.
75. Doherty LS, Kiely JL, Swan V, et al. Long-term effects of nasal continuous positive airway pressure therapy on cardiovascular outcomes in sleep apnea syndrome. Chest 2005; 127(6):2076–2084.
76. Marin JM, Carrizo SJ, Vicente E, et al. Long-term cardiovascular outcomes in men with obstructive sleep apnoea-hypopnoea with or without treatment with continuous positive airway pressure: an observational study. Lancet 2005; 365(9464):1046–1053.
77. Punjabi NM, Shahar E, Redline S, et al. Sleep-disordered breathing, glucose intolerance, and insulin resistance: the Sleep Heart Health Study. Am J Epidemiol 2004; 160(6):521–530.
78. Babu AR, Herdegen J, Fogelfeld L, et al. Type 2 diabetes, glycemic control, and continuous positive airway pressure in obstructive sleep apnea. Arch Intern Med 2005; 165(4):447–452.
79. Guilleminault C, Eldridge FL, Tilkian A, et al. Sleep apnea syndrome due to upper airway obstruction: a review of 25 cases. Arch Intern Med 1977; 137(3):296–300.
80. Mosko S, Zetin M, Glen S, et al. Self-reported depressive symptomatology, mood ratings, and treatment outcome in sleep disorders patients. J Clin Psychol 1989; 45(1):51–60.
81. Ohayon MM. The effects of breathing-related sleep disorders on mood disturbances in the general population. J Clin Psychiatry 2003; 64(10):1195–1200; quiz, 1274–1276.
82. Bednarek M, Plywaczewski R, Jonczak L, et al. There is no relationship between chronic obstructive pulmonary disease and obstructive sleep apnea syndrome: a population study. Respiration 2005; 72(2):142–149.
83. Atwood CW Jr, McCrory D, Garcia JG, et al. Pulmonary artery hypertension and sleep-disordered breathing: ACCP evidence-based clinical practice guidelines. Chest 2004; 126(suppl 1):S72–S77.
84. Resta O, Pannacciulli N, DiGioia G, et al. High prevalence of previously unknown subclinical hypothyroidism in obese patients referred to a sleep clinic for sleep disordered breathing. Nutr Metab Cardiovasc Dis 2004; 14(5):248–253.
85. Sawin CT, Castelli WP, Hershman JM, et al. The aging thyroid. Thyroid deficiency in the Framingham Study. Arch Intern Med 1985; 145(8):1386–1388.
86. Barnes TW, Olsen KD, Morgenthaler TI. Obstructive lingual thyroid causing sleep apnea: a case report and review of the literature. Sleep Med 2004; 5(6):605–607.
87. Mojon DS, Hess CW, Goldblum D, et al. High prevalence of glaucoma in patients with sleep apnea syndrome. Ophthalmology 1999; 106(5):1009–1012.
88. Hallett M, Burden S, Stewart D, et al. Sleep apnea in end-stage renal disease patients on hemodialysis and continuous ambulatory peritoneal dialysis. ASAIO J 1995; 41(3):M435–M441.
89. de Oliveira Rodrigues CJ, Marson O, Tufic S, et al. Relationship among end-stage renal disease, hypertension, and sleep apnea in nondiabetic dialysis patients. Am J Hypertens 2005; 18(2 Pt 1):152–157.
90. Senior BA, Khan M, Schwimmer C, et al. Gastroesophageal reflux and obstructive sleep apnea. Laryngoscope 2001; 111(12):2144–2146.

91. Morse CA, Quan SF, Mays MZ, et al. Is there a relationship between obstructive sleep apnea and gastroesophageal reflux disease? Clin Gastroenterol Hepatol 2004; 2(9):761–768.
92. Sahota PK, Jain SS, Dhand R. Sleep disorders in pregnancy. Curr Opin Pulm Med 2003; 9(6):477–483.
93. Taasan VC, Block AJ, Boysen PG, et al. Alcohol increases sleep apnea and oxygen desaturation in asymptomatic men. Am J Med 1981; 71(2):240–245.
94. Issa FG, Sullivan CE. Alcohol, snoring and sleep apnea. J Neurol Neurosurg Psychiatry 1982; 45(4):353–359.
95. Scanlan MF, Roebuck T, Little PJ, et al. Effect of moderate alcohol upon obstructive sleep apnoea. Eur Respir J 2000; 16(5):909–913.
96. Teschler H, Berthon-Jones M, Wessendorf T, et al. Influence of moderate alcohol consumption on obstructive sleep apnoea with and without AutoSet nasal CPAP therapy. Eur Respir J 1996; 9(11):2371–2377.
97. Wetter DW, Young TB, Bidwell TR, et al. Smoking as a risk factor for sleep-disordered breathing. Arch Intern Med 1994; 154(19):2219–2224.
98. Kashyap R, Hock LM, Bowman TJ. Higher prevalence of smoking in patients diagnosed as having obstructive sleep apnea. Sleep Breath 2001; 5(4):167–172.
99. Redline S, Tishler PV, Tosteson TD, et al. The familial aggregation of obstructive sleep apnea. Am J Respir Crit Care Med 1995; 151(3 Pt 1):682–687.
100. Wu H, Yan-Go F. Self-reported automobile accidents involving patients with obstructive sleep apnea. Neurology 1996; 46(5):1254–1257.
101. Lander ES, Schork NJ. Genetic dissection of complex traits. Science 1994; 265(5181): 2037–2048.
102. Moreno CR, Carvalho FA, Lorenzi C, et al. High risk for obstructive sleep apnea in truck drivers estimated by the Berlin questionnaire: prevalence and associated factors. Chronobiol Int 2004; 21(6):871–879.
103. Pagel JF. Medications and their effects on sleep. Prim Care 2005; 32(2):491–509.
104. Canova CR, Downs SH, Knoblauch A, et al. Increased prevalence of perennial allergic rhinitis in patients with obstructive sleep apnea. Respiration 2004; 71(2):138–143.
105. Hla KM, Young TB, Bidwell T, et al. Sleep apnea and hypertension. A population-based study. Ann Intern Med 1994; 120(5):382–388.
106. Lavie P, Herer P, Hoffstein V. Obstructive sleep apnoea syndrome as a risk factor for hypertension: population study. BMJ 2000; 320(7233):479–482.
107. Nieto FJ, Young TB, Lind BK, et al. Association of sleep-disordered breathing, sleep apnea, and hypertension in a large community-based study. Sleep Heart Health Study. JAMA 2000; 283(14):1829–1836.
108. Young T, Peppard P, Palta M, et al. Population-based study of sleep-disordered breathing as a risk factor for hypertension. Arch Intern Med 1997; 157(15):1746–1752.
109. Grote L, Ploch T, Heitmann J, et al. Sleep-related breathing disorder is an independent risk factor for systemic hypertension. Am J Respir Crit Care Med 1999; 160(6): 1875–1882.
110. Bixler EO, Vgontzas AN, Lim HM, et al. Association of hypertension and sleep-disordered breathing. Arch Intern Med 2000; 160(15):2289–2295.
111. Zonato AI, Bittencourt LR, Martinho FL, et al. Association of systematic head and neck physical examination with severity of obstructive sleep apnea-hypopnea syndrome. Laryngoscope 2003; 113(6):973–980.
112. Zonato AI, Martinho FL, Bittencourt LR, et al. Head and neck physical examination: comparison between nonapneic and obstructive sleep apnea patients. Laryngoscope 2005; 115(6):1030–1034.
113. Liistro G, Rombaux P, Belge C, et al. High Mallampati score and nasal obstruction are associated risk factors for obstructive sleep apnoea. Eur Respir J 2003; 21(2):248–252.
114. Kushida CA, Efron B, Guilleminault C. A predictive morphometric model for the obstructive sleep apnea syndrome. Ann Intern Med 1997; 127(8 Pt 1):581–587.
115. Lofaso F, Coste A, d'Ortho MP, et al. Nasal obstruction as a risk factor for sleep apnoea syndrome. Eur Respir J 2000; 16(4):639–643.
116. Rombaux P, Liistro G, Hamoir M, et al. Nasal obstruction and its impact on sleep-related breathing disorders. Rhinology 2005; 43(4):242–250.

117. Friedman M, Tanyeri H, La Rosa M, et al. Clinical predictors of obstructive sleep apnea. Laryngoscope 1999; 109(12):1901–1907.
118. Schellenberg JB, Maislin G, Schwab RJ. Physical findings and the risk for obstructive sleep apnea. The importance of oropharyngeal structures. Am J Respir Crit Care Med 2000; 162(2 Pt 1):740–748.
119. Min YG, Jang YJ, Rhee CK, et al. Correlation between anthropometric measurements of the oropharyngeal area and severity of apnea in patients with snoring and obstructive sleep apnea. Auris Nasus Larynx 1997; 24(4):399–403.
120. Tsai WH, Remmers JE, Brant R, et al. A decision rule for diagnostic testing in obstructive sleep apnea. Am J Respir Crit Care Med 2003; 167(10):1427–1432.
121. Ipsiroglu OS, Fatemi A, Werner I, et al. Prevalence of sleep disorders in school children between 11 and 15 years of age. Wien Klin Wochenschr 2001; 113(7–8):235–244.
122. Stein MA, Mendelsohn J, Obermeyer WH, et al. Sleep and behavior problems in school-aged children. Pediatrics 2001; 107(4):E60.
123. Hultcrantz E, Lofstrand-Tidestrom B, Ahlquist-Rastad J. The epidemiology of sleep related breathing disorder in children. Int J Pediatr Otorhinolaryngol 1995; 32(suppl):S63–S66.
124. Owen GO, Canter RJ, Robinson A. Overnight pulse oximetry in snoring and non-snoring children. Clin Otolaryngol Allied Sci 1995; 20(5):402–406.
125. Ferreira AM, Clemente V, Gozal D, et al. Snoring in Portuguese primary school children. Pediatrics 2000; 106(5):E64.
126. Kotagal S. Sleep disorders in childhood. Neurol Clin 2003; 21(4):961–981.
127. Gozal D, Wang M, Pope DW Jr. Objective sleepiness measures in pediatric obstructive sleep apnea. Pediatrics 2001; 108(3):693–697.
128. Chan J, Edman JC, Koltai PJ. Obstructive sleep apnea in children. Am Fam Physician 2004; 69(5):1147–1154.
129. Doherty MJ, Spence DP, Young C, et al. Obstructive sleep apnoea with Arnold-Chiari malformation. Thorax 1995; 50(6):690–691; discussion 696–697.

2 Screening and Case Finding

Charles F. P. George
University of Western Ontario, London Health Sciences Centre,
London, Ontario, Canada

INTRODUCTION

Obstructive sleep apnea (OSA) is becoming increasingly recognized. OSA with daytime impairment is estimated to occur in one of 20 adults but is often unrecognized or undiagnosed. Minimally symptomatic or asymptomatic OSA is estimated to occur in one of five adults (1). A primary goal of screening is the detection of a risk factor or disease at an early stage, when it can be corrected or cured. Disorders with a long latency period increase the potential gains associated with detection; however, in many cases early detection does not necessarily influence survival. Screening techniques must be cost-effective, if they are to be applied to large populations. Costs include not only the expense of testing but also time away from work and potential risks. When the risk-to-benefit ratio is less favorable, it is useful to provide information to patients and factor their perspectives into the decision-making process.

In the case of sleep apnea, while the prevalence is high, it remains unclear exactly which cases will develop significant cardiovascular disease, or which will be victims of increased accidents. Because it may be the minority of cases that actually develop morbidity, widespread screening cannot yet be considered for patients with sleep apnea.

Case finding on the other hand mirrors clinical practice more closely and for this reason this chapter will focus on case finding in clinical practice and the tools at the disposal of the sleep medicine physician.

DIAGNOSIS OF SLEEP APNEA

Modern diagnosis of sleep apnea has its roots in the landmark descriptions by Gastaut (2,3), Jung and Kuhlo (4), and others (5,6). Since these early descriptions of polygraphic recordings, the nocturnal, attended in-lab polysomnogram has become the standard for diagnosing OSA. In the early days of our understanding of the condition, the patient presented at advanced stages with severe symptoms, cardiovascular comorbidities, and a prominent history of loud snoring and witnessed apneic episodes. Over the years, a wider spectrum of disease severity has emerged and it is clear that many patients are minimally affected or not symptomatic at all. These patients are usually brought to attention because of their bed partner's descriptions of snoring and concerns about not breathing. This has increased the demands on in-lab polysomnography, still a limited resource, and prompted alternative strategies for diagnosing sleep apnea.

DEFINITIONS OF SLEEP-DISORDERED BREATHING

Apnea was first defined by Guilleminault et al. (7) as a cessation of air flow at the nose and mouth for at least 10 seconds and a sleep apnea syndrome was diagnosed if during seven hours of nocturnal sleep, at least 30 apneic events are observed in both rapid eye movement (REM) and non-rapid eye movement (NREM) sleep, some of which must appear repetitively in NREM sleep. The International Classification of Sleep Disorders (second edition) (ICSD-2) includes both clinical and polysomnographic (PSG) features for defining OSA with "five or more scorable respiratory events per hour of sleep" as the PSG cut-off for disease (8). The concept of hypopnea [as a reflection of an increased but not complete (i.e., apnea) upper airway obstruction] was first highlighted by Gould (9) and the subsequent demonstration of an increased spectrum of upper airways resistance by Guilleminault (10) has led to a more inclusive term of sleep-disordered breathing that includes apneas, hypopneas, and respiratory effort-related arousals (RERA) from sleep. The ICSD-2 and updated practice parameters of the American Academy of Sleep Medicine both highlight the lack of clinical consensus for hypopnea and RERA definitions, although research definitions have been established. More recently, these definitions have been consistent amongst studies but such consistency is missing from some of the early literature (vide infra).

CLINICAL PREDICTION MODELS

Well-established sleep apnea is characterized by loud snoring, witnessed apneic episodes, disturbed nocturnal sleep, daytime sleepiness, and impaired cognition and is typically associated with obesity and (in men) a large neck size. Given this profile, it is not surprising that clinical prediction models would arise in an effort to diagnose OSA in larger populations. Virtually all of these studies have been done in sleep clinic populations rather than in the general population. One of the earliest studies showed that witnessed apneic episodes combined with loud snoring predicted an apnea-hypopnea index (AHI) > 10 with a sensitivity of 78% and specificity of 67% (11). Crocker et al. (12) used an alternative approach and developed a statistical model using clinical data to predict disturbance of sleep-disordered breathing in 114 consecutive patients. Witnessed apneic episodes, hypertension, body mass index (BMI), and age provided a sensitivity of 92% but a specificity of only 51% for an AHI > 15. Using 410 clinic patients, Viner et al. (13) developed a model incorporating snoring, BMI, age, and sex and came up with sensitivity and specificity of 94% and 28%, respectively. The higher the pretest probability of sleep apnea, the better the positive predictive value of their model. Maislin et al. (14) added to this and developed the multivariable apnea prediction index, which includes questions about frequency of symptoms of apnea as well as measurements of BMI, age, and gender. Using this tool, at a BMI > 40, the likelihood of apnea is very high with or without symptoms, while at lower values of BMI, the likelihood of sleep apnea is much more dependent on whether or not the individual has symptoms. Predictive abilities assessed using receiver operating characteristic (ROC) curves noted that for BMI alone the ROC value was 0.73, and for an index measuring a self-report of apnea symptoms it was 0.7. Many other papers have demonstrated varying degrees of variability and specificity with their clinical prediction models (15–17).

Netzer et al. (18) assessed the utility of the Berlin Questionnaire to diagnose sleep apnea in a primary care setting. This questionnaire asks about risk factors for sleep apnea, namely snoring behavior, wake time sleepiness or fatigue, and the presence of obesity or hypertension. A subset of patients underwent overnight portable recording using a six-channel recorder (EdenTrace® Recording System, vide infra). This approach resulted in a sensitivity of 86%, a specificity of 77%, and a positive predictive value of 89% for OSA. This questionnaire appears to be a useful tool but needs to be tested in other populations with neck circumference, age, and race added to the predictive model.

Rodsutti et al. (19) derived and validated a clinical decision rule to assess risk of sleep apnea and prioritized those for polysomnography. Five variables—age, sex, BMI, snoring, and stopped breathing during sleep—were significantly associated with sleep apnea. ROC analysis for both derivation and validation sets gave area under the curve (AUC) values of 0.81 and 0.79, respectively.

The uses of neural networks for predicting or excluding sleep apnea have been demonstrated in a few studies. Artificial neural networks (ANNs) are computer programs modeled after the nervous system and are capable of recognizing complex patterns in data. ANNs are "trained" by presenting a set of data together with the outcomes that the trainer wishes the network to learn. The trained ANN can then be evaluated by inputting similar but previously unseen data. This approach for outcome prediction has been used successfully in medical applications, including the prediction of acute myocardial infarction in patients presenting to an emergency room physician (20), the diagnosis of pulmonary embolism (21,22), and the predicted length of stay of patients in an intensive care unit (23).

El-Solh et al. (24) utilized a back-propagation ANN algorithm on 189 patients as a training set and validated it prospectively on 80 additional patients. Predictive accuracy at different AHI thresholds was assessed by the c-index, which is equivalent to the area under the ROC curve. The c-index for predicting OSA in the validation set was 0.96, 0.95, and 0.935 using thresholds of > 10, > 15, and > 20/hour, respectively. They suggested that ANN may be useful as a predictive tool for OSA. Using a backward error propagation ANN with 23 clinical variables and a leave-k-out strategy, Kirby et al. (25) found the positive predictive value that a patient would not have sleep apnea to be 98%, with a negative predictive value the patient would have sleep apnea (AHI > 10) to be 89%. In that study the use of the ANN would have reduced the number of PSGs performed by 22%.

Additional approaches have also been taken. Kushida et al. (26) incorporated oral cavity measures into a morphometric model of OSA, using a degree of maxillary overjet, intermolar distance, and maxillary mandibular planes and palatal height, combined with neck circumference and BMI. This model had a sensitivity of 98%, specificity of 100% and a positive predictive value of 100% for an AHI > 5. Despite these impressive results, this technique has not been replicated in other centers, possibly because it is somewhat labor intensive. More recently, Tsai et al. (27) noted the three main reliable clinical symptoms of sleep apnea (snoring, witnessed apneas, and hypertension) and three signs of sleep apnea (thyro-mental space less than 1.5 cm, pharyngeal grade > 2, and the presence of an overbite) provided a positive predictive value of 95%. A thyro-mental space of > 1.5 cm excluded sleep apnea with a negative predictive value of 100%.

Rowley et al. (28) prospectively studied the utility of four clinical prediction models for predicting the presence of sleep apnea or prioritizing patients for a split-night protocol. They took four clinical prediction formulae of Crocker, Viner, Flemons, and Maislin to calculate the probability of sleep apnea for each model in each of 370 clinic patients. For an AHI > 10, their sensitivity ranged using these models from 76% to 96%, specificity of only 13% to 54%, and a positive predictive value ranging between 69% and 77%. They concluded that clinical prediction models are not sufficiently accurate to discriminate between patients with or without sleep apnea but could be useful in prioritizing patients for split-night polysomnography.

LABORATORY DIAGNOSIS OF SLEEP APNEA

Attended laboratory-based polysomnography has been and remains a de facto gold standard for diagnosis of sleep-disordered breathing, even though the utility of a single overnight recording for diagnosis or exclusion of significant sleep has never been clearly addressed in the literature. It is clear that there is considerable night-to-night variability in AHI particularly, when the AHI is low (29–32). Standard overnight polysomnography involves: (*i*) recordings of sleep-related electroencephalography (EEG), electromyography (EMG) of the chin and leg muscles, electrooculography (EOG), and electrocardiography (ECG); (*ii*) oxygen saturation; and (*iii*) measures of respiratory effort and airflow. Examples of typical polysomnography are shown in Figure 1. This figure shows clear-cut repetitive obstructive apneic events and for these

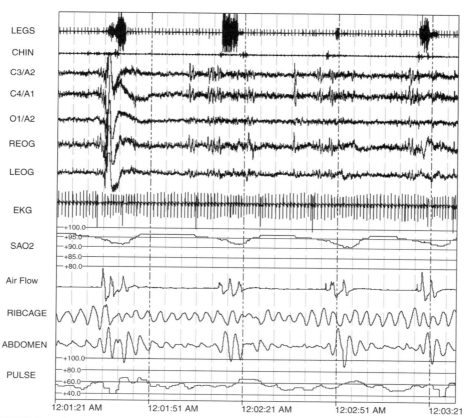

FIGURE 1 Overnight polysomnogram showing repetitive obstructive apneas. Channels recorded: both legs (on single channel); electroencephalogram (EEG) from standard locations left central/right auricular reference EEG (C3/A2), right central/left auricular reference EEG (C4/A1), left occipital/right auricular reference EEG (O1/A2); left (LEOG) and right (REOG) electrooculogram; electrocardiogram (EKG); oxygen saturation (SaO$_2$); airflow, measured by oro-nasal pressure transducer; respiratory effort of ribcage and abdomen; and pulse rate. In this 3-minute example, there are at least five apneas with only modest oxygen desaturation, none below 90%.

patients a diagnosis of sleep apnea may be established on more simple recordings. This has led to a number of recording devices ranging from simple oximetry, snoring sound, respiratory effort, and airflow to full portable attended PSG devices.

PORTABLE MONITORING (SEE ALSO CHAPTER 3)

A number of portable monitoring techniques have been developed over the past 20 years in an attempt to simplify the ambulatory diagnosis of sleep apnea. Some showing initial promises are either no longer available [i.e., Nightwatch™, Respironics, Murrysville, Pennsylvania, U.S. (33,34)] or no longer marketed for a diagnostic purpose [i.e., AutoSet®, ResMed, Poway, California, U.S. (35,36)]. Currently available devices range from comprehensive portable polysomnography to simple oximetry. A committee of the American Academy of Sleep Medicine, American Thoracic Society, and American College of Chest Physicians (37) classified portable monitors into three categories: (*i*) Type 2 monitors include a minimum of seven channels, including EEG, EOG, chin EMG, ECG or heart rate, airflow, respiratory effort, and oxygen saturation; (*ii*) Type 3 monitors include a minimum of four channels, including ventilation or airflow (at least two channels of respiratory movement, or respiratory movement and airflow), heart rate or ECG and oxygen saturation; and (*iii*) Type 4 monitors, where most monitors of this type measure a single parameter or two parameters. For comparison, Type 1 monitoring is in-laboratory, attended polysomnography.

Type 2 Monitors

A comprehensive monitor has been successfully used in the large-scale Sleep Heart Health Study (P-Series PS2, Compumedics Limited, Victoria, Australia). Where home and in-lab PSG were compared, median respiratory disturbance index (RDI) was similar in the unattended home and attended laboratory setting with differences of small magnitude in some sleep parameters (38). Differences in RDI between settings resulted in a rate of disease misclassification that is similar to repeated studies in the same setting.

The DigiTrace Home Sleep System (DHSS, SleepMed, Inc., Columbia, South Carolina, U.S.) can acquire, store, and analyze full polysomnographic data in the ambulatory setting as illustrated in the study by Fry (39). In this study of 77 subjects, more than 95% of all epochs were scorable for sleep and breathing parameters. While these data suggest that full polysomnography can be extended to large patient populations, potentially freeing up valuable lab resources, such an approach has not yet become widely accepted. One likely reason is the need for much technical expertise. Therefore simpler, patient-friendly, even patient-applied devices are more desirable.

Type 3 Monitors

The EdenTrace® II Recording System (Nellcor Puritan Bennett Ltd., Kanata, Ontario, Canada) is a portable monitor that measures nasal and oral air flow via thermistry, chest wall impedance, snoring intensity, oxygen saturation via finger pulse oximetry, heart rate, and body position. Movement is detected by electrical comparison of the signals from the ECG and the pulse oximetry, and discrepancies between these channels are indicated as "motion" on the saturation channel. Several studies have been performed comparing either the ambulatory device only in the laboratory with simultaneously recorded polysomnography, or both home and laboratory recordings (40–43). In all studies there is good agreement between the AHI measured in the laboratory and with the EdenTrace device in the ambulatory setting. Ten percent or more of studies required repetition because of difficulty with recordings; the study by Whittle et al. (43) suggested that home sleep studies have benefits in terms of time and cost, but for diagnostic reliability, an in-laboratory sleep study may be required in more than half of the cases.

The Embletta® Recording System (Medcare, Reykjavik, Iceland) consists of a nasal pressure detector using a nasal cannulae/pressure transducer system (recording the square root of pressure as an index of flow), thoracoabdominal movement detection through two piezoelectric belts, a finger pulse oximeter, and a body position detector. This technology is part of the parent in-lab PSG system (Embla®). Dingli et al. (44) performed a synchronous comparison to polysomnography in 40 patients and a comparison of home Embletta studies with in-laboratory polysomnography in 61 patients. Sleep apnea was classified as definite (AHI > 20), possible (AHI 10–20), and not present (AHI < 10) based on Embletta results in symptomatic patients. Using this classification, all nine patients categorized as not having sleep apnea AHI ≤ 15 on PSG and all 23 with definite sleep apnea on Embletta had an AHI ≥ 15 on polysomnography. Eighteen patients fell into the possible sleep apnea category potentially requiring further investigation and 11 home studies failed. Most patients were satisfactorily classified by home Embletta studies but 29 out of 61 required further investigations. The study suggested a 42% saving in diagnostic costs over polysomnography if this approach were adopted.

The Stardust® Sleep Recorder (Respironics, Murrysville, Pennsylvania, U.S.) detects nasal airflow and snoring (pressure sensor); thoracic or abdominal movement (one strain gauge); arterial oxygen saturation and pulse rate (finger probe); and body position. There are limited published data with this device. One in-lab study from Japan found that Stardust and PSG AHI correlated well with a mean bias of 3.7 ± 13.1/hour (45). Specificity was lowest (25%) in patients with milder sleep apnea (AHI < 15) increasing to 97% with AHI > 50. Sensitivity was high (> 90%) at any level of PSG-derived AHI. We found similar results (K Ferguson, personal communication) but much more data are needed to properly determine the role of this and similar devices.

Type 4 Monitors
Oximetry
Changes in oxygen saturation occur with most, if not all, apneic events. The magnitude of desaturation depends on a number of factors including end-expiratory lung volume at the time of the event, baseline saturation, degree of respiratory effort during the event, and degree of upper airway obstruction (complete or partial). While changes in saturation can result from obstructive apnea, obstructive hypopnea, or central apnea, oximetry cannot by itself provide details of the type of sleep-disordered breathing. Nonetheless, it does give some indication of the frequency and severity of the sleep-disordered breathing. Many laboratory-based studies comparing oximetry to full polysomnography have been published with varying degrees of sensitivity and specificity (46–50). However, they do not provide any information on the utility of such simple measurements in the ambulatory setting. The study of Series et al. (51) is one of few comparing ambulatory oximetry with subsequent polysomnography. Although home oximetry detected only 108 of 176 patients with OSA (positive predictive value, 61.4%), it correctly excluded 62 of

64 patients (negative predictive value, 96.9%). In a more recent albeit smaller study by Hussain and Fleetham (52) all (12 of 30) patients with sleep apnea had a 2% oxygen desaturations index of less than 10/hour. The sensitivity of oximetry increased at lower desaturations indices but this was associated with decreased specificity. Review of oximetry waveform pattern, by experienced physicians, did not improve the diagnostic accuracy. Combining oximetry with a clinical prediction rule would have reduced the need for polysomnography by 30%. The authors concluded that many patients, who present with snoring and/or witnessed apnea and are referred to a sleep disorder clinic for suspected OSA, may have significant OSA even if they deny EDS.

Despite the extensive literature on oximetry, there is no uniformity in the results. This can be explained by the fact that different devices record at different sampling rates, store and analyze the data in different ways. Moreover, and perhaps more importantly, the definition of sleep apnea-hypopnea is not uniform amongst studies.

Oximetry and Snoring

The Calgary group has added a measurement of snoring to saturation detection in an attempt to improve the ambulatory diagnosis of sleep apnea. In an initial report, they compared the SnoreSat® (SagaTech Electronics, Calgary, Alberta, Canada; now known as the Remmers Sleep Recorder) with standard overnight polysomnography (53). Depending on the severity of apnea and the referral population, the sensitivity and specificity of the monitor in detecting OSA ranged between 84% and 90% (sensitivity) and 95% and 98% (specificity). In subsequent studies comparing both at-home with simultaneous in-laboratory measurements (54), the PSG-derived AHI and oximeter-derived RDI were highly correlated ($R = 0.97$). The mean (2SD) of the differences between AHI and RDI was 2.18 (12.34)/hour. The sensitivity and specificity of the algorithm depended on the AHI and RDI criteria selected for OSA case designation. Using a cut-off of 15/hour for AHI and RDI, the sensitivity and specificity were 98% and 88%, respectively. If the PSG-derived AHI included EEG-based arousals as part of the hypopnea definition, the mean (2SD) of the differences between RDI and AHI was −0.12 (15.62)/hour and the sensitivity and specificity profile did not change significantly. While these data suggest that oximetry, or oximetry combined with snoring measurement, may be used in identifying patients with OSA, it is important to remember that not all oximeters are made equally and that some events may not be detected by some devices in some situations (55–57). Indeed, the same group found that oximetry is not useful in a pediatric population (58). Using different devices with different algorithms have shown different results and clinicians need to be aware of these limitations when interpreting the literature.

Snoring is added to oximetry in a number of other devices included MESAM IV® (Madaus Medizin-Elektronik, Cologne, Germany) and the newer ARES™ Unicorder (Apnea Risk Evaluation System, Advanced Brain Monitoring, Inc., Carlsbad, California, U.S.) (heart rate is also recorded; thus these do not technically fit with the classification but are included for completeness). The MESAM IV recording device, widely used in Europe, evaluates sleep-disordered breathing based on an analysis of snoring and saturation change as well as heart rate. Cyclical variation of heart rate in association with decreases in saturation and snoring are taken into account at the same time to determine sleep apnea. Several previous studies evaluating the diagnostic validity of MESAM IV have had conflicting results (59–63). This is because not all studies have the same design, patient populations varied and diagnostic criteria were different.

The ARES™ Unicorder is easily affixed to the forehead by the user and acquires data on oxygen saturation, airflow (nasal pressure), pulse rate, snoring level (microphone), and head position/movement (accelerometers). Proprietary ARES™ software uses oxygen saturation measured by pulse oximetry (SpO_2) as the primary signal, and analyzes changes in pulse rate, snoring sounds, head movement, and the slope of the resaturation curve to identify behavioral markers of arousal that follow desaturation events. The analysis algorithm assumes that desaturation events are terminated by arousal due to sleep apnea. A study by Westbrook (64) reported 284 valid comparisons of in-laboratory simultaneous polysomnography and ARES™ and 187 valid comparisons of in-laboratory polysomnography with a separate two nights of unattended self-applied ARES™ recording. Using a diagnostic AHI cut-off > 10 to establish the accuracy and validity of the ARES™, the concurrent in-laboratory comparison yielded a sensitivity of 97.4%, a specificity of 85.6%, a positive predictive value of 93.6%, and a negative predictive value of 93.9%; in-home comparison sensitivity, specificity, positive predictive value, and negative predictive value were 91.5, 85.7, 91.5, and 85.7%, respectively. The authors concluded that the ARES™ demonstrates a consistently high sensitivity and specificity for both in-laboratory and in-home recordings; and that for patients at risk for sleep apnea who do not a priori need an attended study, the ARES™ could provide a low-cost alternative to traditional polysomnography.

Oximetry and Peripheral Arterial Tonometry

A wrist-worn device, Watch-PAT 100 System (Itamar Medical Ltd., Caesarea, Israel) has been developed to detect OSA. The peripheral arterial tonometry (PAT) technology is based on the principle that episodic vasoconstriction of digital vascular beds from sympathetic stimulation (mediated by alpha receptors) causes attenuation of the PAT signal and that discrete obstructive airway events (e.g., apneas, hypopneas, and upper airway resistance) cause arousals from sleep, sympathetic activation, and peripheral vasoconstriction (65). Thus, this represents a noninvasive measurement of variable sympathetic activation that occurs as part of sleep-disordered breathing events. Two finger probes extend from the main body of the device: one is the pneumo-optical sensor that detects the PAT signal; the other measures arterial oxygen saturation. The body of the device also contains an actigraph, which is used to estimate sleep. The finger-mounted pneumo-optical sensor eliminates venous pulsations and continuously measures the pulse volume of the digit. An automated computerized algorithm is used to calculate the frequency of respiratory events per hour of actigraphy-measured sleep. This algorithm also incorporates the PAT signal attenuation and the oxygen desaturation. Ayas et al. (66) found good correlation between the Watch-PAT 100 System and the gold standard PSG. Schnall et al. (67) found a high correlation between standard polysomnography-scored apnea-hypopnea events and PAT-vasoconstriction events with concurrent tachycardia in an initial study with the bedside version of the system. Bar et al. (68) showed that detection of apnea and hypopnea events based on combined data from PAT and pulse oximetry was highly correlated with standard polysomnography-scored results, a finding confirmed by Pittman et al. (69) using both manual and automatic analysis. A more recent study from Sweden compared the Watch-Pat 100 System with simultaneous in-home unattended full PSG (70). Subjects were instrumented in the lab for full PSG (using the Embla system, Medcare, Reykjavik, Iceland) and the Watch-Pat 100 System and sent home for overnight study. The accuracy of the Watch-Pat 100 System in RDI, AHI, oxygen desaturation index (ODI), and sleep-wake detection was assessed by comparison with data from simultaneous PSG recordings. The mean PSG-AHI in this population was 25.5 ± 22.9 events per hour. The Watch-Pat 100 System RDI, AHI, and ODI correlated closely at 0.88, 0.90, and 0.92, respectively ($p < 0.0001$) with the corresponding indexes obtained by PSG. The AUC for the ROC curves for Watch-Pat 100 System AHI and RDI were 0.93 and 0.90 for the PSG-AHI and RDI thresholds 10 and 20, respectively ($p < 0.0001$). The agreement of the Sleep-Wake assessment based on 30-second bins between the two systems was 82 ± 7%. The authors concluded that the Watch-Pat 100 System was reasonably accurate for unattended home diagnosis of OSA in a population sample not preselected for OSA symptoms. Moreover, they proposed simultaneous home PSG recordings in population-based cohorts as a reasonable validation standard for assessment of simplified recording tools for OSA diagnosis.

Oximetry and Flow
A number of devices combining airflow measurement with oximetry are available primarily in Europe. These include the Reggie (oximetry, airflow, actigraphy (71); Camtech Ltd., Sandvika, Norway) and the SOMNOcheck® (oximetry, flow, snoring, heart rate and position (72); Weinmann Diagnostics GmbH and Co. KG, Hamburg, Germany). As with other devices reasonable agreement with in-lab PSG have been reported but limited data prevent widespread use or endorsement at this time.

Tracheal Sound Analysis
Recognizing that a suprasternal pressure transducer can accurately reflect respiratory efforts (73), Nakano et al. (74) have developed a novel method of using tracheal sound analysis for the diagnosis of sleep apnea-hypopnea syndrome. In a retrospective study involving 383 patients for suspected sleep apnea-hypopnea syndrome, overnight polysomnography with simultaneous tracheal sound recording was performed. The AHI was calculated as the number of apnea and hypopnea events per hour of sleep. Tracheal sounds were digitized and recorded as power spectra. An automated computer program detected transient falls (TS-dip) in the time series of moving average of the logarithmic power of tracheal sound. Tracheal sound-respiratory disturbance index (TS-RDI) was reported as the number of TS-dips per hour of examination and the ODI was calculated as the number of SaO_2 dips of at least 4% per hour of examination. The TS-RDI highly correlated with AHI ($r = 0.93$). The mean (± SD) difference between the TS-RDI and AHI was −8.4 ± 10.4. The diagnostic sensitivity and specificity of the TS-RDI when the same cut-off value was used as for AHI were 93% and 67% for the AHI cut-off value of 5, and 79% and 95% for the AHI cut-off value of 15, respectively. The agreement between the TS-RDI and AHI was better than that between the ODI and AHI. The authors concluded that fully automated tracheal sound analysis is useful for the portable monitoring of the sleep apnea-hypopnea syndrome.

OTHER DIAGNOSTIC APPROACHES

Actigraphy refers to methods using miniaturized computerized wristwatch-like devices to monitor and collect data generated by movements. Most actigraphs contain an analog system to detect movements. In some devices, a piezoelectric beam detects movement in two or three axes and the detected movements are translated to digital counts accumulated across predesigned epoch intervals (e.g., 1 minute) and stored in the internal memory. While these have been very useful in determining disorders of the sleep-wake rhythm (75) and are even quite good in estimating sleep time in patients with sleep apnea (76), they cannot really be used to diagnose sleep apnea (77).

Other surrogate markers have been used to detect sleep apnea including cyclical changes in heart rate on 24-hour Holter monitoring (78) and pulse transit time (79–81). While both of these reflect physiologic changes accompanying obstructive events, the sensitivity and specificity of these are insufficient (owing to wide extremes in spectrum of disease) to warrant routine use.

In assessing the validity and applicability of any ambulatory diagnostic system, several standards should be met (82). These include: (*i*) an independent blind comparison with a reference standard; (*ii*) an appropriate spectrum of patients; (*iii*) avoidance of work-up bias; (*iv*) methods for performing the test described in detail, allowing for duplication of the study; (*v*) adequate description of study population; (*vi*) adequate sample size (conservative estimate is that there should be greater than or equal to 200 patients in the study, approximately equally divided between those with and without the condition. This allows for confidence intervals of approximately ± 10% for estimates of sensitivity and specificity); (*vii*) avoidance of a selection bias—in the case of patients with sleep apnea, this means a consecutive sample of patients referred to a sleep clinic rather than those referred to a sleep laboratory, avoiding filtering of patients; and (*viii*) adequate description of study setting and appropriate setting—for instance, basic descriptors of the study should include whether it is a tertiary referral sleep clinic or a community sleep clinic, types of physicians referring to the sleep clinic, population base, types of patients, and so on.

Because most portable monitors are intended for use outside of the sleep laboratory, this is the setting in which they should be studied. Still, there are very few studies that meet these criteria.

CONCLUSIONS

Polysomnography remains the standard for diagnosis of sleep apnea and other disorders of sleep. However, depending on the prevalence of sleep apnea in the population in question and the diagnostic device used, an ambulatory strategy could easily be adopted. Patients can be stratified according to history (symptoms), physical examination, and clinical prediction strategies. The probability of sleep apnea can be estimated, and when there is a moderate-to-high probability, portable monitoring can confirm the suspicion and subjects can immediately go on to treatment. If there is no sleep apnea and patients are asymptomatic, it can be argued that no further testing is necessary and only follow-up is required. Symptomatic patients, regardless of their pretest probability, would go on to polysomnography. If the pretest probability for sleep apnea is low, polysomnography would be used only for symptomatic patients. While we await long-term outcome studies of such an approach, individual clinicians will have to apply this algorithm within the confines of the local resources, patient expectations, and clinical practice.

REFERENCES

1. Young T, Peppard PE, Gottlieb DJ. Epidemiology of obstructive sleep apnea: a population health perspective. Am J Respir Crit Care Med 2002; 165:1217–1239.
2. Gastaut H, Tassinari CA, Duron B. Etude polygraphique des manifestations épisodiques (hypniques et respiratoires) diurnes et nocturnes, du syndrome de Pickwick. Rev Neurol (Paris) 1965; 112:568–579.

3. Gastaut H, Tassinari CA, Duron B. Polygraphic study of the episodic diurnal and nocturnal (hypnic and respiratory) manifestations of the Pickwick syndrome. Brain Res 1967; 1:167–186.
4. Jung R, Kuhlo W. Neurophysiological studies of abnormal night sleep and the Pickwickian syndrome. Prog Brain Res 1965; 18:140–159.
5. Duron B, Tassinari CA. Syndrome de Pickwick et syndrome cardiorespiratore d l'obesite (a propos d'une observation). J Fr Med Chir Thorac 1966; 20:207–222.
6. Tassinari B, Bernardina D, Cirignotta F. Apnoeic periods and the respiratory related arousal patterns during sleep in the Pickwickian syndrome. A polygraphic study. Bulletin de Physio-Pathologie Respiratoire 1972; 8:1087–1102.
7. Guilleminault C, Dement WC, eds. Sleep Apnea Syndromes. New York, NY: Alan R. Liss, 1978.
8. The International Classification of Sleep Disorders; Diagnostic and Coding Manual. 2nd ed. Westchester, IL 60154, U.S.A.: American Academy of Sleep Medicine, One Westbrook Corporate Center, 2005.
9. Gould GA, Whyte KF, Rhind GB, et al. The sleep hypopnea syndrome. Am Rev Respir Dis 1988; 137:895–898.
10. Guilleminault C, Stooks R, Dunear S, et al. Snoring: daytime sleepiness in regular heavy snorers. Chest 1995; 99:40–49.
11. Kapuniai LE, Andrew DJ, Crowell DH, et al. Identifying sleep apnea from self reports. Sleep 1988; 11:430–436.
12. Crocker BD, Olson LG, Saunders NA, et al. Estimation of the probability of disturbed breathing during sleep before a sleep study. Am Rev Respir Dis 1990; 142:14–18.
13. Viner S, Szalai JP, Hoffstein V. Is history and physical examination a good screening test for obstruction sleep apnea? Ann Intern Med 1991; 115:356–359.
14. Maislin G, Pack AI, Kribbs NB, et al. A survey screen for prediction of apnea. Sleep 1995; 18:158–166.
15. Hoffstein V, Szalai JP. Predictive value of clinical features in predicting obstructive sleep apnea. Sleep 1993; 16:118–122.
16. Kump K, Whalen C, Tishler PV, et al. Assessment of the validity and utility of a sleep symptoms questionnaire. Am J Respir Crit Care Med 1994; 150:735–741.
17. Flemons WW, Whitelaw WA, Brant R, et al. Likelihood ratio for sleep apnea clinical prediction rule. Am J Respir Crit Care Med 1994; 150:1279–1985.
18. Netzer NC, Stoohs RA, Netzer CM, et al. Using the Berlin questionnaire to identify patients at risk for the sleep apnea syndrome. Ann Intern Med 1999; 131:485–491.
19. Rodsutti J, Hensley M, Thakkinstian A, et al. A clinical decision rule to prioritize polysomnography in patients with suspected sleep apnea. Sleep 2004; 27:694–699.
20. Baxt WG. Use of an artificial neural network in the diagnosis of myocardial infarction. Ann Intern Med 1991; 115:843–848.
21. Scott JA. Neural network analysis of ventilation perfusion lung scans. Radiology 1993; 186:661–664.
22. Patil S, Henry JW, Rubenfire M, et al. Neural network in the clinical diagnosis of acute pulmonary embolism. Chest 1993; 104:1685–1689.
23. Danter WR, Wood T, Morrison NJ, et al. Artificial neural network prediction of survival or death following admission to ICU. Clin Invest Med 1996; 19:S14.
24. El-Solh AA, Mador MJ, Ten-Brock E, et al. Validity of neural network in sleep apnea. Sleep 1999; 22:105–111.
25. Kirby SD, Eng P, Danter W, et al. Neural network prediction of obstructive sleep apnea from clinical criteria. Chest 1999; 116:409–415.
26. Kushida CA, Littner MR, Morgenthaler T, et al. Practice parameters for the indications for polysomnography and related procedures: an update for 2005. Sleep 2005; 28(4):499–521.
27. Tsai WH, Remmers JE, Brant R, et al. A decision rule for diagnostic testing in obstructive sleep apnea. Am J Respir Crit Care Med 2003; 167:1427–1432.
28. Rowley JA, Aboussouan LS, Badr MS. The use of clinical prediction formulas in the evaluation of obstructive sleep apnea. Sleep 2000; 23:929–938.
29. Wittig RM, Romaker A, Zorick FJ, et al. Night to night consistency of apneas during sleep. Am Rev Respir Dis 1984; 129:244–246.

30. Bliwise DL, Benkert RE, Ingham RH. Factors associated with nightly variability in sleep disordered breathing in the elderly. Chest 1991; 100:973–976.
31. Meyer TJ, Eveloff SE, Kline LR, et al. One negative polysomnogram does not exclude obstructive sleep apnea. Chest 1993; 103:756–760.
32. Lord S, Sawyer B, O'Connell D, et al. Night to night variability of disturbed breathing during sleep in an elderly community sample. Sleep 1991; 14:252–258.
33. Gugger M, Mathis J, Bassetti C. Accuracy of an intelligent CPAP system with inbuilt diagnostic abilities in detecting apnoeas: a comparison with polysomnography. Thorax 1995; 50:1199–1201.
34. Mayer P, Meurice J.-C, Philip-Joet F, et al. Simultaneous laboratory-based comparison of ResMed Autoset with polysomnography in the diagnosis of sleep apnoea/hypopnoea syndrome. Eur Respir J 1998; 12:770–775.
35. White DP, Gibb TJ, Wall JM, et al. Assessment of accuracy and analysis time of a novel device to monitor sleep and breathing in the home. Sleep 1995; 18:115–126.
36. Ancoli-Israel S, Mason W, Coy TV, et al. Evaluation of sleep disordered breathing with unattended recording: the Nightwatch system. J Med Eng Technol 1997; 21:10–14.
37. Practice parameters for the use of portable monitoring devices in the investigation of suspected obstructive sleep apnea in adults. A joint project sponsored by the American Academy of Sleep Medicine, the American Thoracic Society, and the American College of Chest Physicians. Sleep 2003; 26(7):907–913.
38. Iber C, Redline S, Kaplan Gilpin AM, et al. Polysomnography performed in the unattended home versus the attended laboratory setting-Sleep Heart Health Study methodology. Sleep 2004 May 1; 27(3):536–540.
39. Fry JM, DiPhillipo MA, Curran K, et al. Full polysomnography in the home. Sleep 1998; 21:635–642.
40. Emsellem H, Corson W, Rappaport B, et al. Verification of sleep apnea using a portable sleep apnea screening device. South Med J 1990; 83:748–752.
41. Redline S, Tosteson T, Boucher MA, et al. Measurement of sleep related breathing disturbances in epidemiologic studies: assessment of the validity and reproducibility of a portable monitoring device. Chest 1991; 100:1281–1286.
42. Parra O, Garcia-Esclasans N, Montserrat JM, et al. Should patients with sleep apnoea/hypopnoea syndrome be diagnosed and managed on the basis of home sleep studies? Eur Respir J 1997; 10:1720–1724.
43. Whittle AT, Finch SP, Mortimore IL, et al. Use of home sleep studies for diagnosis of the sleep apnoea/hypopnoea syndrome. Thorax 1997; 52:1068–1073.
44. Dingli K, Coleman EL, Vennelle M, et al. Evaluation of a portable device for diagnosing the sleep apnoea/hypopnoea syndrome. Eur Respir J 2003; 21:253–259.
45. Yin M, Miyazaki S, Ishikawa K. Evaluation of type 3 portable monitoring in unattended home setting for suspected sleep apnea: factors that may affect its accuracy. Otolaryngol Head Neck Surg 2006; 134:204–209.
46. George CF, Millar TW, Kryger MH. Identification and quantification of apneas by computer-based analysis of oxygen saturation. Am Rev Respir Dis 1988; 137:1238–1240.
47. Rauscher H, PoppW, Zwick H. Quantification of sleep disordered breathing by computerized analysis of oximetry, heart rate and snoring. Eur Respir J 1991; 4:655–659.
48. Williams AJ, Yu G, Santiago S, et al. Screening for sleep apnea using pulse oximetry and a clinical score. Chest 1991; 100:631–635.
49. Levy P, Pepin JL, Deschaux-Blanc C, et al. Accuracy of oximetry for detection of respiratory disturbances in sleep apnea syndrome. Chest 1996; 109:395–399.
50. Golpe R, Jimenez A, Carpizo R, et al. Utility of home oximetry as a screening test for patients with moderate to severe symptoms of obstructive sleep apnea. Sleep 1999; 22:932–937.
51. Series F, Marc I, Cormier Y, et al. Utility of nocturnal home oximetry for case finding in patients with suspected sleep apnea hypopnea syndrome. Ann Intern Med 1993; 119:449–453.
52. Hussain SF, Fleetham JA. Overnight home oximetry: can it identify patients with obstructive sleep apnea-hypopnea who have minimal daytime sleepiness? Respir Med 2003; 97(5):537–540.

53. Issa FG, Morrison D, Hadjuk E, et al. Digital monitoring of sleep disordered breathing using snoring sound and arterial oxygen saturation. Am Rev Respir Dis 1993; 148:1023–1029.
54. Vazquez J, Tsai W, Flemons W, et al. Automated analysis of digital oximetry in the diagnosis of obstructive sleep apnoea. Thorax 2000; 55:302–307.
55. West P, George CFP, Kryger MH. Dynamic in vivo response characteristics of three oximeters: Hewlettpackard 47201A, Biox III, and Nellcor N-100. Sleep 1987; 10:263–271.
56. Severinghaus JW, Naifeh KH, Koh SO. Errors in 14 pulse oximeters during profound hypoxia. J Clin Monit 1989; 5:72–81.
57. Vegfors M, Lindberg L.-G, Lennmarken C. The influence of changes in blood flow on the accuracy of pulse oximetry in humans. Acta Anaesthesiol Scand 1992; 36:346–349.
58. Kirk VG, Bohn SG, Flemons WW, et al. Comparison of home oximetry monitoring with laboratory polysomnography. Chest 2003; 124:1702–1708.
59. Stoohs R, Guilleminault C. MESAM 4: an ambulatory device for the detection of patients at risk for obstructive sleep apnea syndrome (OSAS). Chest 1992; 101:1221–1227.
60. Koziej M, Cieslicki J, Gorzelak K, et al. Hand-scoring of MESAM 4 recordings is more accurate than automatic analysis in screening for obstructive sleep apnoea. Eur Respir J 1994; 7:1771–1775.
61. Esnaola S, Duran J, Infante-Rivard C, et al. Diagnostic accuracy of a portable recording device (MESAM IV) in suspected obstructive sleep apnea. Eur Respir J 1996; 9:2597–2605.
62. Cirignotta F, Mondini S, Gerardi R, et al. Unreliability of automatic scoring of MESAM 4 in assessing patients with complicated obstructive sleep apnea syndrome. Chest 2001; 119:1387–1392.
63. Fietze I, Dingli K, Diefenbach K, et al. Night-to-night variation of the oxygen desaturation index in sleep apnoea syndrome. Eur Respir J 2004; 24:987–993.
64. Westbrook PR, Levendowski DJ, Cvetinovic M, et al. Description and validation of the apnea risk evaluation system: a novel method to diagnose sleep apnea-hypopnea in the home. Chest 2005; 128:2166–2175.
65. Pillar G, Bar A, Shlitner A, et al. Autonomic arousal index: an automated detection based on peripheral arterial tonometry. Sleep 2002; 25:543–549.
66. Ayas NT, Pittman S, MacDonald M, et al. Assessment of a wrist-worn device in the detection of OSA. Sleep Med 2003; 4(5):435–442.
67. Schnall RP, Shlitner A, Sheffy J, et al. Periodic, profound peripheral vasoconstriction: a new marker of obstructive sleep apnea. Sleep 1999; 22:939–946.
68. Bar A, Pillar G, Dvir I, et al. Evaluation of a portable device based on peripheral arterial tone for unattended home sleep studies. Chest 2003; 123:695–703.
69. Pittman S, Tal N, Pillar G, et al. Automatic detection of obstructive sleep-disordered breathing events using peripheral arterial tonometry and oximetry. J Sleep Res 2000; 9(suppl):309.
70. Zou D, Grote L, Peker Y, et al. Validation a portable monitoring device for sleep apnea diagnosis in a population based cohort using synchronized home polysomnography. Sleep 2006; 29(3):367–374.
71. Øverland B, Bruskeland G, Akre H, et al. Evaluation of a portable recording device (Reggie) with actimeter and nasopharyngeal/esophagus catheter incorporated. Respiration 2005; 72:600–605.
72. Ficker JH, Wiest GH, Wilpert J, et al. Evaluation of a portable recording device (Somnocheck) for use in patients with suspected obstructive sleep apnoea. Respiration 2001; 68:307–312.
73. Meslier N, Simon I, Kouatchet A, et al. Validation of a suprasternal pressure transducer for apnea classification during sleep. Sleep 2002; 25:753–757.
74. Nakano H, Hayashi M, Ohshima E, et al. Validation of a new system of tracheal sound analysis for the diagnosis of sleep apnea-hypopnea syndrome. Sleep 2004; 27:951–957.
75. Sadeh A, Hauri PJ, Kripke DF, et al. The role of actigraphy in the evaluation of sleep disorders. Sleep 1995; 18:288–302.
76. Hedner J, Pillar G, Pittman SD, et al. A novel adaptive wrist actigraphy algorithm for Sleep-Wake assessment in sleep apnea patients. Sleep 2004; 27:1560–1566.

77. Middelkoop HA, Knuistingh Neven A, van Hilten. Wrist actigraphic assessment of sleep in 116 community based subjects suspected of obstructive sleep apnoea syndrome. Thorax 1995; 50:284–289.

78. Guilleminault C, Connoly S, Winkle R, et al. Cyclical variation of the heart rate in sleep apnea syndrome. Mechanisms and usefulness of 24h electrocardiography as screening technique. Lancet 1984; 1:126–131.

79. Pitson DJ, Sandell A, van der Hout R, et al. Use of pulse transit time as a measure of inspiratory effort in patients with obstructive sleep apnoea. Eur Respir J 1995; 8:1669–1674.

80. Argod J, Pepin JL, Smith RP, et al. Comparison of esophageal pressure with pulse transit time as a measure of respiratory effort for scoring obstructive. Nonapneic respiratory events. Am J Respir Crit Care Med 2000; 162:87–93.

81. Schwartz DL. The pulse transit time arousal index in obstructive sleep apnea before and after CPAP. Sleep Med 2005; 6:199–203.

82. Guyatt G, Tugwell P, Feeny D, et al. The framework for clinical evaluation of diagnostic technologies. CMAJ 1986; 134:587–594.

3 Polysomnography and Cardiorespiratory Monitoring

Michael R. Littner
*VA Greater Los Angeles Healthcare System, Sulpulveda, California and
David Geffen School of Medicine, University of California, Los Angeles,
California, U.S.A.*

INTRODUCTION

The obstructive sleep apnea-hypopnea syndrome (OSA) is recognized pre-dominantly by daytime somnolence and night-time snoring often in obese individuals (1,2). The diagnosis is confirmed by demonstrating a sufficient number of obstructive apneas (absence of airflow with continued respiratory effort) and/or obstructive hypopneas (reduction in airflow despite sufficient respiratory effort to produce normal airflow) (1). The daytime somnolence appears to result, in large part, from short, amnestic arousals that fragment and reduce the efficiency of sleep. OSA appears to affect about 4% of men and 2% of women between 30 and 60 years of age (3). OSA is associated with systemic hypertension, myocardial infarction, motor vehicle accidents, and cerebrovascular accidents (4–7).

Daytime somnolence is a nonspecific symptom and may be due to narcolepsy, insufficient sleep, and idiopathic hypersomnia among other conditions (2). In addition, snoring is a nonspecific finding; for example, 67% of obese patients [body mass index (BMI) ≥ 30] who snored loudly (patient report) had OSA (8). The general non-specificity of daytime sleepiness and snoring requires objective measurement of apneas and hypopneas during sleep for confirmation of OSA.

In general, confirmation involves an overnight sleep study while monitoring a number of respiratory channels (nasal and oral airflow, chest wall and abdominal movement, and oximetry), sleep staging by electroencephalogram (EEG) (central and occipital electrodes usually referenced to the ear), electro-oculogram (right and left eye movement) and chin electromyogram, at least a one-lead electrocardiogram, as well as leg movements (bilateral anterior tibialis electrodes) which may also produce frequent arousals (9). The study is attended by a technician (polysomnographic or sleep technologist) to perform and observe the study, ensure quality and safety, and make needed interventions including application of the most frequently used therapy, continuous positive airway pressure (CPAP). This approach is called polysomnography (PSG).

The number of potential patients usually exceeds the number of sleep laboratory facilities capable of performing the test in a timely fashion. The labor intensity of the attendant, scoring and interpretation of the study, and cost of the space and equipment make PSG relatively expensive, typically costing $1000 or more per study (10).

To increase access to diagnosis and potentially reduce cost, there has been an effort to produce systems that incorporate part or all of the PSG but make it portable and ideally usable without an attendant technician. The ideal system would measure the minimum number of channels necessary, be self-contained and self-administered by the patient, be amenable to rapid and accurate scoring, and provide information that would confirm OSA with identical specificity and sensitivity to the PSG. This review will evaluate the ability of various methods to achieve this goal in adults.

PATHOPHYSIOLOGY

Patients with OSA experience intermittent upper airway obstruction above the epiglottis generally of the pharynx. The pharyngeal musculature attempts to keep the upper airway open to permit ventilation and opposes subatmospheric pressure in the pharynx that results from turbulent flow during partial upper airway obstruction. The genioglossus muscles also keep the upper airway clear of obstruction by pulling it forward. Anatomic factors (e.g., adipose tissue, tongue size, mandibular configuration, uvula, and tonsils) as well as neuromuscular factors (e.g., sleep state affecting the pharyngeal muscles and alcohol) contribute to increasing, maintaining or reducing upper airway patency (11).

Obstructive events result from the completely or partially obstructed upper airway during sleep may lead to cessation (apnea) (Fig. 1) or reduction (hypopnea) (Fig. 2) of airflow. Partial obstruction can also lead to snoring without a reduction in airflow. Partial or complete cessation of respiratory effort leads to central apneas (Fig. 3) or hypopneas. Mixed events start with a central component and end with an obstructive component. Mixed apneas (Fig. 4) and hypopneas are considered to be obstructive in behavior.

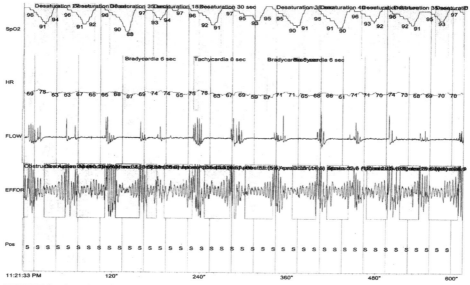

FIGURE 1   A series of obstructive apneas (no airflow with continued respiratory effort) from a Level III portable monitoring system used unattended in the patient's home. Note the severe cyclical arterial oxygen desaturations associated with the apneas. The patient was instructed in the outpatient area of the medical center, took home the system, attached it to himself just before retiring for the night, and brought the system back the next day for analysis. The epoch is 10 minutes in duration. Note that the events were occurring so frequently that the labels "Desaturation" and "Obstructive Apnea" are partially obscured on the record. *Abbreviations*: SpO2, pulse oximetry; HR, heart rate; FLOW from a nasal/oral pressure cannula; EFFOR(T) from the movement of a chest wall belt; POS(ition) is supine (S).

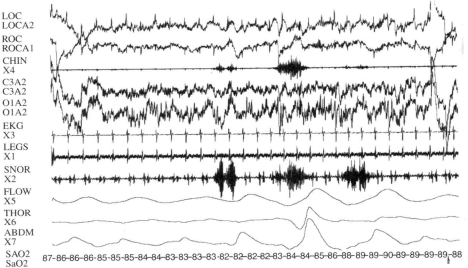

FIGURE 2   An obstructive hypopnea associated with snoring and ending in an arousal. The airflow is reduced but not absent and is associated with continued respiratory effort with a paradox of the abdominal and thoracic movement (respiratory excursions are out of phase) and an arterial oxygen desaturation to 82%. The hypopnea is occurring in rapid eye movement (REM) sleep (REMs seen at the beginning and end of the epoch). The hypopnea ends with a snore associated with a brief arousal noted by an increase in chin electromyogram tone and an increase in the electroencephalogram signal frequency. The record also demonstrates electrocardiogram artifact in several leads. The epoch is 30 seconds in duration. *Abbreviations*: LOCA2, left eye electro-oculogram referenced to the right (A2) ear; ROCA1, right eye electro-oculogram referenced to the left (A1) ear; CHIN, electromyogram recorded from chin muscles; C3A2, O1A2, electroencephalogram electrodes placed centrally or occipitally, respectively, and referenced to the right (A2) ear; EKG, electrocardiogram; LEGS, sensors placed on each leg and linked to provide a single signal for leg movement; SNOR, snoring intensity by microphone; FLOW, airflow measured by oronasal thermistor; THOR and ABDM, thoracic and abdominal movement, respectively, measured by strain gauges; SaO_2, pulse oximetry from a finger sensor.

Although the above distinctions are made, the vast majority of patients with sleep apnea have predominantly obstructive apneas and hypopneas (continued respiratory effort with absence or reduction in airflow, respectively) even if there are elements of central or mixed events. Central apneas are seen more commonly in patients with congestive heart failure (in association with Cheyne-Stokes respiration), underlying neurologic disorders (such as stroke), or in individuals who reside at higher altitudes (1,12).

A variant is known as the upper airway resistance syndrome (UARS) (1), in which the pathologic events are respiratory effort-related arousals (RERAs). RERAs as defined by the American Academy of Sleep Medicine (AASM) (13) are due to partial upper airway obstruction with an increase in amplitude of negative intrathoracic pressure (increase in respiratory effort), leading to minimal reduction in airflow and arterial oxygen saturation but terminating in an arousal. The gold standard for assessing RERAs is by esophageal manometry (i.e., pressure measurements), which typically uses either a water-filled catheter or balloon placed in the esophagus inserted via the nose. Esophageal pressure assesses respiratory effort or work of breathing by estimating transmitted intrathoracic pressure, and can be useful in

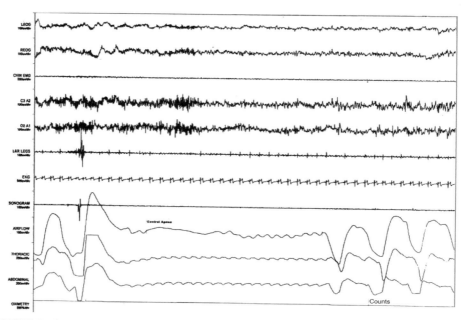

FIGURE 3 A central apnea, probably from a postarousal hyperventilation apnea from an in-laboratory polysomnogram. The chest and abdominal effort are lacking, there is no airflow and there are cardiac oscillations observed on the airflow channel from small amounts of airflow resulting from contraction and relaxation of the heart causing the lungs to slightly compress and decompress. The patient had a modest 4% reduction in arterial saturation (not labeled except as "Desat"). The sleep stage is non-rapid eye movement stage 1 with a frequency of electroencephalogram (EEG) activity of 4 to 6 cycles/second after the arousal (EEG frequency ≥ 8 cycles/second, a subtle increase in chin electromyogram activity and a leg movement from the arousal) that occurred at the beginning of the epoch. The epoch is 60 seconds in duration. *Abbreviations*: LEOG, left eye electro-oculogram; REOG, right eye electro-oculogram; CHIN EMG, electromyogram recorded from chin muscles; C3A2, O2A1, electroencephalogram electrodes placed centrally or occipitally and referenced to the right (A2) or left (A1) ear, respectively; L&R LEGS, sensors placed on each leg and linked to provide a single signal for leg movement; EKG, electrocardiogram; SONOGRAM, snoring intensity by microphone; AIRFLOW, airflow measured by oronasal thermistor; THORACIC and ABDOMINAL, thoracic and abdominal movement, respectively, measured by strain gauges; OXIMETRY, pulse oximetry from a finger sensor.

helping the sleep specialist to identify and distinguish abnormal breathing events (Figs. 5 and 6). Alternatively, a RERA may be inferred from repetitive snoring increasing in amplitude followed by an arousal (Fig. 7). An arousal is an EEG event characterized as an abrupt shift in EEG frequency (excluding delta waves and spindles) lasting more than three seconds and preceded by at least 10 seconds of sleep. An arousal is frequently accompanied by an increase in chin muscle tone, particularly during rapid eye movement (REM) sleep (14).

Cardiac arrhythmias are common in patients with OSA. The most common is sinus arrhythmia but atrial fibrillation, bradycardia, premature atrial and ventricular contractions, and nonsustained and sustained ventricular tachycardia occur more frequently than in control patients (15).

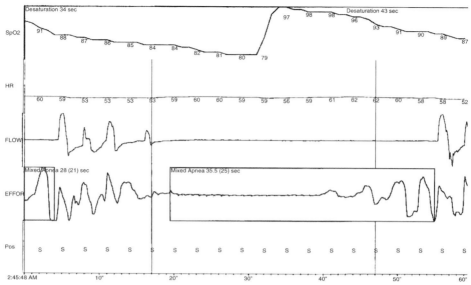

FIGURE 4 A mixed apnea with a central component (no airflow or respiratory effort) followed by an obstructive component (no airflow with continued respiratory effort) from Level III portable monitoring system used unattended in the patient's home. The patient was instructed in the outpatient area of the medical center, took home the system, attached it to himself just before retiring for the night and brought the system back the next day for analysis. The epoch is 60 seconds in duration. Note that the start of arterial oxygen desaturation occurs at about 20 seconds after the start of the apnea. This time delay is due to a combination of arterial circulation lag time from lungs to finger and the oximetry machine electronic lag time from time of sensing to display. *Abbreviations*: SpO2, pulse oximetry; HR, heart rate; FLOW from a nasal/oral pressure cannula; EFFOR(T) from the movement of a chest wall belt; Pos(ition) is supine (S).

DIAGNOSIS OF OBSTRUCTIVE SLEEP APNEA

According to the International Classification of Sleep Disorders (second edition) (ICSD-2) (2), the diagnosis is based on PSG and clinical criteria in adults and children. The following is a brief overview of the diagnostic criteria.

In adults, the patient complains of daytime sleepiness, unrefreshing sleep, fatigue, insomnia, awaking with breath holding, gasping, or choking, or there is a bed partner that notes loud snoring or breathing pauses during sleep. If the patient is not symptomatic, for example the patient has only snoring during sleep, then a PSG showing ≥ 15 obstructive apneas, obstructive hypopneas, and/or RERAs per hour of sleep can be confirmatory. If the patient is symptomatic, for example the patient has daytime sleepiness, OSA is confirmed by a PSG showing ≥ 5 obstructive apneas, obstructive hypopneas, and/or RERAs per hour of sleep.

A child may not be able to give a history and the parent or other caregiver may note snoring, labored or obstructed breathing, or both during the child's sleep. There are a number of witnessed sleep events that may indicate OSA, which include paradoxical inward rib cage motion during inspiration, movement arousals, sweating, or neck hyperextension. In addition, the parent or caregiver may note that the child is excessive sleepy during the day, has hyperactivity or aggressive behavior, has a slow rate of growth, has morning headaches and/or enuresis. This is confirmed by a PSG

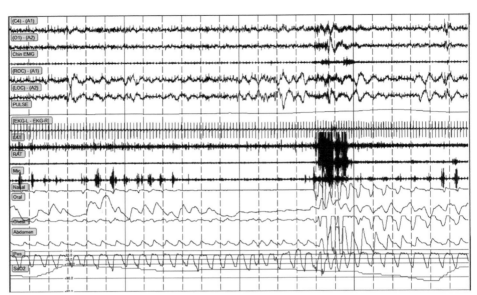

FIGURE 5   An obstructive apnea with a crescendo increase in esophageal pressure (Pes). Snoring intensity, observed in the Mic channel, parallels the changes in esophageal pressure until the start of the apnea. The apnea ends in an arousal, noted by an increase in chin and leg electromyogram tone and an increase in the electroencephalogram signal frequency. There is a paradox of the abdominal and thoracic movement (respiratory excursions are out of phase) and an arterial oxygen desaturation to 87%. The apnea occurs in rapid eye movement sleep, and the epoch is two minutes in duration. *Abbreviations*: C4A1, O1A2, electroencephalogram electrodes placed centrally or occipitally and referenced to the left (A1) and right (A2) ear, respectively; Chin EMG, electromyogram recorded from chin muscles; ROCA1, right eye electro-oculogram referenced to the left (A1) ear; LOCA2, left eye electro-oculogram referenced to the right (A2) ear; PULSE, pulse rate; EKG, electrocardiogram; LAT and RAT, leg movements measured from left and right anterior tibialis, respectively; Mic, snoring intensity by microphone; Nasal and Oral, airflow assessed by pressure transducer and thermistor, respectively; Chest and Abdomen, thoracic and abdominal movement, respectively, measured by impedance bands; Pes, esophageal pressure measurements; SaO2, pulse oximetry from a finger sensor. *Source*: Courtesy of Clete A. Kushida, M.D., Ph.D.

that demonstrates during sleep one or more apneas or hypopneas of at least two respiratory cycles in duration, or frequent RERAs, arterial oxygen desaturation with apnea, or hypercapnia, or frequent arousals and snoring associated with periods of hypercapnia and/or arterial oxygen desaturation or frequent arousals associated with paradoxical breathing (abdominal and thoracic movement out of phase).

CLASSIFICATION OF METHODS FOR DIAGNOSIS OF SLEEP-DISORDERED BREATHING

The AASM, formerly known as the American Sleep Disorders Association, in 1994 (16,17) classified diagnostic sleep equipment into four levels (Table 1). Attended PSG has already been described and is Level I. Unattended PSG is Level II. Measurement of a minimum of four channels, which must include oximetry, one channel each of respiratory effort or movement and airflow or two channels of respiratory effort or movement, and heart rate is Level III. A single or two-channel system typically including oximetry is Level IV. For purposes of this review, traditional systems that do not

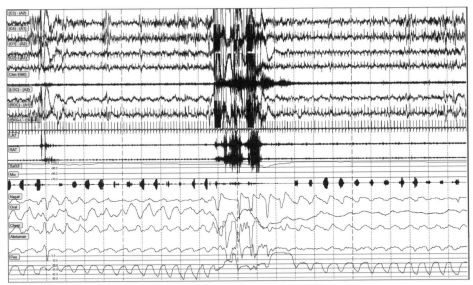

FIGURE 6 A respiratory effort-related arousal (RERA) with a crescendo increase in esophageal pressure (Pes) is depicted in the first half of the epoch. There is a decrease in nasal but not oral airflow, so the abnormal respiratory event does not meet criteria for a hypopnea. Snoring is observed, and the RERA culminates in an arousal, noted by an increase in chin and leg electromyogram tone and an increase in the electroencephalogram signal frequency. The RERA occurs in non-rapid eye movement stage 1 sleep, and the arterial oxygen desaturates to 90%. Following the RERA, there is a resumption of snoring and a crescendo increase in esophageal pressure, and the decrease in both the nasal and oral airflow is more compatible with a hypopnea. The epoch is two minutes in duration. *Abbreviations*: C3A2 and C4A1, left and right electroencephalogram electrodes placed centrally and referenced to the right (A2) and left (A1) ear, respectively; O1A2 and O2A1, left and right electroencephalogram electrodes placed occipitally and referenced to the right (A2) and left (A1) ear, respectively; Chin EMG, electromyogram recorded from chin muscles; LOCA2, left eye electro-oculogram referenced to the right (A2) ear; ROCA1, right eye electro-oculogram referenced to the left (A1) ear; EKG, electrocardiogram; LAT and RAT, leg movements measured from left and right anterior tibialis, respectively; SaO2, pulse oximetry from a finger sensor; Mic, snoring intensity by microphone; Nasal and Oral, airflow assessed by pressure transducer and thermistor, respectively; Chest and Abdomen, thoracic and abdominal movement, respectively, measured by impedance bands; Pes, esophageal pressure measurements. *Source*: Courtesy of Clete A. Kushida, M.D., Ph.D.

meet minimum criteria for a Level III will be classified as Level IV. The classification is essentially one of lesser and lesser channels that are typically part of the PSG.

Portable monitoring systems are generally designed to be used unattended usually in the patient's home. However, the systems can also be used attended in the sleep laboratory and this will also be reviewed. For purposes of this paper, attended PSG will be the reference for comparison of portable monitoring systems.

WHAT IS THE PROPER STUDY DESIGN TO VALIDATE A PORTABLE MONITOR?

As discussed in a review published in 2003 (18), validation of a particular device involves comparison to attended PSG with determination of the sensitivity and specificity of the portable monitor. This comparison should be made in a patient population that is representative of the population in which the method is to be

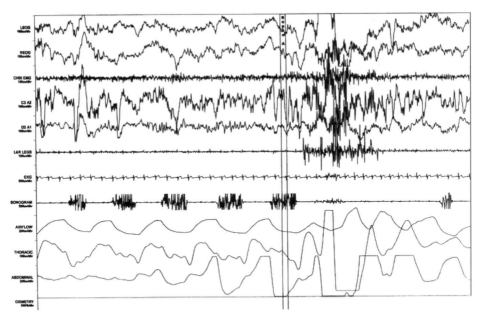

FIGURE 7   A series of increasing snores (noted as increasing duration of activity on the sonogram channel), followed by an arousal marked by an increase in the frequency of the electroencephalogram activity, a leg movement and an increase in chin electromyogram activity. The sleep stage is non-rapid eye movement stage 2 with K complexes prior to the arousal. There is no obvious reduction in airflow or a decrease in arterial oxygen saturation. The epoch is 30 seconds in duration. *Abbreviations*: LEOG, left eye electro-oculogram; REOG, right eye electro-oculogram; CHIN EMG, electromyogram recorded from chin muscles; C3A2, O2A1, electroencephalogram electrodes placed centrally or occipitally and referenced to the right (A2) or left (A1) ear, respectively; L&R LEGS, sensors placed on each leg and linked to provide a single signal for leg movement; EKG, electrocardiogram; SONOGRAM, snoring intensity by microphone; AIRFLOW, airflow measured by oronasal thermistor; THORACIC and ABDOMINAL, thoracic and abdominal movement, respectively, measured by strain gauges; OXIMETRY, pulse oximetry from a finger sensor.

used. Patient selection should be consecutive without undue referral biases or at least with the referral bias clearly defined and uninfluenced by the investigator or a small group of providers. In addition, the prevalence of OSA in the study population should be typical of the population for which the device is ultimately to be used. For example, if a method tests only high probability patients for validation, the results cannot be confidently extrapolated to populations of moderate or low probability.

There are two approaches that should be used to validate a portable monitor. First, the sensitivity and specificity under ideal conditions should be determined in a simultaneous comparison with attended PSG. This must be done blinded. The question of whether a technician should intervene depends, in part, on the intended use of the portable monitor. If there is consideration to use the portable monitor with a technician to attend the study, then intervention is appropriate. If the consideration is only for unattended use, then there should be no intervention to repair or correct possible data loss from the portable monitor. This provides the sensitivity and specificity for the diagnosis in direct comparison during the same real-time period as the PSG. The

TABLE 1 American Academy of Sleep Medicine Classification of Levels of Sleep Apnea Testing (Modified)

	Level I Attended PSG recording	Level II Unattended PSG	Level III Modified portable sleep apnea testing	Level IV[a] Continuous single or dual bioparameter recording
Measures	Minimum of 7, including EEG, EOG, chin EMG, ECG, ventilation, respiratory effort, oxygen saturation	Minimum of 7, including EEG, EOG, chin EMG, ECG or heart rate, ventilation, respiratory effort, oxygen saturation	Minimum of 4, including ventilation, heart rate or ECG, oxygen saturation	Minimum of 1: oxygen saturation, ventilation, or chest movement
Body position	Yes	Possible	Possible	No
Leg movement	EMG or motion sensor desirable but optional	Optional	Optional	No
Personnel	Yes	No	No	No
Interventions	Possible	No	No	No

[a]Level IV may also include any device that does not meet criteria for a higher level.
Abbreviations: ECG, electrocardiography; EEG, electroencephalography; EMG, electromyography; EOG, electrooculography; PSG, polysomnography; patterned after Reference 16. Six hours overnight recording minimum.
Source: Ref. 16

report should include the apneas and hypopneas during various patient positions for the PSG and for the portable system and whether there was intervention and if so, details of the intervention. Ideally, the portable system should have a position monitor. If the system does not perform well in this setting, the system is of questionable use. This comparison is of benefit in validation for attended in-laboratory use only.

The second step in the validation process is to compare the in-laboratory PSG to the portable monitor used in the intended environment, usually unattended in the patient's home. The study should be blinded, randomized and the PSG and portable monitor should be applied in every patient. The interval between studies should be short, preferably a week or less. Variables that may affect the results are body position, total sleep time, REM sleep time, and environmental conditions such as room temperature and extraneous noise. These contribute to normal night-to-night variability (19), which may differ between the laboratory and portable monitoring environment.

A strategy to deal with variability that is not an intrinsic characteristic of the portable monitoring device is to also conduct the PSG on a second night in the laboratory. Ideally, a fourth night should also be performed outside the laboratory in order to determine the night-to-night variability of the unattended portable monitor. This information would help separate the effects of night-to-night variability on the results from those due to intrinsic differences between the PSG and portable monitor. To date, one study of a Level III monitor has adopted much of this approach (20).

The methods should include full disclosure of the PSG and portable monitor sensors and channels, definition of apneas and hypopneas for both the PSG and portable monitor, epoch length for scoring of sleep and respiratory variables, oximeter sampling and recording rates, and funding for the study.

WHAT CAN BE EXPECTED FROM A COMPARISON OF A PORTABLE MONITOR TO POLYSOMNOGRAPHY?

The concept that portable monitoring can be as diagnostically effective as PSG rests on the assumption that not all of the PSG monitored channels are necessary to make a diagnosis of OSA. That is, some of the channels are either redundant or measure variables that are not essential to the diagnosis. For this to be valid, the definition of what constitutes a confirmatory study for OSA is important. The typical definition of an apnea is the cessation of airflow (i.e., a decrease of 90% or greater from baseline levels) for 10 seconds or more that cannot be attributed to another cause or artifact. A report of a task force of the AASM on research methods (13) provided an alternative definition that did not distinguish between an apnea and a hypopnea; the obstructive apnea/hypopnea event was defined as a reduction in airflow (50% or greater from baseline levels) lasting 10 seconds or greater or a decrease in airflow that does not meet this criterion but is accompanied by an arterial oxygen desaturation (greater than 3%) or an EEG arousal. In addition, a RERA was included as a respiratory event consistent with OSA that does not meet criteria for an apnea or hypopnea. The Centers of Medicare and Medicaid Services (CMS) (i.e., Medicare) requires a 4% desaturation during sleep in addition to airflow reduction (21). The Medicare criteria require that sleep be measured using traditional sensors in a facility-based sleep laboratory making most if not all portable systems currently unacceptable as diagnostic devices for Medicare purposes.

The design of a portable system is potentially limited by the goals of measurement. For example, if the goal is to define OSA by a combination of hypopneas associated with oxygen desaturations and clear-cut apneas, a two-channel system may be sufficient if the issues of sleep, central apneas, (apneas without continued respiratory effort) and body position are not clinically relevant. On the other hand, the two-channel system is totally inadequate to detect hypopneas with arousals or RERAs. These types of considerations have not been well-evaluated in most previous studies. Some studies are weighted to favor the portable system by defining respiratory events identically between the PSG and portable monitor with the exception of use of sleep time in the PSG and recording time (often minus artifact) in the portable monitor. In summary, the more types of events that are deemed necessary to make a diagnosis of OSA, the less likely that the portable monitor will detect most of the events. With these considerations in mind, the following section evaluates the evidence to support or not to support the use of portable monitors to diagnose OSA.

WHAT IS THE EVIDENCE TO DATE? (SEE ALSO CHAPTER 2)

There are a large number of studies that have used portable monitors without direct comparison to PSG for a variety of epidemiologic and diagnostic purposes. However, these will not be reviewed since they provide little or no insight into the sensitivity and specificity of portable monitoring compared to PSG in an individual patient. Based on the evidence to be discussed, Level II and IV portable monitors are not sufficiently accurate or validated to recommend for use at this time, particularly unattended in the home. Level III monitors are useful attended in the laboratory and of possible usefulness unattended in either the laboratory or the home.

In October 2003, a joint task force of the AASM, the American College of Chest Physicians (ACCP) and the American Thoracic Society (ATS) published an evidence-based review (Joint Review) of portable monitors (18). Fifty-one publications with 54 studies were reviewed. Sensitivities and specificities were calculated in 49 of these studies. Since then there have been at least 24 publications (1 Level II, 9 Level III, 11 Level IV, and 3 of a hybrid Level IV system) with 29 studies (5 had both simultaneous laboratory as well as home to laboratory studies). In what follows, the apnea/hypopnea index (AHI) per hour of sleep is designated as AHI for PSG and the respiratory disturbance index (RDI) per hour of recording or equivalent is designated as RDI for portable monitors unless otherwise indicated.

Many studies, particularly Level IV, required different thresholds for AHI and/or RDI to achieve the highest possible sensitivity and specificity pairs (best sensitivity and sensitivity). This left many patients with a nondiagnostic RDI, which would require a subsequent evaluation including potentially an attended PSG. Despite the use of best values, many studies failed to achieve an acceptable pair for diagnostic purposes. This was defined in the Joint Review as a likelihood ratio (LR) pair of ≥ 5 to increase post-test probability (i.e., increasing the positive predictive value) of OSA with a positive test and ≤ 0.2 to decrease post-test probability (i.e., increasing the negative predictive value) with a negative test. These LR values indicate a modest improvement in diagnostic accuracy (22) over no test at all. The reader is referred to Reference (18) for a more detailed discussion of LRs.

The Joint Review classified evidence based on the following grades:

1. Blinded comparison, consecutive patients, reference standard (i.e., PSG) performed on all patients;
2. Blinded comparison, nonconsecutive patients, reference standard performed on all patients;
3. Blinded comparison, consecutive patients, reference standard not performed on all patients;
4. Reference standard was not applied blindly or independently.

The definition of hypopnea and the threshold AHI to define OSA varied from study-to-study but was consistent within each study. That is, the evidence can be used to determine the performance of portable monitors compared to PSG but cannot easily be used to define what is an acceptable AHI or RDI to identify OSA across all studies.

There were a total of three papers on Level II monitors of evidence grades II, IV and IV (23–25). In addition, there is one study published since the Joint Review of grade II evidence (26). The study suggests that similar data can be obtained from home compared to a telemetry monitored and partially attended in-hospital study but the failure rate of home monitoring was unacceptably high at 23.4%. In addition, the telemetry-monitored studies had an 11.2% failure rate. Of 99 subjects, evaluable data were available in 65 for both nights. Using the telemetry-monitored studies as the reference standard, the sensitivity and specificity were 94.9% and 80.8% with LRs of 4.95 and 0.063, respectively, for the 65 subjects (calculated from data presented in the publication). The paucity of data does not allow one to reach any conclusion regarding the utility of these systems in the diagnosis of OSA. In concept, Level II should be the most accurate. In practice, as indicated by one of the publications (26), the complexity of these systems makes patient setup and subsequent data loss a potential problem.

Of nine studies of a Level III monitor done simultaneously attended in the sleep laboratory nine had an acceptable LR pair from the Joint Review (18). Only one of the studies had a group of nondiagnostic RDIs (36%). Of four studies comparing home to laboratory, two had an acceptable LR pair with 22% and 37% nondiagnostic RDIs. Data loss, when reported, was under 10% for those with an acceptable LR pair.

Table 2 summarizes the data for simultaneously attended Level III monitors (20,27–40), which includes the nine simultaneous studies (28–36) from the Joint

TABLE 2 Studies of Level III Portable Monitors Simultaneous with In-Laboratory Tests

Study	AHI	RDI	Prev (%)	Sens	Spec	LR(H)	LR(L)	Non (%)	PPV	NPV	Evid	Comment
28	10	6	24	89	92	11.1	0.12	0	78	96	II	Red in airflow plus 3% red in sat or an arousal used to determine AHI. Red in airflow plus 3% red in sat used to determine RDI.
29	15	15	50	86	95	17	0.15	0	94	87	IV	Red in airflow plus 4% red in sat or an arousal used to determine AHI.
30	5	5	62	95	96	24	0.05	0	98	92	I	Red in airflow used to determine AHI and RDI. Compressed time frame for scoring RDI but not AHI.
31	10	10	57	97	100	[a]	0.03	0	100	96	II	Red in thoracoabdominal movement of 50% plus 4% red in sat for AHI. Discernable red in airflow plus 4% red in sat for RDI.
32	15	15	27	86	95	17	0.15	0	86	95	II	Red in airflow used to determine AHI and RDI.
33	10	10	84	95	100	[a]	0.05	0	100	80	II	Red in airflow plus 4% red in sat or 2% red in sat plus arousal for AHI. Red in airflow plus 2% red in sat for RDI.
34	10	10	47	92	96	25	0.08	0	93	95	I	Red in airflow used to determine AHI and RDI.
35	10 for sens, 20 for spec	10 for sens, 20 for spec	63.3 for sens, 43.3 for spec	100 (64 corr spec)	88 (77 corr sens)	6.5	0	36	83	100	II	Red in airflow plus 4% red in sat (Denver) or 2% red in sat (Los Angeles) or arousal for AHI and RDI. Arousals were measured indirectly with PM. Compressed time frame for scoring RDI but not AHI.
36	10	10	66	100	100	[a]	0	0	100	100	I	Red in airflow used to determine AHI and RDI. Sleep stages not used for either PSG or PM.
20 (new study)	15	15	48 (est)	95	91	10.6	0.06	0	91	96	I	Red in airflow and 2% desaturations with automatic scoring for AHI and RDI. 12% data loss for PM.
37 (new study)	15	10 for sens, 20 for spec	62	100 (corr spec 67)	93 (corr sens 88)	12.6	0	18	95	100	II	RDI red in thoracoabdominal movement and red in nasal pressure. AHI red in thoracoabdominal movement for hypopneas. 3% data loss.

27 (new study)	5 levels (5, 10, 15, 20, 30)	6.7 for sens, 27.6 for spec	86 for AHI 5 (RDI 6.7), 44 for AHI 30 (RDI 27.6)	97.1 (corr spec 90.9)	90.9 (corr sens 88.6)	7.97	0.0319	41	98.5	90.9	IV	Automatic scoring had unacceptable results. PSG scoring used arousals. Data loss under 10%. Evidence grade IV since blinding of scoring not reported.
38 (new study)	?5 for sens, 10 for spec	5 for sens, 10 for spec	?86 for sens, 84 for spec	100 (corr spec 71.4)	100 (corr sens, 95.2 or 92.9, unclear from paper)	a	0	12	based on text of results	100	I	Scoring same for apneas and hypopneas for PSG and PM without arousals. No prevalence data for AHI ≥ 5. Oximetry sampling rates not given. Time in bed used for PM RDI was 35% longer than total sleep time used for AHI.
39 (new study)	10	10	38.6	79.3	97.8	36	0.212	0	95.8	88.2	II	AHI of 10 gives best pair of NPV and PPV. Patients with heart failure. Arousals included in AHI for PSG. Oximeter sampling rate of five seconds on PM and PSG.
40 (new study)	5 for sens, 15 for spec	5 for sens, 15 for spec	83.3 for sens, 51.6 for spec	98 (corr spec 40)	75.9 (corr sens 83.9)	3.48	0.05	32	78.8	80	I	Scoring same for apneas and hypopneas for PSG and PM without arousals. Oximeter sampling rate not disclosed. AHI of five gave best PPV (89.1%) due to high prevalence although high LR was minimally increased at 1.63.

Note: Data obtained with portable monitor simultaneous with polysomnography. Apnea/hypopnea index per hour of sleep with polysomnography. Respiratory disturbance index, apnea/hypopnea index per hour of recording unless otherwise indicated for portable monitor.

aCannot be calculated due to division by 0.

Abbreviations: AHI, apnea/hypopnea index; corr, corresponding sensitivity or specificity when best sensitivity and specificity at different RDI or AHI thresholds (when this occurs, there are a number of nondiagnostic tests); est, estimate; Evid, evidence grade; H, high; LR, likelihood ratio; L, low; NPV, negative predictive value = true negatives/true negatives plus false negatives (%); Non (%), percent of nondiagnostic tests; PM, portable monitor; PSG, attended polysomnography; Prev (%), prevalence in percent; PPV, positive predictive value = true positives/true positives plus false positives (%); red, reduction; RDI, respiratory disturbance index; Sens, sensitivity (%); Spec, specificity (%); sat, arterial oxygen desaturation.

Review (18). In addition, Table 2 includes six studies not yet published at the time the Joint Review was closed (20,27,37–40). All but one had acceptable LRs and the studies had a spectrum of grades I, II and IV evidence. In the new studies, there were 12%, 18%, 32%, and 41% nondiagnostic studies, and 12% data loss in one study.

Table 3 summarizes data for home to laboratory Level III monitors (20,35,37, 41–44) including four home to laboratory studies from the Joint Review (18). Table 3 includes two studies (20,37) not yet published at the time that the Joint Review was closed. These two studies had acceptable LRs but data loss was 14% and 18% and one had 36% nondiagnostic studies. In addition, there is an unpublished Level III study in manuscript form available on the Internet (44). The LRs were acceptable at AHI thresholds of five and 15.

Of 25 studies of a Level IV monitor done simultaneously in the sleep laboratory, 14 had an acceptable LR pair (18). Nine of the 14 studies had nondiagnostic RDIs ranging from 11% to 67%. Of eight studies comparing home to laboratory, one had an acceptable LR pair with 49% nondiagnostic RDIs. Data loss, when reported, was under 10% for those with an acceptable LR pair.

Since the Joint Review, at least 11 Level IV monitor publications with 12 studies have been published (45–55), six simultaneous, one on different nights for oximetry and PSG in the laboratory, and five home to laboratory. The results of these 12 studies had a spectrum of sensitivities and specificities with PSG. One simultaneous laboratory study (46) using a fast Fourier analysis of the spectrum of the heart rate and saturation from the pulse oximeter had acceptable LRs and, if reproducible in a home to laboratory study, may show promise. Another prospective study using oximetry simultaneous with PSG had acceptable LRs for severe sleep apnea ($AHI \geq 30$). The low prevalence (4.7%) led to an excellent negative predictive value (99%) with an LR of 0.122 but an unacceptable positive predictive value (estimated from the publication at about 50%) despite an LR estimated at 16 (53). On the other hand, in one study (49), 40% of patients with a normal home oximetry had significant OSA ($AHI > 15$) on PSG. However, this study used a 12-second oximeter recording setting, which has been documented to substantially underestimate the number of arterial oxygen desaturations (56–58). In another Level IV home to laboratory study, of 31 subjects using a system that records oronasal sound and airflow, eight normal PSG studies were classified as positive by portable monitor, and one classified as moderate and one as severe on PSG were normal on the portable study (55).

There is at least one system that uses an alternative technology. This monitor is a hybrid with an oximeter, an actigraph, and a measurement of radial artery pulse volume. The studies to date on this monitor show promise (59–61) and one validation study comparing both in-laboratory and home monitoring with sensitivity and specificity at specific thresholds is available (61). The LRs in this study are acceptable at several AHI thresholds but it is unclear if this is a consistent finding (Tables 4 and 5).

To reiterate, almost all attended Level III portable monitors have acceptable high and low LRs making them potentially useful to diagnose OSA. However, the number of nondiagnostic studies and the inherent insensitivity to measure subtle hypopneas requires careful follow-up and, usually, a PSG to fully evaluate the patient with a negative or nondiagnostic study. Level II and IV portable monitors do not appear to have sufficient diagnostic accuracy and/or reliability to be recommended for the diagnosis of OSA.

TABLE 3 Studies of Level III Portable Monitors Home to Laboratory Tests

Study	AHI	RDI	Prev (%)	Sens	Spec	LR(H)	LR(L)	Non (%)	PPV	NPV	Evid	Comment
35	10 for sens, 20 for spec	10 for sens, 20 for spec	61.4 for sens, 41.4 for spec	91 (corr spec 70.4)	82.9 (corr sens 86)	5.1	0.13	22	78	83	II	Red in airflow plus 4% red in sat (Denver) or 2% red in sat (Los Angeles) or arousal for AHI and RDI. Arousals were measured indirectly with PM. Compressed time frame for scoring RDI but not AHI.
41	10	10	74	100	66	2.9	0	0	89	100	IV	Red in airflow for AHI and RDI. Two min epochs used for PM.
42	15	10 for sens, 20 for spec	55	94 (corr spec 35)	89 (corr sens 38)	3.26	0.179	55	64	54	IV	Red in thoracoabdominal movement of AHI. Red in chest movement for RDI. Only patients with RDI < 30 included in analysis.
43	10	8 for sens, 23 for spec	84	95 (corr spec 33)	93 (corr sens 63)	9	0.15	37	98	55	II	Red in airflow or thoracoabdominal paradox with an arousal or cyclical red in sat for AHI. Same with cyclical 2% red in sat and no arousals criteria. One month between studies.
20 (new study)	15	15	48 (est)	91	83	5.35	0.11	0	83	91	I	Red in airflow and 2% desaturations with automatic scoring for AHI and RDI. 14% data loss for PM. 91% split-night studies in sleep laboratory, up to three nights averaged for home.
37 (new study)	10 for sens, 20 for spec	15	76	100 (corr spec 75)	100 (corr sens 61)	a	0	36	100	100	I	RDI and AHI red in thoracoabdominal movement. Manual scoring better than automatic. 18% data loss for PM.
44 (new study)	5	5	80	100	100	a	0	0	100	100	IV	Not obviously blinded. Automatic scoring with review for the portable device. Patient selection not well described.
	15	15	70	86	100	a	0.14	0	100	75		

Note: Laboratory, data obtained from polysomnography; Home, data obtained with portable monitor unattended in the home; Apnea/hypopnea index per hour of sleep with PSG; Respiratory disturbance index, apnea/hypopnea index per hour of recording unless otherwise indicated for portable monitor.

[a]Cannot be calculated due to division by 0.

Abbreviations: AHI, apnea/hypopnea index; corr, corresponding sensitivity or specificity when best sensitivity and specificity at different RDI or AHI thresholds (when this occurs, there are a number of nondiagnostic tests); est, estimate; Evid, evidence grade; H, high; LR, likelihood ratio; L, low; Non (%), percent of nondiagnostic tests; NPV, negative predictive value = true negatives/true negatives plus false negatives; PM, portable monitor; PSG, attended polysomnography; Prev (%), prevalence in percent; PPV, positive predictive value = true positives/true positives plus false positives; RDI, respiratory disturbance index; red, reduction; sat, arterial oxygen desaturation; Sens, sensitivity (%); Spec, specificity (%).

TABLE 4 Peripheral Arterial Tonometry Simultaneous with Polysomnography in the Laboratory

Study	AHI	RDI	Prev (%)	Sens	Spec	LR(H)	LR(L)	Non (%)	PPV	NPV	Evid	Comment
61 (Chicago criteria for AHI)	5	5	100	100	100	a	a	0	100	100	I	High prevalence makes generalization difficult. Oximeter sampling rates identical between PSG and PM with a sampling rate of one second.
61 (Medicare criteria for AHI)	10	9.5	48	100	100	a	a	0	100	100	I	RDI was oxygen desaturation index for PAT (i.e., functioned as an oximeter). Oximeter sampling rates identical between PSG and PM with a sampling rate of one second.
59	15 for sens 30 for spec	NA	50% for 15 20% for 30	93.3 (corr spec 73.3)	91.7 (corr sens 83.3)	3.49	0.1	30	77.8	95.6	II	Oximeter sampling rates not disclosed. Oximeter model on PM not disclosed. PSG hypopneas included arousals.
60	20	20	NA	85 (est)	82 (est)	4.72	0.183	NA	NA	NA	II	Oximeter sampling rates not disclosed. Oximeter model on PM not disclosed. PSG hypopneas included arousals. Sensitivity and specificity estimated from receiver operating characteristic (ROC) curves.
	10	10		75 (est)	82 (est)	4.17	0.305					

Note: Data obtained with portable monitor simultaneous with polysomnography; Chicago, apnea/hypopnea index (AHI) and respiratory disturbance index (RDI) calculated from criteria proposed in Reference (16); Medicare, AHI and RDI calculated from criteria required by Medicare (17); AHI per hour of sleep with polysomnography; RDI, AHI per hour of recording unless otherwise indicated for portable monitor.

aCannot be calculated due to division by 0.

Abbreviations: corr, corresponding sensitivity or specificity when best sensitivity and specificity at different RDI or AHI thresholds (when this occurs, there are a number of nondiagnostic tests); est, estimated from receiver operating characteristic (ROC) curves; Evid, evidence grade; H, high; LR, likelihood ratio; L, low; NA, not available; Non (%), percent of nondiagnostic tests; NPV, negative predictive value = true negatives/true negatives plus false negatives; PAT, peripheral arterial tonometry; PSG, attended polysomnography; PM, portable monitor; Prev (%), prevalence in percent; PPV, positive predictive value = true positives/true positives plus false positives; red, reduction; Sens, sensitivity (%); Spec, specificity (%).

TABLE 5 Peripheral Arterial Tonometry Laboratory Vs. Home

Study	AHI	RDI	Prev (%)	Sens	Spec	LR(H)	LR(L)	Non (%)	PPV	NPV	Evid	Comment[b,c]
61 (Chicago criteria for AHI)	5	5	100	100	100	a	a	0	100	100	—	—
61 (Medicare criteria for AHI)	5	4.7	55	100	100	a	a	0	100	100	—	—

Note: Laboratory, data obtained from polysomnography; Home, data obtained with portable monitor unattended in the home; Chicago, apnea/hypopnea index (AHI) and respiratory disturbance index (RDI) calculated from criteria proposed in Reference (16); Medicare, AHI and RDI calculated from criteria required by Medicare (17); AHI per hour of sleep with polysomnography; RDI and AHI per hour of recording unless otherwise indicated for portable monitor.

aCannot be calculated due to division by 0.

bHigh prevalence (100%) makes generalization difficult. Oximeter sampling rates identical between PSG and PM with a sampling rate of one second.

cRDI was oxygen desaturation index for PAT (i.e., essentially functioned as an oximeter). Oximeter sampling rates identical between PSG and PM with a sampling rate of one second.

Abbreviations: Evid, evidence grade; H, high; L, low; LR, likelihood ratio; Non (%), percent of nondiagnostic tests; NPV, negative predictive value = true negatives/true negatives plus false negatives; PAT, peripheral arterial tonometry; PSG, attended polysomnography; PM, portable monitor; Prev (%), prevalence in percent; PPV, positive predictive value = true positives/true positives plus false positives; Sens, sensitivity (%); Spec, specificity (%).

WHAT ARE LIMITATIONS OF POLYSOMNOGRAPHY AS A REFERENCE STANDARD?

There are limitations to PSG implementation and interpretation. Sleep staging is reasonably well-standardized according to published rules (62) but these were developed before OSA was well-recognized. For example, arousals were not well-defined (62) and while there are subsequent published recommendations (14), there are no universally accepted or easily reproducible definitions, making inter-scorer reliability potentially poor between clinical centers.

Scoring of hypopneas is in evolution. Although research definitions have been proposed (13), the correlation between these definitions and clinical outcomes is essentially unknown at this time. This leads to difficulty in determining a threshold AHI to confirm OSA.

Night-to-night variability of the AHI or RDI can be substantial and is due to a number of factors, including body position and the amount of REM sleep (supine and REM AHIs are almost always higher than non-rapid eye movement [NREM] and lateral position AHIs). Although the mean AHI in a group of OSA patients does not change substantially, individual patients may have large increases or decreases (19). For this reason, more than one night of PSG may be necessary to clarify whether a patient has OSA. This variability also makes it difficult to know how much of the difference between a portable monitor and PSG result is normal variability and how much is from the limited set of monitored variables attended or unattended during sleep.

The use of a single AHI to characterize the entire night's study is simplistic. For example, the classification of OSA by overall AHI does not take into account a number of variables that may well have clinical relevance such as supine and REM AHIs and the degree of arterial oxygen desaturation.

SLEEP STAGING

Portable monitors do not generally provide a measure of REM sleep and many do not provide body position. This makes it difficult to fully characterize the RDI result. For example, a patient who snores and has severe daytime sleepiness may sleep mostly in stages 2 to 4 of NREM sleep and have a RDI of four on one night but have normal REM on a second night with a RDI of 15. Most portable monitors do not have sleep staging and the interpretation of these two RDIs would be difficult. On the other hand, a PSG with sleep stages would provide important information in the interpretation of the study. In particular, an AHI of four in the first case would potentially prompt a second baseline study but in the case of the portable monitor it might be interpreted as nonsignificant and the patient may not be properly evaluated.

WHAT IS THE APPROPRIATE APNEA-HYPOPNEA INDEX DEFINITION OF OBSTRUCTIVE SLEEP APNEA BY PORTABLE MONITORING?

Historically, hypopneas (decreased airflow) have been used to characterize OSA and studies have suggested that hypopneas may have the same clinical significance as apneas in many patients (63). However, the standard method of measuring air-flow with a thermistor may leave many hypopneas unrecognized by this technique (13). In addition, partial upper airway obstruction that leads to increased amplitude of intrathoracic pressure can trigger an arousal (i.e., a RERA) and such arousals may produce daytime sleepiness (13,64).

Methods to capture more subtle hypopneas and measure airflow more quantitatively have become available. These currently focus around nasal pressure measurement which is an indirect measure of airflow and more sensitive than thermistors (13). Nasal pressure has been favorably compared against pneumotachograph airflow in OSA and appears more accurate than thermistor airflow (65,66). In addition, the use of an esophageal balloon or tube to measure intrathoracic pressure swings is recommended to determine the presence of RERAs (13).

Based on this newer technology, definitions of hypopnea and respiratory events for research purposes have been proposed including syndrome definition using a composite AHI ≥ 5 for confirmation of OSA (13). However, almost all previous OSA studies used thermistors and none of the new definitions have been adequately validated against thermistors in patients with OSA or against non-OSA controls. Given the newer, more sensitive technology to detect respiratory events, it is possible, even likely, that a diagnostic AHI will be much higher than previously observed and many individuals who were considered with a combination of clinical evaluation and PSG results not to have OSA will now have an AHI in the OSA range of at least five and possibly much higher.

PSG is potentially capable of capturing all of the currently recommended respiratory events whereas portable monitors, in general, capture only disturbances in airflow and saturation leading to a RDI that frequently underestimates the number of potential respiratory disturbances during sleep (i.e., apneas, hypopneas, desaturations, arousals, and RERAs). Depending on the technology and definitions used, RDI may vary considerably on the same night in the same patient.

To confuse the matter further, Medicare as mentioned, has published criteria for scoring hypopneas on PSG for purposes of qualifying for CPAP (21). These require a ≥ 30% decrease in airflow associated with a 4% desaturation from baseline during recorded sleep ≥ 2 hours duration. The PSG must be performed in a facility-based sleep study laboratory and not in the home or in a mobile facility. Without the sleep requirement, it is likely that a portable monitor could more readily replicate this definition. Of note, several Local Medical Review Policies (LMRP) may have substituted recording time for sleep time (e.g., http://www.tricenturion.com). Medicare criteria require an AHI of at least five patients with symptoms of OSA such as daytime sleepiness or an AHI of 15, irrespective of symptoms.

The user of a portable monitor should be aware of the operating characteristics of the monitor and not rely on computer-generated scoring. In addition, since the portable monitor does not measure a number of events that may be recorded on the PSG and does not usually measure sleep and may not measure position, a negative study should not be accepted to exclude a diagnosis of OSA. On the other hand, since the portable monitor is generally less sensitive than the PSG, a positive study with a properly validated monitor, if technically adequate, should generally be accepted as confirmatory in the appropriate clinical setting.

WHAT ARE DIFFERENTIAL DIAGNOSTIC CONSIDERATIONS?

Patients with Cheyne-Stokes respiration may mimic OSA but with a combination of airflow, respiratory movement, and saturation measurements; this should be apparent on a portable monitor. Patients with chronic obstructive pulmonary disease (COPD) may have periods of desaturation that typically occur during REM sleep (67). Since the portable monitor does not measure REM sleep, studies in patients with severe COPD should be avoided if attempting to diagnose OSA.

As mentioned, daytime sleepiness can occur in sleep disorders other than OSA (2). The typical Level III portable monitor is of little use in these cases and patients with daytime sleepiness and a negative portable monitor study should have the cause of the daytime sleepiness characterized. This will often require a PSG and possibly a multiple sleep latency test, which requires measurement of sleep staging (2,68).

TECHNICAL CONSIDERATIONS

The type of sensors may impact the results. For example, use of a thermistor is excellent for detection of apneas but relatively insensitive for detection of modest reductions in airflow (13). Thoracoabdominal movement by inductance plethysmography appears more sensitive for detection of hypopneas but the belts may lose calibration or shift during the study. Nasal pressure appears to be very sensitive to reductions in airflow but data loss may be a problem due to loss of signal or mouth breathing (13).

Several studies have documented that the method of sampling the saturation signal with an oximeter is important in accurately measuring reductions in arterial oxygen saturation (56–58). For example, an oximeter set at a three-second recording rate produced almost twice as many 3% desaturations as a 12-second recording rate (56). Furthermore, desaturations stored in oximeter memory substantially underestimate desaturations displayed in real time on-line at any recording rate (57).

The method of scoring, manual versus computer is also a consideration. Without the ability to manually review data, results will always be suspect since artifact may often mimic respiratory events. In general, computer scoring has been less accurate than manual scoring but the time involved is considerably greater with manual scoring (69). In addition, the ability to independently calibrate and test the equipment is desirable to ensure that equipment failure is not producing erroneous results.

WHAT CAN BE SUPPORTED BY THE EVIDENCE?

As discussed previously, based on the current evidence, an attended Level III system with a minimum of airflow, oximetry, respiratory movement, and heart rate can be recommended under certain conditions. Strongly recommended is an additional sensor to measure body position. Also recommended is a sensor to measure snoring.

The use of an attended Level III portable monitor to diagnose OSA would appear from both evidential and strategic analyses to be more appropriate rather than to exclude patients with OSA since:

1. A positive portable study, if properly performed in a patient with clinical features of OSA, has a high degree of specificity and positive predictive value.
2. A negative or nondiagnostic portable study should be followed, usually with an attended PSG, since the portable monitor study
   a. is less likely to detect other evidence of OSA including RERAs and subtle hypopneas and will not allow the determination of REM AHI;
   b. will not diagnose other disorders contributing to the patient's clinical presentation such as periodic limb movement disorder.

Based on considerations similar to the above, the AASM/ATS/ACCP task force guidelines (69) recommend that attended Level III studies are acceptable for diagnosis with careful follow-up of negative studies including, in most cases, a PSG for confirmation.

This review at this point has concentrated on the diagnosis of OSA without considering that PSG is used to monitor CPAP titration during sleep. To date, there appears to be only one study that examined a Level III portable monitoring montage to titrate CPAP during an attended study (70). In addition, the use of an attended portable monitor to make a diagnosis during the first half of the night followed by a CPAP titration during the second half of the night (split-night study) has not been examined. For these reasons, use of a portable monitor to both diagnose and titrate CPAP cannot be well-supported by evidence.

WHAT OTHER OPTIONS MAY BE CONSIDERED?

The evidence is lacking to support unattended use of a portable monitor in the patient's home as a stand-alone approach to diagnosis of OSA. However, in the proper setting, with appropriate patient selection, and careful follow-up including ready access to attended PSG, unattended Level III home portable studies are feasible. Based on an integration of the evidence available, the following conditions would appear to be necessary:

1. A high pretest probability (i.e., a high prevalence of OSA in the patient population), ideally to exceed 70%. There are a number of equations that use readily available data such as BMI, sex, history of snoring, neck circumference, and so on, or more complicated data such as X-rays of the upper airway with cephalometric measurements (68,71–76).
2. The availability of attended PSG for patients with a strong clinical history and a negative or nondiagnostic portable monitoring study.
3. The availability of treatment including PSG titration for CPAP.
4. An experienced sleep practitioner who is capable of evaluating both the clinical and portable monitoring information.

The approach to CPAP titration is beyond the scope of this chapter; there has been a trend to use auto-titrating positive airway pressure (APAP) machines unattended in the patient's home (see also Chapter 8). The reader is referred to an evidence-based review of the topic and guidelines published by the AASM (77,78) and a Canadian technology review (79), which indicate that unattended use for CPAP titration is not established for CPAP naïve patients. Subsequent to publication of the guidelines, at least one study has provided evidence that APAP can lead to favorable outcomes in CPAP naïve patients (80). In general, such an approach should only be carried out with the knowledge that the evidence for the efficacy of unattended home CPAP titration in CPAP naïve patients is in evolution.

COST EFFECTIVENESS

This is a complicated topic since the costs must be weighed against the accessibility of patients to diagnostic studies. If there are sufficient resources to study all patients who are identified as candidates, then the cost of the attended PSG, often a split-night study, must be balanced against the cost of the portable study and the potential need for a second study for CPAP treatment. The lower sensitivity of the portable study for OSA, particularly if the research criteria (13) are used for comparison, and the night-to-night variability of any test for OSA require careful evaluation of negative and nondiagnostic studies with strong consideration given to proceeding to a subsequent attended PSG. In addition, local reimbursements are also an issue and the Medicare rules essentially exclude portable monitoring attended or unattended as an option for confirming a diagnosis of OSA.

If there are not sufficient resources, then unattended Level III portable monitoring with the possibility of APAP becomes a potential option, recognizing all the limitations of portable monitoring and the use of APAP machines to titrate and determine treatment for patients.

Of note, the use of a Level III portable monitor attended in the laboratory is another potential addition to the overall diagnostic strategy and at least one analysis suggests that this may be more cost-effective than performing attended PSGs on all patients (81).

Although a comprehensive answer cannot be given, the following, at a minimum, should be assessed:

1. What is the cost of the PSG equipment, supplies, space, utilities, technician time, physician time, etc?
2. What is the cost of portable monitoring equipment, supplies, time spent with patient, interpretation time, etc?
3. What are the numbers of studies that are nondiagnostic and require follow-up PSG?
4. What is the strategy for CPAP titration? Does it include an attended PSG, a portable monitoring titration, an APAP, or some combination?
5. What are the acceptance and adherence with CPAP with any of the strategies?
6. What is an acceptable wait time for a test and if too long, how does this impact the quality of life of the patients?
7. Based on the acceptable wait time, what are the resources necessary for each of the possible strategies?
8. What is the patient population to be studied? What is the prevalence of OSA? What is the likelihood that other diagnoses are present such as periodic limb movement disorder or narcolepsy?

CONCLUSIONS

At the present time, the typical procedure for confirmation of the diagnosis of OSA and its management is an in-laboratory PSG with application of CPAP. Portable monitoring systems have arisen to increase access to the diagnosis of OSA and to potentially reduce costs. A RDI ≥ 5 in adults is used to confirm OSA unless the patient is asymptomatic, in which case a RDI ≥ 15 is used to confirm OSA. For children, one or more apneas or hypopneas of at least two respiratory cycles in duration, or other evidence of respiratory disturbance (i.e., RERAs, arterial oxygen desaturation, snoring, hypercapnia, arousals) confirm OSA. Validation of a portable monitoring device should involve the assessment of sensitivity and specificity of the OSA diagnosis using the device under ideal conditions as well as in the intended environment (typically the patient's home) versus simultaneous comparison with attended PSG. At the present time, Level II and IV portable monitors are not sufficiently accurate or validated to recommend for use, particularly unattended in the home, while Level III monitors are useful attended in the laboratory and of possible usefulness unattended in either the laboratory or the home, with the proviso that careful follow-up and usually a PSG is necessary to fully evaluate the patient with a negative or nondiagnostic study. The role of PSG as a reference standard is limited given issues such as the lack of standardized scoring of hypopneas and the night-to-night variability of the AHI or RDI; however, features such as sleep stage, body position, and all currently recommended respiratory event data are typically found in PSG systems but are lacking in portable monitors. Complicating these issues is the fact that current Medicare guidelines make it difficult for portable monitors to adhere to Medicare criteria for OSA diagnostic devices, and portable monitors are not the best choice for confirming the OSA diagnosis in patients with COPD or who have significant daytime sleepiness from causes other than OSA. The type of electrodes or sensors, oximeter sampling rate, and manual versus computerized scoring are technical factors that should be considered in the selection of the portable monitoring device. The most appropriate use of an attended Level III portable monitor appears to be the diagnosis of OSA rather than the exclusion of patients with OSA based on both evidential and strategic analyses. Lastly, the cost effectiveness of portable monitoring compared to in-laboratory PSG studies is a complex issue that at the present time has not been resolved.

REFERENCES

1. Bassiri AG, Guilleminault C. Clinical features and evaluation of obstructive sleep apnea-hypopnea syndrome. In: Kryger MH, Roth T, Dement WC eds, Principles and Practice of Sleep Medicine 3rd ed. Philadelphia, PA: W.B. Saunders, 2000:869–878.
2. American Sleep Disorders Association. International classification of sleep disorders. 2nd ed. Diagnostic and Coding Manual. Westchester, Illinois: American Academy of Sleep Medicine, 2005.
3. Young T, Palta M, Dempsey J, Skatrud J, Weber S, Badr S. The occurrence of sleep-disordered breathing among middle-aged adults. N Engl J Med 1993; 328: 1230–1235.
4. Findley LJ, Unverzagt ME, Suratt PM. Automobile accidents involving patients with obstructive sleep apnea. Am Rev Respir Dis 1988; 138:337–340.
5. Peppard PE, Young T, Palta M, Skatrud J. Prospective study of the association between sleep-disordered breathing and hypertension. N Engl J Med 2000; 342:1378–1384.
6. Hung J, Whitford EG, Parsons RW, Hillman DR. Association of sleep apnoea with myocardial infarction in men. Lancet 1990; 336:261–264.
7. Dyken ME, Somers VK, Yamada T, Ren ZY, Zimmerman MB. Investigating the relationship between stroke and obstructive sleep apnea. Stroke 1996; 27:401–407.
8. Resta O, Foschino-Barbaro MP, Legari G, et al. Sleep-related breathing disorders, loud snoring and excessive daytime sleepiness in obese subjects. Int J Obes Relat Metab Disord 2001; 25:669–675.
9. Hening WA, Allen RP, Earley CJ, Picchietti DL, Silber MH. Restless Legs Syndrome Task Force of the Standards of Practice Committee of the American Academy of Sleep Medicine. An update on the dopaminergic treatment of restless legs syndrome and periodic limb movement disorder. Sleep 2004; 27(3):560–583.
10. Chervin RD, Murman DL, Malow BA, Totten V. Cost-utility of three approaches to the diagnosis of sleep apnea: polysomnography, home testing, and empirical therapy. Ann Intern Med 1999; 130:496–505.
11. Rama A, Tekwani S, Kushida C. Sites of obstruction in obstructive sleep apnea. Chest 2002; 122:1139–1147.
12. Leung RS, Bradley TD. Sleep apnea and cardiovascular disease. Am J Respir Crit Care Med 2001; 164:2147–2165. PMID: 11751180.
13. American Academy of Sleep Medicine. Sleep-related breathing disorders in adults: recommendations for syndrome definition and measurement techniques in clinical research. The Report of an American Academy of Sleep Medicine Task Force. Sleep 1999; 22:667–689.

14. Anonymous. EEG arousals: scoring rules and examples: a preliminary report from the Sleep Disorders Atlas Task Force of the American Sleep Disorders Association. Sleep 1992; 15:173–184.

15. Mehra R, Benjamin EJ, Shahar E, et al. Sleep Heart Health Study. Association of nocturnal arrhythmias with sleep-disordered breathing: The Sleep Heart Health Study. Am J Respir Crit Care Med 2006; 173:910–916.

16. Ferber R, Millman R, Coppola M, et al. Portable recording in the assessment of obstructive sleep apnea. Sleep 1994; 17:378–392.

17. Standards of Practice Committee of the American Sleep Disorders Association. Practice parameters for the use of portable recording in the assessment of obstructive sleep apnea. Sleep 1994; 17:372–377.

18. Flemons WW, Littner MR, Rowley JA, et al. Home diagnosis of sleep apnea: a systematic review of the literature: an evidence review cosponsored by the American Academy of Sleep Medicine, the American College of Chest Physicians, and the American Thoracic Society. Chest 2003; 124:1543–1579.

19. Le Bon O, Hoffmann G, Tecco J, et al. Mild to moderate sleep respiratory events: one negative night may not be enough. Chest 2000; 118:353–359.

20. Reichert JA, Bloch DA, Cundiff E, Votteri BA. Comparison of the NovaSom QSG, a new sleep apnea home-diagnostic system, and polysomnography. Sleep Med 2003; 213–218.

21. http://www.aptweb.org/pdf/cmscpap.pdf last accessed 7-18-06.

22. Flemons W, Littner MR. Measuring agreement between diagnostic devices. Chest 2003; 124:1535–1542.

23. Orr WC, Eiken T, Pegram V, et al. A laboratory validation study of a portable system for remote recording of sleep related respiratory disorders. Chest 1994; 105(1):160–162.

24. Mykytyn IJ, Sajkov D, Neill AM, et al. Portable computerized polysomnography in attended and unattended settings. Chest 1999; 115:114–122.

25. Portier F, Portmann A, Czernichow P, et al. Evaluation of home versus laboratory poly-somnography in the diagnosis of sleep apnea syndrome. Am J Respir Crit Care Med 2000; 162:814–818.

26. Gagnadoux F, Pelletier-Fleury N, Philippe C, Rakotonanahary D, Fleury B. Home unat-tended vs. hospital telemonitored polysomnography in suspected obstructive sleep apnea syndrome: a randomized crossover trial. Chest 2002; 121:753–758. PMID: 11888956.

27. Calleja JM, Esnaola S, Rubio R, Duran J. Comparison of a cardiorespiratory device versus polysomnography for diagnosis of sleep apnoea. Eur Respir J 2002; 20:1505–1510.

28. Ballester E, Solans M, Vila X, et al. Evaluation of a portable respirator recording device for detecting apneas and hypopnoeas in subjects from a general population. Eur Respir J 2000; 16:123–127.

29. Claman D, Murr A, Trotter K. Clinical validation of the Bedbugg in detection of obstructive sleep apnea. Otolaryngol Head Neck Surg 2001; 125:227–230.

30. Emsellem H, Corson W, Rappaport B, et al. Verification of sleep apnea using a portable sleep apnea screening device. South Med J 1990; 83:748–752.

31. Ficker JH, Wiest GH, Wilpert J, Fuchs FS, Hahn EG. Evaluation of a portable recording device (Somnocheck) for use in patients with suspected obstructive sleep apnoea. Respiration 2001; 68:307–312.

32. Man G, Kang B. Validation of a portable sleep apnea monitoring device. Chest 1995; 108:388–393.

33. Redline S, Tosteson T, Boucher M, et al. Measurement of sleep-related breathing distur-bances in epidemiologic studies. Assessment of the validity and reproducibility of a por-table monitoring device. Chest 1991; 100:1281–1286.

34. Verse T, Pirsig W, Junge-Hulsing B, et al. Validation of the POLY-MESAM seven-channel ambulatory recording unit. Chest 2000; 117:1613–1618.

35. White D, Gibb T, Wall J, et al. Assessment of accuracy and analysis time of a novel device to monitor sleep and breathing in the home. Sleep 1995; 18:115–126.

36. Zucconi M, Ferini-Strambi L, Castronovo V, et al. An unattended device for sleep-related breathing disorders: validation study in suspected obstructive sleep apnoea syndrome. Eur Respir J 1996; 9:1251–1256.

37. Dingli K, Coleman EL, Vennelle M, et al. Evaluation of a portable device for diagnosing the sleep apnoea/hypopnoea syndrome. Eur Respir J 2003; 21:253–259.

38. Marrone O, Salvaggio A, Insalaco G, Bonsignore MR, Bonsignore G. Evaluation of the POLYMESAM system in the diagnosis of obstructive sleep apnea syndrome. Monaldi Arch Chest Dis 2001; 56(6):486–490.
39. Quintana-Gallego E, Villa-Gil M, Carmona-Bernal C, et al. Home respiratory polygraphy for diagnosis of sleep-disordered breathing in heart failure. Eur Respir J 2004; 24(3): 443–448.
40. Su S, Baroody FM, Kohrman M, Suskind D. A comparison of polysomnography and a portable home sleep study in the diagnosis of obstructive sleep apnea syndrome. Otolaryngol Head Neck Surg 2004; 131(6):844–850.
41. Ancoli-Israel S, Mason W, Coy T, et al. Evaluation of sleep disordered breathing with unattended recording: the Nightwatch System. J Med Eng Technol 1997; 21:10–14.
42. Whittle AT, Finch SP, Mortimore IL, et al. Use of home sleep studies for diagnosis of the sleep apnoea/hypopnoea syndrome. Thorax 1997; 52:1068–1073.
43. Parra O, Garcia-Esclasans N, Montserrat J, et al. Should patients with sleep apnoea/ hypopnoea syndrome be diagnosed and managed on the basis of home sleep studies? Eur Respir J 1997; 10:1720–1724.
44. Carter GS, Coyle MA, Mendelson WB. Validity of a portable cardio-respiratory system to collect data in the home environment in patients with obstructive sleep apnea. http:// www.cms.hhs.gov/coverage/download/id110a.pdf, last accessed 7-18-06.
45. Golpe R, Jimenez A, Carpizo R. Home sleep studies in the assessment of sleep apnea/ hypopnea syndrome. Chest 2002; 122:1156–1161.
46. Zamarron C, Gude F, Barcala J, Rodriguez JR, Romero PV. Utility of oxygen saturation and heart rate spectral analysis obtained from pulse oximetric recordings in the diagnosis of sleep apnea syndrome. Chest 2003; 123:1567–1576.
47. Raymond B, Cayton RM, Chappell MJ. Combined index of heart rate variability and oximetry in screening for the sleep apnoea/hypopnoea syndrome. J Sleep Res 2003; 1:53–61.
48. Roche N, Herer B, Roig C, Huchon G. Prospective testing of two models based on clinical and oximetric variables for prediction of obstructive sleep apnea. Chest 2002; 12:747–752.
49. Hussain SF, Fleetham JA. Overnight home oximetry: can it identify patients with obstructive sleep apnea-hypopnea who have minimal daytime sleepiness? Respir Med 2003; 97:537–540.
50. Shochat T, Hadas N, Kerkhofs M, et al. The SleepStrip: an apnoea screener for the early detection of sleep apnoea syndrome. Eur Respir J 2002; 19:121–126.
51. Westbrook PR, Levendowski DJ, Cvetinovic M, et al. Description and validation of the apnea risk evaluation system: a novel method to diagnose sleep apnea-hypopnea in the home. Chest 2005; 128(4):2166–2175.
52. Nakano H, Hayashi M, Ohshima E, Nishikata N, Shinohara T. Validation of a new system of tracheal sound analysis for the diagnosis of sleep apnea-hypopnea syndrome. Sleep 2004; 27(5):951–957.
53. Gurubhagavatula I, Maislin G, Nkwuo JE, Pack AI. Occupational screening for obstructive sleep apnea in commercial drivers. Am J Respir Crit Care Med 2004 15; 170:371–376.
54. Fietze I, Dingli K, Diefenbach K, et al. Night-to-night variation of the oxygen desaturation index in sleep apnoea syndrome. Eur Respir J 2004; 24(6):987–993.
55. Liesching TN, Carlisle C, Marte A, Bonitati A, Millman RP. Evaluation of the accuracy of SNAP technology sleep sonography in detecting obstructive sleep apnea in adults compared to standard polysomnography. Chest 2004; 125:886–891.
56. Davila DG, Richards KC, Marshall BL, et al. Oximeter's acquisition parameter influences the profile of respiratory disturbances. Sleep 2003; 26:91–95.
57. Davila DG, Richards KC, Marshall BL, et al. Oximeter performance: the influence of acquisition parameters. Chest 2002; 122:1654–1660.
58. Wiltshire N, Kendrick A, Catterall J. Home oximetry studies for diagnosis of sleep apnea/hypopnea syndrome. Limitation of memory storage capabilities. Chest 2001; 120:384–389.
59. Ayas NT, Pittman S, MacDonald M, White DP. Assessment of a wrist-worn device in the detection of obstructive sleep apnea. Sleep Med 2003; 4(5):435–442.
60. Bar A, Pillar G, Dvir I, Sheffy J, Schnall RP, Lavie P. Evaluation of a portable device based on peripheral arterial tone for unattended home sleep studies. Chest 2003; 123:695–703.

61. Pittman SD, Ayas NT, MacDonald MM, Malhotra A, Fogel RB, White DP. Using a wrist-worn device based on peripheral arterial tonometry to diagnose obstructive sleep apnea: in-laboratory and ambulatory validation. Sleep 2004; 27:923–933.
62. Rechtschaffen A, Kales A. A manual of standardized terminology, techniques, and scoring system for sleep stages of human subjects. Los Angeles: Brain Information Service, 1968.
63. Gould GA, Whyte KF, Rhind GB, et al. The sleep hypopnea syndrome. Am Rev Respir Dis 1988; 137:895–898.
64. Guilleminault C, Stoohs R, Clerk A, Cetel M, Maistros P. A cause of excessive daytime sleepiness. The upper airway resistance syndrome. Chest 1993; 104:781–787.
65. Heitman SJ, Atkar RS, Hajduk EA, Wanner RA, Flemons WW. Validation of nasal pressure for the identification of apneas/hypopneas during sleep. Am J Respir Crit Care Med 2002; 166:386–391.
66. Norman RG, Ahmed MM, Walsleben JA, Rapoport DM. Detection of respiratory events during NPSG: nasal cannula/pressure sensor versus thermistor. Sleep 1997; 20:1175–1184.
67. Littner MR, McGinty DJ, Arand DL. Determinants of oxygen desaturation in the course of ventilation during sleep in chronic obstructive pulmonary disease. Am Rev Respir Dis 1980; 122:849–857.
68. Chesson AL, Ferber RA, Fry JM, et al. Standards of Practice Committee Task Force. Practice parameters for the indications for polysomnography and related procedures. Sleep 1997; 20:406–422.
69. Chesson AL Jr, Berry RB, Pack A. Practice parameters for the use of portable monitoring devices in the investigation of suspected obstructive sleep apnea in adults. Sleep 2003; 26:907–913.
70. Montserrat JM, Alarcón A, Lloberes P, Ballester E, Fornas C, Rodriguez-Roisin R. Adequacy of prescribing nasal continuous positive airway pressure therapy for the sleep apnoea/hypopnoea syndrome on the basis of night time respiratory recording variables. Thorax 1995; 50:969–971.
71. Gurubhagavatula I, Maislin G, Pack AI. An algorithm to stratify sleep apnea risk in a sleep disorders clinic population. Am J Respir Crit Care Med 2001; 164:1904–1909.
72. Flemons WW, Whitelaw WA, Brant R, Remmers JE. Likelihood ratios for a sleep apnea clinical prediction rule. Am J Respir Crit Care Med 1994; 150:1279–1285.
73. Viner S, Szalai JP, Hoffstein V. Are history and physical examination a good screening test for sleep apnea? Ann Intern Med 1991; 115:356–359.
74. Netzer NC, Stoohs RA, Netzer CM, et al. Using the Berlin Questionnaire to identify patients at risk for the sleep apnea syndrome. Ann Intern Med 1999; 131:485–536.
75. Kushida CA, Efron B, Guilleminault C. A predictive morphometric model for the obstructive sleep apnea syndrome. Ann Intern Med 1997; 127:581–587.
76. Tsai WH, Remmers JE, Brant R, Flemons WW, Davies J, Macarthur C. A decision rule for diagnostic testing in obstructive sleep apnea. Am J Respir Crit Care Med 2003; 167:1427–1432.
77. Berry RB, Parish JM, Hartse KM. The use of auto-titrating continuous positive airway pressure for treatment of adult obstructive sleep apnea. An American Academy of Sleep Medicine review. Sleep 2002; 25:148–173.
78. Littner M, Hirshkowitz M, Davila D, et al. Standards of Practice Committee of the American Academy of Sleep Medicine. Practice parameters for the use of auto-titrating continuous positive airway pressure devices for titrating pressures and treating adult patients with obstructive sleep apnea syndrome. An American Academy of Sleep Medicine report. Sleep 2002; 25:143–147.
79. Hailey D, Jacobs P, Mayers I, Mensinkai S. Auto-titrating nasal continuous positive airway pressure systems in the management of obstructive sleep apnea. Ottawa: Canadian Coordinating Office for Health Technology Assessment; 2003. Technology report no. 39. http://www.ccohta.ca, last accessed 3/5/06.
80. Senn O, Brack T, Matthews F, Russi EW, Bloch KE. Randomized short-term trial of two autoCPAP devices versus fixed continuous positive airway pressure for the treatment of sleep apnea. Am J Respir Crit Care Med 2003; 168:1506–1511.
81. Reuven H, Schweitzer E, Tarasiuk A. A cost-effectiveness analysis of alternative at-home or in-laboratory technologies for the diagnosis of obstructive sleep apnea syndrome. Med Decis Making. 2001; 21:451–458.

Upper Airway Imaging

Nirav P. Patel
Division of Pulmonary, Critical Care, and Allergy, Center for Sleep & Respiratory Neurobiology, University of Pennsylvania Medical Center, Philadelphia, Pennsylvania, U.S.A.

Richard J. Schwab
Division of Sleep Medicine, Pulmonary, Allergy, and Critical Care Division; University of Pennsylvania Medical Center, Philadelphia, Pennsylvania, U.S.A.

INTRODUCTION

Although obstructive sleep apnea (OSA) is a major public health problem in the US and the rest of the world we have not unraveled the pathogenesis of this disorder. Nonetheless, the level of understanding and treatment of this disorder has escalated dramatically in the last 20 years. Several upper airway imaging techniques have provided important insight into the anatomical basis of OSA and its treatment. OSA appears to result from a combination of abnormal upper airway anatomy and changes in neural activation mechanisms intrinsic to sleep. Regardless of the fundamental initiating event, the final pathway in patients with OSA is obstruction of the airway during sleep and therefore upper airway assessment is vital to further understanding of the disorder.

This chapter reviews upper airway imaging modalities and how they relate airway morphology to the understanding of OSA and its therapeutic interventions. First, a review of the normal upper airway is provided.

NORMAL UPPER AIRWAY ANATOMY AND PHYSIOLOGY

The upper airway extends from the posterior margin of the nasal septum to the larynx. It is divided into four anatomical regions (Fig. 1):

- Nasopharynx: between the nares and hard palate.
- Retropalatal: between the hard palate and caudal margin of the soft palate.
- Retroglossal: between the distal margin of the soft palate and the base of the epiglottis.
- Hypopharynx: from the base of the tongue to the larynx.

The physiologic functions of the upper airway include ventilation, phonation, and deglutition. The evolutionary adaptations necessary to allow for such functional diversity have resulted in a structure that is heavily dependent on muscle activity and intrinsic airway collapsibility to maintain airway patency. The collapsibility of the upper airway represents a balance between opposing forces. The negative intraluminal pressure generated by the diaphragm during inspiration and the positive extraluminal pressure from surrounding tissue constitute the collapsing factors. The action of the upper airway pharyngeal dilator muscles counteracts the collapsing forces.

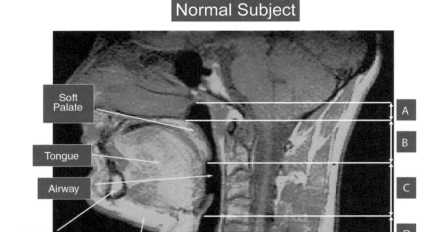

FIGURE 1   Mid-sagittal magnetic resonance imaging (MRI) in a normal subject highlighting the four upper airway regions: (**A**) nasopharynx; (**B**) retropalatal; (**C**) retroglossal; and (**D**) hypopharynx. Fat is white on an MRI scan.

Several surrounding tissue and craniofacial structures contribute to the morphology of the airway. A majority of patients with OSA experience narrowing or closure in the retropalatal and retroglossal regions. For this reason, the boundaries discussed below pertain specifically to these regions of the upper airway. The anterior oropharyngeal wall is formed mainly by the soft palate and tongue, while the posterior wall is bounded by the superior, middle, and inferior pharyngeal constrictor muscles. These lie anterior to the cervical spine. The lateral walls are complex structures that constitute muscles (hyoglossus, styloglossus, stylohyoid, stylopharyngeus, palatoglossus, palatopharyngeus, and the pharyngeal constrictors), lymphoid tissue, and adipose tissue (parapharyngeal fat pads). The lateral wall tissue is bounded by the parapharyngeal fat pads in the retropalatal region and by the mandibular rami in the retroglossal region (Fig. 2). The biomechanical relationships between the upper airway soft tissue and craniofacial structures are complicated and not fully understood. Nonetheless, upper airway imaging studies have begun to unravel these relationships.

TECHNIQUES AND MODES OF IMAGING THE UPPER AIRWAY

A wide array of options exists to image the upper airway. In the past, the upper airway was examined by measuring pressure at different levels to obtain data pertaining to airway compliance and collapsibility (1–4). Investigators have also examined electromyographic activity of various upper airway muscles such as genioglossus, levator palatini, alae nasi, tensor palatini, geniohyoid, sternohyoid, palatoglossus, and the pharyngeal constrictors (1,5–11). These studies have

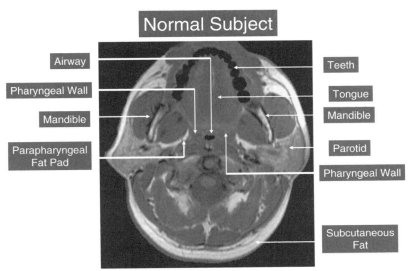

FIGURE 2 Retropalatal axial magnetic resonance imaging (MRI) in a normal subject. The tongue, soft palate, parapharyngeal fat pads, lateral parapharyngeal walls (muscles between the airway and lateral parapharyngeal fat pads), parotid, subcutaneous fat, teeth, and mandibular rami are all highlighted on this axial MRI. *Source*: From Ref. 23.

provided collectively important information pertaining to the maintenance of airway patency and pathogenesis of airway collapse. During wakefulness, pharyngeal patency is maintained predominantly by activation of pharyngeal dilator muscles (11). During apnea, it has been demonstrated that genioglossus and tensor palatine activation is primarily influenced by negative pressure in the airway (7,11). The negative pressure milieu is amplified during apnea due to greater inspiratory effort and increased tonic muscular activity (11). Further evidence demonstrates that administration of nasal continuous positive airway pressure (CPAP) reduces the accentuated genioglossus response to apnea to normal levels (7). However, the accentuated genioglossus electromyographic activation in apneics does not necessarily indicate that the tongue is moving since electromyographic activity does not correlate with mechanical action. Newer imaging techniques such as computed tomography (CT) and magnetic resonance imaging (MRI) have allowed for a greater depth of understanding of the mechanical behavior of the soft-tissue structures.

The list of upper airway imaging techniques includes: cephalography (cephalometric radiography), nasopharyngoscopy, acoustic reflection, conventional and electron beam CT, three-dimensional CT, MRI/volumetric MRI, and optical coherence tomography. Together, these imaging modalities have greatly improved our understanding of OSA; however, each has its limitations. Fluoroscopy, an older imaging technique, involves significant radiation exposure and is time-consuming; it has been replaced by newer imaging modalities that can also provide dynamic images with the capability to obtain more precise anatomic measurements. The ideal imaging technique would provide safe, accurate, and repetitive measurements in the supine position. Such a modality would allow for three-dimensional volumetric reconstructions of the upper airway and its surrounding tissues/craniofacial structures and allow for measurements during wakefulness and sleep. A critique of the different imaging modalities is provided below beginning with the most recent development.

Optical Coherence Tomography

Armstrong et al. (12) utilized an endoscopic optical technique (optical coherence tomography) that generates quantitative, real-time images of the upper airway that enables accurate determination of shape and size. Optical coherence tomography involves the insertion into the nares of an optical probe (3 mm diameter) that is housed in a catheter. Rotation of this probe within the catheter provides a 360-degree profile of surrounding tissue, and longitudinal movement allows the upper airway to be scanned at multiple sites without irritation of the airway mucosa thereby avoiding waking a potentially sleeping subject. A similar technique has been used to examine microscopic tissue anatomy in the specialties of ophthalmology, dermatology, vascular medicine, gastroenterology, and urology. Simultaneous optical coherence tomography and CT images of the upper airway in five healthy subjects at three different levels of the airway showed comparable airway dimensions within 0.8 mm of each on average. The cross-sectional area derived from optical coherence tomography was on average 14.1 mm^2 smaller than CT-derived images. The authors describe their validation of this technique with CT in five healthy subjects (12). Intraobserver and interobserver variability was assessed and the correlation coefficients were stated to be 0.99 and 0.99, respectively. In addition to the capacity to continuously measure changes in the airway dimensions under a variety of conditions, other advantages cited by the group using optical coherence tomography include patient comfort, minimal effect on sleep quality or architecture, and lack of radiation. Early shortcomings appear to be the limited capacity to view the complete circumference of the airway at all sites in all subjects and the inability to track changes in airway caliber when breathing is rapid (12). In addition, this imaging modality examines the airway lumen; it cannot evaluate craniofacial or soft tissue structures that are not adjacent to the airway.

Magnetic Resonance Imaging

MRI may be the best current mode of imaging for assessment of the upper airway and surrounding soft tissue and craniofacial structures (Figs. 1–4) (13–25). Advantages of MRI include that it: (*i*) achieves high resolution images of the upper airway and soft tissue; (*ii*) provides precise and accurate measurements of the upper airway and surrounding tissue; (*iii*) obtains multiplanar images in the axial, sagittal, and coronal planes; (*iv*) permits volumetric data analysis including three-dimensional reconstruction images of the upper airway and surrounding structures; (*v*) permits state-dependent imaging; and (*vi*) avoids radiation exposure allowing for repeat measurements. The shortcomings of MRI include that it: (*i*) is costly and not widely available; (*ii*) cannot be performed on patients with metallic implants such as pacemakers; (*iii*) has noise related to the machine that can be disturbing to sleep; and (*iv*) is difficult to perform in patients with claustrophobia and morbid obesity. Nonetheless, MRI studies have advanced our understanding of the pathophysiology of OSA as well as the mechanisms underlying effective treatments such as weight loss, CPAP, oral appliances, and upper airway surgery (13–16,18–20,23–27). The advent of ultrafast MRI techniques has

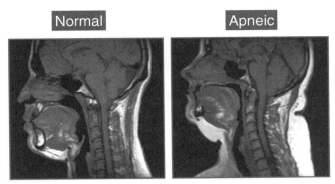

FIGURE 3 Mid-sagittal magnetic resonance imaging of a normal subject (*left*) and a patient with sleep apnea (*right*). The upper airway is smaller in both the retropalatal and retroglossal region in the apneic patient. The soft palate is longer in the apneic patient. The amount of subcutaneous fat (white area at the back of the neck) is greater in the apneic. *Source*: From Ref. 23.

provided multiple images at multiple sites with sufficient image quality and temporal resolution to allow a dynamic assessment of the pharyngeal musculature (14,16,28).

Volumetric MRI appears to be a powerful tool to assess and measure anatomic risk factors for OSA. Schwab et al. (29) demonstrated that the volume of upper airway soft tissue structures is enlarged in patients with sleep apnea, even after controlling for volume of the parapharyngeal fat pads (Fig. 5). Furthermore, the volume of the tongue and lateral pharyngeal walls were shown to be particularly important independent risk factors for sleep apnea (29).

Computed Tomography
CT is a noninvasive technique that permits a thorough evaluation of the entire upper airway. CT techniques employed to study the upper airway include standard axial CT images with the option to three-dimensionally reconstruct the upper airway

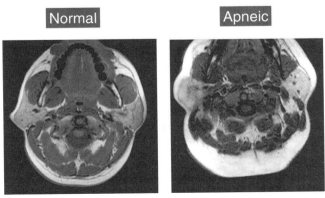

FIGURE 4 Axial magnetic resonance imaging in the retropalatal region of a normal subject (*left*) and a patient with sleep apnea (*right*). The upper airway is smaller in the lateral dimension in the patient with sleep apnea. The apneic patient has more subcutaneous fat than the normal subject. *Source*: From Ref. 23.

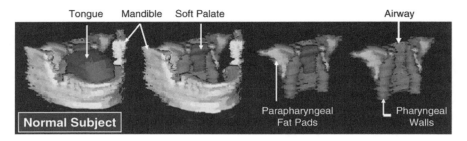

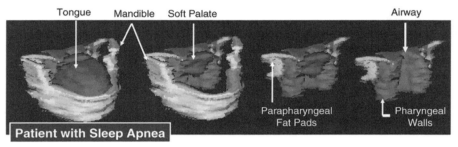

FIGURE 5 (*See color insert.*) Volumetric reconstruction of axial magnetic resonance images in a normal subject (*top panel*) and a patient with sleep apnea (*bottom panel*). The mandible is depicted in gray, the tongue in orange/rust, the soft palate in purple, the lateral parapharyngeal fat pads in yellow, and the lateral/posterior pharyngeal walls in green. Both subjects had an elevated body mass index (32.5 kg/m²). The airway is larger in the normal subject than in the patient with sleep apnea. The tongue, soft palate, and lateral pharyngeal walls are all larger in the patient with sleep apnea than in the normal subject. *Source*: From Ref. 29.

structures (30,31), electron beam CT that permits dynamic evaluation, and helical CT scanners (32,33) that have the ability to provide volumetric images. CT scanning, however, has limited soft-tissue contrast resolution compared with MRI scanning. This is particularly relevant to evaluating upper airway adipose tissue. Other limitations of CT scanning include expense and the radiation exposure patients receive each time they are studied. Nonetheless, upper airway imaging studies with CT scanning has enhanced our understanding of upper airway anatomy and its relationship to OSA (30–49).

Most of the studies using CT have evaluated airway dimension during states of wakefulness and sleep and have shown narrowing predominantly in the retropalatal region in patients with OSA (31,34–49). In addition, the degree of narrowing has been correlated directly with OSA severity (40). Volumetric CT studies have demonstrated smaller airway caliber and larger tongue volume in obese patients with OSA (31,50). Three-dimensional CT has shown that the most important parameter associated with sleep-disordered breathing appears to be narrowing at the retropalatal area (30) and that lateral airway caliber compromise correlates with the apnea-hypopnea index (AHI). CT studies have also been employed to try to identify favorable surgical candidates for uvulopalatopharyngoplasty (UPPP) and to examine dynamic changes of the upper airway and surrounding soft tissue structures during respiration (15,20,51–53). These dynamic CT imaging studies have shown that the upper airway is narrowest at end-expiration and early-inspiration in both normal and apneic subjects (15,20,52,53).

Cephalometry

Lateral cephalometry is a simple and well-standardized technique involving radiographs of the head and neck with focus on bony and soft tissue structures. Several cephalometric studies have been performed in OSA patients and have provided important insights (54–64). Most of these studies have investigated the airway with the subject in the upright position, although comparisons between upright and supine postures have been made (54,55). An upright lateral cephalograph is obtained while the subject is seated with gaze parallel to the floor and teeth together. Investigators have used radiopaque material to enhance the outline of the oropharyngeal structures (56). The cephalometric images are used to study measurements of many set points, planes or distances within the head and neck region. The cephalometric technique has highlighted important differences between sleep apneics and normal subjects, sleep apneics and snorers, and obese and nonobese subjects. OSA patients have been shown to have a small posteriorly-placed mandible, a narrow posterior airway space, an enlarged tongue and soft palate, and an inferiorly located hyoid (58,59,64). All five of the above variables have been shown to be significant determinants of apnea severity. The craniofacial abnormalities in OSA patients are reported more frequently in the subgroup of patients who are not obese (60). OSA patients compared with snorers have been demonstrated to have a longer soft palate in addition to an inferiorly positioned hyoid bone and posteriorly displaced mandible. Interestingly, when subdivided for age or body mass index (BMI), it was found that the significant differences between upper airway dimensions of OSA patients and snorers in the overall population were almost exclusively derived from the younger (age < 52 years) and leaner (BMI < 27 kg/m^2) subgroups. The upper airway measurements studied in obese or older OSA patients were not different from obese or older snorers (61). More recent work with supine cephalometry has shown that the transition from upright to supine position in sleep apneics is associated with a significant narrowing of the oropharyngeal sagittal dimension (54,62,63). Cephalometry has also been employed to assess and optimize the efficacy of mandibular advancement oral appliances based on the anatomical changes in supine imaging (62).

Limitations of cephalometry pertain to the two-dimensional nature of the image and to the examination of soft tissue. Cephalometry provides two-dimensional static images in the sagittal plane and therefore cannot provide information about transverse dimensions, cross-sectional shape or volume, or dynamic changes of the airway during sleep. The patient is required to be awake and therefore extrapolation to the sleep state may be inaccurate.

Acoustic Reflection

Acoustic reflection is an imaging technique that employs analysis of the phase and amplitude of sound waves reflected from surrounding airway structures. The information derived is used to calculate the upper airway cross-sectional area at defined distances from the mouth (52,65–67). Subjects hold a device in their mouth that is connected to the acoustic reflection apparatus. Using this modality, reproducible measurements can be obtained to assess the airway with a noninvasive and radiation-free technique. The effect of posture (sitting versus supine position) on the upper airway can be studied with this technique. Acoustic reflection has demonstrated that sleep apnea subjects have a smaller cross-sectional airway area when compared to normal subjects (40,52). It has also shed light on differences in airway dimension between genders, confirming that men have a larger upper airway than women when seated (68).

In the last decade, there have been only a few studies employing acoustic reflection as an upper airway imaging technique. This is probably a result of inherent limitations of the technique and the availability of better imaging options. The use of a mouthpiece (which requires opening of the mouth) alters upper airway morphology: the soft palate is no longer contiguous with the posterior tongue and the craniofacial structures alter their position. This limits not only the clinical applicability to an apneic event but also the comparison to data derived from other modes of imaging where the mouth is closed. In addition, acoustic reflection does not provide direct imaging of the airway, soft tissues or craniofacial structures since it derives upper airway cross-sectional area from a reflected wave. Moreover, it only provides information about the airway lumen not the surrounding structures that influence its morphology.

Nasopharyngoscopy

Otolaryngologists employ this technique to assess the upper airway beginning from the nasal passage. Nasopharyngoscopy is a relatively inexpensive method that allows a direct real-time view of the upper airway without radiation. Although it is invasive, it is well-tolerated and safely performed in the outpatient setting. It allows static and dynamic anatomical assessment, when coupled with a Müller maneuver. A Müller maneuver is performed in awake subjects and involves voluntary inspiration against a closed mouth and obstructed nares. It is thought to simulate the upper airway collapse that occurs during the negative airway pressure of apneic episodes although it is a voluntary maneuver. The limitation of extrapolation from an awake subject attempting to simulate a negative pressure-induced apnea to a sleep-induced apnea is well recognized. Nonetheless, valuable information on the intrinsic soft tissue tone and collapsibility can be derived from nasopharyngoscopy with a Müller maneuver.

Nasopharyngoscopy has been employed to examine the physiological changes in the hypotonic airway (69,70); state-dependent changes in patients with obstructive and central sleep apnea (25,71–73); and changes in upper airway caliber after weight loss (74), UPPP (70), laser-assisted uvulopalatoplasty (LAUP) (75), and while using mandibular repositioning oral appliances (76,77). Several studies have been performed to evaluate OSA patients for the suitability of UPPP using endoscopy with the Müller maneuver (78). These studies were based on semi-quantitative techniques for estimation of airway collapse. Upper airway videoendoscopy during sleep has been shown to predict a favorable response to UPPP, although this is not feasible in clinical outpatient practice (72). Unfortunately, data during wakefulness is not convincing in its predictive power for surgical success (78,79). More recent work with awake nasopharyngoscopy has validated the precision of quantitative measurements against MRI and has shown good correlation of retropalatal area collapsibility with OSA severity. This work may permit surgeons to target suitable UPPP patients with higher accuracy (80,81). Despite this work, it must be noted that nasopharyngoscopy offers insight to the luminal side of the airway only and not the surrounding tissue and bony structures. This may well explain the limited predictability for surgical success on subjects who appear to have airway substrate that should benefit from UPPP.

PATHOGENESIS OF OBSTRUCTIVE SLEEP APNEA—INSIGHTS FROM UPPER AIRWAY IMAGING

The imaging modalities described in the previous section have examined the pathogenesis of obstructive apneas by assessing airway morphology in different states: awake, asleep, and during respiration. Awake imaging studies examine the static factors (craniofacial and soft tissue structures) that predispose subjects to obstructive apnea. Imaging during sleep provides insight into the state-dependent anatomico-physiological changes in the airway. Dynamic imaging permits examination of the airway during inspiration and expiration and have allowed us to understand the narrowing or occlusion of the airway that can occur during expiration (28).

Upper Airway During Wakefulness

Individuals with normal upper airway anatomy do not suffer from obstructive apneas or hypopneas even though they experience reductions in muscle tone and airway caliber during sleep. What anatomic factors predispose an individual to sleep apnea? Why are the upper airway structures enlarged in patients with OSA? This section will first highlight the differences between normal and apneic upper airways and then discuss the factors that confer/influence these differences.

The overwhelming majority of imaging studies have demonstrated that the upper airway of apneic subjects is smaller than that of the normal population (7,14, 23,29,37,41,43,52,66,67,82–84). The minimum caliber of the upper airway has been shown to be primarily located in the retropalatal oropharynx (23,39,43,49) and therefore this has become the main area of interest for studying airway collapse. In a minority of patients, the initial site of collapse is the retroglossal region (85). OSA patients in general demonstrate an excess of upper airway soft tissue for the space available bounded by the bony structures, which envelop the pharyngeal lumen. Studies have suggested that the reduction in aperture of the airway of OSA patients is a result of a relative or actual excess soft tissue and/or an altered bony cage (29,83). The craniofacial features (primarily determined with cephalometric techniques) of OSA patients include reduction in the length of the mandible, an inferiorly-positioned hyoid bone, and a retroposition of the maxilla (58,67,86–90). Shorter, posteriorly displaced mandibles have been observed in up to two-thirds of OSA patients and correlate with decreased pharyngeal size (27,90). Several soft tissue abnormalities have also been shown to narrow the upper airway in patients with sleep apnea when compared to normals including an increase in the volume of the tongue, soft palate, parapharyngeal fat pads, and the lateral walls surrounding the pharynx (14,15,22,23,29,31,36,91). The larger the volume of the lateral pharyngeal walls, tongue, and total soft tissue (Fig. 5), the greater is the likelihood of developing OSA (29). Although the lateral parapharyngeal fat pads are enlarged in OSA patients when compared with controls, they do not necessarily affect the airway lumen (23).

The airway configuration also appears to be an important factor in apneic subjects. In contrast to normals, who have the major axis of the pharyngeal airway in the lateral dimension, OSA patients have an axis oriented anteroposteriorly. This type of narrowing is believed to be due to thickening of the lateral pharyngeal wall (29) and indeed, may compromise the pharyngeal dilator muscles' ability to maintain airway patency (92). Attention has also focused on airway length as another important anatomical variable influencing airway patency. Using finite element analysis modeling and MRI, it has been shown that normal men have significantly increased pharyngeal airway length (even after normalizing for body size), greater soft palate cross-sectional area, and increased pharyngeal volume compared to females (17). Based on this observed gender differences in airway anatomy, the investigators demonstrated that the male airway is more collapsible at any given negative airway pressure than the female airway. Cephalometry techniques have also demonstrated a lengthening of the pharynx in men with OSA compared to controls. This could increase the risk of upper airway collapse by lengthening the "at risk" portion of the airway lumen (55). In addition, cephalometric studies have shown inferior displacement of the hyoid bone in OSA patients compared with controls, and it is accompanied by an inferior displacement of the tongue into the hypopharynx (93). The distance between the hyoid bone and the mandibular plane has been shown to predict the critical collapsing pressure of an airway and the airway resistance in awake apnea patients (94,95). Furthermore, the extent of inferior hyoid displacement is correlated to the AHI (96).

It is thought that these soft tissue and craniofacial abnormalities predispose the patient with sleep apnea to have upper airway collapse during sleep. Several factors (obesity, edema, muscular dysfunction, gender, ethnicity, genetics) have been proposed to explain these abnormalities of upper airway soft tissue and craniofacial structures. These factors will be discussed below. It is important to note that these factors may be additive and interact conferring enhanced overall risk for the development of obstructive apneas. For example, a male who is obese is more likely to have OSA than a woman of similar body mass.

Factors Influencing Upper Airway Soft Tissue Structures
Obesity

The best-studied factors that alter upper airway dimensions are obesity (97,98) and increased neck circumference. Obesity of the centripetal type (more common in men) where fat distribution predominates in the regions of the abdominal viscera, upper body, and neck is significantly more correlated with OSA than the peripheral pattern of obesity (more common in women) where fat locates to the hips and thighs (99,100). Neck circumference is a strong predictor of sleep apnea among anthropometric variables (98). Population studies have also demonstrated that neck circumference is an important predictor of sleep apnea (51,101). The enlarged neck size in apneics may be secondary to the increased centripetal fat deposition in the neck region of OSA patients. The strength of the association between obesity and sleep apnea should lead us to believe a causal relation. However, the mechanisms of obesity-induced apneas still are being unraveled. Nonobese individuals with sleep apnea have more total body fat and fat deposited in the upper airway than age-, BMI-, and neck circumference-matched controls (102).

Upper airway imaging studies have provided important data to enable investigators to try to better understand the relationship between sleep apnea and obesity. Imaging studies have shown increased adipose tissue surrounding the upper airway in obese patients with sleep apnea (23,24,27,41,102,103). MRI has allowed accurate quantification of fat tissue since fat has a short relaxation time and therefore has a higher intensity than other soft tissues in T1 weighted spin echo MRI. Fat has been proposed to alter upper airway structure through either loading of the pharynx or by luminal encroachment from fat deposits (53). Abdominal and chest wall fat reduces lung volume which, in turn, causes a decrease in upper airway caliber and an increase in compliance from loss of caudal traction on the trachea (53,104).

A majority of the imaging investigations pertaining to the role of obesity have reported increased fat deposition in the lateral pharyngeal fat pads. This finding has consequently been linked to the reduction of airway caliber of sleep apneics. This may not be the case. It has not been proven that increased fat deposition in the parapharyngeal fat pads directly narrows the upper airway. Studies have shown that after controlling for BMI the volume of the parapharyngeal fat pads is not different in apneics and normals (29). Nonetheless, this does not mean that fat deposited around the upper airway is not important. Fat deposition in other sites such as the tongue, soft palate, and uvula or under the mandible may be important (21,27,105). Furthermore, the total amount of fat surrounding the upper airway has been proposed to be more pertinent than fat localized to a specific site. In fact, a correlation between the fat enclosed by the mandibular rami and AHI has been demonstrated (27). Finally, weight gain is known to increase muscle mass in addition to fat (106–108). Approximately 25% to 30% of the increased weight in obese patients is attributable to fat-free tissue (107,109). Therefore, weight gain may directly increase the size of the muscular soft tissue structures surrounding the airway in addition to the fat deposition in the fat pads.

Upper Airway Edema/Trauma
Chronic trauma or repetitive exposure to negative pressures during snoring or apnea also appears to be important factors leading to enlargement of upper airway soft tissue structures. The repetitive apneic events are thought to result in two consequences: edema and muscular dysfunction. The soft palate is especially at risk for the development of edema due to caudal tugging during apneic events. MRI has demonstrated this edema (39) and CPAP is thought to reduce it (43). Quantitative magnetic resonance mapping has demonstrated increased edema and/or fat in the genioglossus muscles of apneics compared to controls (110). Uvulas of OSA patients histologically have shown increased edema (70). Tobacco abuse may also play a role in provoking inflammatory edema and therefore compromise upper airway diameter (111,112). Thus, there is emerging evidence that edema may be important in the pathogenesis of upper airway soft tissue enlargement in apneics.

Muscular Dysfunction/Sensory Neuropathy
Experiments measuring two-point discrimination and vibratory sensation thresholds have shown that snorers and apneics have compromised upper airway mucosal sensory function compared to controls supporting the presence of a sensory neuropathy in the upper airway of such patients (113). Muscular dysfunction has also been shown in OSA patients (114). Histological investigations have demonstrated inflammatory cell infiltration in skeletal muscle of apneics, which leads to contractile dysfunction (114). An abnormally high ratio of type-IIa fatigable to type I fatigue-resistant muscle fibers has been observed in apneic subjects and this finding is used to support the notion that there is a myopathy of the pharyngeal dilators that compromises their ability to maintain patency of the airway. English bulldogs, an animal model for sleep apnea, also have increased type II fibers in the genioglossus muscle (115). The myopathy, however, has been shown to be a consequence of sleep apnea rather than a cause based on a study that showed reversal of the histological changes with the use of CPAP (115). Nonetheless, the myopathic changes in apneics may alter the structure/function of the muscles that surround the upper airway.

Gender (See Also Chapter 14)
Gender-related differences have been reported in relation to upper airway structures (17,52,68,98,116–125). The prevalence and severity of sleep-disordered

breathing is markedly increased in men (98,116). Explanations of these gender-related differences are multi-factorial and include differences in body fat distribution, hormones, control of breathing, upper airway dimensions, and abnormalities in the upper airway mechanics. Investigators have compared normal males and females using acoustic reflection, cephalometry, CT, and MRI and have found many anatomical differences. Women have been shown to have a smaller upper airway (52,117), smaller neck size (118,119), more fat distributed to the lower body and extremities (peripheral fat distribution) (120–122), smaller airway soft tissue structures/volume (17,122,123), and shorter upper airway length (17). The differences listed above are not widely established findings except for body fat distribution. Men with OSA have demonstrated a more collapsible upper airway during non-rapid eye movement (NREM) sleep when compared to BMI-matched women with OSA (125). Inconsistent data exist with regard to differences in pharyngeal mechanics between men and women; however, it appears that women "defend" their airway better in the supine position than men (68). Some investigators argue that the gender difference in collapsibility can be attributed to differences in neck circumference since the increased airway compliance observed in males is not observed when corrected for neck circumference (124). Gender differences in upper airway structure and function may also be explained by sex hormones, that is, postmenopausal women have a higher prevalence of OSA compared to premenopausal and postmenopausal women receiving hormone replacement therapy (116). In addition, new onset of OSA has been reported in a woman who received exogenous testosterone (126). Thus, it is likely that multiple factors explain the gender differences that exist between men and women in OSA.

Genetics/Race

Emerging evidence suggests that sleep apnea can be explained on the basis of genetics (127–132). Sleep apnea has been shown to cluster in families: relatives of an afflicted patient exhibit increased relative risk of OSA (127,128) even after adjusting for BMI. A single major gene inherited in an autosomal recessive fashion has been shown to account for approximately 20% of the variance among Caucasians and African-Americans in the Cleveland Family Study (129). Preliminary linkage studies have shown specific areas of the genome that are linked to sleep apnea as a quantitative trait (130,131). A more recent investigation used volumetric MRI to address the question of familial aggregation with regard to size of upper airway structures (132). These data demonstrated heritability for the size of tongue, lateral walls, and total soft tissue independent of obesity, age, gender, craniofacial size, and ethnicity. Further, it was demonstrated that the increased volume of the soft palate, lateral pharyngeal walls, and total soft tissue volume was associated with increased likelihood of having a sibling with apnea after adjusting for gender, age, ethnicity, craniofacial size, and visceral neck fat (132). These data suggest that genetic factors have an important role in the pathogenesis of the enlargement of the upper airway soft tissue structures in apneics.

Factors Influencing Craniofacial Morphology

Several studies have also demonstrated family aggregation of craniofacial morphology in patients with OSA (119,133). A study on first-degree relatives of probands with sleep apnea showed that family members had retroposed mandibles and inferiorly displaced hyoid bones (119). Cephalometric data also support craniofacial differences (retroposed maxillae and mandibles, shorter mandibles, longer soft palates, and wider uvulas) in first-degree relatives of nonobese OSA patients compared to age-, sex-, height-, and weight-matched controls (133). Craniofacial morphology is also influenced by gender and race similar to upper airway soft tissue structures. Bimaxillary prognathism is more frequent in African-Americans than Hispanics and Caucasians (134). Asians have shorter maxillae and mandibles, smaller anterior-posterior facial dimensions, and lower BMIs than Caucasians (135–137). Therefore, many of the factors that modify the size of the upper airway soft tissue structures also modify the size of the craniofacial structures.

Upper Airway During Sleep

Abnormal upper airway anatomy predisposes to airway collapse during sleep. The onset of sleep is associated with a number of changes in the factors affecting pharyngeal patency including neuromuscular activity, ventilation, chemical, and load responses. Central drive to the respiratory muscle apparatus and upper airway dilators is reduced at the transition from wakefulness to NREM sleep. This leads to reduced upper airway cross-sectional area and increased airway resistance, which together compromise the airway's ability to remain patent. Sites of upper airway narrowing in wakefulness do not necessarily correlate with the site of obstruction during sleep (2,25). Several studies employing nasopharyngoscopy, CT, and MRI have shown that the narrowing/closure site in the airway during sleep is most commonly in the retropalatal area (14,25,41,48,138). Studies have also demonstrated that reductions in airway dimensions occur in the lateral and/or anteroposterior axes in apneics and normals (14,25,41,71,72,138) (Fig. 6) The reason for the former is thought to be secondary to thickening of the lateral pharyngeal walls and the latter is thought to be secondary to posterior displacement of the soft palate (138). Videoendoscopy during sleep has shown that pharyngeal occlusion appears to be due to a combination of inspiratory and expiratory narrowing in the breaths that precede an apnea. Expiratory narrowing renders the lumen vulnerable to complete collapse during the

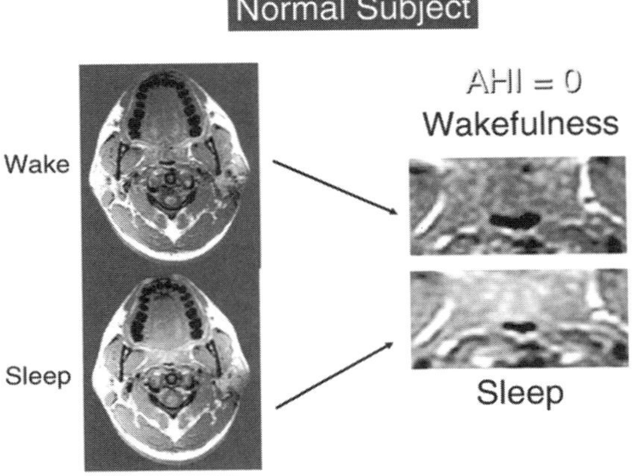

FIGURE 6 State-dependent magnetic resonance imaging in the retropalatal region of a normal subject (apnea-hypopnea index = 0 events/hour). Airway area is smaller during sleep in this normal subject. The state-dependent change in airway caliber is secondary to reductions in the lateral and anterior-posterior airway dimensions. *Source*: From Ref. 138.

subsequent inspiratory effort (72). Contrary to prior beliefs, the airway is not a homogeneous tube that collapses uniformly (Fig. 7). It behaves more like a Starling resistor where pharyngeal occlusion occurs once the intraluminal pressure decreases below the surrounding pressure. Airflow limitation occurs despite continued increases in driving pressure as a result of the upstream segment (e.g., nose) and the transmural pressure surrounding the collapsible segment. Studying the upper airway anatomical differences between apneics and normals during sleep is necessary to eliminate the confounding effects of muscle activity. One such study used endoscopic techniques to assess pharyngeal size in OSA patients and controls under general anesthesia with full paralysis (69). Results obtained showed a smaller airway caliber, especially in the retropalatal area and increased collapsibility in apnea patients (69). An MRI study confirmed this differential narrowing by quantifying volume reduction in the retropalatal (19% volume reduction) compared with the retroglossal (4% volume reduction) regions during sleep in normal patients (138) (Fig. 7). The specific mechanisms explaining the predominance of narrowing in the retropalatal region during sleep remain to be unraveled. Nonetheless, such data indicate that during sleep, normals, in addition to apneics, narrow their upper airway primarily in the retropalatal region.

Upper Airway During Respiration
Although static and state-dependent upper airway imaging modalities have provided valuable information regarding the mechanisms that affect the airway morphology, examination of the airway during respiration provides data to understand the dynamic behavior of the upper airway. Dynamic upper airway imaging modalities including CT, MRI, and nasopharyngoscopy have been employed to study the upper airway during inspiration, expiration, and simulated apneas via a Müller maneuver (14,35,43,45,72,84,139–141).

Geometrical changes in the airway during respiration have been well-characterized (7,84) (Fig. 8). In inspiration the upper airway area is relatively constant inferring a balance between muscle dilator activity and negative airway lumen pressure. Early expiration exhibits airway maximal enlargement, which is likely linked to positive intraluminal pressure. At end-expiration there is significant decline in airway caliber. The finding that the upper airway is at its minimal caliber

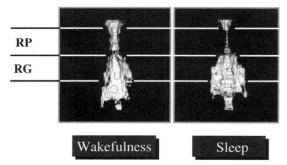

FIGURE 7 (*See color insert.*) Volumetric state-dependent airway imaging in a normal subject using magnetic resonance imaging. Airway volume during sleep is smaller in the retropalatal (RP) region but not the retroglossal (RG) region. Such images suggest that the upper airway during sleep does not narrow as a homogenous tube. *Source*: From Ref. 138.

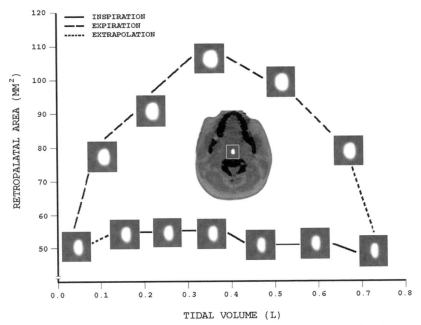

FIGURE 8 Changes in upper airway area as a function of tidal volume during the respiratory cycle. Airway caliber is relatively constant in inspiration. Airway size increases in early expiration and decreases in late expiration. *Source*: From Ref. 43.

at end-expiration, along with other studies demonstrating apneics events during expiration, has led to the conclusion that airway closure can occur in both inspiration and expiration (23,71,72,142,143).

Nasopharyngoscopy combined with a Müller maneuver has provided an awake simulation of an apnea event when a subject is requested to inspire against a closed mouth and occluded nose. Studying airway narrowing at graded negative intraluminal pressures generated by the subject has reaffirmed that airway collapse is not homogeneous (144). More recent work has demonstrated a good correlation between AHI and retropalatal narrowing during a Müller maneuver (80,81).

It appears based on comparisons between apneic patients and controls that the former have greater decrements in airway dimension during a Müller maneuver suggesting an increased compliance in the apneic upper airway (144). In general, studies examining the dynamic behavior of the upper airway have provided a framework for understanding the pathogenesis of airway closure.

TREATMENT OF OBSTRUCTIVE SLEEP APNEA AND UPPER AIRWAY IMAGING

Imaging studies have also allowed us to understand the effect of sleep apnea treatment on upper airway anatomy. The following section reviews the information attained from imaging studies pertaining to the effect of weight loss, CPAP, oral appliances and surgery upon upper airway size, and the surrounding soft tissue and craniofacial structures.

Weight Loss (See Also Chapter 13)

The importance of obesity in OSA patients has been discussed in prior sections of this chapter. Several predominantly uncontrolled studies have been performed to investigate the effect of various methods of nonsurgical weight loss (diet, behavior, and activity) on sleep apnea (53,145–147). In general, such studies have shown that significant weight loss (approximately 10%) is associated with varying degrees of improvement in sleep apnea (53,145). Importantly, weight loss is challenging to sustain and therefore re-emergence of apnea may occur. Examining the effect of weight loss on airway properties, investigators have reported that OSA patients who achieved a mean reduction of 17% in body weight demonstrated significant decreases in airway collapsibility [i.e., critical closing pressure (Pcrit)] and, in turn, significant decreases (greater than a 50% decrement) in disordered breathing (74). Three-dimensional MRI in obese normal women (AHI < 5 events per hour) has demonstrated that a 17.7% weight loss increased the volume of the upper airway and significantly decreased the volume of the lateral pharyngeal walls and para-pharyngeal fat pads (148) (Figs. 9 and 10). The volume of the soft palate and tongue also decreased but these changes did not achieve statistical significance. The explanation of these upper airway geometry changes with weight loss has not been completely elucidated. It is possible that decrements in fat pad volume could lead to a lateral traction effect upon the lateral pharyngeal walls. In addition, adipose tissue within the lateral pharyngeal walls, tongue, uvula, and under the mandible could decrease with weight loss and hence contribute to the overall increase in volume of the upper airway. Finally, weight loss may affect the muscular tissue surrounding the airway thereby altering airway biomechanical properties. It is well documented that weight gain in obese patients is not solely due to increased fat but also muscle (107,109). Further investigation is required to clarify the anatomic

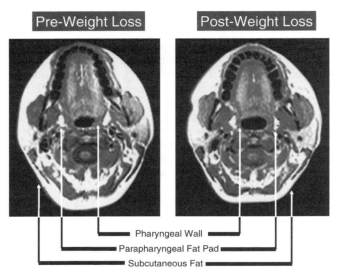

FIGURE 9 Axial retropalatal magnetic resonance imaging of a normal woman, before and after a 17% weight loss. Airway area and lateral airway dimensions increase and the thickness of lateral pharyngeal walls and the size of the parapharyngeal fat pads decrease with weight loss.

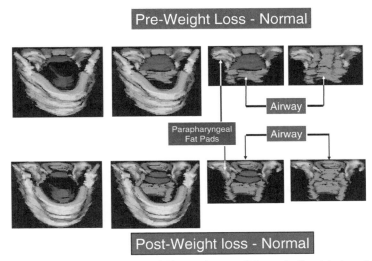

FIGURE 10 (*See color insert.*) Upper airway soft tissue [soft palate (purple), the tongue (orange/rust), the lateral pharyngeal walls (green), parapharyngeal fat pads (yellow)] and craniofacial [mandible (gray)] magnetic resonance imaging reconstructions before and after a 17% weight loss in a normal woman. The size of the upper airway increases with weight loss. The largest reductions in the size of the upper airway soft tissue structures with weight loss were in the lateral pharyngeal walls and the parapharyngeal fat pads. *Source*: From Ref. 148.

relationship between weight loss and sleep apnea. The extent of weight loss required for improved outcomes in patients with sleep apnea and the effects on the airway configuration require more study.

Continuous Positive Airway Pressure Therapy (See Also Chapter 6)

CT and MRI techniques have shown significant increases in upper airway caliber during wakefulness with the use of CPAP in normals and patients with OSA (19,26,42,149,150). The predominant change in airway dimension with the application of CPAP is an increase in the airway's lateral axis (Figs. 11–14). A dose–dependent relationship between increasing CPAP settings (up to 15 cm H_2O) and airway volume, airway area, and lateral airway dimension has been observed in normal subjects (42). Thinning of the lateral walls has shown in an MRI study to be inversely related to the CPAP level used (26). The administration of CPAP has little influence on the anteroposterior configuration of the airway. But CPAP significantly increases upper airway caliber and decreases airway edema.

Oral Appliances (See Also Chapter 12)

The evidence assessing the role of oral appliances in the treatment of OSA continues to grow in both quantity and quality with several randomized placebo-controlled and cross-over trials having been completed (151). The efficacy of oral appliances in successfully treating mild-to-moderate OSA (defined as less than or equal to 10 apneas or hypopnea per hour of sleep) is approximately 50% (151). The oral appliances can be broadly divided into two types: devices that reposition the mandible

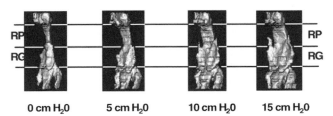

CPAP - Airway 3D Volumes

0 cm H₂0   5 cm H₂0   10 cm H₂0   15 cm H₂0

FIGURE 11 (*See color insert.*) Volumetric magnetic resonance imaging reconstruction of the upper airway in a normal subject with progressively greater continuous positive airway pressure (CPAP) (0 to 15 cm H$_2$O) settings. Upper airway volume increases significantly in both the retropalatal (RP) and retroglossal (RG) regions with higher levels of CPAP. *Source*: From Ref. 26.

and devices which advance the tongue. In general, their mechanism of action is thought to be related to anterior displacement of the jaw/tongue increasing the cross-sectional diameter of the airway and/or reducing the collapsibility of the upper airway (152). Upright lateral (153,154) and supine cephalometry studies (155–157), CT, and MRI have shown that mandibular repositioning appliances can increase the following: posterior airway space (153,154), airway cross-sectional area (153–157) at multiple levels, pharyngeal size (153,158), and pharyngeal volume (159). However, the specific biomechanical change in airway configuration produced by the oral appliances remains unclear and may be device dependent. Some

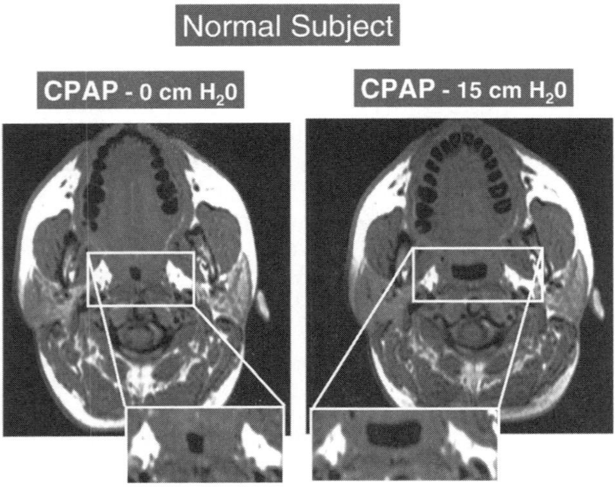

FIGURE 12 Axial retropalatal magnetic resonance imaging in a normal subject at two levels of continuous positive airway pressure (CPAP) (0 and 15 cm H$_2$O). Airway area is significantly greater at 15 cm H$_2$O than without CPAP. The airway enlargement with the application of CPAP is predominantly in the lateral dimension. *Source*: From Ref. 26.

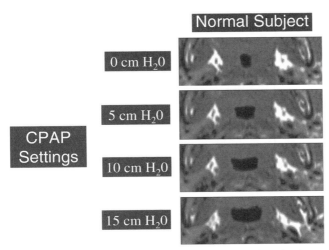

FIGURE 13 Axial retropalatal magnetic resonance imaging in a normal subject (the same subject as in Fig. 12) with continuous positive airway pressure (CPAP) ranging from 0 to 15 cm H_2O. Significant lateral airway enlargement with progressive increase in CPAP results in thinning of the lateral pharyngeal walls but the parapharyngeal fat pads are not displaced. The increase in airway size with greater levels of CPAP is primarily in the lateral dimension; the anterior-posterior dimensions of the airway do not change significantly with CPAP. *Source*: From Ref. 26.

investigators report increased diameter of the retroglossal region in an anterior-posterior orientation (154,160), while others report greater changes in the retropalatal region (153,161) and lateral dimension (161). Videoendoscopy techniques provide further support to the latter findings, revealing that mandibular repositioning appliances lead to greater changes in the retropalatal region (77,161). Overall, these disparate findings suggest that the effect of oral appliances on airway configuration

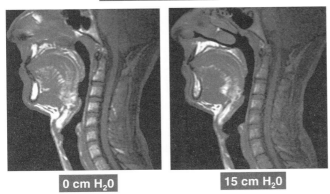

FIGURE 14 Mid-sagittal magnetic resonance imaging of a normal subject (the same subject as in Figs. 12 and 13) at two levels of continuous positive airway pressure (CPAP) (0 and 15 cm H_2O). There is very little change in airway caliber with the application of CPAP since CPAP does not significantly affect the anterior-posterior structures. *Source*: From Ref. 26.

is complex. To predict the success of oral appliances, investigators are beginning to use upper airway imaging techniques to access the size and position of the upper airway (77).

Upper Airway Surgery (See Also Chapter 11)

There are several surgical options for sleep apnea patients including UPPP (tonsillectomy and removal of the uvula, distal margin of soft palate, and any excessive tissue), uvulopalatopharyngo-glossoplasty (UPPGP—combines UPPP with limited resection of the tongue), transpalatal advancement pharnyngoplasty (TPAP—resection of the posterior hard palate with advancement of the soft palate to enlarge the retropalatal airway), sliding genioplasty or genioglossus advancement (advancing the tongue forward by displacing its attachment to the genial tubercle forward), hyoid advancement (displacement of the hyoid bone forward to enlarge the retroglossal airway), and maxillary-mandibular advancement (forward displacement of the maxillae and mandible to advance the soft tissue structures) (162). Typically, surgical options to treat sleep apnea are invasive and may require a staged approach. Since the upper airway obstruction may not be at one site, selecting the appropriate sleep apnea patient and a suitable surgical approach is important.

Surgical selection may be achieved by examining data from clinical, fiberoptic, and radiologic sources. The Müller maneuver (voluntary inspiration against a closed mouth and obstructed nares) permits visualization of the airway structures during a simulated apneic event and has been used to identify surgical candidates (78). CT and MRI can also be employed to provide detailed information about structural dimensions during wakefulness and sleep (28,163) and may predict surgical outcome (70).

UPPP, the most common upper airway surgical procedure, was introduced in 1981 and although there have been many studies in OSA patients examining this surgical technique its failure rate exceeds 50% (162). UPPP only corrects one vulnerable upper airway site, the retropalatal pharynx. Patients with retropalatal obstruction have been shown to have a 52% success rate with UPPP whereas patients with retroglossal obstruction have a 5% success rate with UPPP (164). CT and MRI studies have demonstrated that UPPP results in enlargement of the airway only in the operated area (162). Upper airway narrowing in the unresected portion of the soft palate post-UPPP is a recognized problem and likely explains the limited efficacy of UPPP. A further issue, highlighted by a study of LAUP, is that anatomical improvements in the airway postsurgery, as documented by videoendoscopy measurements during wakefulness, are not necessarily indicative or predictive of objective improvements in apnea severity during sleep (75).

Patients with craniofacial abnormalities should be considered for surgical techniques such as mandibular and/or maxillary advancement and sliding genioplasty (24). Cephalometry and nasopharyngoscopy have shown that maxillomandibular advancement increases upper airway caliber in the retroglossal and retropalatal regions by physically expanding the skeletal boundaries of the upper airway (165). Maxillomandibular advancement is reported as the most effective surgical treatment for sleep apnea with success rates between 75% and 100% (165).

Bariatric Surgery (See Also Chapter 13)

Bariatric surgery has the potential for improving patients with sleep apnea secondary to weight loss (166). Although significant weight loss is expected after bariatric surgery, limited data exist regarding the effect of gastric surgery on OSA (167). That significant improvement occurs in the AHI (greater than 50% decrease) even in the long-term is promising; however, large-scale studies examining polysomnography pre- and postgastric bypass surgery need to be performed (167,168). Furthermore, it is necessary to re-evaluate after surgery for the presence of persistent sleep apnea requiring CPAP treatment. Currently, no data are available regarding the anatomic changes in the upper airway associated with this surgery.

CONCLUSIONS

Upper airway imaging techniques employed to study the human upper airway have significantly advanced our understanding of OSA. Important determinants of airway geometry have been identified: volume of tongue, lateral pharyngeal wall thickness, and total amount of soft tissue surrounding the airway. The sleep apneic airway has been characterized as an elliptical or circular shape that is oriented in the anteroposterior axis. Static imaging studies have shown that soft tissue and cranio-facial structures are influenced by important factors such as body mass, neck circumference, gender, and genetics. The effects of sleep apnea treatments have also been clarified through imaging techniques. Upper airway imaging is not routinely indicated in the assessment of a sleep apnea patient. If CPAP therapy is efficacious, then upper airway imaging is not warranted. However, imaging does have role in the preoperative (and postoperative) evaluation of patients undergoing upper airway surgery to characterize the airway geometry. The likelihood of success of UPPP is related to the site of airway obstruction and this can be assessed by MRI (preferably three-dimensional) or by nasopharyngoscopy with the Müller maneuver. Imaging should also be considered when utilizing an oral appliance to determine if upper airway caliber increases with the appliance (especially if the AHI does not improve). Upper airway imaging studies have provided important new insights into the pathogenesis, genetics, and treatment of OSA.

REFERENCES

1. Horner RL. Motor control of the pharyngeal musculature and implications for the pathogenesis of obstructive sleep apnea. Sleep 1996; 19(10):827–853.
2. Hudgel DW. Variable site of airway narrowing among obstructive sleep apnea patients. J Appl Physiol 1986; 61(4):1403–1409.
3. Schwartz AR, Smith PL, Wise RA, Gold AR, Permutt S. Induction of upper airway occlusion in sleeping individuals with subatmospheric nasal pressure. J Appl Physiol 1988; 64(2):535–542.
4. Suratt PM, Wilhoit SC, Cooper K. Induction of airway collapse with subatmospheric pressure in awake patients with sleep apnea. J Appl Physiol 1984; 57(1):140–146.
5. Kuna ST, Smickley JS, Vanoye CR. Respiratory-related pharyngeal constrictor muscle activity in normal human adults. Am J Respir Crit Care Med 1997; 155(6):1991–1999.
6. Mathew OP. Upper airway negative-pressure effects on respiratory activity of upper airway muscles. J Appl Physiol 1984; 56(2):500–505.
7. Mezzanotte WS, Tangel DJ, White DP. Waking genioglossal electromyogram in sleep apnea patients versus normal controls (a neuromuscular compensatory mechanism). J Clin Invest 1992; 89(5):1571–1579.
8. Stanchina ML, Malhotra A, Fogel RB, et al. Genioglossus muscle responsiveness to chemical and mechanical stimuli during non-rapid eye movement sleep. Am J Respir Crit Care Med 2002; 165(7):945–949.
9. Wheatley JR, White DP. The influence of sleep on pharyngeal reflexes. Sleep 1993; 16(suppl 8):S87–S89.

10. Wiegand DA, Latz B, Zwillich CW, Wiegand L. Upper airway resistance and geniohyoid muscle activity in normal men during wakefulness and sleep. J Appl Physiol 1990; 69(4):1252–1261.
11. Fogel RB, Malhotra A, Pillar G, et al. Genioglossal activation in patients with obstructive sleep apnea versus control subjects. Mechanisms of muscle control. Am J Respir Crit Care Med 2001; 164(11):2025–2030.
12. Armstrong JJ, Leigh MS, Sampson DD, Walsh JH, Hillman DR, Eastwood PR. Quantitative upper airway imaging with anatomic optical coherence tomography. Am J Respir Crit Care Med 2006; 173(2):226–233.
13. Abbey NC, Block AJ, Green D, Mancuso A, Hellard DW. Measurement of pharyngeal volume by digitized magnetic resonance imaging. Effect of nasal continuous positive airway pressure. Am Rev Respir Dis 1989; 140(3):717–723.
14. Ciscar MA, Juan G, Martinez V, et al. Magnetic resonance imaging of the pharynx in OSA patients and healthy subjects. Eur Respir J 2001; 17(1):79–86.
15. Do KL, Ferreyra H, Healy JF, Davidson TM. Does tongue size differ between patients with and without sleep-disordered breathing? Laryngoscope 2000; 110(9):1552–1555.
16. Jager L, Gunther E, Gauger J, Reiser M. Fluoroscopic MR of the pharynx in patients with obstructive sleep apnea. AJNR Am J Neuroradiol 1998; 19(7):1205–1214.
17. Malhotra A, Huang Y, Fogel RB, et al. The male predisposition to pharyngeal collapse: importance of airway length. Am J Respir Crit Care Med 2002; 166(10):1388–1395.
18. Rodenstein DO, Dooms G, Thomas Y, et al. Pharyngeal shape and dimensions in healthy subjects, snorers, and patients with obstructive sleep apnoea. Thorax 1990; 45(10): 722–727.
19. Ryan CF, Lowe AA, Li D, Fleetham JA. Magnetic resonance imaging of the upper airway in obstructive sleep apnea before and after chronic nasal continuous positive airway pressure therapy. Am Rev Respir Dis 1991; 144(4):939–944.
20. Schoenberg SO, Floemer F, Kroeger H, Hoffmann A, Bock M, Knopp MV. Combined assessment of obstructive sleep apnea syndrome with dynamic MRI and parallel EEG registration: initial results. Invest Radiol 2000; 35(4):267–276.
21. Schwab RJ. Imaging for the snoring and sleep apnea patient. Dent Clin North Am 2001; 45(4):759–796.
22. Schwab RJ, Goldberg AN. Upper airway assessment: radiographic and other imaging techniques. Otolaryngol Clin North Am 1998; 31(6):931–968.
23. Schwab RJ, Gupta KB, Gefter WB, Metzger LJ, Hoffman EA, Pack AI. Upper airway and soft tissue anatomy in normal subjects and patients with sleep-disordered breathing. Significance of the lateral pharyngeal walls. Am J Respir Crit Care Med 1995; 152(5 Pt 1):1673–1689.
24. Shelton KE, Woodson H, Gay S, Suratt PM. Pharyngeal fat in obstructive sleep apnea. Am Rev Respir Dis 1993; 148(2):462–466.
25. Suto Y, Matsuo T, Kato T, et al. Evaluation of the pharyngeal airway in patients with sleep apnea: value of ultrafast MR imaging. AJR Am J Roentgenol 1993; 160(2):311–314.
26. Schwab RJ, Pack AI, Gupta KB, et al. Upper airway and soft tissue structural changes induced by CPAP in normal subjects. Am J Respir Crit Care Med 1996; 154(4 Pt 1):1106–1116.
27. Shelton KE, Gay SB, Hollowell DE, Woodson H, Suratt PM. Mandible enclosure of upper airway and weight in obstructive sleep apnea. Am Rev Respir Dis 1993; 148(1):195–200.
28. Schwab RJ. Upper airway imaging. Clin Chest Med 1998; 19(1):33–54.
29. Schwab RJ, Pasirstein M, Pierson R, et al. Identification of upper airway anatomic risk factors for obstructive sleep apnea with volumetric magnetic resonance imaging. Am J Respir Crit Care Med 2003; 168(5):522–530.
30. Li HY, Chen NH, Wang CR, Shu YH, Wang PC. Use of 3-dimensional computed tomography scan to evaluate upper airway patency for patients undergoing sleep-disordered breathing surgery. Otolaryngol Head Neck Surg 2003; 129(4):336–342.
31. Ryan CF, Lowe AA, Li D, Fleetham JA. Three-dimensional upper airway computed tomography in obstructive sleep apnea. A prospective study in patients treated by uvulopalatopharyngoplasty. Am Rev Respir Dis 1991; 144(2):428–432.
32. Aksoz T, Akan H, Celebi M, Sakan BB. Does the oropharyngeal fat tissue influence the oropharyngeal airway in snorers? Dynamic CT study. Korean J Radiol 2004; 5(2):102–106.
33. Akan H, Aksoz T, Belet U, Sesen T. Dynamic upper airway soft-tissue and caliber changes in healthy subjects and snoring patients. AJNR Am J Neuroradiol 2004; 25(10):1846–1850.

34. Burger CD, Stanson AW, Daniels BK, Sheedy PF, II, Shepard JW, Jr. Fast-CT evaluation of the effect of lung volume on upper airway size and function in normal men. Am Rev Respir Dis 1992; 146(2):335–339.

35. Burger CD, Stanson AW, Sheedy PF, II, Daniels BK, Shepard JW, Jr. Fast-computed tomography evaluation of age-related changes in upper airway structure and function in normal men. Am Rev Respir Dis 1992; 145(4 Pt 1):846–852.

36. Caballero P, Alvarez-Sala R, Garcia-Rio F, et al. CT in the evaluation of the upper airway in healthy subjects and in patients with obstructive sleep apnea syndrome. Chest 1998; 113(1):111–116.

37. Ell SR, Jolles H, Galvin JR. Cine CT demonstration of nonfixed upper airway obstruction. AJR Am J Roentgenol 1986; 146(4):669–677.

38. Ell SR, Jolles H, Keyes WD, Galvin JR. Cine CT technique for dynamic airway studies. AJR Am J Roentgenol 1985; 145(1):35–36.

39. Galvin JR, Rooholamini SA, Stanford W. Obstructive sleep apnea: diagnosis with ultrafast CT. Radiology 1989; 171(3):775–778.

40. Haponik EF, Smith PL, Bohlman ME, Allen RP, Goldman SM, Bleecker ER. Computerized tomography in obstructive sleep apnea. Correlation of airway size with physiology during sleep and wakefulness. Am Rev Respir Dis 1983; 127(2):221–226.

41. Horner RL, Shea SA, McIvor J, Guz A. Pharyngeal size and shape during wakefulness and sleep in patients with obstructive sleep apnoea. Q J Med 1989; 72(268):719–735.

42. Kuna ST, Bedi DG, Ryckman C. Effect of nasal airway positive pressure on upper airway size and configuration. Am Rev Respir Dis 1988; 138(4):969–975.

43. Schwab RJ, Gefter WB, Hoffman EA, Gupta KB, Pack AI. Dynamic upper airway imaging during awake respiration in normal subjects and patients with sleep disordered breathing. Am Rev Respir Dis 1993; 148(5):1385–1400.

44. Shepard JW, Jr, Garrison M, Vas W. Upper airway distensibility and collapsibility in patients with obstructive sleep apnea. Chest 1990; 98(1):84–91.

45. Shepard JW, Jr, Stanson AW, Sheedy PF, Westbrook PR. Fast-CT evaluation of the upper airway during wakefulness in patients with obstructive sleep apnea. Prog Clin Biol Res 1990; 345:273–279; discussion 280–282.

46. Stanford W, Galvin J, Rooholamini M. Effects of awake tidal breathing, swallowing, nasal breathing, oral breathing and the Muller and Valsalva maneuvers on the dimensions of the upper airway. Evaluation by ultrafast computerized tomography. Chest 1988; 94(1):149–154.

47. Stauffer JL, Zwillich CW, Cadieux RJ, et al. Pharyngeal size and resistance in obstructive sleep apnea. Am Rev Respir Dis 1987; 136(3):623–627.

48. Stein MG, Gamsu G, de Geer G, Golden JA, Crumley RL, Webb WR. Cine CT in obstructive sleep apnea. AJR Am J Roentgenol 1987; 148(6):1069–1074.

49. Shepard JW, Jr, Thawley SE. Evaluation of the upper airway by computerized tomography in patients undergoing uvulopalatopharyngoplasty for obstructive sleep apnea. Am Rev Respir Dis 1989; 140(3):711–716.

50. Fleetham JA. Upper airway imaging in relation to obstructive sleep apnea. Clin Chest Med 1992; 13(3):399–416.

51. Davies RJ, Ali NJ, Stradling JR. Neck circumference and other clinical features in the diagnosis of the obstructive sleep apnoea syndrome. Thorax 1992; 47(2):101–105.

52. Brown IG, Zamel N, Hoffstein V. Pharyngeal cross-sectional area in normal men and women. J Appl Physiol 1986; 61(3):890–895.

53. Strobel RJ, Rosen RC. Obesity and weight loss in obstructive sleep apnea: a critical review. Sleep 1996; 19(2):104–115.

54. Ingman T, Nieminen T, Hurmerinta K. Cephalometric comparison of pharyngeal changes in subjects with upper airway resistance syndrome or obstructive sleep apnoea in upright and supine positions. Eur J Orthod 2004; 26(3):321–326.

55. Pae EK, Lowe AA, Fleetham JA. A role of pharyngeal length in obstructive sleep apnea patients. Am J Orthod Dentofacial Orthop 1997; 111(1):12–17.

56. Ferguson KA, Ono T, Lowe AA, Ryan CF, Fleetham JA. The relationship between obesity and craniofacial structure in obstructive sleep apnea. Chest 1995; 108(2):375–381.

57. Bacon WH, Turlot JC, Krieger J, Stierle JL. Cephalometric evaluation of pharyngeal obstructive factors in patients with sleep apneas syndrome. Angle Orthod 1990; 60(2):115–122.

58. deBerry-Borowiecki B, Kukwa A, Blanks RH. Cephalometric analysis for diagnosis and treatment of obstructive sleep apnea. Laryngoscope 1988; 98(2):226–234.
59. Shepard JW, Jr, Gefter WB, Guilleminault C, et al. Evaluation of the upper airway in patients with obstructive sleep apnea. Sleep 1991; 14(4):361–371.
60. Nelson S, Hans M. Contribution of craniofacial risk factors in increasing apneic activity among obese and nonobese habitual snorers. Chest 1997; 111(1):154–162.
61. Mayer P, Pepin JL, Bettega G, et al. Relationship between body mass index, age and upper airway measurements in snorers and sleep apnoea patients. Eur Respir J 1996; 9(9):1801–1809.
62. Tsuiki S, Lowe AA, Almeida FR, Kawahata N, Fleetham JA. Effects of mandibular advancement on airway curvature and obstructive sleep apnoea severity. Eur Respir J 2004; 23(2):263–268.
63. Pae EK, Lowe AA, Sasaki K, Price C, Tsuchiya M, Fleetham JA. A cephalometric and electromyographic study of upper airway structures in the upright and supine positions. Am J Orthod Dentofacial Orthop 1994; 106(1):52–59.
64. Bacon WH, Krieger J, Turlot JC, Stierle JL. Craniofacial characteristics in patients with obstructive sleep apneas syndrome. Cleft Palate J 1988; 25(4):374–378.
65. Bradley TD, Brown IG, Grossman RF, et al. Pharyngeal size in snorers, nonsnorers, and patients with obstructive sleep apnea. N Engl J Med 1986; 315(21):1327–1331.
66. Hoffstein V, Zamel N, Phillipson EA. Lung volume dependence of pharyngeal cross-sectional area in patients with obstructive sleep apnea. Am Rev Respir Dis 1984; 130(2):175–178.
67. Rivlin J, Hoffstein V, Kalbfleisch J, McNicholas W, Zamel N, Bryan AC. Upper airway morphology in patients with idiopathic obstructive sleep apnea. Am Rev Respir Dis 1984; 129(3):355–360.
68. Martin SE, Mathur R, Marshall I, Douglas NJ. The effect of age, sex, obesity and posture on upper airway size. Eur Respir J 1997; 10(9):2087–2090.
69. Isono S, Remmers JE, Tanaka A, Sho Y, Sato J, Nishino T. Anatomy of pharynx in patients with obstructive sleep apnea and in normal subjects. J Appl Physiol 1997; 82(4):1319–1326.
70. Launois SH, Feroah TR, Campbell WN, et al. Site of pharyngeal narrowing predicts outcome of surgery for obstructive sleep apnea. Am Rev Respir Dis 1993; 147(1):182–189.
71. Badr MS, Toiber F, Skatrud JB, Dempsey J. Pharyngeal narrowing/occlusion during central sleep apnea. J Appl Physiol 1995; 78(5):1806–1815.
72. Morrell MJ, Arabi Y, Zahn B, Badr MS. Progressive retropalatal narrowing preceding obstructive apnea. Am J Respir Crit Care Med 1998; 158(6):1974–1981.
73. Woodson BT, Wooten MR. Comparison of upper-airway evaluations during wakefulness and sleep. Laryngoscope 1994; 104(7):821–828.
74. Schwartz AR, Gold AR, Schubert N, et al. Effect of weight loss on upper airway collapsibility in obstructive sleep apnea. Am Rev Respir Dis 1991; 144(3 Pt 1):494–498.
75. Ryan CF, Love LL. Unpredictable results of laser assisted uvulopalatoplasty in the treatment of obstructive sleep apnoea. Thorax 2000; 55(5):399–404.
76. Isono S, Tanaka A, Sho Y, Konno A, Nishino T. Advancement of the mandible improves velopharyngeal airway patency. J Appl Physiol 1995; 79(6):2132–2138.
77. Johal A, Battagel JM, Kotecha BT. Sleep nasendoscopy: a diagnostic tool for predicting treatment success with mandibular advancement splints in obstructive sleep apnoea. Eur J Orthod 2005; 27(6):607–614.
78. Sher AE, Thorpy MJ, Shprintzen RJ, Spielman AJ, Burack B, McGregor PA. Predictive value of Muller maneuver in selection of patients for uvulopalatopharyngoplasty. Laryngoscope 1985; 95(12):1483–1487.
79. Crumley RL, Stein M, Gamsu G, Golden J, Dermon S. Determination of obstructive site in obstructive sleep apnea. Laryngoscope 1987; 97(3 Pt 1):301–308.
80. Hsu PP, Han HN, Chan YH, et al. Quantitative computer-assisted digital-imaging upper airway analysis for obstructive sleep apnoea. Clin Otolaryngol Allied Sci 2004; 29(5):522–529.
81. Hsu PP, Tan BY, Chan YH, Tay HN, Lu PK, Blair RL. Clinical predictors in obstructive sleep apnea patients with computer-assisted quantitative videoendoscopic upper airway analysis. Laryngoscope 2004; 114(5):791–799.
82. Bohlman ME, Haponik EF, Smith PL, Allen RP, Bleecker ER, Goldman SM. CT demonstration of pharyngeal narrowing in adult obstructive sleep apnea. AJR Am J Roentgenol 1983; 140(3):543–548.

83. Schwab RJ. Pro: sleep apnea is an anatomic disorder. Am J Respir Crit Care Med 2003; 168(3):270–271; discussion 273.
84. Schwab RJ, Gefter WB, Pack AI, Hoffman EA. Dynamic imaging of the upper airway during respiration in normal subjects. J Appl Physiol 1993; 74(4);1504–1514.
85. Bhattacharyya N, Blake SP, Fried MP. Assessment of the airway in obstructive sleep apnea syndrome with 3-dimensional airway computed tomography. Otolaryngol Head Neck Surg 2000; 123(4):444–449.
86. Lyberg T, Krogstad O, Djupesland G. Cephalometric analysis in patients with obstructive sleep apnoea syndrome. I. Skeletal morphology. J Laryngol Otol 1989; 103(3):287–292.
87. Lyberg T, Krogstad O, Djupesland G. Cephalometric analysis in patients with obstructive sleep apnoea syndrome: II. Soft tissue morphology. J Laryngol Otol 1989; 103(3):293–297.
88. Partinen M, Guilleminault C, Quera-Salva MA, Jamieson A. Obstructive sleep apnea and cephalometric roentgenograms. The role of anatomic upper airway abnormalities in the definition of abnormal breathing during sleep. Chest 1988; 93(6):1199–1205.
89. Pracharktam N, Hans MG, Strohl KP, Redline S. Upright and supine cephalometric evaluation of obstructive sleep apnea syndrome and snoring subjects. Angle Orthod 1994; 64(1):63–73.
90. Riley R, Guilleminault C, Herran J, Powell N. Cephalometric analyses and flow-volume loops in obstructive sleep apnea patients. Sleep 1983; 6(4):303–311.
91. Lowe AA, Gionhaku N, Takeuchi K, Fleetham JA. Three-dimensional CT reconstructions of tongue and airway in adult subjects with obstructive sleep apnea. Am J Orthod Dentofacial Orthop 1986; 90(5):364–374.
92. Leiter JC. Upper airway shape: Is it important in the pathogenesis of obstructive sleep apnea? Am J Respir Crit Care Med 1996; 153(3):894–898.
93. Riha RL, Brander P, Vennelle M, Douglas NJ. A cephalometric comparison of patients with the sleep apnea/hypopnea syndrome and their siblings. Sleep 2005; 28(3):315–320.
94. Sforza E, Bacon W, Weiss T, Thibault A, Petiau C, Krieger J. Upper airway collapsibility and cephalometric variables in patients with obstructive sleep apnea. Am J Respir Crit Care Med 2000; 161(2 Pt 1):347–352.
95. Verin E, Tardif C, Buffet X, et al. Comparison between anatomy and resistance of upper airway in normal subjects, snorers and OSAS patients. Respir Physiol 2002; 129(3): 335–343.
96. Young JW, McDonald JP. An investigation into the relationship between the severity of obstructive sleep apnoea/hypopnoea syndrome and the vertical position of the hyoid bone. Surgeon 2004; 2(3);145–151.
97. Bliwise DL, Feldman DE, Bliwise NG, et al. Risk factors for sleep disordered breathing in heterogeneous geriatric populations. J Am Geriatr Soc 1987; 35(2):132–141.
98. Young T, Palta M, Dempsey J, Skatrud J, Weber S, Badr S. The occurrence of sleep-disordered breathing among middle-aged adults. N Engl J Med 1993; 328(17):1230–1235.
99. Vgontzas AN, Papanicolaou DA, Bixler EO, et al. Sleep apnea and daytime sleepiness and fatigue: relation to visceral obesity, insulin resistance, and hypercytokinemia. J Clin Endocrinol Metab 2000; 85(3):1151–1158.
100. Young T, Shahar E, Nieto FJ, et al. Predictors of sleep-disordered breathing in community-dwelling adults: the Sleep Heart Health Study. Arch Intern Med 2002; 162(8):893–900.
101. Davies RJ, Stradling JR. The relationship between neck circumference, radiographic pharyngeal anatomy, and the obstructive sleep apnoea syndrome. Eur Respir J 1990; 3(5):509–514.
102. Mortimore IL, Marshall I, Wraith PK, Sellar RJ, Douglas NJ. Neck and total body fat deposition in nonobese and obese patients with sleep apnea compared with that in control subjects. Am J Respir Crit Care Med 1998; 157(1):280–283.
103. Horner RL, Mohiaddin RH, Lowell DG, et al. Sites and sizes of fat deposits around the pharynx in obese patients with obstructive sleep apnoea and weight matched controls. Eur Respir J 1989; 2(7):613–622.
104. Brown IG, Bradley TD, Phillipson EA, Zamel N, Hoffstein V. Pharyngeal compliance in snoring subjects with and without obstructive sleep apnea. Am Rev Respir Dis 1985; 132(2):211–215.
105. Stauffer JL, Buick MK, Bixler EO, et al. Morphology of the uvula in obstructive sleep apnea. Am Rev Respir Dis 1989; 140(3):724–728.

106. Hill JO, Sparling PB, Shields TW, Heller PA. Effects of exercise and food restriction on body composition and metabolic rate in obese women. Am J Clin Nutr 1987; 46(4): 622–630.
107. Wadden TA, Foster GD, Letizia KA, Mullen JL. Long-term effects of dieting on resting metabolic rate in obese outpatients. JAMA 1990; 264(6):707–711.
108. Series F, Cote C, Simoneau JA, et al. Physiologic, metabolic, and muscle fiber type characteristics of musculus uvulae in sleep apnea hypopnea syndrome and in snorers. J Clin Invest 1995; 95(1):20–25.
109. Foster GD, Wadden TA, Mullen JL, et al. Resting energy expenditure, body composition, and excess weight in the obese. Metabolism 1988; 37(5):467–472.
110. Schotland HM, Insko EK, Schwab RJ. Quantitative magnetic resonance imaging demonstrates alterations of the lingual musculature in obstructive sleep apnea. Sleep 1999; 22(5):605–613.
111. Stradling JR, Crosby JH. Predictors and prevalence of obstructive sleep apnoea and snoring in 1001 middle aged men. Thorax 1991; 46(2):85–90.
112. Stradling JR, Crosby JH, Payne CD. Self reported snoring and daytime sleepiness in men aged 35–65 years. Thorax 1991; 46(11):807–810.
113. Kimoff RJ, Sforza E, Champagne V, Ofiara L, Gendron D. Upper airway sensation in snoring and obstructive sleep apnea. Am J Respir Crit Care Med 2001; 164(2):250–255.
114. Boyd JH, Petrof BJ, Hamid Q, Fraser R, Kimoff RJ. Upper airway muscle inflammation and denervation changes in obstructive sleep apnea. Am J Respir Crit Care Med 2004; 170(5):541–546.
115. Petrof BJ, Pack AI, Kelly AM, Eby J, Hendricks JC. Pharyngeal myopathy of loaded upper airway in dogs with sleep apnea. J Appl Physiol 1994; 76(4):1746–1752.
116. Bixler EO, Vgontzas AN, Lin HM, et al. Prevalence of sleep-disordered breathing in women: effects of gender. Am J Respir Crit Care Med 2001; 163(3 Pt 1):608–613.
117. Brooks LJ, Strohl KP. Size and mechanical properties of the pharynx in healthy men and women. Am Rev Respir Dis 1992; 146(6):1394–1397.
118. Dancey DR, Hanly PJ, Soong C, Lee B, Shepard J, Jr, Hoffstein V. Gender differences in sleep apnea: the role of neck circumference. Chest 2003; 123(5):1544–1550.
119. Guilleminault C, Partinen M, Hollman K, Powell N, Stoohs R. Familial aggregates in obstructive sleep apnea syndrome. Chest 1995; 107(6):1545–1551.
120. Legato MJ. Gender-specific aspects of obesity. Int J Fertil Womens Med 1997; 42(3):184–197.
121. Millman RP, Carlisle CC, McGarvey ST, Eveloff SE, Levinson PD. Body fat distribution and sleep apnea severity in women. Chest 1995; 107(2):362–366.
122. Whittle AT, Marshall I, Mortimore IL, Wraith PK, Sellar RJ, Douglas NJ. Neck soft tissue and fat distribution: comparison between normal men and women by magnetic resonance imaging. Thorax 1999; 54(4):323–328.
123. Mohsenin V. Gender differences in the expression of sleep-disordered breathing: role of upper airway dimensions. Chest 2001; 120(5):1442–1447.
124. Rowley JA, Sanders CS, Zahn BR, Badr MS. Gender differences in upper airway compliance during NREM sleep: role of neck circumference. J Appl Physiol 2002; 92(6):2535–2541.
125. Guilleminault C, Quera-Salva MA, Partinen M, Jamieson A. Women and the obstructive sleep apnea syndrome. Chest 1988; 93(1):104–109.
126. Johnson MW, Anch AM, Remmers JE. Induction of the obstructive sleep apnea syndrome in a woman by exogenous androgen administration. Am Rev Respir Dis 1984; 129(6):1023–1025.
127. Palmer LJ, Redline S. Genomic approaches to understanding obstructive sleep apnea. Respir Physiol Neurobiol 2003; 135(2–3):187–205.
128. Redline S, Tishler PV, Tosteson TD, et al. The familial aggregation of obstructive sleep apnea. Am J Respir Crit Care Med 1995; 151(3 Pt 1):682–687.
129. Buxbaum SG, Elston RC, Tishler PV, Redline S. Genetics of the apnea hypopnea index in Caucasians and African Americans: I. Segregation analysis. Genet Epidemiol 2002; 22(3):243–253.
130. Palmer LJ, Buxbaum SG, Larkin E, et al. A whole-genome scan for obstructive sleep apnea and obesity. Am J Hum Genet 2003; 72(2):340–350.

131. Palmer LJ, Buxbaum SG, Larkin EK, et al. Whole genome scan for obstructive sleep apnea and obesity in African-American families. Am J Respir Crit Care Med 2004; 169(12):1314–1321.

132. Schwab RJ, Pasirstein M, Kaplan L, et al. Family aggregation of upper airway soft tissue structures in normal subjects and patients with sleep apnea. Am J Respir Crit Care Med 2006; 173(4):453–463.

133. Mathur R, Douglas NJ. Family studies in patients with the sleep apnea-hypopnea syndrome. Ann Intern Med 1995; 122(3):174–178.

134. Will MJ, Ester MS, Ramirez SG, Tiner BD, McAnear JT, Epstein L. Comparison of cephalometric analysis with ethnicity in obstructive sleep apnea syndrome. Sleep 1995; 18(10):873–875.

135. Lam B, Ip MS, Tench E, Ryan CF. Craniofacial profile in Asian and white subjects with obstructive sleep apnoea. Thorax 2005; 60(6):504–510.

136. Li KK, Kushida C, Powell NB, Riley RW, Guilleminault C. Obstructive sleep apnea syndrome: a comparison between Far-East Asian and white men. Laryngoscope 2000; 110(10 Pt 1):1689–1693.

137. Liu Y, Zeng X, Fu M, Huang X, Lowe AA. Effects of a mandibular repositioner on obstructive sleep apnea. Am J Orthod Dentofacial Orthop 2000; 118(3):248–256.

138. Trudo FJ, Gefter WB, Welch KC, Gupta KB, Maislin G, Schwab RJ. State-related changes in upper airway caliber and surrounding soft-tissue structures in normal subjects. Am J Respir Crit Care Med 1998; 158(4):1259–1270.

139. Burger CD, Stanson AW, Daniels BK, Sheedy PF, II, Shepard JW, Jr. Fast-computed tomographic evaluation of the effect of route of breathing on upper airway size and function in normal men. Chest 1993; 103(4):1032–1037.

140. Ritter CT, Trudo FJ, Goldberg AN, Welch KC, Maislin G, Schwab RJ. Quantitative evaluation of the upper airway during nasopharyngoscopy with the Muller maneuver. Laryngoscope 1999; 109(6):954–963.

141. Welch KC, Ritter CT, Gefter WB, et al. Dynamic respiratory related upper airway imaging during wakefulness in normal subjects and patients with sleep-disordered breathing using MRI. Am J Respir Crit Care Med 1998; 157:A54.

142. Sanders MH, Kern N. Obstructive sleep apnea treated by independently adjusted inspiratory and expiratory positive airway pressures via nasal mask. Physiologic and clinical implications. Chest 1990; 98(2):317–324.

143. Sanders MH, Moore SE. Inspiratory and expiratory partitioning of airway resistance during sleep in patients with sleep apnea. Am Rev Respir Dis 1983; 127(5):554–558.

144. Ritter CT, Trudo FJ, Goldberg AN, et al. Quantitative evaluation of the upper airway changes in normals and apneics during Muller maneuver. Am J Respir Crit Care Med 1998; 157:A54.

145. Smith PL, Gold AR, Meyers DA, Haponik EF, Bleecker ER. Weight loss in mildly to moderately obese patients with obstructive sleep apnea. Ann Intern Med 1985; 103(6 Pt 1):850–855.

146. Suratt PM, McTier RF, Findley LJ, Pohl SL, Wilhoit SC. Changes in breathing and the pharynx after weight loss in obstructive sleep apnea. Chest 1987; 92(4):631–637.

147. Loube DI, Loube AA, Mitler MM. Weight loss for obstructive sleep apnea: the optimal therapy for obese patients. J Am Diet Assoc 1994; 94(11):1291–1295.

148. Welch KC, Foster GD, Ritter CT, et al. A novel volumetric magnetic resonance imaging paradigm to study upper airway anatomy. Sleep 2002; 25(5):532–542.

149. Brown IB, McClean PA, Boucher R, Zamel N, Hoffstein V. Changes in pharyngeal cross-sectional area with posture and application of continuous positive airway pressure in patients with obstructive sleep apnea. Am Rev Respir Dis 1987; 136(3):628–632.

150. Collop NA, Block AJ, Hellard D. The effect of nightly nasal CPAP treatment on underlying obstructive sleep apnea and pharyngeal size. Chest 1991; 99(4):855–860.

151. Ferguson KA, Cartwright R, Rogers R, Schmidt-Nowara W. Oral appliances for snoring and obstructive sleep apnea: a review. Sleep 2006; 29(2):244–262.

152. Ferguson KA, Love LL, Ryan CF. Effect of mandibular and tongue protrusion on upper airway size during wakefulness. Am J Respir Crit Care Med 1997; 155(5):1748–1754.

153. Ishida M, Inoue Y, Suto Y, et al. Mechanism of action and therapeutic indication of prosthetic mandibular advancement in obstructive sleep apnea syndrome. Psychiatry Clin Neurosci 1998; 52(2):227–229.

154. Schmidt-Nowara WW, Meade TE, Hays MB. Treatment of snoring and obstructive sleep apnea with a dental orthosis. Chest 1991; 99(6):1378–1385.

155. Johal A, Battagel JM. An investigation into the changes in airway dimension and the efficacy of mandibular advancement appliances in subjects with obstructive sleep apnoea. Br J Orthod 1999; 26(3):205–210.

156. Liu Y, Park YC, Lowe AA, Fleetham JA. Supine cephalometric analyses of an adjustable oral appliance used in the treatment of obstructive sleep apnea. Sleep Breath 2000; 4(2):59–66.

157. Tsuiki S, Lowe AA, Almeida FR, Fleetham JA. Effects of an anteriorly titrated mandibular position on awake airway and obstructive sleep apnea severity. Am J Orthod Dentofacial Orthop 2004; 125(5):548–555.

158. Gale DJ, Sawyer RH, Woodcock A, Stone P, Thompson R, O'Brien K. Do oral appliances enlarge the airway in patients with obstructive sleep apnoea? A prospective computerized tomographic study. Eur J Orthod 2000; 22(2):159–168.

159. Cobo J, Canut JA, Carlos F, Vijande M, Llamas JM. Changes in the upper airway of patients who wear a modified functional appliance to treat obstructive sleep apnea. Int J Adult Orthodon Orthognath Surg 1995; 10(1):53–57.

160. Bonham PE, Currier GF, Orr WC, Othman J, Nanda RS. The effect of a modified functional appliance on obstructive sleep apnea. Am J Orthod Dentofacial Orthop 1988; 94(5):384–392.

161. Ryan CF, Love LL, Peat D, Fleetham JA, Lowe AA. Mandibular advancement oral appliance therapy for obstructive sleep apnoea: effect on awake calibre of the velopharynx. Thorax 1999; 54(11):972–977.

162. Sher AE. Upper airway surgery for obstructive sleep apnea. Sleep Med Rev 2002; 6(3):195–212.

163. Welch KC, Goldberg AN, Trudo FJ, et al. Upper anatomic changes with magnetic resonance imaging in uvulopalatopharyngoplasty patients. Am J Respir Crit Care Med 1997; 155:A938.

164. Sher AE, Schechtman KB, Piccirillo JF. The efficacy of surgical modifications of the upper airway in adults with obstructive sleep apnea syndrome. Sleep 1996; 19(2):156–177.

165. Li KK. Surgical therapy for obstructive sleep apnea syndrome. Semin Respir Crit Care Med 2005; 26(1):80–88.

166. Schirmer B, Watts SH. Laparoscopic bariatric surgery. Surg Endosc 2003; 17(12):1875–1878.

167. Verse T. Bariatric surgery for obstructive sleep apnea. Chest 2005; 128(2):485–487.

168. Dixon JB, Schachter LM, O'Brien PE. Polysomnography before and after weight loss in obese patients with severe sleep apnea. Int J Obes (Lond) 2005; 29(9):1048–1054.

5   Alertness and Sleepiness Assessment

Max Hirshkowitz
*Sleep Center, VA Medical Center and Departments of Medicine and Psychiatry,
Baylor College of Medicine, Houston, Texas, U.S.A.*

INTRODUCTION

Excessive sleepiness represents a major, albeit poorly recognized public safety and health problem (1). Countless motor vehicle and work-related accidents directly result from sleepiness. Sleepiness contributes to such accidents via inattention, response slowing, or unexpected lapses into sleep. Sleepiness is the normal physiological consequence of sleep loss, sleep disruption, or diminished sleep integrity. Sleepiness can also arise from central nervous system alterations produced by brain lesions, medications, or disease. Severe sleepiness is the hallmark symptom of several sleep disorders, including narcolepsy, obstructive sleep apnea, behaviorally induced insufficient sleep syndrome, and idiopathic hypersomnia with or without long sleep time (2). Excessive sleepiness may occur secondary to psychiatric, neurological, medical, and substance abuse conditions. Therefore, a careful evaluation of sleepiness is both clinically relevant and important. Results of such evaluation must be interpreted within the context of sleep schedule, napping, diet, comorbid illnesses, and concurrent medication.

As a hypothalamic physiologically motivated state, sleepiness may be viewed as an appetite. This appetite promotes a behavioral action designed to alleviate a "drive" state. Thus, in response to hunger we eat, in response to thirst we drink, and in response to sleepiness we sleep. Sleepiness, however, has an additional layer of complexity in as much as it is the net balance between physiological systems promoting sleep and other systems promoting wakefulness. The two-factor model, as proposed by Borbély (3) posits increasing sleepiness in response to sustained wakefulness (Factor S) and fluctuating sleepiness in response to an internal biological clock (Factor C). At least one current model views the circadian (C) factor as an alerting signal opposing the wakefulness-driven rising sleep load. The alerting signal is further countered by oscillating melatonin levels (that provide the brain an internal signal for darkness) but melatonin itself can be suppressed by bright light. These interwoven systems governing sleepiness and alertness are further complicated by autonomic nervous system (ANS) influences. ANS sympathetic activation can increase alertness and reduce sleepiness. Thus, sleepiness may be viewed as a composite of at least three (and maybe more) physiological systems. Consequently, it is easy to appreciate the difficulty encountered when attempts are made to measure it as a unitary phenomenon.

When we ask, "how sleepy are you?" are we asking (*i*) how do you feel? (*ii*) how quickly could you fall asleep? or (*iii*) how difficult would it be for you to remain awake? To better delineate issues, Carskadon and Dement (4) proposed characterizing sleepiness as introspective, physiological, and manifest. This approach provides a potentially useful framework for understanding measurement similarities and differences (Fig. 1). "Introspective sleepiness" indexes an individual's self-assessment of their internal state, or more simply, how they feel. By contrast,

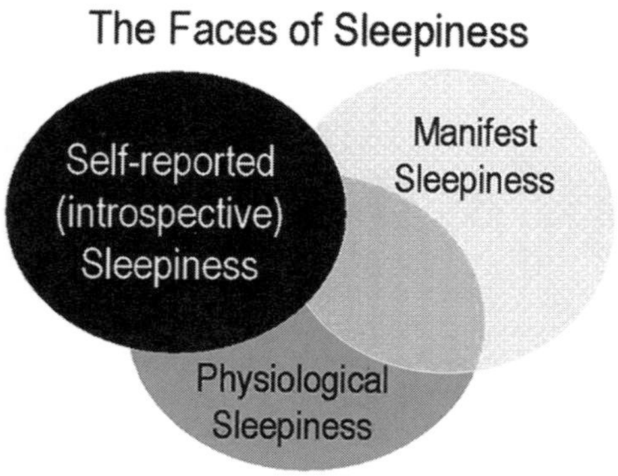

The Faces of Sleepiness

FIGURE 1 Venn diagram for introspective, physiological, and manifest sleepiness.

"physiological sleepiness" can be thought of as the underlying biologic drive to sleep indexed by the amount of time it takes to fall asleep, given the opportunity. Finally, "manifest sleepiness" reflects an individual's inability to volitionally remain awake. This state can be indexed by behavioral signs of sleepiness or sleep onset (eye closure, head bobbing, snoring) or by performance deficit on a wide variety of psychomotor and cognitive tasks. Although introspective, physiological, and manifest sleepiness levels may stem from a common source, tests assessing sleepiness in these different realms cannot be used interchangeably. Furthermore, attempts to use these measures interchangeably miss the importance of the differences between them.

At extreme ends of the spectrum, sleepiness measures may be concordant. That is, a male soldier who has remained awake continuously for 48 hours, when asked at 4:00 A.M. if he is sleepy will most likely respond affirmatively. If provided the opportunity to lie down on a comfortable bed in a dark, quiet room he would probably fall asleep rapidly (in 5 minutes, or less). Furthermore, if he sits down in a comfortable chair in a nonstimulating environment (a dark, quiet, and warm room), he may be unable to remain awake (unless provided strong coffee or other stimulants). In such a circumstance, introspective, physiological, and manifest sleepiness measures would all agree. Conversely, a woman on vacation who has caught up on her sleep to the point that she spontaneously awakens in the morning and feels alert all day will typically not fall asleep at 7:00 P.M., even if she lays down on a comfortable bed. Nor does she have any difficulty remaining awake sitting in a comfortable chair in a darkened, quiet environment. Thus, at this other end of the spectrum, there is a convergence in measures indicating full alertness.

It is the state in between full alertness and maximal sleepiness that provide a challenge for understanding test measurement. For example, if a couple has stayed up all night (24 hours) and is watching the sunrise at 7:00 A.M. they may not feel sleepy. However, 2.5 hours ago at 4:30 A.M., they could barely rally enough to stay awake, but that feeling of overwhelming sleepiness has dissipated. Nonetheless, if given the opportunity to lie down in a comfortable bed in a dark and quiet room, they would fall asleep instantly (unless they have been drinking coffee all night or taking stimulants). Depending on their individual ability to maintain alertness, they may be able to stay awake for more than 20 minutes if seated in a dark and quiet room. Thus, the introspective and manifest measures of sleepiness are negative, while the physiological measure is positive. Furthermore, even though they are now awake longer, 2.5 hours ago, introspective and physiological measures were positive but manifest sleepiness level was not. This illustrates the importance of understanding the differences between measurements and not generalizing results from one to another.

INTROSPECTIVE SLEEPINESS
Overview
There is an assortment of instruments available to assess introspective sleepiness (Table 1). These questionnaires are all self-administered and request the individual either to make a prediction about their behavior, estimate what they have done in the recent past, or to assess how they feel "right now" with respect to one or another descriptor. The instruments asking for self-report "right now" fall into a general category of testing called "momentary assessment." Such instruments are sensitive to oscillation occurring over the course of a day and can be extremely useful in scientific investigations. By contrast, assessment of how one felt during "the past month" provide more global estimates that may be more useful clinically.

Introspective sleepiness evaluation instruments rely on self-report. Thus, all of the advantages and disadvantages inherent in self-reported information apply. In one sense, when it comes to rating how sleepy someone is, there is no one in a better position to have knowledge than the person in question. Furthermore, when it comes to indicating how one feels, the person is the only one who can render an accurate judgment. However, the resultant index is inherently subjective. Sleepiness reduces self-awareness and has been shown to interfere with the ability to accurately judge internal states (i.e., it produces alexithymia). Self-reported sleepiness tends to follow an adaptation curve such that high levels over a long duration may regress toward the mean. This may be related to a resetting of an individual's reference point over time, develop from memory impairment, or both. Moreover, some individuals are minimizers or may even be in denial. They will report low values for everything, including sleepiness. By contrast, others are augmenters and generally provide high scores and extreme values, regardless of the specifics in question. Finally, responses are directly controlled by the individuals. If they have an agenda, they can further that agenda. For example, if an individual wants his motor vehicle driver license reinstated, he is unlikely to affirm excessive sleepiness when asked.

Epworth Sleepiness Scale
Clinically, the most widely used test for sleepiness is probably the Epworth sleepiness scale (ESS). The popularity of ESS stems in part from its brevity. This, in conjunction with open access for use, its simplicity, and validation studies, has cemented its place in the clinical arena. Developed by Murray Johns (5) at the Epworth Hospital in Melbourne, Australia, the ESS is an eight-item, validated questionnaire asking for a self-reported expectation of "dozing" in different situations. The response set for chance of dozing is: (0) none, (1) slight, (2) moderate, or (3) high. The situations asked about on ESS are: (1) sitting and reading, (2) watching television, (3) sitting and inactive in a public place (e.g., a theater or a meeting), (4) as a passenger in a car

TABLE 1 Instruments Used to Assess Introspective Sleepiness

Test name	Abbreviation	Creator
Epworth sleepiness scale	ESS	Johns
Stanford sleepiness scale	SSS	Hoddes et al.
Karolinska sleepiness scale	KSS	Akerstedt
Pictorial sleepiness scale	PSS	Maldonado
Profile of mood states	POMS	McNair
Visual analog scales	VAS	Assorted versions
Side effect checklists	SEC	Assorted versions

for an hour without a break, (5) lying down to rest in the afternoon when circumstances permit, (6) sitting and talking to someone, (7) sitting quietly after a lunch without alcohol, and (8) in a car, while stopped for a few minutes in traffic. Johns conducted reliability and validity studies on patients with sleep apnea and medical student control subjects (6). In Johns' study, student control subjects had a mean ESS total score of 7.6. Adult respondents in our hospital (942 patients waiting at outpatient dermatology, audiology, and ophthalmology clinics) had a mean ESS of 8.1 compared to a mean of 5.2 found from 1120 healthy people attending health fairs or community health lectures (7). Based on these data, we categorize ESS score 0 to 8 as normal, 9 to 12 as mild, 13 to 16 as moderate, and greater than 16 as severe. ESS is a popular treatment outcome measure for assessing the benefit of positive airway pressure for treating sleep apnea (8), and an ESS score above 10 is often used to indicate significant sleepiness.

Stanford Sleepiness Scale

The Stanford sleepiness scale (SSS) is a momentary assessment scale developed by Hoddes et al. (9) in the early 1970s. It is very brief and easy to use. It can be administered repeatedly at short intervals (e.g., hourly) and is sensitive to sleepiness as it waxes and wanes over the course of a day in response to circadian factors. It is also responsive to sleep deprivation; however, normative data do not exist. For many years, SSS was the standard measure of introspective sleepiness. It produces a single score chosen by the individual to reflect or best describe how they feel. Choices are: (1) feeling active and vital, alert, wide awake, (2) functioning at a high level but not at peak; able to concentrate, (3) relaxed, awake, responsive, not at full alertness, (4) a little foggy, not at peak; let down, (5) fogginess, beginning to lose interest in remaining awake; slowed down, (6) sleepiness, prefer to be lying down, fighting sleep, woozy, and (7) almost in a reverie, sleep onset soon, lost struggle to remain awake.

Karolinska Sleepiness Scale

The Karolinska sleepiness scale (KSS) has been gaining popularity for use in research studies over the past five years. It consists of a nine-point scale that ranges from (1) very alert to (9) very sleepy, great effort to stay awake or fighting sleep. Any score of 7 or above is considered pathological. The KSS has been used to assess sleepiness in drug trials, and in aircrews, oil-rig workers, train engineers, and professional drivers. Its brevity combined with now proven sensitivity to expected changes is bringing KSS onto equal footing with the SSS. Furthermore, KSS has been validated against electrophysiologic (EEG) and behavioral parameters (10).

Pictorial Sleepiness Scale

Maldonado et al. (11) sought to develop a nonverbal sleepiness scale that could be used to test young children or poorly educated adults. Subject groups were asked to rank in order seven cartoon faces designed to depict different sleepiness levels. Results were used to transform rankings into linear measures that eliminated two faces. A new subject group ranked the remaining five cartoons and a scale was constructed. The scale correlated significantly with KSS and SSS when tested in groups of normal control adults, sleep apnea patients, shift workers, and school children. The authors envision using this scale clinically and for research. It remains to be seen whether this scale will gain popularity.

Profile of Mood States

As the name implies, the profile of mood states (POMS) was originally designed to assess mood (12). However, over the years POMS gained significant popularity among sleep researchers. Ironically, early versions of the test included a dimension for sleepiness that was eliminated as part of psychometric test purification (because it was not an independent factor). Sleepiness loads several subscales, including Vigor (negative), Confusion, and Fatigue. The Confusion scale appears to be responsive to severe sleepiness while the Vigor scale may be more responsive to partial sleep deprivation (13). Similarly, subscales of the Medical Outcomes Study Short Form-36 (SF-36) have been used to assess sleepiness, particularly in drug trials.

Visual Analog Scales and Side Effect Checklists

Any number of visual analog scales and side effect checklists are available to assess sleepiness (Fig. 2). These tests are popular because of their simplicity, ease of administration, and face validity. Formal validation studies have not been conducted on these tests. However, these types of tests are generally sensitive to changes within an individual in response to an intervention. For example, sleepiness reliably increases in response to sleep deprivation and decreases in response to stimulant administration. Nonetheless, absolute values of the scores are difficult to compare meaningfully across subjects. This limits these tests' utility for clinical purposes.

PHYSIOLOGICAL SLEEPINESS
Overview

The three most common methods for indexing physiological sleepiness use: (*i*) the multiple sleep latency test (MSLT), (*ii*) pupillometry, and (*iii*) quantitative electroencephalography (EEG) analysis. Measuring sleepiness using physiological indices provides the clinician an objective technique that does not have the disadvantages inherently associated with self-report. Falling asleep represents an involuntary process. Therefore, appraising the biological substrate either during this process or under conditions conducive to falling asleep can minimize psychological, psychiatric, and intentional confounds. However, one should be aware that the results derived from such testing are not necessarily above manipulation by a test subject. In as much as the test procedure relies on cooperation, there is room for intentional alteration, within limits. For example, individuals attempting to prove they are not sleepy may engage in a mental arithmetic task when asked to close their eyes and relax during an

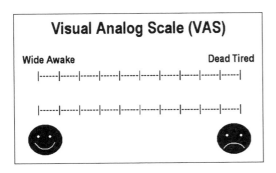

FIGURE 2 Example of a visual analog scale.

EEG baseline sample. Physiological measures may be more reliable for demonstrating sleepiness than proving alertness (i.e., if a positive test is one that affirms sleepiness, physiological tests are more prone to false negative than false positive results).

Multiple Sleep Latency Test

MSLT provides a direct, objective, quantitative measure indexing sleepiness. It is generally thought that nonsleepy individuals cannot make themselves fall asleep. Thus, if a positive MSLT is one that indicates sleepiness, then false-positive test liability is minimal. The MSLT consists of a series of nap opportunities (4–6) presented across the day. The series begins approximately two hours after the morning awaking from an in-laboratory polysomnographic study and continues with successive trials at two-hour intervals (14). Testing includes polysomnographic sleep monitoring during the nap opportunities. Recordings include: (1) left or right central EEG (C3 or C4), (2) left or right occipital EEG (O1 or O2), (3) left horizontal or oblique electrooculogram (EOG), (4) right horizontal or oblique EOG, (5) sub-mentalis (chin) electromyogram (EMG), (6) electrocardiogram (ECG), (7) respiratory flow (if needed), and (8) respiratory sounds (if needed). Subjects may not remain in bed between test sessions and should wear normal street clothing. Rooms must be dark and quiet during nap opportunities. Two MSLT protocols have evolved, one for clinical use and one for research. In the clinical protocol, a subject that falls asleep on a nap opportunity is allowed an additional 15 minutes of sleep to see whether rapid eye movement (REM) sleep occurs. The presence of REM sleep on two or more naps is used to confirm narcolepsy. In the research protocol, sleep accumulation is minimized. The test session is terminated when either (*i*) unequivocal sleep occurs (one epoch of stage 2, 3, 4, or REM) or (*ii*) three successive epochs of stage 1 sleep occur. In both clinical or research protocols, the nap opportunity is terminated after 20 minutes if sleep onset fails to occur. At the beginning of each nap opportunity, the subject is instructed to "let yourself fall asleep" or "do not resist falling asleep." The speed with which an individual falls asleep (defined by polysomnographic criteria) is used to index the level of sleepiness. Changes in sleep latency associated with age, circadian factors, sleep deprivation, sleep extension, and sleep disorders have been described (15–18). The MSLT provides a sensitive index for evaluating response to treatment and is a favorite outcome measure in drug trials (19–21) and other treatment outcome studies (8). Therefore, the MSLT should not be conducted after a night of profoundly disturbed sleep, during drug withdrawal, or while a patient is under the influence of sedating medication. The American Academy of Sleep Medicine (AASM) Standards of Practice Committee published new practice parameters for the clinical use of MSLT (22). Recommendations were based on a comprehensive evidence-based medicine literature review; however, expert consensus was used to bridge areas where data were insufficient (23). Recommendations are summarized in Table 2.

Pupillometry

In a dark room, an individual's pupils dilate in order to allow more light to enter the eye. This process is part of dark adaptation. However, when a person is sleepy and begins to fall asleep, the pupils constrict in response to the ANS increasing parasympathetic tone associated with sleep. Thus, recording changes in pupil size can physiologically index sleep tendency (24,25). Thus, a wide-awake individual's pupils will dilate and remain dilated over time in a dark room. By contrast, an individual with

TABLE 2 Summary of American Academy of Sleep Medicine Standards of Practice Committee Recommendations for Clinical Use of the Multiple Sleep Latency Test

---

The MSLT is indicated as part of the clinical evaluation for patients with suspected narcolepsy (two or more SOREMPs has a 0.78 sensitivity and a 0.93 specificity for diagnosing narcolepsy).
The MSLT may be helpful for clinical assessment of patients with suspected idiopathic hypersomnia.
The MSLT is not indicated for routine evaluation of obstructive sleep apnea, insomnia, circadian rhythm disorders, or dyssomnia associated with medical, psychiatric, or neurological disorders (other than narcolepsy and idiopathic hypersomnia).
The MSLT is not indicated for routine re-evaluation of patients with sleep apnea treated with positive airway pressure therapy.
Repeat MSLT may be indicated when:
  Study conditions were inappropriate during initial testing
  Results are ambiguous
  Earlier MSLT did not confirm narcolepsy.

Abbreviations: MSLT, multiple sleep latency test; SOREMP, sleep-onset REM period.

excessive sleepiness will not maintain pupil dilation as he or she drifts from alertness to drowsiness to sleep. Pupillometry provides an objective method for recording changes in the pupil and has been used to study narcolepsy (26). Pupillometry has also been correlated with MSLT and SSS indices (27). Changes occurring within subjects are sensitive and reliable; however, comparisons across subjects can be difficult. Additionally, normative data are not available.

Quantitative Electroencephalographic Analysis

It would seem obvious that the EEG should change as sleepiness increases. With widely available computerized waveform analysis one would expect there to be a recognizable marker in brain activity. EEG delta activity seems a strong candidate and was found to increase in response to sleep deprivation (28). Other EEG markers have also been reported (29). It is also classic knowledge that EEG alpha disappears at sleep onset (first noted by Hans Berger almost 100 years ago). Furthermore, just before alpha activity disappears, its frequency decreases and its amplitude increases. Santamaria and Chiappa (30) filled an entire book with illustrations of the EEG of drowsiness. Nonetheless, the interlocking piece reliably connecting EEG and sleepiness has been elusive. Even simple observation by a trained observer remains more sensitive than the most sophisticated measures for predicting sleepiness (31) and sleepiness-related performance deficits (32).

MANIFEST SLEEPINESS
Overview

Measurements of manifest sleepiness are actually designed to index the point at which alertness fails. An individual may be very sleepy but nonetheless can maintain wakefulness. However, at some point, even the most heroic attempts to stay awake are to no avail and it is at this point the individual lapses into sleep. There is usually some response slowing and lapsing even before frank sleep onset occurs. For many years the notion of "functional deafferentation" was considered; however, most data point toward inattention and slowing of information processing. Another controversial issue involves the concept of microsleep (brief sleep episodes lasting 5–15 seconds).

Industrial psychology and human factors research attempting to design better man–machine interfaces (ergonomics) avoided issues surrounding microsleep because an equipment operator's performance cannot be improved by rearranging a panel's switches, keyboards, and indicator lights if he or she has fallen asleep. Another issue concerning microsleep involves the locus of its generation. Attempts to externalize the cause of microsleep have led to blaming rural motor vehicle accidents on things such as "highway hypnosis." The problem, however, is internal. The driver is sleepy and when sleepiness reaches a threshold that exceeds the alertness system's ability to offset, manifest sleepiness occurs and sleep onset soon follows.

Observation and Observer Scales

Yawning has long been a traditional sign of sleepiness. Simple observation of eyelid closure, wandering direction of gaze, and eyes rolling upward are among the strongest indicators of sleepiness. Head nodding with eyes closed strongly suggests sleep onset. These observable events testify to manifest sleepiness. Some of the earliest attempts to index sleepiness involved the development of observer scales, one of which was used to grade individuals undergoing prolonged sleep deprivation. Studies conducted at Walter Reed Hospital in the 1960s employed the "Cognitive Disorganization Scale" (33). This five-point observer rating scale ranges from (1) slowing of mental processes, some difficulty thinking of words (no undue interference with normal communication) all the way to (5) rambling incoherent speech for brief periods, with failure to recognize errors, unable to straighten out jumble of incoherent thoughts when challenged.

Maintenance of Wakefulness Test

The maintenance of wakefulness test (MWT) is procedurally similar to the MSLT. The major differences are: (*i*) the person being tested is told to "attempt to remain awake" at the beginning of each test session, (*ii*) the individual is seated rather than laying down in bed, (*iii*) each test session is 40 minutes in duration, and (*iv*) polysomnography the night before testing is not required. Thus, the MWT is used to assess an individual's capability to not be overwhelmed by sleepiness. In a sense, this test is gauging the strength of the wakefulness system (34). If the wakefulness system fails, sleepiness becomes manifest. In the MWT there is no other task than remaining awake and concurrent EEG–EOG–EMG monitoring is conducted to verify success or failure (35,36). In some ways the MWT is a simulation of sedentary inactivity in a nonstimulating environment. Like the MSLT, there are four to six sessions, scheduled at two-hour intervals beginning approximately two hours after awakening from the previous night's sleep. Until standardization at 40 minutes recommended by the AASM Standards of Practice Committee, individual test session durations on the MWT varied from 20 to 60 minutes in different studies. The MWT has proven useful as an outcome measure in clinical trials (37) and is recognized for evaluating noncommercial pilot relicensing after sleep apnea treatment (38). Practice guidelines for MWT were developed along with those for the MSLT. MWT testing is indicated for evaluating individuals whose inability to remain alert constitutes a safety hazard. MWT testing is also recommended to determine treatment response in patients with narcolepsy (or idiopathic hypersomnia). The practice parameter emphasizes the critical importance of clinical judgment and stresses the fact that normal MWT values do not guarantee safety. Recommendations are summarized in Table 3.

TABLE 3 Summary of American Academy of Sleep Medicine Standards of Practice Committee Recommendations for Clinical Use of the Maintenance of Wakefulness Test

The 40-minute MWT protocol should be used.
MWT is indicated for assessing an individual's ability to remain awake when sleepiness constitutes a public or personal safety issue.
MWT may be used to assess response to treatment.
On a 40-minute MWT, 59% of normal subjects remain awake the entire time across all four trials.
On the 40-minute MWT
A sleep latency less than eight minutes is abnormal
A sleep latency between 8 and 40 minutes is of unknown significance
The mean ($\pm$ SD) sleep latency is 30.4 ($\pm$ 11.2)
The upper 95% confidence interval is 40 minutes.

Abbreviation: MWT, maintenance of wakefulness test.

Vigilance and Performance Tests

Impaired vigilance and performance decrements accompany sleepiness and an increase in response to sleep deprivation. Inattention, cognitive slowing, and lapses represent manifestations of sleepiness. Experimenter-paced, monotonous, time-keeping tasks with low target presentation rates generally fall into the category of "vigilance tests." Tests with higher throughput and greater intrinsic stimulation are classed as "performance tests." Vigilance tests do not require much skill, are less sensitive to educational level, and have little in the way of learning curves compared to performance tests. Landmark studies of sleep deprivation pioneered the use of vigilance and performance testing to assess sleepiness (39,40). These studies are collectively known as the Walter Reed experiments because they were conducted at Walter Reed Army Hospital. Results indicated that time-on-task, response slowing, and response lapsing were essential factors in sustained attention tasks [for an excellent review, see Dinges and Kribbs (41)]. Several vigilance and performance tests are in standard use in sleepiness research (42–44). Perhaps, the most popular is the psychomotor vigilance test (PVT) developed by David Dinges et al. at the University of Pennsylvania (45,46). This hand-held device measures response speed and accuracy in a signal detection algorithm. The PVT has been cross-validated with the SSS and MSLT and data are reported from normal controls, sleep-deprived individuals, and sleep disorder patient groups. Another test system that has been used in several studies is the Oxford sleep resistance (OSLER) test (47,48). The OSLER test consists of four 40-minute-long trials during which there are multiple signal presentations. The subject is instructed to respond to each signal with a simple button press. Trials are ended after 40 minutes or after a failure to respond (which is thought to indicate sleep onset).

CONCLUSIONS

Sleepiness is a cardinal symptom for some sleep disorders. Consequently, assessing sleepiness and alertness is a crucial part of a clinical evaluation. There is an assortment of techniques available to measure sleepiness. Sleepiness, however, represents an interaction of physiological systems that increase sleep tendency and other systems opposing sleep drive. These complementary factors provide a dynamic equilibrium that oscillates over the course of a day depending on homeostatic sleep debt and circadian phase. Furthermore, the internal state individuals interpret as indicating sleepiness can be influenced by other factors. The net result is that different measures may not correlate well with one another in some individuals. Understanding the differences between introspective, physiological, and manifest sleepiness metrics is useful to interpret results. The ESS is a widely used self-report instrument in general clinical practice. By contrast, the MWT is a recommended objective evaluation technique when personal and public safety concerns arise. This test measures the ability to sustain wakefulness in a soporific environment. Recommendations for the use of the MSLT and the MWT are summarized in this chapter. Unfortunately, no simple blood test or assay is available for indexing sleepiness. The difficulty in measuring sleepiness poses a significant challenge in the regulatory arena. Nonetheless, sleepiness is a serious, noncommunicable, potentially life-threatening condition.

REFERENCES

1. National Commission on Sleep Disorders Research: Wake up America: A national sleep alert. Executive Summary and Executive Report, Report of the National Commission on Sleep Disorders Research. Washington, DC, National Institutes of Health, U.S. Government Printing Office, 1993; 1:45.
2. American Academy of Sleep Medicine. The International Classification of Sleep Disorders, revised: diagnostic and coding manual. 2nd ed. Rochester: American Academy of Sleep Medicine, 2004.
3. Borbély AA, Achermann P. Concepts and models of sleep regulation: an overview. J Sleep Res 1992; 1:63.
4. Carskadon MA, Dement WC. The multiple sleep latency test: what does it measure? Sleep 1982; 5:S67–S72.
5. Johns MW. A new method for measuring daytime sleepiness: the Epworth Sleepiness Scale. Sleep 1991; 14:540–545.
6. Johns MW. Reliability and factor analysis of the Epworth Sleepiness Scale. Sleep 1992; 15:376–381.
7. Sharafkhaneh A, Hirshkowitz M. Contextual factors and perceived self-reported sleepiness: a preliminary report. Sleep Med 2003; 4:327–331.
8. Patel SR, White DP, Malhotra A, Stanchina ML, Ayas NT. Continuous positive airway pressure therapy for treating sleepiness in a diverse population with obstructive sleep apnea: results of a meta-analysis. Arch Intern Med 2003; 163(5):565–571.
9. Hoddes E, Zarcone V, Smythe H, et al. Quantification of sleepiness: a new approach. Psychophysiology 1973; 10:431–436.
10. Kaida K, Takahashi M, Akerstedt T, et al. Validation of the Karolinska sleepiness scale against performance and EEG variables. Clin Neurophysiol 2006; 117(7):1574–1581.
11. Maldonado CC, Bentley AJ, Mitchell D. A pictorial sleepiness scale based on cartoon faces. Sleep 2004; 27(3):541–548.
12. McNair DM, Lorr M, Droppleman LF. Manual of the Profile of Mood States. San Diego, California: Educational and Industrial Testing Service, 1992.
13. Horne J. Dimensions to sleepiness. In: Monk TM, ed. Sleep, Sleepiness and Performance. Chichester, England: John Wiley, 1991:169–196.
14. Carskadon MA, Dement WC, Mitler MM, et al. Guidelines for the multiple sleep latency test (MSLT): a standard measure of sleepiness. Sleep 1986; 9:519–524.
15. Carskadon MA, Dement WC. Cumulative effects of sleep restriction on daytime sleepiness. Psychophysiology 1981; 18:107–113.
16. Carskadon MA, Dement WC. Daytime sleepiness: quantification of behavioral state. Neurosci Biobehav Rev 1987; 11:307–317.
17. Mitler MM, Nelson S, Hajdukovic R. Narcolepsy: diagnosis, treatment, and management. Psychiatr Clin North Am 1987; 10:593–606.
18. Richardson GS, Carskadon MA, Orav EJ, et al. Circadian variation in sleep tendency in elderly and young adult subjects. Sleep 1982; 5:S82–S94.
19. Lamphere J, Roehrs T, Wittig R, et al. Recovery of alertness after CPAP in apnea. Chest 1989; 96:1364–1367.

20. U.S. Narcolepsy Study Group (USMNSG). Randomized trial of for the treatment of pathological somnolence in narcolepsy. Ann Neurol 1998; 43:88–97.
21. Zorick F, Roehrs T, Conway W, et al. Effects of uvulopalatopharyngoplasty on the daytime sleepiness associated with sleep apnea syndrome. Bull Eur Physiopathol Respir 1983; 19:600–603.
22. Standards of Practice Committee of the American Academy of Sleep Medicine. Practice parameters for clinical use of the multiple sleep latency test and the maintenance of wakefulness test. Sleep 2005; 28:113–121.
23. A Review by the MSLT and MWT Task Force of the Standards of Practice Committee of the American Academy of Sleep Medicine. The clinical use of the MSLT and MWT. Sleep 2005; 28:123–144.
24. Schmidt HS, Fortin L. Electronic pupillography in disorders of arousal. In: Guilleminault C, ed. Sleeping and Waking Disorders: Indications and Techniques. Menlo Park, California: Addison-Wesley, 1982:127–143.
25. Morad Y, Lemberg H, Yofe N, Dagan Y. Pupillography as an objective indicator of fatigue. Curr Eye Res 2000; 21:535–542.
26. Yoss RE, Moyer NJ, Ogle KN. The pupillogram and narcolepsy: a method to measure decreased levels of wakefulness. Neurology 1969; 19:921–928.
27. Danker-Hopfe H, Kraemer S, Dorn H, et al. Time-of-day variations in different measures of sleepiness (MSLT, pupillography, and SSS) and their interrelations. Psychophysiology 2001; 38:828–835.
28. Borbely AA, Baumann F, Brandeis D, et al. Sleep deprivation: effect on sleep stages and EEG power density in man. Electroencephalogr Clin Neurophysiol 1981; 51:483–493.
29. Hasan J, Hirvonen K, Varri A, et al. Validation of computer analyzed polygraphic patterns during drowsiness and sleep onset. Electroencephalogr Clin Neurophysiol 1993; 87:117–127.
30. Santamaria J, Chiappa KH. The EEG of Drowsiness. New York: Demos, 1987.
31. Mitler MM, Miller JC, Lipsitz JJ, et al. The sleep of long-haul truck drivers. N Engl J Med 1997; 337:755–761.
32. Dinges DF, Mallis MM. Managing fatigue by drowsiness detection: can technological promises be realized? Third International Conference on Fatigue in Transportation: Coping with the 24-Hour Society. Fremantle, Western Australia, February 9–13, 1998.
33. Morris GO, Williams HL, Lubin A. Misperception and disorientation during sleep deprivation. Arch Gen Psychiat 1960; 2:247–254.
34. Sangal RB, Thomas L, Mitler MM. Disorders of excessive sleepiness: treatment improves ability to stay awake but does not reduce sleepiness. Chest 1992; 102:699–703.
35. Doghramji K, Mitler MM, Sangal RB, et al. A normative study of the Maintenance of Wakefulness Test (MWT). Electroencephalogr Clin Neurophysiol 1997; 103:554–562.
36. Mitler MM, Miller JC. Methods of testing for sleepiness. Behav Med 1996; 21:171–183.
37. Mitler MM, Gujavarty KS, Browman CP. Maintenance of wakefulness test: a polysomnographic technique for evaluation of treatment efficacy in patients with excessive somnolence. Electroencephalogr Clin Neurophysiol 1982; 53:658–661.
38. Federal Aviation Administration (FAA). Sleep Apnea Evaluation Specifications. Federal Aviation Administration specification letter dated October 6, 1992. U.S. Department of Transportation, 1992.
39. Lubin A. Performance under sleep loss and fatigue. In: Kety SS, Evarts EV, Williams HL, eds. Sleep and Altered States of Consciousness. Baltimore, MD: Williams and Wilkins; 1967:506–513.
40. Williams HL, Lubin A, Goodnow JJ. Impaired performance and acute sleep loss. Psychol Monogr 1959; 73(Pt 14):1–26.
41. Dinges DF, Kribbs NB. Performing while sleepy: effects of experimentally induced sleepiness. In: Monk TM, ed. Sleep, Sleepiness and Performance. Chichester, England: John Wiley, 1991:97–128.
42. Wilkinson RT. Sleep deprivation: performance tests for partial and selective sleep deprivation. In: Abt LA, Reiss BF, eds. Progress in Clinical Psychology. Vol. 3. London: Grune & Stratton, 1968:28–43.
43. Hirshkowitz M, De La Cueva L, Herman JH. The multiple vigilance test. Behav Res Methods Instrum Comput 1993; 25:272–275.

44. Findley L, Unverzagt M, Guchu R, et al. Vigilance and auto-mobile accidents in patients with sleep apnea or narcolepsy. Chest 1995; 108:619–624.
45. Kribbs NB, Pack AI, Kline LR, et al. Effects of one night without nasal CPAP treatment on sleep and sleepiness in patients with obstructive sleep apnea. Am Rev Respir Dis 1993; 147:1162–1168.
46. Doran SM, Van Dongen HP, Dinges DF. Sustained attention performance during sleep deprivation: evidence of state instability. Arch Ital Biol 2001; 139:253–267.
47. Bennett LS, Stradling JR, Davies RJ. A behavioural test to assess daytime sleepiness in obstructive sleep apnoea. J Sleep Res 1997; 6:142–145.
48. Priest B, Brichard C, Aubert G, et al. Microsleep during a simplified maintenance of wakefulness test: a validation study of the OSLER test. Am J Respir Crit Care Med 2001; 163:1619–1625.

Continuous Positive Airway Pressure

Peter R. Buchanan and Ronald R. Grunstein
*Royal Prince Alfred Hospital, Woolcock Institute of Medical Research and
The University of Sydney, Sydney, Australia*

INTRODUCTION

Continuous positive airway pressure (CPAP), usually nasally applied, is the established treatment for moderate-to-severe obstructive sleep apnea (OSA) (1). Nasal CPAP therapy for sleep apnea was first described in 1981 (2). Although there was initial skepticism of its efficacy and concern regarding its potential adverse effects on breathing (3,4), there was also early recognition of the importance of having a treatment that could essentially prevent disordered breathing during sleep in OSA patients. This is in contrast to the efficacy of other alternatives available, including partial or variable response to surgery (5). By 1985, more than 100 patients were using this therapy on a regular basis (6). Over the past 20 years, the evidence base supporting the use of CPAP has improved both in quantity and quality, driven at least in part by the demands of government funding authorities and health maintenance organizations and the availability of industry sponsorship with the increasing commercial success of companies selling CPAP equipment (7).

There are methodological problems designing studies to assess and validate a mechanical device such as CPAP, compared with those required for medications. Performing true double-blind randomized controlled trials (RCTs) of CPAP treatment or variants are technically and logistically difficult. "Sham CPAP" by its nature will have less efficacy on unavoidably observable variables such as snoring or apnea with consequent difficulties to truly "blind" study participants. Due to the requisite modification to the equipment, it is also quite difficult to effectively blind a CPAP therapist or doctor involved in such studies compared with pharmaceutical trials involving placebo medications. Also the advent of automatically titrating CPAP devices (see Chapter 8) has major implications for the delivery of healthcare to patients with sleep apnea and for the traditional sleep laboratory–patient relationship.

CPAP is currently the "gold standard" treatment for moderate-to-severe OSA because of its demonstrated efficacy. Even so, many patients do not use it, or use it irregularly, reducing the delivered effectiveness of the therapy. Comparative, double-blind intention-to-treat trials in all degrees of OSA severity are needed to delineate treatment pathways in this condition. Currently, studies focusing on comparative treatments and ways in which there are better effectiveness of CPAP, including timely and economical initiation of therapy, are forming the next phase in the historical development of this treatment modality. Although there are tremendous interest and active research in potential pharmacotherapy for OSA, the absence of any currently available viable pharmacological therapy for sleep apnea (8–10) suggests that CPAP will remain the appropriate therapy standard in the foreseeable future for OSA of more than mild degree.

CONTINUOUS POSITIVE AIRWAY PRESSURE
Mode of Action

The concept of CPAP in managing respiratory failure is relatively old (11). However, the original experiments using CPAP in sleep apnea followed from the notion that closure of the oropharynx in OSA results from an imbalance of the forces (12) that normally keep the upper airway open. In the first description of CPAP use for treatment of OSA in 1981 (2), it was suggested that nasal CPAP acts as a pneumatic splint to prevent collapse of the pharyngeal airway, by elevating the pressure in the oropharyngeal airway and reversing the transmural pressure gradient across the pharyngeal airway (Fig. 1). This notion has been subsequently confirmed by a number of studies which either demonstrate the "pneumatic splint" effect by endoscopic or other imaging, or show that CPAP does not increase upper airway muscle activity by reflex mechanisms (13). Detailed magnetic resonance imaging has confirmed that CPAP increases airway volume and airway area, and reduces lateral pharyngeal wall thickness and upper airway edema secondary to chronic vibration and occlusion of the airway (14). The apparatus providing the pressure at the nasal

WAKE

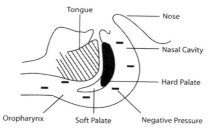

SLEEP

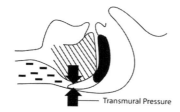

SLEEP + CPAP

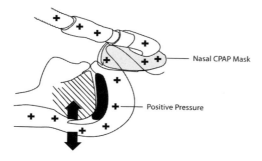

FIGURE 1 Mechanism of upper airway occlusion in obstructive sleep apnea and its prevention by continuous positive airway pressure: "pneumatic splint" effect. *Source*: From Ref. 2.

airway must have the "capacity" to maintain any given pressure during inspiration. Early embodiments of the technology failed to respond rapidly to the airflow challenge at early inspiration, with an attendant pressure drop and consequently requiring a higher "set" pressure to compensate for such drops. The simplest CPAP systems involve an air blower with sufficient pressure-flow characteristics to provide CPAP while also accommodating both a fixed resistive leak in the system (typically adjacent to the mask) as well as unintentional leaks at the patient/delivery interface (Fig. 2). Such contemporary devices are generally microprocessor-controlled in order to meet rapid changes in the flow demands presented by the patient as well as the dynamics of variable leak often seen in clinical use of CPAP.

Continuous Positive Airway Pressure and Central Apnea

Regardless of the mechanism, nasal CPAP has been documented to be effective in eliminating both mixed and obstructive apneas (15). Some central apneas (see Chapter 19), particularly those observed in patients with predominantly obstructive events, are also eliminated by nasal CPAP (15). Clearly, some central apneas are associated with increased upper airway resistance and it could be argued that it is better to consider apnea classification as being CPAP responsive or CPAP nonresponsive. CPAP may also be effective in controlling central apneas associated with cardiac failure (see section: Continuous Positive Airway Pressure and Cardiac Failure). In some instances, CPAP alone will not control severe mixed central and obstructive apneas and adjunctive entrainment of low concentrations of carbon dioxide, with CPAP, or the use of other noninvasive ventilatory techniques, may further reduce the respiratory disturbance index (RDI) in such individuals (16).

PRACTICAL ASPECTS OF TREATMENT

Originally, most patients commenced CPAP under supervision, usually in a hospital-based sleep laboratory. The purposes of this supervision included ensuring that the patient was appropriately educated about the therapy, to select the best interface (mask) for the individual, and determine the adequacy of CPAP across the night. Such observation also allowed an evaluation of the immediate acceptance of or problems with the therapy. Economic pressures within health systems however

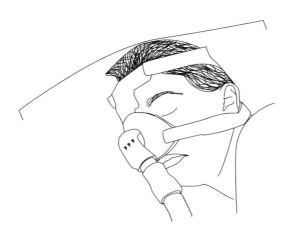

FIGURE 2 Subject wearing nasal continuous positive airway pressure.

have challenged this approach. Alternative nonlaboratory-based approaches to initiating CPAP are being applied in numerous health systems. For example, in 2004, throughout New Zealand nearly all (> 90% in some centers) CPAP initiation was implemented via either an attended in-laboratory split-night or unattended home auto-CPAP titration (Neill A, personal communication). Similarly, in the United Kingdom full in-laboratory CPAP titration studies are not routinely undertaken in many centers. Economic drivers have been of major importance in the adoption of these practices in these and other health services. As part of the drive toward economic rationalization, health authorities expect some evidence base for clinical CPAP titration strategies. Some such evidence has been accumulated; however, findings are somewhat contradictory.

Irrespective of the location or method of CPAP titration, there is a clear demand for proper patient assessment (e.g., does the patient have awake respiratory failure or marked hypoxemia in sleep?), which in turn requires specific physician training and experience. Until recently there was no evidence for the safety and efficacy of CPAP titration outside of a medically supervised process (17). Current evidence supports the use of trained technologists to provide patient education, technical aspects of titration, and follow-up. However, data from studies of small patient samples have challenged the presumption of close medical supervision during the initiation of therapy. Clearly this area requires further major research focus before a consensus may be derived (18–20).

The First Night

Sleeping with a nasal mask applied to the face, along with feeling the pressure sensation of CPAP, although not necessarily uncomfortable, are certainly novel experiences for most patients. Physician explanation, video programs, and mask "acclimatization" sessions prior to commencing CPAP are routine in many centers. Although the benefits of these approaches have not been fully scientifically evaluated, it would seem obvious that patient education about CPAP will reduce anxiety and improve acceptance. Current evidence provides some support for the benefit of more intensive patient education in CPAP usage (17,21). Thus, patient exposure to CPAP actually may begin prior to the first full night of therapy.

On the first night of treatment, it is important to ensure that the CPAP level that is identified as most therapeutically effective is sufficient not only to prevent apnea and oxyhaemoglobin desaturation (Fig. 3) but also to prevent respiratory-related arousals in all sleep stages and postures of sleep. Thus, simple apnea prevention is not the sole endpoint of CPAP titration. It is important to ensure that the airflow-CPAP pressure measurement is competent so as to avoid residual partial airway obstruction (7). An abnormal or technically challenged tracing (e.g., amplifier saturation, clipped signals) presents an opportunity for failure in detection of flow limitation and snoring. It is important to treat residual flow limitation as it may indicate upper airway obstruction, potentially causing arousal (22). Studies have emphasized the importance of proper airflow measurement in CPAP titration using pressure-based airflow transducers rather than thermistors or other more indirect airflow measures (23). Proper airflow measurement could help determine the optimal CPAP level by providing insights regarding the etiology of arousals; whether they are related to respiratory events (respiratory-related arousals) and if increasing pressure has a beneficial effect on sleep continuity. Although acute (one-night) studies suggest that flow limitation correction may be the preferred endpoint of CPAP

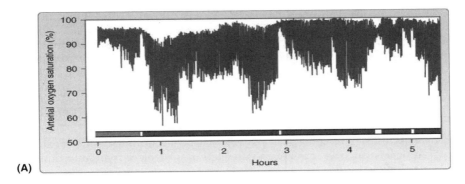

(A)

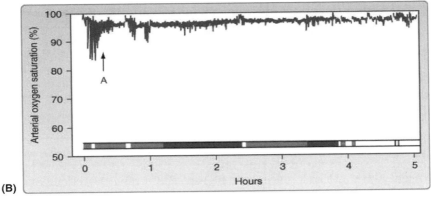

(B)

FIGURE 3   All-night recordings of arterial hemoglobin saturation in one of the earliest patients to use home continuous positive airway pressure (CPAP). (**A**) Control night. (**B**) CPAP trial night. A CPAP of 7 cm H_2O was applied at *arrow* A and continued for the rest of the night. *Source*: From Ref. 2.

titration, long-term data are sparse (24). Furthermore, pursuing normalization of the RDI may not be the only or even optimal goal in CPAP titration strategies in some OSA patients, who exhibit a cyclic alternating pattern non-rapid eye movement (NREM) sleep stage respiratory instability and who are relatively nonresponsive to CPAP (25). Prediction equations for starting pressures may enhance the success of titration studies (26) and also potentially offer the option of an effective outpatient setting titration strategy for CPAP-providing health services (27–30). Heated humidification appears not to offer any advantages during nasal CPAP titration studies (31).

When the correct CPAP level is reached and the airway is open, sleep should no longer be fragmented by repetitive arousals. There is often substantial "rebound" augmentation of slow-wave and rapid eye movement (REM) sleep (32). This rebound phase of recovery from prior severe sleep fragmentation lasts about a week; the duration and intensity of this rebound decrease quickly after the first night of treatment (32). The improvement in basic aspects of sleep architecture is usually immediate and can be used as a sign of an effective CPAP level. Also, following the time course of more detailed analysis of sleep pattern reorganization beyond the first night of treatment under the influence of CPAP therapy may provide a novel adjunct to conventional CPAP titration (33).

Continued frequent arousals may indicate that a critical level of upper airway resistance persists, especially if associated with flow limitation. Continued snoring is another sign of inadequate CPAP pressure. There are data demonstrating that hysteresis exists in the CPAP-upper airway resistance relationship. In other words, to eliminate inspiratory flow limitation, higher pressures are required during upward titration of CPAP compared with downward titration from higher pressures (34). This means that an OSA patient may actually normalize their breathing during sleep at a lower CPAP level if manual or automatic titration involves both upward titration till airflow is sinusoidal in shape, and downward titration till obstructed events recur. This may be an important concept in patients with complications of CPAP due to higher CPAP levels (such as mask or mouth leak) or a problem if an auto-titrating CPAP does not allow for this "up-then-down" titration approach.

Considering the length of time CPAP has been used to treat patients with sleep apnea, there are surprisingly little published data on the variability in CPAP pressure with posture or sleep stage. Some evidence exists for higher pressure requirements with the supine posture (35) and REM sleep (36). It appears that a CPAP level accurately set on one night is generally effective on subsequent nights (37). Early work and clinical experience suggested this was the case, but the use of auto-titrating CPAP (auto-CPAP) technology in the home has provided the research methodology to support this view (38). Clinically, in patients who respond immediately to CPAP but then report continued daytime sleepiness on home treatment, it may be appropriate to empirically increase CPAP pressure, assuming that the laboratory study underestimated the subsequent "domiciliary" CPAP pressure requirement. However, this has not been specifically studied. There is also a range of factors which may have an impact on the therapeutic efficacy of a given CPAP pressure in the home. Weight gain may lead to a need for a higher CPAP setting (39). Heavy, but not moderate, alcohol consumption may affect CPAP pressure, presumably owing to the effect of alcohol in depressing upper airway neuromuscular tone (40). Nasal congestion, alterations in levels of daily fatigue, or a different posture in the home may also lead to different pressure requirements but this has not been well researched.

Initiation of Treatment in Decompensated Patients with Cardiorespiratory Failure

Patients with carbon dioxide retention, heart failure, and extreme nocturnal hypoxemia (i.e., SaO_2 50% or less), require close supervision when commencing CPAP. Such patients may have confusion at night from delirium (due to their blood gas derangement) that may be exacerbated by someone trying to place a mask on their face. The nurse or technician needs to provide close attention throughout the night, in case the patient tries to repeatedly pull off the mask. After the first few nights, these patients typically settle down and sleep with CPAP without the need for intensive monitoring or intervention. The previous choice of therapy for these patients was endotracheal intubation or urgent tracheostomy. Intubation may still be the appropriate option; however, in trained hands, nasally applied CPAP or noninvasive ventilation (see Chapter 10) will readily control the breathing disturbance during sleep. CPAP may not adequately normalize gas exchange in many of these patients, as they may have both upper airway obstruction and hypoventilation (41). Increasingly, the clinical approach in these patients is to employ bilevel positive airway pressure therapy (BPAP). Auto-CPAP approaches are inappropriate in such patients. Newer auto-bilevel pressure devices have been introduced, but prospective trials of their efficacy in this population have not yet been performed and this technology remains unproven. Hospitalization would be the most reasonable approach in management of patients with severe CO_2 retention due to a hypoventilation syndrome and/or chronic lung disease (see Chapters 10 and 20), until studies showing the safety of unattended or domiciliary approaches are available.

The Split-Night Study

It has been suggested that CPAP can be successfully initiated on the same night the diagnosis is established (42,43). However, in these studies patient selection was not randomized and split-night studies tended to be performed in patients with more severe disease, who had been waiting a shorter time for their CPAP titration. Others have identified a subset of patients for whom a split-night study provided insufficient time for CPAP titration to achieve a satisfactory prescription (44). Patients with milder degrees of sleep-disordered breathing (SDB) [apnea–hypopnea index (AHI) less than 20 events per hour] in whom the titration is initiated later in the night (because prolonged monitoring was required to establish a diagnosis) were more likely to have unsuccessful split-night titrations. CPAP can also potentially be titrated during the day (45). With these approaches, both daytime and nocturnal CPAP titration studies yielded sufficient amounts of REM and NREM sleep to help determine CPAP settings. The diurnal and nocturnal CPAP titrations resulted in comparable therapeutic pressures, resolution of SDB, and one-week adherence. Split-night or day studies may appear attractive from a cursory economic point of view. The full economic impact of such techniques must, necessarily, include the ultimate costs of improper or inadequate titration (both in retitration, cost of untreated sleep-disordered breathing, and attendant preventable comorbidity). Data in larger numbers of unselected patients are required before these ultimate economic consequences are known and this approach is routinely accepted. It is possible but speculative at this stage, depending on outcome studies, whether a combination of split-night titration and subsequent home auto-titration may provide an adequate and cost-effective strategy.

Initiation of Continuous Positive Airway Pressure in the Home Setting

There may be theoretical economic advantages from starting CPAP at home and avoiding a formal in-laboratory polysomnographic (PSG) CPAP titration. However, outcome studies showing true cost versus benefit analyses are not available. Current reviews and guidelines do not advocate home commencement of CPAP, particularly using auto-titrating devices (46). This is a controversial area as it implies a major change of practice in sleep centers. One study has observed poorer CPAP adherence in patients assessed only with respiratory monitoring (47); another study has shown poorer adherence outcomes with patients having initial unattended CPAP PSG at home (48). Conversely, equivalence of outcomes between in-laboratory and home-based studies have also been reported (19,30,49). Other workers have found reasonable utility with unattended in-hospital CPAP titration in patients with mild-to-moderate disease but not severe OSA (50). Some studies have suggested that equations can be determined which would allow an empirical CPAP level to be set, potentially preventing the need for any investigation of CPAP efficacy (30,44). Data from a small group of patients support an empirical method of home CPAP titration instead of laboratory initiation (18). A further multicenter three-month trial involving 360 CPAP-naïve OSA patients has shown equivalence of some key outcomes (AHI, subjective daytime sleepiness, adherence, dropout rates) whether CPAP was titrated in-laboratory, by auto-CPAP or by using a prediction formula (29). A six-month assessment of outcomes has shown equivalence for three methods of CPAP initiation including auto-CPAP as a long-term therapy, fixed-pressure CPAP with pressure calculated using an algorithm, or after one week of auto-CPAP to determine therapeutic fixed CPAP levels (30). Thus, even though long-term outcome data are lacking, there is a growing body of evidence supporting effective alternatives to in-laboratory CPAP titration in selected groups of OSA patients.

PROBLEMS AND SIDE EFFECTS (SEE ALSO CHAPTER 9)

Side effects reported by the patient are usually, but not exclusively, related to pressure or airflow or the mask-face interface. The minimization of side effects is important for effective CPAP usage; patients who complain of side effects use CPAP less frequently than those without side effects (51). A nonspecific claustrophobic feeling may be reported by patients but this often involves either mask/interface problems, nasal congestion, or exhalation difficulties that are discussed below. Dangerous complications of nasal CPAP therapy are extremely rare and represent isolated case reports in the literature including: pulmonary barotrauma, pneumocephalus, increased intraocular pressure, tympanic membrane rupture, cerebrospinal fluid (CSF) leak and meningitis (52), massive epistaxis, and subcutaneous emphysema after facial trauma (53). It is clear that caution should be used when implementing CPAP therapy post-neuro, -airway, or -facial surgery. Irritating side effects such as aerophagy and musculoskeletal chest discomfort have also been reported (53).

Nasal Congestion

Nasal congestion is a common side effect of CPAP therapy (53). Although most patients experience initial self-limiting nasal congestion, at least 10% complain of persistent nasal stuffiness of some degree after six months of therapy (54). There appear to be many possible reasons for nasal symptoms. CPAP may provoke pressure-sensitive mucosal receptors, leading to vasodilation and increased mucus production. In some patients, it may unmask allergic rhinitis by restoring the nasal route of breathing after years of "mouth breathing." In others, fixed nasal obstruction with polyps or a deviated septum may produce symptoms. Mouth leaks also cause increased nasal resistance (55).

Brief CPAP exposure reduces saccharin transit times in healthy subjects but mucous transportability was not affected (56). Histologic changes of nasal mucosa vary between untreated OSA patients and those treated with CPAP, and further vary according to the duration of CPAP treatment; rhinitic symptoms can be correlated with these changes (57). On the other hand, in a small study of nasal mechanics and function in OSA patients treated for six months with nonhumidified CPAP, measures of nasal resistance, mucociliary clearance, and ciliary beat frequency did not change over time (58).

Treatment of nasal congestion will depend on the exact cause. Mouth leak producing increased nasal flow may be minimized by ensuring that the mask interface selection is ideal and the correct CPAP pressure is used. Sometimes, it may be necessary to use chin straps. However, these may be uncomfortable and acclimatization is often necessary. Nasal congestion can be treated with antihistamines, topical steroids, or topical saline sprays. Added humidification of the circuit will improve nasal dryness. Heated, rather than cold, pass-over humidification is necessary to treat nasal congestion (55,59,60). Intranasal ipratropium bromide can be helpful in abating CPAP-induced rhinorrhea.

Patients with persistent symptoms of nasal congestion or those with obvious nasal obstruction should have nasopharyngoscopy performed. In such patients there is some limited evidence of benefit from corrective surgery for an obstructive lesion such as polyps, marked mucosal thickening, or deviated septum (61). Oral masks may also be of value in managing a few patients with nasal side effects (62).

The Interface

Initially, masks were custom-made from silastic compounds. In the mid-1980s new forms of plastic self-sealing masks that were more convenient to use were commercially available. Mask technology has improved greatly, and this is important as mask comfort remains a pivotal influence on CPAP acceptance and adherence. Poorly-fitting masks permit air leakage and a drop in pressure leading to persistent "breakthrough" OSA and sleep fragmentation. The leak is usually the source of considerable discomfort; for example, if it is directed toward the eye, it may cause conjunctivitis (63). A potential problem with a poorly fitting mask is the development of bruising or even ulceration of the bridge of the nose.

There are few studies comparing different mask types despite the constant availability of new designs. Anecdotally, the newer generation of mask types is associated with fewer mask-fit problems. Nevertheless, certain patients become claustrophobic when using nasal CPAP with any mask. Changing the interface prescription from a nasal mask to less confining nasal prongs or "pillows" may correct that problem. However, nasal prongs may cause irritation in the nares and long-term use data is needed. Newer interfaces are constantly being developed to address mask problems but for some patients, particularly younger patients with mild disease, perceived aesthetic problems with CPAP, regardless of interface, preclude this treatment modality.

An infrequent but difficult problem is the patient who has no upper front teeth. The upper teeth provide the rigid structure against which the lower part of the mask can be pulled. If there is no dentition, the mask simply rolls around the top gums into the mouth, with loss of an adequate seal. The problem may be rectified by providing a denture (64) or possibly an oronasal (i.e., "full face") mask.

Pressure Level and Airflow

Although frequently mentioned as a problem, there is no convincing evidence that the CPAP pressure level actually impairs adherence. Some patients may complain of initial increased resistance to exhalation or the sensation of too much pressure in the nose. For these patients, a CPAP unit with a pressure ramp may be considered. Ramp is a standard feature on most contemporary CPAP devices. The ramp allows the pressure to increase gradually over a set time interval (usually 5–30 minutes) to the optimal CPAP pressure. No studies have been performed to show that a ramp feature improves acceptance or adherence with CPAP; however, interestingly, a case of "ramp abuse" has been reported where continuous patient application of the ramp function led to undertreatment of sleep apnea (65). Alternatively, a BPAP system, in which inspiratory and expiratory positive airway pressure (PAP) can be adjusted independently, may be used, as this approach lowers mean airway pressure and resistance to expiration. Again, it is not clear whether these approaches will improve adherence. Limited data indicate that use of bilevel devices does not affect positive pressure usage in OSA patients (66) (see also Chapter 7). More recently, a novel type of CPAP with reduced expiratory compared to inspiratory pressure has been marketed (C-Flex™, Respironics, Inc., Murrysville, Pennsylvania, U.S.) with no evidence in one study for increased patient adherence using this modality at one month compared to conventional CPAP (67). The researchers report some adherence and other modest advantage in another study at three months follow-up (68). Interim reports [published as abstracts at the Associated Professional Sleep Societies (APSS) Meeting in 2005] of further studies of this device suggest equivalence or marginally better outcomes compared to conventional CPAP (69–73). Further large-scale clinical trials are necessary to determine any definite advantage.

Patients occasionally find the air generated by the CPAP unit too warm or too cold. Initial correction attempts may involve moving the machine from the floor to a bedside table, heating the bedroom, placing tubing under the blankets or the use of a specifically-designed insulated wrap. If these do not correct the problem, incorporating a heated humidifier into the circuit may help. Bed partners may also experience cold air on their bodies from the expiratory port of the device. Employment of an alternative mask or interface may help redirect the stream of air away from the bed partner. Another complaint, also usually from the bed partner is that the CPAP machine generates too much noise. With the newest generation of CPAP devices, the majority of noise is aerodynamic, being generated either through the tubing, or at the patient interface. However, for noisy machines, removing the machine from the bedside or placing it in a closet may remedy the problem. Extra tubing may be needed but it is important to recheck pressures if nonstandard tubing is used. Excessive noise, or a changing level of noise intensity or quality may be a problem in some auto-CPAP devices, as well as in CPAP with expiratory pressure relief, due to the nature of their motor control.

COMPARISON WITH OTHER TREATMENTS

One of the great advantages of nasal CPAP is that it is immediately and demonstrably efficacious in relieving OSA (2,74). Although that effect is often clinically obvious as early as the CPAP titration night, this beneficial effect of reducing or normalizing the RDI has been convincingly demonstrated in follow-up PSG studies between two weeks and three months after CPAP initiation. This normalization is in contrast to other treatments including sham CPAP, other placebo, conservative management and positional therapy (75–78). Another advantage is that it can be offered on a "trial" basis and withdrawn if not tolerated, in contrast to surgical options. This is particularly important in milder cases of OSA, or where the contribution of OSA to the patient's symptomatology is unclear. A few studies have attempted to compare CPAP with other treatments for OSA using formal protocols. There is a dearth of adequate studies comparing the results of surgical interventions for OSA and those that exist do not support widespread surgical intervention as a satisfactory method of treating OSA (79). The conclusion of most of these studies is that CPAP is the appropriate therapy for patients with moderate-to-severe sleep apnea (80–83). This view is also supported by the 2006 American Academy of Sleep Medicine Standards of Practice Committee Task

Force practice parameters and review of the use of PAP treatment in adults with sleep-disordered breathing (1,84) .

ADHERENCE (SEE ALSO CHAPTER 9)
General Issues
It is widely acknowledged that CPAP is an effective treatment for OSA but just as readily recognized that there are significant limitations to patients' effective use of this treatment modality. In addition to adherence, various other terms such as compliance, acceptance, and others have been used by authors when reporting studies describing utilization of prescribed CPAP treatment. These terms need standardized definitions and use to allow valid across-studies interpretation of results (85). True "efficacy" studies have yet to be performed. Such studies would need to measure not only the CPAP usage and residual "breakthrough" respiratory events, but also the total amount of sleep. Thus, a measure of not only protected sleep (as measured on the CPAP device), but also the amount of "unprotected" sleep, without CPAP therapy. Nevertheless, when one looks at all the CPAP usage data currently available, adherence with CPAP devices compares favorably with medication use in various other chronic medical conditions.

Several specific factors can potentially affect CPAP initial acceptance and long-term adherence, including machine cost, the technical characteristics of the equipment, and prescriber motivation. Current machines are quieter compared to those of past years, with a ramp facility to slowly increase the pressure over the first period of sleep, and there are more comfortable masks. Many earlier CPAP usage studies used equipment that has been replaced by newer devices (for example, the "C-Flex" CPAP device; see above section: Pressure Level and Airflow) and adherence data need to be continually updated to verify whether these technical changes do actually influence CPAP use or are purely "cosmetic" in the intense marketing environment of CPAP equipment sales. This situation is somewhat analogous to clinical trials of new medications within the same drug class, for example, comparative studies of beta-blockers.

Most contemporary CPAP equipment includes some mechanism for adherence monitoring. Many feature the ability to detect ventilation, and record "mask-on-face" time. If a CPAP mask is taken off the face, there is detectable drop in pressure and loss of the predictable ventilatory pattern. This can be recorded on devices with data storage capability. So, if patients simply switch on their machine and leave the mask on the floor, then there would be a major discrepancy between "machine-on" time and "mask-on-face" time. A simultaneous study of CPAP use and pressure delivery at the mask revealed a reasonable correlation between claimed usage and measured adherence (86).

"Dosage" studies are not available for CPAP. The question *do patients have to use CPAP every night to receive beneficial therapeutic effects?* remains incompletely answered. Even average CPAP use of less than four hours per night produces a demonstrable reduction in sleepiness (87). Another study showed that one night off CPAP in adherent CPAP users led to a recurrence in daytime sleepiness (88). At this stage all criteria set for CPAP usage or nonusage or adherence or nonadherence (86,87) are essentially arbitrary. Newer studies are anticipated that may help define these criteria according to meaningful physiologic or neurocognitive outcomes.

Furthermore, it is clear that even partial-night CPAP use can lead to measurable clinical improvement. Some sleep apnea patients use CPAP for only part of the night because they derive a satisfactory degree of symptomatic benefit from that limited application (81). This possibly reflects interindividual variation of function with sleep loss or fragmentation, with some patients "needing" to obtain less sleep to function at a reasonable level during wakefulness (82). Given the evidence that shortened sleep hours are associated with significant performance deficit, patients need to be warned about the risk of persisting problems with alertness, which may accompany limited hours of use of CPAP. Newer-generation CPAP devices that allow monitoring of more precise patterns of use and efficacy will give us insight into the minimal duration of CPAP use that is needed to maintain normal daytime neurobehavioral function and, possibly, to modify the vascular consequences of sleep apnea.

Acceptance and Purchase

We do not know how many people with moderate-to-severe OSA avoid initial consultation with a sleep physician, or seek primary referral to surgeons or dentists, because they will not entertain even the possibility of using CPAP. The percentage of patients who refuse CPAP after an in-hospital trial is variable (89). CPAP purchase rates after PSG CPAP titration are over 50%, based on a calculation comparing new CPAP machine sales provided by manufacturers with national insurance data on multiple sleep study frequency (90). In other words, over 50% of patients completing a sleep laboratory trial end up purchasing a CPAP machine or having one purchased for them by the health system.

Long-Term Use of Continuous Positive Airway Pressure

Covert objective monitoring of CPAP has demonstrated that adherence with nasal CPAP is substantially less than in studies where adherence is reported on the basis of subjective patient data (86), with only 46% of patients having used nasal CPAP equal to or greater than four hours for 70% of the observed nights. Adherence at one month predicted adherence at three months (86,91). Other studies have generally confirmed this degree of usage.

Published CPAP follow-up cohorts are biased by the same factors that affect clinical trials of pharmaceuticals. Patient populations are often highly selected for intellectual capacity, geographical access, health consciousness, and lack of comorbidities—all factors that may affect adherence in the real world. More large "open" studies from a variety of sleep clinics (92) would provide better information on true CPAP adherence.

Attempts to improve CPAP adherence have involved technical refinements of devices, including the implementation of microprocessor-controlled blowers, ramp features, integrated heated humidification, use of auto-CPAP, and adjunctive supportive measures. A flexible PAP device (see section: Pressure Level and Airflow) may prove advantageous for some patients (68). Video education at the outset may enhance CPAP usage and clinic attendance at one month postinitiation (93).

A Cochrane review of interventions to improve CPAP adherence did not report a clear-cut advantage of increased hours of use in favor of auto-CPAP over fixed CPAP in pooled data of unselected patients though, where measured, patient preference was for auto-CPAP. In the same review, two of six studies of educational/ psychological interventions demonstrated improved hours of use (94).

Baseline Indicators Influencing Continuous Positive Airway Pressure Usage

Identification of claustrophobia prior to initiating CPAP using a 15-item Fear and Avoidance Scale predicted lower CPAP adherence at three months (95). Remedial measures to address such identified claustrophobia, logically, may improve adherence in those subjects. A patient's reporting "initial problems" after the first night of CPAP (using auto-titration) was the most powerful predictor of lower hours of CPAP "on time" at one-month follow-up (88). "Recent life events" and "living alone" were less robust predictors of adherence. In the same study, pretreatment measures of anxiety or depression failed to predict one-month adherence. Contrariwise, in another study low CPAP adherence predicted high anxiety scores, and low CPAP adherence and excessive daytime sleepiness predicted high depression scores in a questionnaire-based study of OSA patients (96). Predominant nose breathing rather than mouth breathing at outset predicted better adherence with CPAP at one year follow-up in moderate–severe OSA (97).

Progressing from diagnosis to titration to purchase of CPAP requires manifold interlocking promoting elements. Such progression, in many healthcare delivery systems requiring co-payment for CPAP, is facilitated by higher socioeconomic status, is correlated with higher measures of subjective sleepiness and severity of OSA (e.g., as quantified by RDI or AHI), and is abetted by support from the bed partner, referring physician and sleep lab staff (21).

Several other studies have confirmed that the pretreatment severity of sleepiness is correlated with the likelihood of greater usage of CPAP—that is, that patients with good objective usage or reported adherence are sleepier at baseline (53,86,92,98,99). Although daytime sleepiness as measured by the multiple sleep latency test (MSLT) improves following CPAP (87), baseline MSLT scores do not appear to predict CPAP adherence and it is controversial whether the amount of improvement in MSLT scores will predict adherence (86,98). It is possible that the maintenance of wakefulness test may be a better predictor of CPAP usage in patients with sleep apnea, but this is untested. Sleep fragmentation measured by an electroencephalographic neural network analysis or movement events on video recordings are reasonably correlated with CPAP adherence (100). Improved adherence has also been linked to the degree of improvement in sleep efficiency and quality between diagnostic and treatment studies (101). Other factors that may be related to reduced usage include previous palatal surgery and fewer years of education. Surprisingly, as mentioned above, considering the potential discomfort and potential mask leak, having a higher CPAP pressure level has not been shown to have a negative influence on adherence (12,17,18,53). In fact, it may be associated with improved adherence, though these data could be confounded by more marked symptoms (and thus a greater potential for symptom improvement) in patients requiring higher pressures (92).

Role of Physician or Technologist Motivation/Support

It would seem obvious that with greater positive reinforcement given to patients, the more likely the patient will use CPAP as prescribed. Various studies have shown the value of patient education although it is unclear as to the quantum of education and support that is necessary to improve adherence (17,18,21,102). Early experience with cognitive behavior therapy approaches as an adjunct to standard CPAP education practices shows promise.

MANAGEMENT OF CONTINUOUS POSITIVE AIRWAY PRESSURE FAILURE

What constitutes CPAP failure? This is a subjective issue and, in the absence of hard data addressing the diverse health consequences of varying "exposures" of CPAP for sleep apnea, practice varies from center to center. CPAP failure certainly includes those cases with continuing significant sleepiness or other sequelae of sleep apnea. An objective measure of CPAP failure (as measured by usage of the CPAP therapy) has been defined (a priori) as the "use of CPAP for less than four hours per night on 70% of the nights and/or lack of symptomatic improvement" (86). This figure equates to a minimum acceptable average usage of only 2.7 hours per night. This figure was essentially an arbitrary threshold, based on the authors' expert clinical opinion (86). Some have adopted a policy of reclaiming loaned CPAP machines if use is less than two hours per night (92). Sometimes patients will use CPAP effectively but only for part of their total sleep time. This may represent CPAP failure depending on the endpoint of therapy (103,104).

Clearly, it is important to identify the cause of CPAP failure. Some of the commonest side effects and potential solutions have been mentioned. Ear, nose, and throat assessment may be appropriate in looking for any structural reasons to explain CPAP failure. It is important also to consider if there has been a misdiagnosis or if there is coexistent sleepiness from other causes (104). Residual sleepiness in CPAP-treated subjects should be subjected to rigorous review including, if necessary, the use of esophageal pressure balloons to detect subtle episodes of upper airway obstruction. A proportion of such patients will be shown to have been undertreated rather than having truly failed treatment.

Some attempts to overcome true CPAP treatment failures have involved the use of PAP devices other than CPAP, such as bilevel PAP, but supporting evidence is limited (84).

HEALTH OUTCOMES AND CONTINUOUS POSITIVE AIRWAY PRESSURE

Over the past decade, there have been a number of RCTs that have demonstrated the effectiveness of CPAP in improving neurobehavioral outcomes such as daytime sleepiness and blood pressure, in patients with moderate-to-severe OSA (99,105,106). Benefits have also been demonstrated in OSA subgroups such as those patients with coincident Alzheimer's disease and OSA (107). Different parameters of sleep patterns improve over a defined time scale but mostly within one month of establishing CPAP in severe OSA patients (33). Depression symptoms associated with untreated OSA may ameliorate with successful institution of CPAP therapy (108). However, the evidence for benefits is less clear in patients with more severe disease without significant sleepiness (98) or in patients with mild disease (109).

Researchers have employed either an oral placebo or sham/sub-therapeutic CPAP as control arms in RCTs examining the effects of CPAP. There is no "perfect placebo" for CPAP and each approach has limitations and obvious difficulties in blinding. Even a patient on sham CPAP may be made aware of persisting snoring or observed apneas by a bed partner. However, existing studies have clearly defined a role for CPAP in moderate-to-severe symptomatic OSA. The treatment of the asymptomatic patient with milder disease remains controversial (109). One study compared (humidified) CPAP to sham CPAP in mild OSA and showed improvement in subjective sleepiness and a trend toward improved objective wakefulness in the treatment group along with improvement in PSG indices of OSA, but other outcomes (mood, quality of life, psychomotor vigilance task reaction times) were similar in the two groups as were adherence and treatment preference (110). A meta-analysis of RCTs in mild–moderate OSA suggests quite modest benefit from CPAP treatment on both subjective and objective measures of daytime sleepiness (111).

CONTINUOUS POSITIVE AIRWAY PRESSURE AND CARDIOVASCULAR OUTCOMES

The present evidence for a significant protective or ameliorating effect of CPAP against adverse cardiovascular outcomes in OSA is mixed, especially in the management of mild OSA. In a large observational cohort study, there was an increased risk of stroke and death, which persisted after allowing for other risk factors including hypertension; however, CPAP use did not appear to provide protection against adverse outcomes in this study (112). In contrast, in case-control studies, there is some evidence of cardiovascular benefit from nasal CPAP therapy in severe sleep apnea. Long-term CPAP therapy seemed to provide a protective benefit against death from established cardiovascular disease though there was no difference in the development of new cases of hypertension, cardiac disorder or stroke between CPAP-treated and untreated groups (113). In a large Spanish study patients with untreated severe OSA had a higher incidence of both fatal and nonfatal cardiovascular events than untreated patients with mild–moderate OSA, simple snorers, healthy subjects, and patients treated with CPAP (114). CPAP also appears to provide a protective benefit against new vascular events after stroke or transient ischaemic attack in moderate–severe OSA subjects (115). These results suggest a protective benefit of CPAP against these adverse cardiovascular outcomes, but better designed RCTs are needed to convincingly demonstrate this benefit.

Cardiovascular-protective benefits of CPAP have been demonstrated mainly against hypertension. Short-term improvements in hypertension control have been shown in a randomized parallel trial of CPAP-treated OSA patients when compared to sub-therapeutic-CPAP, and cardiovascular risk benefits imputed therefrom (106). In a RCT of CPAP, sham-CPAP and nocturnal oxygen, two weeks of CPAP therapy resulted in a significant reduction in daytime mean arterial and diastolic blood pressure and night-time systolic, mean, and diastolic blood pressure (116). In a small study of nonrandomized OSA subjects measures of muscle sympathetic traffic were improved over time with CPAP treatment although blood pressure did not change (117). However, recent data question the ability of CPAP to decrease blood pressure over longer time periods, particularly in nonsleepy patients (118).

Although acute auto-CPAP use did not alter systolic nor diastolic blood pressure, nor heart rate, from diagnostic (pretreatment) values in 12 OSA patients, CPAP treatment was associated with a stabilizing effect by reducing night-time but not daytime variability of pressure parameters (119). Nearly half of a group of moderate–severe OSA patients experienced severe, mainly nocturnal, cardiac arrhythmia documented by use of an insertable loop recorder (but largely not documented by Holter monitor); and long-term CPAP treatment was associated with marked reduction of arrhythmia (120).

Preeclamptic women exhibited sleep-induced decrements of heart rate, stroke volume and cardiac output, and exacerbated increase of total peripheral resistance, and these changes were minimized and reduced, respectively in subjects treated with CPAP (121). There is an apparent linkage between untreated OSA and left-to-right cardiac shunt (LRS) via a patent foramen ovale, and a case report documents reversal of wake LRS with institution of CPAP therapy (122).

In summary, although there is tantalizing evidence from small physiological and case studies of potential cardiovascular benefit from treating OSA patients with CPAP, and epidemiological evidence of significant cardiovascular and mortality risk from OSA, there is a continuing need for large-scale RCTs to support the idea that we provide cardiovascular benefit to our OSA patients on CPAP, beyond merely reducing the level of respiratory disturbances.

CONTINUOUS POSITIVE AIRWAY PRESSURE AND CARDIAC FAILURE

Sleep apnea of both central and obstructive nature is common in patients with cardiac failure (123). It has been suggested that OSA may cause or exacerbate ventricular dysfunction by a number of mechanisms. These include increasing left ventricular afterload through the combined effects of elevations in systemic blood pressure and the generation of exaggerated negative intrathoracic pressure, and by activating the sympathetic nervous system through the influence of hypoxia and arousals from sleep (124). Use of nasal CPAP in OSA and in cardiac failure patients for one month (125) and three months (126), respectively, leads to improvement in left ventricular function.

A number of studies have reported the presence of central sleep apnea in patients with ventricular dysfunction. Central apnea appears to be an adverse prognostic factor in such patients (127). Studies, including some with a randomized controlled design, have demonstrated improvement in various endpoints, including reduced mitral regurgitant fraction, atrial natriuretic factor secretion, inspiratory muscle strength, reduced left ventricular afterload, tendency to normalization of $PaCO_2$, and norepinephrine concentrations, with CPAP treatment in patients with cardiac failure and central apnea (127). However, recently published research, while confirming small physiological changes with active treatment, has shown no advantage on survival or transplant-free interval in such patients treated with CPAP (128). That study included several methodological issues which, in retrospect, may have led to the reported outcomes. It is also possible changes in effective cardiac failure therapy over time and during the life of this study may have influenced the essentially negative results of the Canadian Continuous Positive Airway Pressure Trial for Congestive Heart Failure Patients with Central Sleep Apnea (CANPAP) study (129). It is also possible that further sub-group analysis may demonstrate a particular type of patient with cardiac failure and central apneas who may benefit from CPAP therapy.

CONTINUOUS POSITIVE AIRWAY PRESSURE COST AND REIMBURSEMENT ISSUES

In Australia, for the majority of those requiring it, the cost of CPAP is borne directly by the patient, or indirectly by the patient through his/her coverage in a health insurance fund. Such funds, and wherein medical devices such as CPAP are covered under the specific scheme, reimburse approximately 30% to 50% of retail cost. Percentage reimbursement can be significantly better, even 100%, in smaller "boutique" health insurance schemes. Approximately 43% of Australians (2006 statistics) carry some level of private health insurance.

Australian patients requiring CPAP who do not carry private health insurance must meet the full cost of purchase; costs approximate AUD$1300 to 1500 (CPAP machine, mask with tubing). Many patients will not readily acquire CPAP because of this financial hurdle. For impecunious patients requiring CPAP, there are schemes across all states in Australia, administered by state health departments through public hospitals, whereby after medical criteria for CPAP are seen to have been met, and there has been strict financial means testing, patients will be provided with CPAP equipment at subsidized cost (often the full machine costs are covered but "ancillary" equipment such as mask, tubing, humidifier, are not). Such schemes have a limited annually recurring financial budget, provide other medical devices against which CPAP provision must compete, and have a waiting time dictated by an available budget for CPAP under which these schemes may vary considerably from region to region. An analogous mixture of public and private purchasing of CPAP equipment, and most notable for controlled limited budgeting and regional variations of availability of supply and consequent waiting times for CPAP therapy in the public sector, applies in the United Kingdom and New Zealand.

CONTINUOUS POSITIVE AIRWAY PRESSURE REIMBURSEMENT IN THE UNITED STATES

Peter C. Gay, MD

For any therapeutic plan to be viable for the patient, it must be accessible and reimbursable. The coverage criterion throughout the world varies but, generally, more socialized governmentally directed care is difficult to access, but is more favorably reimbursed. The opposite is true in the United States where accessibility to care is typically easy, but coverage criteria are usually more cumbersome. Throughout the world, a physician must not only decide the appropriate treatment but also ensure that the patient can access the treatment recommended. The Center for Medicare and Medicaid (CMS) in the United States has unique coverage criteria that for appropriate patient management must be understood. The following is pertinent for patients dependent on CMS coverage criteria, but clinicians worldwide are encouraged to familiarize themselves with similar issues in their area.

Patients with suspected OSA are mandated to undergo a diagnostic study in a "facility-based polysomnography laboratory" with a minimum of 120 minutes of recorded sleep. This stipulation was largely inserted to emphasize the CMS bias against empiric or portable sleep study diagnosis of OSA. An apnea–hypopnea index (AHI) of 15 events per hour is required in order to qualify for coverage, unless the patient has symptoms of hypersomnolence or cardiovascular consequences such as hypertension, in which case they need only demonstrate five events per hour.

Access to alternative treatment such as auto-titration CPAP (APAP) or bilevel PAP (BPAP) is surprisingly easy since the criteria are not specified for APAP at all because the reimbursement is equivalent to simple CPAP and the only stipulation necessary to utilize BPAP is for the physician to stipulate that "CPAP has been tried and proven ineffective." The ineffectiveness of the CPAP can be on the basis of intolerance or poor response and the time period of decision-making is not stipulated, so there is much left to the discretion of the treating physician. Under no circumstance can a BPAP device with a backup rate be prescribed for OSA alone and, if desired, this requires an additional diagnosis, such as central sleep apnea, restrictive lung disease with neuromuscular disease or thoracic cage abnormality or, hypercapnic chronic obstructive lung disease failing BPAP without a BPAP rate. The complete coverage criteria for CPAP and BPAP devices are available online[1].

---

[1]Websites for CPAP and BPAP—must cut and paste into website address to work:
http://www.adminastar.com/Providers/DMERC/MedicalPolicy/Files/CPAPSystemsRev42.pdf
http://www.adminastar.com/Providers/DMERC/MedicalPolicy/Files/RespiratoryAssistDevicesRev42.pdf

CONCLUSIONS

CPAP is the treatment of first choice for management of OSA of moderate or greater severity in adults. Applied via a facial interface it is a very effective and safe method of preventing the upper airway obstructions characteristic of OSA. There remain issues of imperfect patient acceptance and adherence with CPAP, uncertainties regarding the role of CPAP in mild OSA, and whether it achieves the desired cardiovascular benefits. Techniques of diagnosing OSA, selection of appropriate subjects for CPAP therapy, and practical methods of initiating CPAP in a timely and economic manner continue to evolve.

ACKNOWLEDGMENTS

PRB was supported by a Translational Research Fellowship of the Woolcock Institute of Medical Research Centre for Clinical and Research Excellence of the National Health and Medical Research Council (NHMRC) of Australia. RRG was supported by a Practitioner Fellowship from the NHMRC of Australia. Thanks to A. Dawes for assistance with Figures 1 and 2.

REFERENCES

1. Kushida CA, Littner MR, Hirshkowitz M, et al. Practice parameters for the use of continuous and bilevel positive airway pressure devices to treat adult patients with sleep-related breathing disorders. Sleep 2006; 29(3):375–380.
2. Sullivan CE, Issa FG, Berthon-Jones M, Eves L. Reversal of obstructive sleep apnoea by continuous positive airway pressure applied through the nares. Lancet 1981; 317(8225):862–865.
3. Wagner DR, Pollak CP, Weitzman ED. Nocturnal nasal-airway pressure for sleep apnea. N Engl J Med 1983; 308(8):461–462.
4. Krieger J, Weitzenblum E, Monassier JP, Stoeckel C, Kurtz D. Dangerous hypoxaemia during continuous positive airway pressure treatment of obstructive sleep apnoea. Lancet 1983; 2(8364):1429–1430.
5. Bradley D, Phillipson EA. The treatment of obstructive sleep apnea. Separating the wheat from the chaff. Am Rev Respir Dis 1983; 128(4):583–586.
6. Grunstein RR, Dodd MJ, Costas L, Sullivan CE. Home nasal CPAP for sleep apnea-acceptance of home therapy and its usefulness. Aust N Z J Med 1986; 16:635.
7. Grunstein RR. Sleep-related breathing disorders. 5. Nasal continuous positive airway pressure treatment for obstructive sleep apnoea. Thorax 1995; 50(10):1106–1113.
8. Grunstein RR, Hedner J, Grote L. Treatment options for sleep apnoea. Drugs 2001; 61(2):237–251.
9. Buchanan PR, Grunstein RR. Chapter: Neuropharmacology of obstructive sleep apnea and central apnea. Clinical Pharmacology of Sleep. Switzerland: Birkhauser, 2006.
10. Abad VC, Guilleminault C. Pharmacological management of sleep apnoea. Expert Opin Pharmacother 2006; 7(1):11–23.
11. Gregory GA, Kitterman JA, Phibbs RH, Tooley WH, Hamilton WK. Treatment of the idiopathic respiratory-distress syndrome with continuous positive airway pressure. N Engl J Med 1971; 284(24):1333–1340.
12. Remmers JE, deGroot WJ, Sauerland EK, Anch AM. Pathogenesis of upper airway occlusion during sleep. J Appl Physiol 1978; 44(6):931–938.
13. Strohl KP, Redline S. Nasal CPAP therapy, upper airway muscle activation, and obstructive sleep apnea. Am Rev Respir Dis 1986; 134(3):555–558.
14. Schwab RJ, Pack AI, Gupta KB, et al. Upper airway and soft tissue structural changes induced by CPAP in normal subjects. Am J Respir Crit Care Med 1996; 154(4 Pt 1):1106–1116.
15. Issa FG, Sullivan CE. Reversal of central sleep apnea using nasal CPAP. Chest 1986; 90(2):165–171.

16. Thomas RJ, Daly RW, Weiss JW. Low-concentration carbon dioxide is an effective adjunct to positive airway pressure in the treatment of refractory mixed central and obstructive sleep-disordered breathing. Sleep 2005; 28(1):69–77.
17. Zozula R, Rosen R. Compliance with continuous positive airway pressure therapy: assessing and improving treatment outcomes. Curr Opin Pulm Med 2001; 7(6):391–398.
18. Fitzpatrick MF, Alloway CE, Wakeford TM, MacLean AW, Munt PW, Day AG. Can patients with obstructive sleep apnea titrate their own continuous positive airway pressure? Am J Respir Crit Care Med 2003; 167(5):716–722.
19. Hukins C. Comparative study of autotitrating and fixed-pressure CPAP in the home: a randomized, single-blind crossover trial. Sleep 2004; 27(8):1512–1517.
20. Hukins CA. Arbitrary-pressure continuous positive airway pressure for obstructive sleep apnea syndrome. Am J Respir Crit Care Med 2005; 171(5):500–505.
21. Brin YS, Reuveni H, Greenberg S, Tal A, Tarasiuk A. Determinants affecting initiation of continuous positive airway pressure treatment. Isr Med Assoc J 2005; 7(1):13–18.
22. Montserrat JM, Ballester E, Olivi H, et al. Time-course of stepwise CPAP titration. Behavior of respiratory and neurological variables. Am J Respir Crit Care Med 1995; 152(6 Pt 1):1854–1859.
23. Hosselet JJ, Norman RG, Ayappa I, Rapoport DM. Detection of flow limitation with a nasal cannula/pressure transducer system. Am J Respir Crit Care Med 1998; 157(5 Pt 1):1461–1467.
24. Meurice JC, Paquereau J, Denjean A, Patte F, Series F. Influence of correction of flow limitation on continuous positive airway pressure efficiency in sleep apnoea/hypopnoea syndrome. Eur Respir J 1998; 11(5):1121–1127.
25. Thomas RJ, Terzano MG, Parrino L, Weiss JW. Obstructive sleep-disordered breathing with a dominant cyclic alternating pattern—a recognizable polysomnographic variant with practical clinical implications. Sleep 2004; 27(2):229–234.
26. Rowley J, Tarbichi A, Badr M. The use of a predicted CPAP equation improves CPAP titration success. Sleep Breathing 2005; 9(1):26–32.
27. Stradling JR, Hardinge M, Paxton J, Smith DM. Relative accuracy of algorithm-based prescription of nasal CPAP in OSA. Respir Med 2004; 98(2):152–154.
28. Stradling JR, Hardinge M, Smith DM. A novel, simplified approach to starting nasal CPAP therapy in OSA. Respir Med 2004; 98(2):155–158.
29. Masa JF, Jimenez A, Duran J, et al. Alternative methods of titrating continuous positive airway pressure: a large multicenter study. Am J Respir Crit Care Med 2004; 170(11):1218–1224.
30. West SD, Jones DR, Stradling JR. Comparison of three ways to determine and deliver pressure during nasal CPAP therapy for obstructive sleep apnoea. Thorax 2006; 61(3):226–231.
31. Duong M, Jayaram L, Camfferman D, Catcheside P, Mykytyn I, McEvoy RD. Use of heated humidification during nasal CPAP titration in obstructive sleep apnoea syndrome. Eur Respir J 2005; 26(4):679–685.
32. Issa FG, Sullivan CE. The immediate effects of nasal continuous positive airway pressure treatment on sleep pattern in patients with obstructive sleep apnea syndrome. Electroencephalogr Clin Neurophysiol 1986; 63(1):10–17.
33. Parrino L, Thomas RJ, Smerieri A, Spaggiari MC, Felice AD, Terzano MG. Reorganization of sleep patterns in severe OSAS under prolonged CPAP treatment. Clin Neurophysiol 2005; 116(9):2228.
34. Condos R, Norman RG, Krishnasamy I, Peduzzi N, Goldring RM, Rapoport DM. Flow limitation as a noninvasive assessment of residual upper-airway resistance during continuous positive airway pressure therapy of obstructive sleep apnea. Am J Respir Crit Care Med 1994; 150(2):475–480.
35. Pevernagie DA, Shepard JW Jr. Relations between sleep stage, posture and effective nasal CPAP levels in OSA. Sleep 1992; 15(2):162–167.
36. Marrone O, Insalaco G, Bonsignore MR, Romano S, Salvaggio A, Bonsignore G. Sleep structure correlates of continuous positive airway pressure variations during application of an autotitrating continuous positive airway pressure machine in patients with obstructive sleep apnea syndrome. Chest 2002; 121(3):759–767.
37. Jokic R, Klimaszewski A, Sridhar G, Fitzpatrick MF. Continuous positive airway pressure requirement during the first month of treatment in patients with severe obstructive sleep apnea. Chest 1998; 114(4):1061–1069.

38. Willson G, Grunstein R, Doyle J, et al. Domiciliary use of autoset nasal continuous positive airway pressure (nCPAP): feasibility, efficacy and night to night variability. Sleep Res 1996; 25:210.
39. Miljeteig H, Hoffstein V. Determinants of continuous positive airway pressure level for treatment of obstructive sleep apnea. Am Rev Respir Dis 1993; 147(6 Pt 1):1526–1530.
40. Berry RB, Desa MM, Light RW. Effect of ethanol on the efficacy of nasal continuous positive airway pressure as a treatment for obstructive sleep apnea. Chest 1991; 99(2):339–343.
41. Becker HF, Piper AJ, Flynn WE, et al. Breathing during sleep in patients with nocturnal desaturation. Am J Respir Crit Care Med 1999; 159(1):112–118.
42. Sanders MH, Kern NB, Costantino JP, et al. Adequacy of prescribing positive airway pressure therapy by mask for sleep apnea on the basis of a partial-night trial. Am Rev Respir Dis 1993; 147(5):1169–1174.
43. McArdle N, Grove A, Devereux G, Mackay-Brown L, Mackay T, Douglas NJ. Split-night versus full-night studies for sleep apnoea/hypopnoea syndrome. Eur Respir J 2000; 15(4):670–675.
44. Hoffstein V, Mateika S. Predicting nasal continuous positive airway pressure. Am J Respir Crit Care Med 1994; 150(2):486–488.
45. Rosenthal L, Nykamp K, Guido P, et al. Daytime CPAP titration: a viable alternative for patients with severe obstructive sleep apnea. Chest 1998; 114(4):1056–1060.
46. Littner M, Hirshkowitz M, Davila D, et al. Practice parameters for the use of auto-titrating continuous positive airway pressure devices for titrating pressures and treating adult patients with obstructive sleep apnea syndrome. An American Academy of Sleep Medicine report. Sleep 2002; 25(2):143–147.
47. Krieger J, Sforza E, Petiau C, Weiss T. Simplified diagnostic procedure for obstructive sleep apnoea syndrome: lower subsequent compliance with CPAP. Eur Respir J 1998; 12(4):776–779.
48. Means MK, Edinger JD, Husain AM. CPAP compliance in sleep apnea patients with and without laboratory CPAP titration. Sleep Breath 2004; 8(1):7–14.
49. White DP, Gibb TJ. Evaluation of the Healthdyne NightWatch system to titrate CPAP in the home. Sleep 1998; 21(2):198–204.
50. Juhasz J, Schillen J, Urbigkeit A, Ploch T, Penzel T, Peter JH. Unattended continuous positive airway pressure titration. Clinical relevance and cardiorespiratory hazards of the method. Am J Respir Crit Care Med 1996; 154(2 Pt 1):359–365.
51. Engleman HM, Asgari-Jirhandeh N, McLeod AL, Ramsay CF, Deary IJ, Douglas NJ. Self-reported use of CPAP and benefits of CPAP therapy: a patient survey. Chest 1996; 109(6):1470–1476.
52. Kuzniar TJ, Gruber B, Mutlu GM. Cerebrospinal fluid leak and meningitis associated with nasal continuous positive airway pressure therapy. Chest 2005; 128(3):1882–1884.
53. Strollo PJ Jr, Sanders MH, Atwood CW. Positive pressure therapy. Clin Chest Med 1998; 19(1):55–68.
54. Pepin JL, Leger P, Veale D, Langevin B, Robert D, Levy P. Side effects of nasal continuous positive airway pressure in sleep apnea syndrome. Study of 193 patients in two French sleep centers. Chest 1995; 107(2):375–381.
55. Richards GN, Cistulli PA, Ungar RG, Berthon-Jones M, Sullivan CE. Mouth leak with nasal continuous positive airway pressure increases nasal airway resistance. Am J Respir Crit Care Med 1996; 154(1):182–186.
56. de Oliveira LR, Albertini Yagi CS, Figueiredo AC, Saldiva PHN, Lorenzi-Filho G. Short-term effects of nCPAP on nasal mucociliary clearance and mucus transportability in healthy subjects. Respir Med 2006; 100(1):183.
57. Schrodter S, Biermann E, Halata Z. Histologic evaluation of nasal epithelium of the middle turbinate in untreated OSAS patients and during nCPAP therapy. Rhinology 2004; 42(3):153–157.
58. Bossi R, Piatti G, Roma E, Ambrosetti U. Effects of long-term nasal continuous positive airway pressure therapy on morphology, function, and mucociliary clearance of nasal epithelium in patients with obstructive sleep apnea syndrome. Laryngoscope 2004; 114(8):1431–1434.
59. Martins De Araujo MT, Vieira SB, Vasquez EC, Fleury B. Heated humidification or face mask to prevent upper airway dryness during continuous positive airway pressure therapy. Chest 2000; 117(1):142–147.

60. Mador MJ, Krauza M, Pervez A, Pierce D, Braun M. Effect of heated humidification on compliance and quality of life in patients with sleep apnea using nasal continuous positive airway pressure. Chest 2005; 128(4):2151–2158.

61. Friedman M, Tanyeri H, Lim JW, Landsberg R, Vaidyanathan K, Caldarelli D. Effect of improved nasal breathing on obstructive sleep apnea. Otolaryngol Head Neck Surg 2000; 122(1):71–74.

62. Beecroft J, Zanon S, Lukic D, Hanly P. Oral continuous positive airway pressure for sleep apnea: effectiveness, patient preference, and adherence. Chest 2003; 124(6):2200–2208.

63. Stauffer JL, Fayter N, MacLurg BJ. Conjunctivitis from nasal CPAP apparatus. Chest 1984; 86(5):802.

64. Bucca C, Carossa S, Pivetti S, Gai V, Rolla G, Preti G. Edentulism and worsening of obstructive sleep apnoea. Lancet 1999; 353(9147):121–122.

65. Pressman MR, Peterson DD, Meyer TJ, Harkins JP, Gurijala L. Ramp abuse. A novel form of patient noncompliance to administration of nasal continuous positive airway pressure for treatment of obstructive sleep apnea. Am J Respir Crit Care Med 1995; 151(5):1632–1634.

66. Reeves-Hoche MK, Hudgel DW, Meck R, Witteman R, Ross A, Zwillich CW. Continuous versus bilevel positive airway pressure for obstructive sleep apnea. Am J Respir Crit Care Med 1995; 151(2 Pt 1):443–449.

67. Gay PC, Herold DL, Olson EJ. A randomized, double-blind clinical trial comparing continuous positive airway pressure with a novel bilevel pressure system for treatment of obstructive sleep apnea syndrome. Sleep 2003; 26(7):864–869.

68. Aloia MS, Stanchina M, Arnedt JT, Malhotra A, Millman RP. Treatment adherence and outcomes in flexible vs standard continuous positive airway pressure therapy. Chest 2005; 127(6):2085–2093.

69. Ruyak P, Stanchina M, Arnedt J, et al. The efficacy of C-Flex at improving treatment adherence in obstructive sleep apnea (OSA). Sleep 2005; 28(Abstract suppl):A170.

70. Aloia M, Arnedt J, Zimmerman M, et al. Combined therapy to improve adherence to CPAP. Sleep 2005; 28(Abstract suppl):A192.

71. Rosenthal L, Hansbrough J, Zachek M, et al. International multi-center long-term study of treatment satisfaction and compliance in OSA: CPAP with expiratory pressure relief versus conventional CPAP. Sleep 2005; 28(Abstract suppl):A180.

72. Duntley S, Morrissey A, Doerr C, Svoboda J, Duntley L, Kampelman J. Flexible CPAP with expiratory pressure relief: an in-laboratory, polysomnographic comparison with conventional CPAP. Sleep 2005; 28(Abstract suppl):A182.

73. Rosenthal L, Hansbrough J, Zachek M, et al. International multi-center CPAP study of split-night titration and expiratory pressure relief—long-term effect on compliance and subjective satisfaction. Sleep 2005; 28(Abstract suppl):A210.

74. Lojander J, Maasilta P, Partinen M, Brander PE, Salmi T, Lehtonen H. Nasal-CPAP, surgery, and conservative management for treatment of obstructive sleep apnea syndrome. A randomized study. Chest 1996; 110(1):114–119.

75. Henke KG, Grady JJ, Kuna ST. Effect of nasal continuous positive airway pressure on neuropsychological function in sleep apnea-hypopnea syndrome. A randomized, placebo-controlled trial. Am J Respir Crit Care Med 2001; 163(4):911–917.

76. Barnes M, McEvoy RD, Banks S, et al. Efficacy of positive airway pressure and oral appliance in mild to moderate obstructive sleep apnea. Am J Respir Crit Care Med 2004; 170(6):656–664.

77. Becker HF, Jerrentrup A, Ploch T, et al. Effect of nasal continuous positive airway pressure treatment on blood pressure in patients with obstructive sleep apnea. Circulation 2003; 107(1):68–73.

78. Monasterio C, Vidal S, Duran J, et al. Effectiveness of continuous positive airway pressure in mild sleep apnea-hypopnea syndrome. Am J Respir Crit Care Med 2001; 164(6):939–943.

79. Sundaram S, Bridgman SA, Lim J, Lasserson TJ. Surgery for obstructive sleep apnoea. Cochrane Database Syst Rev 2005; (4):CD001004.

80. Grunstein RR, Handelsman DJ, Lawrence SJ, Blackwell C, Caterson ID, Sullivan CE. Neuroendocrine dysfunction in sleep apnea: reversal by continuous positive airways pressure therapy. J Clin Endocrinol Metab 1989; 68(2):352–358.

81. Hers V, Liistro G, Dury M, Collard P, Aubert G, Rodenstein DO. Residual effect of nCPAP applied for part of the night in patients with obstructive sleep apnoea. Eur Respir J 1997; 10(5):973–976.

82. Van Dongen HP, Maislin G, Dinges DF. Dealing with inter-individual differences in the temporal dynamics of fatigue and performance: importance and techniques. Aviat Space Environ Med 2004; 75(3 suppl):A147–A154.
83. Rauscher H, Popp W, Wanke T, Zwick H. Acceptance of CPAP therapy for sleep apnea. Chest 1991; 100(4):1019–1023.
84. Gay P, Weaver T, Loube D, Iber C. Evaluation of positive airway pressure treatment for sleep related breathing disorders in adults. A review by the positive airway pressue task force of the Standards of Practice Committee of the American Academy of Sleep Medicine. Sleep 2006; 29(3):381–401.
85. Grunstein R. Chapter 89. Continuous Positive Airway Pressure Treatment for Obstructive Sleep Apnea-Hypopnea Syndrome, in Principles and Practice of Sleep Medicine. 4th ed. Philadelphia: Elsevier Saunders, 2005.
86. Kribbs NB, Pack AI, Kline LR, et al. Objective measurement of patterns of nasal CPAP use by patients with obstructive sleep apnea. Am Rev Respir Dis 1993; 147(4):887–895.
87. Engleman HM, Martin SE, Deary IJ, Douglas NJ. Effect of continuous positive airway pressure treatment on daytime function in sleep apnoea/hypopnoea syndrome. Lancet 1994; 343(8897):572–575.
88. Kribbs NB, Pack AI, Kline LR, et al. Effects of one night without nasal CPAP treatment on sleep and sleepiness in patients with obstructive sleep apnea. Am Rev Respir Dis 1993; 147(5):1162–1168.
89. Meurice JC, Dore P, Paquereau J, et al. Predictive factors of long-term compliance with nasal continuous positive airway pressure treatment in sleep apnea syndrome. Chest 1994; 105(2):429–433.
90. Grunstein R. Investigation and treatment of sleep apnea in Australia 1991–95. Am J Respir Crit Care Med 1997; 155:A133.
91. Weaver TE, Kribbs NB, Pack AI, et al. Night-to-night variability in CPAP use over the first three months of treatment. Sleep 1997; 20(4):278–283.
92. McArdle N, Devereux G, Heidarnejad H, Engleman HM, Mackay TW, Douglas NJ. Long-term use of CPAP therapy for sleep apnea/hypopnea syndrome. Am J Respir Crit Care Med 1999; 159(4 Pt 1):1108–1114.
93. Jean Wiese H, Boethel C, Phillips B, Wilson JF, Peters J, Viggiano T. CPAP compliance: video education may help! Sleep Med 2005; 6(2):171–174.
94. Haniffa M, Lasserson TJ, Smith I. Interventions to improve compliance with continuous positive airway pressure for obstructive sleep apnoea. Cochrane Database Syst Rev 2004; (4):CD003531.
95. Chasens ER, Pack AI, Maislin G, Dinges DF, Weaver TE. Claustrophobia and adherence to CPAP treatment. West J Nurs Res 2005; 27(3):307–321.
96. Kjelsberg FN, Ruud EA, Stavem K. Predictors of symptoms of anxiety and depression in obstructive sleep apnea. Sleep Med 2005; 6(4):341–346.
97. Bachour A, Maasilta P. Mouth breathing compromises adherence to nasal continuous positive airway pressure therapy. Chest 2004; 126(4):1248–1254.
98. Barbe F, Mayoralas LR, Duran J, et al. Treatment with continuous positive airway pressure is not effective in patients with sleep apnea but no daytime sleepiness. a randomized, controlled trial. Ann Intern Med 2001; 134(11):1015–1023.
99. Patel SR, White DP, Malhotra A, Stanchina ML, Ayas NT. Continuous positive airway pressure therapy for treating sleepiness in a diverse population with obstructive sleep apnea: results of a meta-analysis. Arch Intern Med 2003; 163(5):565–571.
100. Bennett LS, Langford BA, Stradling JR, Davies RJ. Sleep fragmentation indices as predictors of daytime sleepiness and nCPAP response in obstructive sleep apnea. Am J Respir Crit Care Med 1998; 158(3):778–786.
101. Drake CL, Day R, Hudgel D, et al. Sleep during titration predicts continuous positive airway pressure compliance. Sleep 2003; 26(3):308–311.
102. Hoy CJ, Vennelle M, Kingshott RN, Engleman HM, Douglas NJ. Can intensive support improve continuous positive airway pressure use in patients with the sleep apnea/hypopnea syndrome? Am J Respir Crit Care Med 1999; 159(4 Pt 1):1096–1100.
103. Grote L, Hedner J, Grunstein R, Kraiczi H. Therapy with nCPAP: incomplete elimination of sleep related breathing disorder. Eur Respir J 2000; 16(5):921–927.
104. Stepnowsky CJ Jr, Moore PJ. Nasal CPAP treatment for obstructive sleep apnea: developing a new perspective on dosing strategies and compliance. J Psychosom Res 2003; 54(6):599–605.

105. White J, Cates C, Wright J. Continuous positive airways pressure for obstructive sleep apnoea. Cochrane Database Syst Rev 2002; (2):CD001106.
106. Pepperell JC, Ramdassingh-Dow S, Crosthwaite N, et al. Ambulatory blood pressure after therapeutic and subtherapeutic nasal continuous positive airway pressure for obstructive sleep apnoea: a randomised parallel trial. Lancet 2002; 359(9302):204–210.
107. Chong M, Ayalon L, Marler M, et al. Continuous positive airway pressure reduces subjective daytime sleepiness in patients with mild to moderate Alzheimer's disease with sleep disordered breathing. J Am Geriatr Soc 2006; 54(5):777–781.
108. Schwartz DJ, Kohler WC, Karatinos G. Symptoms of depression in individuals with obstructive sleep apnea may be amenable to treatment with continuous positive airway pressure. Chest 2005; 128(3):1304–1309.
109. Barnes M, Houston D, Worsnop CJ, et al. A randomized controlled trial of continuous positive airway pressure in mild obstructive sleep apnea. Am J Respir Crit Care Med 2002; 165(6):773–780.
110. Marshall NS, Neill AM, Campbell AJ, Sheppard DS. Randomised controlled crossover trial of humidified continuous positive airway pressure in mild obstructive sleep apnoea. Thorax 2005; 60(5):427–432.
111. Marshall NS, Barnes M, Travier N, et al. Continuous positive airway pressure reduces daytime sleepiness in mild-moderate obstructive sleep apnoea: meta-analysis. Thorax 2006; 61(5):430–434.
112. Yaggi HK, Concato J, Kernan WN, Lichtman JH, Brass LM, Mohsenin V. Obstructive sleep apnea as a risk factor for stroke and death. N Engl J Med 2005; 353(19):2034–2041.
113. Doherty LS, Kiely JL, Swan V, McNicholas WT. Long-term effects of nasal continuous positive airway pressure therapy on cardiovascular outcomes in sleep apnea syndrome. Chest 2005; 127(6):2076–2084.
114. Marin JM, Carrizo SJ, Vicente E, Agusti AG. Long-term cardiovascular outcomes in men with obstructive sleep apnoea–hypopnoea with or without treatment with continuous positive airway pressure: an observational study. Lancet 2005; 365(9464):1046–1053.
115. Martinez-Garcia MA, Galiano-Blancart R, Roman-Sanchez P, Soler-Cataluna J-J, Cabero-Salt L, Salcedo-Maiques E. Continuous positive airway pressure treatment in sleep apnea prevents new vascular events after ischemic stroke. Chest 2005; 128(4):2123–2129.
116. Norman D, Loredo JS, Nelesen RA, et al. Effects of continuous positive airway pressure versus supplemental oxygen on 24-hour ambulatory blood pressure. Hypertension 2006; 47(5):840–845.
117. Narkiewicz K, Kato M, Phillips BG, Pesek CA, Davison DE, Somers VK. Nocturnal continuous positive airway pressure decreases daytime sympathetic traffic in obstructive sleep apnea. Circulation 1999; 100(23):2332–2335.
118. Robinson GV, Smith DM, Langford BA, Davies RJO, Stradling JR. CPAP does not reduce blood pressure in non-sleepy hypertensive OSA patients. Eur Respir J 2006; 09031936.06.00062805.
119. Dursunoglu N, Dursunoglu D, Cuhadaroglu C, Kilicaslan Z. Acute effects of automated continuous positive airway pressure on blood pressure in patients with sleep apnea and hypertension. Respiration 2005; 72(2):150–155.
120. Simantirakis EN, Schiza SI, Marketou ME, et al. Severe bradyarrhythmias in patients with sleep apnoea: the effect of continuous positive airway pressure treatment: a long-term evaluation using an insertable loop recorder. Eur Heart J 2004; 25(12):1070–1076.
121. Blyton DM, Sullivan CE, Edwards N. Reduced nocturnal cardiac output associated with preeclampsia is minimized with the use of nocturnal nasal CPAP. Sleep 2004; 27(1):79–84.
122. Pinet C, Orehek J. CPAP suppression of awake right-to-left shunting through patent foramen ovale in a patient with obstructive sleep apnoea. Thorax 2005; 60(10):880–881.
123. Javaheri S, Parker TJ, Liming JD, et al. Sleep apnea in 81 ambulatory male patients with stable heart failure. Types and their prevalences, consequences, and presentations. Circulation 1998; 97(21):2154–2159.
124. Bradley TD, Floras JS. Sleep apnea and heart failure: Part I: obstructive sleep apnea. Circulation 2003; 107(12):1671–1678.
125. Kaneko Y, Floras JS, Usui K, et al. Cardiovascular effects of continuous positive airway pressure in patients with heart failure and obstructive sleep apnea. N Engl J Med 2003; 348(13):1233–1241.

126. Mansfield DR, Gollogly NC, Kaye DM, Richardson M, Bergin P, Naughton MT. Controlled trial of continuous positive airway pressure in obstructive sleep apnea and heart failure. Am J Respir Crit Care Med 2004; 169(3):361–366.
127. Bradley TD, Floras JS. Sleep apnea and heart failure: Part II: central sleep apnea. Circulation 2003; 107(13):1822–1826.
128. Bradley TD, Logan AG, Kimoff RJ, et al. Continuous positive airway pressure for central sleep apnea and heart failure. N Engl J Med 2005; 353(19):2025–2033.
129. Somers VK. Sleep—a new cardiovascular frontier. N Engl J Med 2005; 353(19):2070–2073.

7 Bilevel Pressure and Adaptive Servo-Ventilation for Obstructive and Complex Sleep Apnea

Peter C. Gay
Pulmonary, Critical Care, and Sleep Medicine, Mayo Clinic College of Medicine, Rochester, Minnesota, U.S.A.

BACKGROUND

The clinical defect in patients with obstructive sleep apnea (OSA) was primarily described as an inspiratory event four decades ago by Gastaut (1) as both airway closure and increased effort became evident during this phase of breathing. Other earlier studies noted increased total pulmonary resistance in the breaths preceding an apneic event and also reported that airway disturbances occur during both the expiratory and the inspiratory phases of ventilation (2,3). It is known that there must be a balance of opposing forces that either support pharyngeal patency or encourage the pharynx to collapse (4). The genioglossus and other major pharyngeal dilator muscles are phasically activated muscles that show a burst of inspiratory activity followed by a reduction in tone during exhalation. During early exhalation, the elevated lung recoil pressure maintains pharyngeal patency but at end-exhalation when positive pressure is at a minimum, the pharynx is most susceptible to collapse (5). Other elegant imaging studies have also revealed that there is a crucial timing for positive airway pressure (PAP) therapy in patients with OSA and occurs most critically at the end of exhalation (6). The above studies make it easy to recognize that there are important factors occurring throughout all phases of respiration.

It should have been expected that PAP therapy would evolve to include targeted treatment of both inspiratory and expiratory events to eliminate apneas and hypopneas. There are several types of airflow generators that are capable of specifically altering pressure during the inspiratory and expiratory phase including volume or pressure targeted intensive care unit (ICU) ventilators, pressure support ventilation (PSV), proportional assist ventilation (PAV), flexible continuous positive airway pressure (CPAP), adaptive servo-ventilation (ASV), and conventional bilevel PAP (BPAP). Although ICU ventilators, PSV, and PAV have been used to treat patients with OSA, these modes are generally not used or unavailable in the United States and flexible CPAP is discussed elsewhere in this book (see Chapter 6) (7). It has also been suggested that accommodating to flow-dependent changes with PAP designed to adjust proportionately during the respiratory cycle may also be useful but this is also just experimental (8). This chapter will focus on the use of BPAP and ASV for the treatment of patients with primarily OSA as the major concern for their sleep-disordered breathing (SDB).

HISTORICAL

Although it was recognized that the forces governing inspiratory and expiratory flow are of different magnitudes, Sanders and Kern (9) were the first to hypothesize that a different level of expiratory PAP (EPAP) than inspiratory PAP (IPAP) could be used to eliminate SDB events and introduced the first bilevel device for OSA patients called BiPAP® (Respironics, Inc., Murrysville, Pennsylvania, U.S.). They demonstrated resolution of residual hypopneic events with increased IPAP once an adequate EPAP level was established to open the airway as shown in Figure 1. During a comparative evaluation of CPAP versus BiPAP, this study of 13 OSA patients revealed that independent adjustment of EPAP and IPAP could reduce the mean apneic events from 55.5/hour to 1.8/hour and increase the minimum percent oxygen saturation from 47.1 to 87.2. This occurred at a reduced mean EPAP of 8.9 compared to the CPAP pressure of 14 cm H_2O. They concluded that BiPAP may reduce the adverse effects associated with nasal CPAP therapy and possibly improve long-term adherence with PAP therapy.

TITRATION

Although it has never been clearly proven as to precisely how the titration of BPAP should best proceed, the Sander's protocol proposed a workable methodology as shown in Figure 2. A critical opening pressure with EPAP must first be established to create airway patency and then titration of the IPAP level can progress to eliminate whatever degree of hypopnea or flow limitation still exists. The importance of obtaining an adequate EPAP level was highlighted in an anatomic study performed in eight awake patients with OSA using computed tomography to measure minimum and maximum pharyngeal cross-sectional areas of the velopharynx and hypopharynx (10). The pharyngeal areas were measured while breathing without and with either 12 cm H_2O CPAP or BPAP set at an IPAP = 12 cm H_2O and EPAP = 6 cm H_2O. Compared with normal unassisted breathing, CPAP showed a significant increase in the minimum area of both the velopharynx and the hypopharynx but BPAP did not. Although they did not do their evaluation during sleep, they concluded that CPAP at 12 cm H_2O

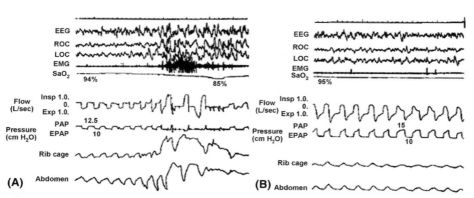

FIGURE 1 Representative tracing demonstrating elimination of apnea in the same patient by increasing inspiratory positive airway pressure (IPAP) during nasal bilevel positive airway pressure (BiPAP®) therapy. (**A**) Obstructive apnea during nasal BiPAP® (IPAP = 12.5 cm H_2O, expiratory positive airway pressure = 10 cm H_2O). (**B**) Elimination of obstructive apnea after increasing IPAP to 15 cm H_2O. *Abbreviations*: EEG, electroencephalogram; EMG, electromyogram; ROC and LOC, right and left outer canthi (eye movements), respectively; SaO_2, oxygen saturation. *Source*: From Ref. 9.

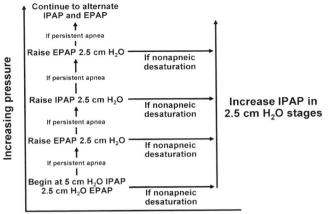

FIGURE 2   Algorithm for adjustment of inspiratory positive airway pressure and expiratory positive airway pressure during the trial of nasal bilevel positive airway pressure (BiPAP®). *Source*: From Ref. 9.

is more effective in splinting the pharynx open than BPAP in patients with OSA. Another study of 10 selected patients with OSA requiring ≥ 10 cm H_2O of CPAP failed to show optimal resolution of SDB at any level of IPAP until a critical level of EPAP was achieved indicating a clear need to select an adequate EPAP level (11).

An alternative approach to BPAP titration has been to optimize all SDB events with CPAP and then to reduce both the EPAP and IPAP as allowed taking advantage of the natural hysteresis that occurs during a typical CPAP titration episode. In one study, a small but significant reduction in the optimal CPAP level occurred when a downward titration followed an initial titration procedure (12).

SELECTION OF PATIENTS
Severe Obesity
The importance of recognizing and addressing the differences in respiratory system loading that occurs during the inspiratory phase in specific subtypes of patients has helped guide which patients might best be considered for BPAP as well. The impact of obesity on the mechanical loading of the respiratory system, neuromuscular control, and the pathogenesis of apnea and related hypoventilation has been known for many years. This issue was more precisely studied in three groups of severely obese patients, who were eucapnic obese without OSA (O), eucapnic obese with OSA (OSA), or hypercapnic obese with sleep apnea (OH), and were compared to nonobese volunteers (NO) who were subjected to abdominal mass loading (13). This was assessed with diaphragmatic electromyogram (EMGdi), a measure of muscle activation, and mouth occlusion pressure (P0.15), an assessment of mechanical drive, during CO_2 stimulation. The authors showed that P0.15 responses were decreased in OSA and OH but the EMGdi responses did not differ from the control subjects. However, when the NO control subjects were subjected to mass loading, the EMGdi and P0.15 responses increased. Their findings showed that both OSA and OH patients did not develop the expected increase in respiratory muscle response for a given level of activation and the impaired mass load compensation predisposes obese patients to develop hypercapnia. These kinds of observations may help

explain why the early BiPAP study focused on patients with a mean body mass index (BMI) of 57.4 kg/m^2 even though they were normocapnic and why severe obesity has emerged as an independent predictor of failed CPAP therapy (9,14).

The unloading of inspiratory muscle activity with BPAP measured as diaphragmatic pressure time product was studied in 18 obese subjects with a BMI $\geq$ 40 kg/m^2 including five healthy controls with simple obesity (SO), seven patients with OSA, and six with obesity-hypoventilation syndrome (OHS) (15). Although the overall ventilation as measured by end-tidal carbon dioxide with BPAP was not changed in SO and OSA, it was decreased in OHS, while the inspiratory muscle activity was reduced by at least 40% in all groups. The authors concluded that BPAP may be particularly effective for improving ventilation in patients with OHS by unloading the inspiratory muscles.

Hypercapnia and Other Factors

Other studies have specifically targeted the presence of hypercapnia in patients with severe OSA as a reason to justify short- or long-term treatment with modes enabled to deliver more aggressive ventilatory capability (13,16,17). In most cases these studies showed marked improvement in daytime $PaCO_2$ levels with treatment of accompanying nocturnal hypoventilation with BPAP, which in some cases allowed resumption of CPAP treatment alone for satisfactory response to the underlying OSA. Patient adherence remained high in these patients (18).

In order to assess the reasons why a BPAP device was provided to a group of moderate-to-severe OSA patients, a study was done to investigate the frequency of BPAP prescription when CPAP was ineffective or not tolerated during titration (19). Of 286 consecutive adult patients referred to two sleep labs, 130 patients were enrolled and 105 (84% males) completed the study. A split-night (diagnostic and therapeutic) polysomnogram (PSG) was done, followed by another PSG with BPAP if CPAP was not tolerated, or failed to correct sleep-related breathing (SRB) abnormalities. There were 24 patients (23% overall) that received BPAP with the highest prevalence (11 of 17) in patients with OSA associated with OHS. The BPAP treated patients were more obese, hypercapnic, had severe SRB desaturations, and also had more obstruction, restriction, and hypoxia.

The prevalence and mechanism of hypercapnia in morbidly obese patients were investigated in a selected group of 285 patients presented to a sleep laboratory without other significant comorbid diseases. There were 89 morbidly obese patients (31.2%) who had a BMI $\geq$ 40 kg/m^2 and surprisingly 59.6% were predominately females (20). This group was further divided into three subgroups who were normocapnic without OSA, normocapnic with OSA, and lastly hypercapnic ($PaCO_2 \geq$ 45 mmHg) with OSA. Their results showed that hypercapnia was found in 27% of the morbidly obese subjects (who were predominately males) but only in 11% of the nonmorbidly obese patients (P < 0.01). Several characteristics were more common in the patients with hypercapnia and OSA than patients with or without OSA including significantly more restriction based on a mean total lung capacity (%predicted) of 63.8% $\pm$ 16.4%, a higher respiratory disturbance index of 46.3 $\pm$ 26.9 events/hour, a longer total sleep time with $SpO_2 < 90\%$ ($TSTSpO_2 < 90\%$) of 63.4 $\pm$ 33.9 minutes, and a lower rapid eye movement (REM) sleep at 9.5 $\pm$ 1.2%. Their conclusion about important factors associated with hypercapnia and OSA allowed them to construct a predictive model for diurnal hypercapnia: $PaCO_2 = -0.03$ FVC %predicted $- 0.05$ FEV1 %predicted $+ 0.036$ $TSTSpO_2 < 90\%$ $- PaO_2 + 57.13$ ($r^2 = 0.44$).

Another small study investigated whether a variety of factors were associated with failure of CPAP therapy to resolve the apnea–hypopnea index (AHI) to < 5 or mean SaO2 > 90% (14). This study of 13 patients with OSA (Group A) over a 15-month period compared to an age- and AHI-matched control group (Group B) successfully treated by CPAP used logistic regression analysis to identify factors associated with initial failure to CPAP. The Group A versus Group B patients were significantly more obese (mean BMI = 44.2 kg/m^2 vs. 31.2 kg/m^2; $P < 0.001$), hypoxic at rest ($P < 0.001$), and at exercise ($P < 0.005$). Hypercapnia at rest ($P < 0.001$) and worsening during exercise was also more likely, and Group A patients also spent significantly ($P < 0.0001$) more time with oxygen saturation < 90%, which was the only factor independently associated with the initial failure of CPAP [odds ratio (OR) 1.13; 95% confidence interval (CI) 1.0–1.2]. The patients' awake blood gases proved that both daytime hypoxemia and hypercapnia improved significantly ($P < 0.05$) after three months of treatment with BPAP.

ADHERENCE

CPAP can produce objective and subjective improvements in patients with OSA and other types of SDB (21–23). Despite its demonstrable efficacy, many OSA patients have difficulty with long-term acceptance of CPAP (24,25). Several intervention strategies have been suggested to improve adherence to CPAP, including use of specialized education and follow-up programs (26,27) and added airway humidification (28). Others have suggested that modifications of the airflow delivery pattern, as with continuously auto-adjusting CPAP (29) or bilevel devices capable of varying inspiratory and expiratory levels (9), may also boost adherence in more difficult-to-treat OSA patients.

As these earlier reports indicated, there was a general reduction in the mean effective PAP level using BPAP compared to CPAP (3,9). It was therefore thought that bilevel devices might prove to be a benefit for improvement in adherence to PAP in OSA patients. There have been two high-level evidence randomized trials that compared the use of BPAP versus CPAP for OSA patients who were first time users without complicating comorbid medical problems. The first study randomized 83 OSA patients to receive either CPAP or BPAP with a primary endpoint of adherence based on mean machine timer hours of CPAP (30). A total of 62 patients were evaluated and followed for one year and of these, 26 received BPAP and 36 CPAP pressures. The groups did not differ for BPAP versus CPAP by age (48 ± 1 years vs. 46 ± 1 years) or BMI (40 ± 1 kg/m^2 vs. 39 ± 1 kg/m^2), but were different by gender (65.5% vs. 52.8% males). Over the 12-month period, the mean machine timer hours of CPAP versus bilevel therapy were not different at 5.0 ± 0.19 (SEM) versus 4.9 ± 0.23 hours per night. There was also no difference between high and low hourly users for the CPAP or BPAP pressures required during therapy. These patients had similar percentages of time that the machine was running at the prescribed effective pressure at 80% in the CPAP group and 82% in the BPAP users with both groups reporting an equal number of complaints with respect to mask discomfort, machine noise, and nasal stuffiness.

The second high-level evidence trial studied newly diagnosed OSA patients without coexisting daytime respiratory disease and compared CPAP with a bilevel device that also employed a prototype flow feature of the presently available Bi-Flex® device (Respironics, Inc., Murrysville, Pennsylvania, U.S.) (31). The primary endpoint was the percentage of nights with at least four hours of use and hours of use per night after 30 days treatment. This was based on objective machine-determined measurement of time at effective pressure beginning after diagnosis and titration by split-night polysomnography (PSG) in a sleep laboratory. There were no significant baseline group differences for the 27 adults (22 men) in age, BMI, AHI (mean ± SD, CPAP vs. BPAP group of 46.1 ± 23.1 events/hour vs. 41.8 ± 25.8 events/hour, respectively), CPAP requirement, or scores on the Epworth sleepiness scale and Functional Outcomes of Sleep Questionnaire. The percentage of nights with ≥ 4 hours/night use was high in both groups but was not significantly different (CPAP vs. BPAP = 80.5 ± 24% vs. 77.6 ± 24.8%). In both of these studies, the BPAP appeared to be as effective as CPAP for the treatment of OSA but offered no advantages in patients receiving first-time therapy for OSA.

A randomized controlled trial published in 2005 investigated whether BPAP with Bi-Flex could prove valuable in patients who were considered nonadherent to CPAP therapy (32). The unique design had two phases that first attempted to improve adherence to a treatment threshold of four hours per night of CPAP. There were 204 adult patients diagnosed with OSA (AHI ≥ 10) by PSG within 24 months who had been titrated to an optimal CPAP level but were not able to adhere to regular CPAP use (nonresponders) at a mean treatment time of 254 ± 333 (SD) days. Patients were questioned about various complaints and these were addressed with a systematic conventional intervention program including further education, CPAP desensitization as needed, alternative mask or resizing, and heated humidification. After two more weeks of CPAP therapy there were 24% (49 patients) who became responders (≥ 4 hours/night), 76% (155 patients) who were still nonresponders or who withdrew. The nonresponders who agreed to proceed on to phase 2 then had a full-night PSG retitration and blinded randomization to either CPAP or Bi-Flex for three months. In the 104 patients initiating the trial, there were no significant differences in baseline characteristics of the Bi-Flex versus CPAP groups for age (51.9 ± 11.3 years vs. 52.5 ± 11.3 years), sex (65% vs. 72% males), BMI (33.4 ± 7.9 kg/m^2 vs. 32.5 ± 6.3 kg/m^2), and AHI (40.4 ± 23.4 events/hour vs. 44.0 ± 26.1 events/hour). At three months, there was a trend to a higher success rate with Bi-Flex versus CPAP treatment (49% vs. 28.3% of patients using PAP therapy > 4 hours/night; $p < 0.05$) but the overall success rate for either PAP treatment was low at near 40%. The authors found no strong clinical predictors to distinguish patients in either arm who become adherent (responders) after conventional intervention techniques and concluded that sleep specialists must be very aggressive at achieving initial CPAP adherence as subsequent efforts to achieve optimal adherence to PAP therapy are less fruitful but consideration could be given to repeat PSG and use of alternative modes of flow delivery to further encourage patients to use PAP treatment.

COMPLEX SLEEP APNEA

Central and obstructive apneas may occur in the same individual, either simultaneously within a single breath as a mixed apnea, or as sequential breathing events (33). The majority of OSA patients can be expected to respond favorably to CPAP but CPAP often initially exaggerates central sleep apnea (CSA) and some patients identified as having OSA, develop frequent central apneas and/or Cheyne-Stokes respiratory (CSR) pattern after application of CPAP. This is an increasingly recognized but not new clinical problem encountered when patients with significant OSA develop CSA when exposed to CPAP (34,35). These patients that develop new or very prominent CSA during CPAP titration are now referred to as complex sleep apnea (CompSA) and from a consecutive series of 133 patients referred to a sleep lab for OSA, 34 (25.6%) proved to have CompSA (36).

In this study, the mean age (near 55 years) and total diagnostic AHI (near 30 events/hour) were similar between the groups but there were a few distinguishing features between the patients with OSA versus CompSA. The CompSA patients were more likely to be males (82.4% vs. 63.9%; p = 0.03) and the OSA patients tended to be slightly heavier (36 ± 10.3 kg/m^2 vs. 33 ± 5.9 kg/m^2; $p < 0.03$). By definition, CompSA patients had a significantly higher AHI during a standard CPAP titration (CompSA vs. OSA AHI on CPAP = 24.6 ± 21.6 events/hour vs. 2.1 ± 2.7 events/hour; $p<0.0001$) with most or all the residual difference related to the central apneas that emerged on CPAP (19.4 ± 19.0 vs. 2.1 ± 2.7 central events/hour; $p < 0.0001$). In a different investigation selecting patients who were chosen to undergo BPAP for a variety of reasons, many patients showed a CompSA like response to BPAP (rarely was a backup rate added) but it was not possible to discern an incidence estimate from the data provided (37).

Treatment of Complex Sleep Apnea with Bilevel Positive Airway Pressure Vs. Adaptive Servo-Ventilation

BPAP and ASV have been shown to improve SDB in patients with CSA (38). The best approach for treatment of CompSA patients remains unclear but one study pursued this issue comparing the response for both BPAP and the newly approved VPAP Adapt™, Adapt Servo Ventilator or ASV (ResMed, Poway, CA) (39). This study investigated 21 adult patients (95% male) with CSA/CSR mixed apnea or CompSA who had previously undergone diagnostic PSG and titration with PAP in a randomized crossover design. Patients with a diagnostic AHI = 54.7 ± 23.8 events/hour, mean age and BMI of 65 ± 12.4 (SD) years and 31.0 ± 4.9 kg/m^2, respectively, were randomly assigned initially to either BPAP or ASV during two full-night PSG studies. Following previously attempted optimal titration with CPAP, the CompSA patients (n = 15) had a mean AHI > 30 but with either BPAP or ASV the AHI improved markedly from baseline to 6.2 ± 7.6 events/hour or 0.8 ± 2.4 events/hour, respectively. The treatment arms were different; however based on the preselected endpoints of the AHI and respiratory arousal index proving to be significantly superior for ASV ($p<0.02$). The authors concluded that both BPAP and ASV seem to be effective in the acute setting for treatment of SDB in patients with CompSA and far more efficacious than CPAP alone but the CompSA patients seemed to respond optimally to ASV. A classic example of a CompSA patient response at baseline, treated with CPAP, and then the improvement with ASV can been seen in Figures 3 to 5, respectively.

REIMBURSEMENT CRITERIA

The delivery of appropriate treatment for any condition may at times become problematic if coverage criteria are not met or are not well-documented for the individual patient. This is especially true in the world of SDB for Medicare patients with respect to PAP therapy. There are separate criteria specifically for BPAP or in Center for Medicare and Medicaid (CMS) vernacular, respiratory assist devices. The coverage criteria are divided into four categories but two of these related to patients with either neuromuscular or chronic obstructive lung disease are not pertinent for this chapter. The specifics can be obtained from any regional durable medical equipment regional carrier (DMERC) web site (40). The new regulations released in March 2006 and retroactive to January 1, 2006 recognize two basic pathways for BPAP treatment

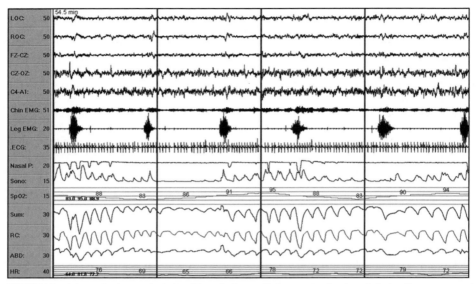

FIGURE 3 A two-minute epoch during Stage 2 sleep with frequent episodes of obstructive apnea and oxygen desaturation. Incidental periodic limb movements are also noted in leg electromyogram channel. *Abbreviations*: ABD, abdominal plethysmogram; C4-A1, right central-left reference EEG; CZ-OZ, midline central-occipital EEG; ECG, electrocardiogram; EEG, electroencephalogram; EMG, electromyogram; FZ-CZ, midline frontal-central EEG; HR, heart rate; LOC and ROC, left and right outer canthi (eye movements), respectively; Nasal P, nasal pressure via transducer; RC, rib cage plethysmogram; Sono, sonogram (snoring intensity); SpO₂, oxygen saturation; Sum, plethysmogram summed signal.

coverage. The simplest avenue to BPAP is for OSA patients who have a "facility-based" diagnostic PSG and meet criteria for CPAP treatment; yet, CPAP "has been tried and proven ineffective." Although this is nonspecific, it can be utilized if the patient has tried CPAP and is intolerant, nonadherent to CPAP, or it does not satisfy the therapeutic goals. A BPAP device without a backup rate (E0470) can be prescribed and covered under these circumstances. The patients with CompSA can obtain BPAP with a backup rate (E0471 and ASV is considered an equivalent device) through the same pathway as the patients with CSA. This approach also requires a diagnostic PSG and failure with CPAP titration with a primary diagnosis of CSA or CompSA which the DMERC web sites specifically define as:

"Complex sleep apnea (CompSA) is a form of central apnea specifically identified by the persistence or emergence of central apneas or hypopneas upon exposure to CPAP (E0601) or an E0470 device once obstructive events have disappeared. These patients have predominately obstructive or mixed apneas during the diagnostic sleep study occurring at greater than or equal to five times per hour. With use of a CPAP or E0470, they show a pattern of apneas and hypopneas that meets the definition of CSA described earlier."

Central apnea is precisely defined as:

1. An AHI greater than five,
2. Central apneas/hypopneas greater than 50% of the total apneas/hypopneas,
3. Central apneas or hypopneas greater than or equal to 5 times per hour, and
4. Symptoms of either excessive sleepiness or disrupted sleep.

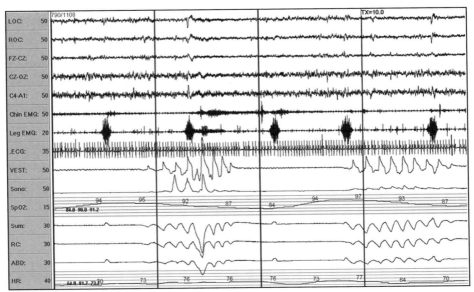

FIGURE 4 Another two-minute epoch during non-rapid eye movement stage 2 sleep now with 10 cm H_2O of continuous positive airway pressure applied. Note the exaggerated periodic breathing with central apnea pattern now predominating. *Abbreviations*: ABD, abdominal plethysmogram; C4-A1, right central-left reference EEG; CZ-OZ, midline central-occipital EEG; ECG, electrocardiogram; EEG, electroencephalogram; EMG, electromyogram; FZ-CZ, midline frontal-central EEG; HR, heart rate; LOC and ROC, left and right outer canthi (eye movements), respectively; Nasal P, nasal pressure via transducer; RC, rib cage plethysmogram; Sono, sonogram (snoring intensity); SpO_2, oxygen saturation; Sum, plethysmogram summed signal; VEST, estimated flow from device.

The last complicating feature regarding reimbursement is that patients must be followed up and proven adherent with the PAP treatment at least four hours per night between 61 and 90 days after initiation. The whole process demands that formal documentation be readily available for patients and although exact follow-up guidelines are not otherwise provided in any literature, some formal and regular follow-up is generally accepted as good clinical practice (23).

CONCLUSIONS

This chapter reviewed the rationale for the design of BPAP to treat patients with SDB primarily due to OSA and additional clinical recommendations from evidence review and practice parameter paper were published in 2006 (23,41). Even though there have been no comparative studies to determine the optimal titration protocol, a few titration techniques were discussed above. There was no evidence found that BPAP improves efficacy or adherence to therapy in OSA patients who are first-time PAP users but studies did at least support equivalency of CPAP and BPAP. There was also no evidence available to support the practice of BPAP use at an arbitrary higher level of CPAP pressure during a routine titration of OSA patients. There may be some role for BPAP treatment in patients who have struggled with CPAP but there is limited data. Special considerations are also needed for patients with mixed apnea or CompSA who respond poorly to CPAP and it seems most appropriate to

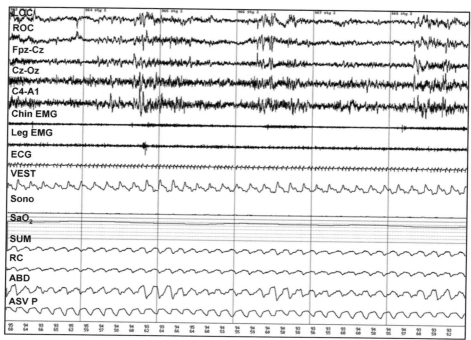

FIGURE 5 This 180-second epoch shows the patient stabilized in non-rapid eye movement stage 2 sleep now using the Adaptive Servo Ventilator (ASV) device. Note the subtle alterations in the ASV pressure (P) as the abdominal excursion is reduced or increased. The ASV P falls during increased abdominal effort and vice versa to create a more uniform breathing pattern. *Abbreviations*: ABD, abdominal plethysmogram; ASV P, mask pressure from ASV device; C4-A1, right central-left reference EEG; CZ-OZ, midline central-occipital EEG; ECG, electrocardiogram; EEG, electroencephalogram; EMG, electromyogram; Fpz-Cz, midline fronto-parietal-central EEG; HR, heart rate; LOC and ROC, left and right outer canthi (eye movements), respectively; Nasal P, nasal pressure via transducer; RC, rib cage plethysmogram; Sono, sonogram (snoring intensity); SaO$_2$, oxygen saturation; SUM, plethysmogram summed signal; VEST, estimated flow from device.

consider treatment with BPAP with a backup rate or an ASV device. It is important to know and document coverage criteria so that the information is available to enable proper reimbursement and some formal follow-up program is encouraged. Lastly, future research should be performed to pursue ways to verify the efficacy and treatment adherence benefits with BPAP or ASV in patients with CSA or CompSA especially over the long term.

REFERENCES

1. Gastaut H, Tassinari A, Duron B. Polygraphic study of the episodic diurnal and nocturnal (hypnic and respiratory) manifestations of the Pickwickian syndrome. Brain Res 1966; 2:167.
2. Martin RJ, Pennock BE, Orr WC, et al. Respiratory mechanics and timing during sleep in occlusive sleep apnea. J Appl Physiol 1980; 48(3):432–437.
3. Sanders MH, Moore SE. Inspiratory and expiratory partitioning of airway resistance during sleep in patients with sleep apnea. Am Rev Respir Dis 1983; 127(5):554–558.

4. Remmers JE, Bartlett D. Reflex control of expiratory airflow and duration. J Appl Physiol 1977; 42:80–87.
5. Malhotra A, White DP. Obstructive sleep apnoea. Lancet 2002; 360:237–245.
6. Schwab RJ, Pasirstein M, Pierson R, et al. Identification of upper airway anatomic risk factors for obstructive sleep apnea with volumetric magnetic resonance imaging. Am J Respir Crit Care Med 2003; 168(5):522–530.
7. Juhasz J, Becker H, Cassel W, et al. Proportional positive airway pressure: a new concept to treat obstructive sleep apnoea. Eur Respir J 2001; 17(3):467–473.
8. Farré R, Peslin R, Montserrat JM, et al. Flow-dependent positive airway pressure to maintain airway patency in sleep apnea–hypopnea syndrome. Am J Respir Crit Care Med 1998; 157:1855–1863.
9. Sanders MH, Kern N. Obstructive sleep apnea treated by independently adjusted inspiratory and expiratory positive airway pressures via nasal mask. Physiologic and clinical implications. Chest 1990; 98(2):317–324.
10. Gugger M, Vock P. Effect of reduced expiratory pressure on pharyngeal size during nasal positive airway pressure in patients with sleep apnoea: evaluation by continuous computed tomography. Thorax 1992; 47(10):809–813.
11. Resta O, Guido P, Picca V, et al. The role of the expiratory phase in obstructive sleep apnoea. Respir Med 1999; 93(3):190–195.
12. Bureau MP, Series F. Comparison of two in-laboratory titration methods to determine effective pressure levels in patients with obstructive sleep apnoea. Thorax 2000; 55:741–745.
13. Lopata M, Onal E. Mass loading, sleep apnea, and the pathogenesis of obesity hypoventilation. Am Rev Respir Dis 1982; 126(4):640–645.
14. Schafer H, Ewig S, Hasper E, et al. Failure of CPAP therapy in obstructive sleep apnoea syndrome: predictive factors and treatment with bilevel-positive airway pressure. Respir Med 1998; 92(2):208–215.
15. Pankow W, Hijjeh N, Schuttler F, et al. Influence of noninvasive positive pressure ventilation on inspiratory muscle activity in obese subjects. Eur Respir J 1997; 10(12):2847–2852.
16. Piper AJ, Sullivan CE. Effects of short-term NIPPV in the treatment of patients with severe obstructive sleep apnea and hypercapnia. Chest 1994; 105:434–440.
17. Waldhorn RE. Nocturnal nasal intermittent positive pressure ventilation with bi-level positive airway pressure (BiPAP) in respiratory failure. Chest 1992; 101:516–521.
18. Laursen SB, Dreijer B, Hemmingsen C, et al. Bi-level positive airway pressure treatment of obstructive sleep apnoea syndrome. Respiration 1998; 65:114–119.
19. Resta O, Guido P, Picca V, et al. Prescription of nCPAP and nBIPAP in obstructive sleep apnoea syndrome: Italian experience in 105 subjects. A prospective two centre study. Respir Med 1998; 92(6):820–827.
20. Resta O, Foschino-Barbaro MP, Bonfitto P, et al. Prevalence and mechanisms of diurnal hypercapnia in a sample of morbidly obese subjects with obstructive sleep apnoea. Respir Med 2000; 94(3):240–246.
21. Engelman HM, Kingshott RN, Wraith PK, et al. Randomized placebo-controlled crossover trial of continuous positive airway pressure for mild sleep apnea/hypopnea syndrome. Am J Respir Crit Care Med 1999; 159:461–467.
22. Jenkinson C, Davies RJ, Mullins R, et al. Comparison of therapeutic and subtherapeutic nasal continuous positive airway pressure for obstructive sleep apnoea: a randomized prospective parallel trial. Lancet 1999; 353:2100–2105.
23. Gay PC, Weaver T, Loube D, et al. Evaluation of positive airway pressure treatment for sleep related breathing disorders in adults. Sleep 2006; 29(3):381–401.
24. Berry RB. Improving CPAP compliance-man more than machine. Sleep Med 2000; 1:175–178.
25. Weaver TE, Kribbs NB, Pack AI, et al. Night-to-night variability in CPAP use over the first three months of treatment. Sleep 1997; 20:278–283.
26. Hoy CJ, Vennelle M, Kingshott RN, et al. Can intensive support improve continuous positive airway pressure use in patients with sleep apnea/hypopnea syndrome? Am J Respir Crit Care Med 1999; 159:1096–1100.
27. Chervin RD, Theut S, Bassetti C, et al. Compliance with nasal CPAP can be improved by simple interventions. Sleep 1997; 20:284–289.

28. Massie CA, Hart RW, Peralez K, et al. Effects of humidification on nasal symptoms and compliance in sleep apnea patients using continuous positive airway pressure. Chest 1999; 116:403–408.
29. Berry RB, Parish JM, Hartse KM. The use of auto-titrating continuous positive airway pressure for treatment of adult obstructive sleep apnea. An American Academy of Sleep Medicine review. Sleep 2002; 25:148–173.
30. Reeves-Hoche MK, Hudgel DW, Meck R, et al. Continuous versus bilevel positive airway pressure for obstructive sleep apnea. Am J Respir Crit Care Med 1995; 151:443–449.
31. Gay PC, Herold DL, Olson EJ. A randomized, double-blind clinical trial comparing continuous positive airway pressure with a novel bilevel pressure system for treatment of obstructive sleep apnea syndrome. Sleep 2003; 26:864–869.
32. Ballard R, Gay PC, Strollo PJ. Interventions to improve compliance in sleep apnea patients previously non-compliant with continuous positive airway pressure. Accepted Chest 2007.
33. Sleep-related breathing disorders in adults: recommendations for syndrome definition and measurement techniques in clinical research. The Report of an American Academy of Sleep Medicine Task Force. Sleep 1999; 22:667–689.
34. Thomas RJ, Terzano MG, Parrino L, et al. Obstructive sleep-disordered breathing with a dominant cyclic alternating pattern—a recognizable polysomnographic variant with practical clinical implications. Sleep 2004; 27:229–234.
35. Gilmartin GS, Daly RW, Thomas RJ. Recognition and management of complex sleep-disordered breathing. Curr Opin Pulm Med 2005; 11:485–493.
36. Pusalavidyasagar SS, Olson EJ, Gay PC, et al. Treatment of complex sleep apnea syndrome: a retrospective comparative review. Sleep Med 2006; 7(6):474–479.
37. Johnson KG, Johnson DC. Bilevel positive airway pressure worsens central apneas during sleep. Chest 2005; 128:2141–2150.
38. Teschler H, Dohring J, Wang YM, et al. Adaptive pressure support servo-ventilation: a novel treatment for Cheyne-Stokes respiration in heart failure. Am J Respir Crit Care Med 2001; 164(4):614–619.
39. Morgenthaler TI, Gay PC, Brown LK. Adaptive servo-ventilation versus noninvasive positive pressure ventilation for central and complex sleep apnea syndromes. Sleep 2007; in press.
40. http://www.palmettogba.com/palmetto/providers.nsf/$$ViewTemplate+for+Docs?ReadForm&Providers/DMERC/Publications/DMEPOS+Supplier+Manual/Current
41. Standards of Practice Committee of the American Academy of Sleep Medicine. Kushida CA, Littner MR, Hirshkowitz M, et al. Practice parameters for the use of continuous and bilevel positive airway pressure devices to treat adult patients with sleep-related breathing disorders. Sleep 2006; 29(3):375–380.

8   Auto-Positive Airway Pressure

Richard B. Berry
Division of Pulmonary, Critical Care, and Sleep Medicine, University of Florida, Gainesville, Florida, U.S.A.

INTRODUCTION

Auto-positive airway pressure (APAP) devices provide a useful alternative for providing positive airway pressure (PAP) treatment for patients with obstructive sleep apnea (OSA) (1–3). One can separate the uses of these devices into two large categories (Table 1). These include: (*i*) auto-titration PAP to determine an effective fixed level of continuous positive airway pressure (CPAP) and (*ii*) auto-adjusting PAP for chronic treatment. When used in the auto-titration mode the devices are used by the patient for a period of time (one night to several weeks). Information stored in the device is transferred to a computer and can be used to select an optimal fixed level of CPAP for chronic treatment. When APAP devices are used for chronic treatment they have the potential advantage of delivering the lowest effective pressure in any circumstance (body position, sleep stage). The mean pressure for the night may be lower than a single pressure that would be effective in all circumstances (the prescription pressure). For example, higher CPAP is usually needed in the supine posture and during rapid eye movement (REM) sleep (4–6). A schematic representation of the delivered pressure profile for a single night on auto-adjusting PAP is shown in Figure 1. In this example, the patient spent only a small portion of the night at the higher pressure required for the supine position. The average pressure is much lower than a single pressure that would be effective throughout the night. A substantial literature now exists evaluating the use of the devices in these modes of operation.

DEVICE CHARACTERISTICS

Many brands and models of APAP devices are currently approved for treatment. The devices differ in the respiratory variables that are monitored and in the algorithms used to adjust the delivered pressure. The devices typically monitor one or more of the following: airflow (or motor speed), airflow profile (flattening), snoring (airway vibration), or airway impedance (forced oscillation technique). The algorithms used to adjust pressure are proprietary but determine if the delivered pressure should be increased or decreased. Depending on the type of respiratory event that is detected the delivered pressure is increased by a certain amount. Typically, pressure changes occur slowly over several minutes to prevent pressure-induced arousals. If no respiratory events are detected within a certain time window the delivered pressure is slowly decreased. Thus, the lowest effective pressure is delivered. In some of the devices machine adjustment is available for various mask types and for the type of humidifier that is being used.

Studies comparing different APAP devices provide evidence that devices from different manufacturers will not deliver the same pressure for a given clinical circumstance (7,8). These studies used a mechanical lung/upper airway with set patterns of apnea or hypopnea to challenge different APAP devices. In Figure 2 the

TABLE 1 Potential Uses of Auto-Positive Airway Pressure

Auto-titrating mode
  Attended auto-titration in CPAP naïve patient (technologist extender)
  Unattended auto-titration in CPAP naïve patient
  Check prescription pressure after weight gain/loss
  Salvage a failed manual CPAP titration
Auto-adjusting mode
  Initial chronic treatment of OSA (no titration needed)
  Chronic treatment in patients not tolerating CPAP
  Chronic treatment in patients with difficult mask/mouth leak

Abbreviations: CPAP, continuous positive airway pressure; OSA, obstructive sleep apnea.

responses of several devices differs markedly in response to apnea. Some of the devices increased the delivered pressure in response to apnea while others did not (7). Kessler et al. (9) compared the 95th percentile pressure of one APAP device based on airflow to another based on the forced oscillation technique using a randomized crossover study design. There was poor agreement between the optimal pressure identified by the two devices. The 95th percentile pressure determined by the APAP machine based on flow was on average 3 cm H_2O higher than that of the other device. Senn et al. (10) compared an APAP device responding to apnea, hypopnea, and snoring with a second device responding to the previous variables as well as airflow limitation (airflow profile flattening). The adherence and clinical outcomes were similar although the median applied pressure was slightly higher with the device that responded to airflow limitation (10). Thus, differences in the devices do not always translate into differences in outcomes.

The problems of mask/mouth leak and central apnea have provided a challenge for the designers of APAP algorithms. However, these two problems are familiar to technologists manually titrating CPAP. Mask/mouth leaks tend to raise the baseline flow delivered by blower units and diminish the variations in flow during inspiration and expiration. The resulting airflow signal may be interpreted as an apnea or hypopnea and prompt an increase in pressure that may further increase leak. Teschler and Berthon-Jones (3) reported on their clinical experience in 1000 patients using the AutoSet T™ (ResMed, North Ryde, Australia) APAP device and estimated that leak exceeds 0.4 L/s (considered high leak) on average for 10% of an attended APAP night and 15% on an unattended APAP night. To handle the leak problem many APAP units have algorithms that limit pressure increases when leak exceeds certain values or when increases in blower speed no longer result in increases

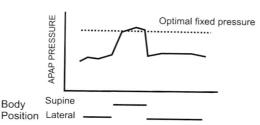

FIGURE 1 This schematic tracing of delivered pressure over an entire night illustrates that the patient slept at a lower pressure for most of the night than a single fixed pressure that would be effective in all body positions. The APAP device increased pressure when the patient was supine. *Abbreviation*: APAP, auto-positive airway pressure.

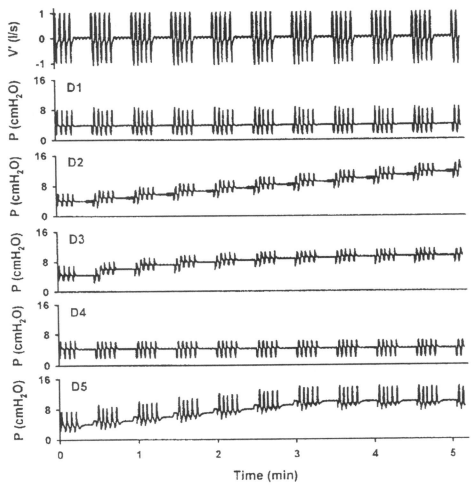

FIGURE 2 Response of the auto-positive airway pressure (APAP) devices (D1–D5) when subjected to a disturbed flow (V') breathing pattern consisting of repetitive apneas. P and V' are the actual pressure and flow, respectively, measured at the entrance of the APAP device (V' > 0: inspiration). *Source*: From Ref. 7.

in mask pressure. Other units have leak alarms that can prompt the patient to adjust the mask. Mouth leaks can be approached by using a chin strap or full-face mask.

Central apnea during APAP treatment/titration is another difficult problem in some patients (1). Central apneas of the Cheyne-Stokes type are common in patients in congestive heart failure. Other patients with OSA may have central apneas during CPAP titration (treatment-emergent central apneas). Algorithms often include limits on upward titration of pressure for apnea to avoid the delivery of high pressure for central apneas. For example, pressure is not increased above 10 cm H_2O unless apnea is associated with snoring or airflow profile flattening. Of note, many published studies of APAP excluded patients with congestive heart failure or frequent central apneas on the preceding diagnostic sleep study.

Recently, expiratory pressure relief (C-Flex™, Respironics, Inc., Murrysville, Pennsylvania, U.S.) is now available for one brand of APAP devices. This mode allows a reduction in pressure during early expiration with a return to the current set pressure at end expiration. This feature could improve patient tolerance to pressure. However, only one published study has demonstrated an advantage for CPAP with C-Flex compared to traditional CPAP treatment (11). Another recent development is the availability of APAP machines providing automatic adjustment of bilevel PAP (BPAP) (Fig. 3). These devices vary inspiratory positive airway pressure (IPAP) and expiratory positive airway pressure (EPAP) according to a proprietary algorithm. The physician sets the minimum EPAP, maximum IPAP, and maximum IPAP–EPAP difference. The option of using inspiratory and expiratory pressure relief (Bi-Flex®, Respironics, Inc., Murrysville, Pennsylvania, U.S.) is currently available for one device brand. Inspiratory pressure relief allows a drop in pressure at end inhalation (IPAP) while expiratory pressure relief allows a pressure drop at the start of exhalation (EPAP). The superiority of APAP devices with either C-Flex or the ability to deliver bilevel positive pressure (with or without Bi-Flex) remains to be demonstrated. These new features do increase treatment alternatives.

AUTO-TITRATION

The gold standard for the titration of PAP is attended polysomnography with full-electroencephalogram (EEG) monitoring to detect the presence and stage of sleep (12). Respiratory monitoring allows classification of apneas (obstructive, mixed, and central) and detection of hypopnea or drop in arterial oxygen saturation. Snoring and evidence of airflow limitation or leak can also be detected with the proper monitoring equipment. Body position is identified by technologist documentation or by position sensors. Manual PAP titration is labor intensive and usually a single technologist can titrate only two patients at a time. Patients in some geographical areas may have limited or delayed access to a sleep laboratory offering polysomnography. In addition, the gold standard PAP titration method may result in suboptimal titrations due to a number of problems including poor sleep, lack of supine REM sleep, high mask leak, or uncorrected mouth leak. Patient characteristics such as weight gain may also render previously selected pressures inadequate. Auto-titrating PAP devices can be used to address some of these problems.

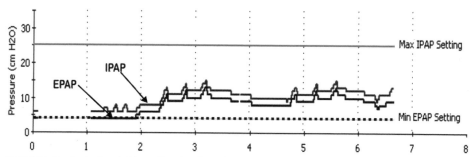

FIGURE 3 A single night profile showing changes in inspiratory positive airway pressure and expiratory positive airway pressure over the night with auto-bilevel positive airway pressure.

Evidence of Efficacy of Auto-Titrating Positive Airway Pressure

One important use of APAP devices is selection of a fixed CPAP pressure as an alternative to traditional manual (attended) PAP titration (1,2,10–19). Information stored in the device memory can be analyzed and a pressure can be chosen for fixed CPAP treatment. A common method is to choose the 90th or 95th percentile pressure (pressure exceeded only 10% or 5% of the time, respectively) as the prescription pressure. This assumes periods of high leak have been eliminated from the analysis.

There is considerable evidence that APAP devices can be successfully used to establish a fixed CPAP pressure. However, in reviewing the literature it is important to note whether the studies were attended or unattended and the proportion of patients excluded. There are really two methods with which to judge APAP selection of a fixed CPAP pressure. First, will APAP titration allow selection of a fixed level of CPAP resulting in acceptable treatment [apnea–hypopnea index (AHI) < 10/hour] and/or good clinical outcome? A second approach is to determine if APAP titration can identify an optimal pressure for fixed CPAP treatment that is similar to the pressure chosen by manual titration.

Several studies found that APAP titration could select a fixed CPAP pressure that was effective. For example, Gagnadoux et al. (13) performed an attended APAP titration followed by treatment with fixed CPAP chosen as the P95 (i.e., 95th percentile pressure). After three months of treatment a sleep study on the fixed pressure found the AHI < 10/hour in 21 of 24 patients. Two other attended studies (14,15) reached similar conclusions. Unattended APAP titration also appears to be effective. Berkani et al. (16) found that unattended APAP was successful at identifying an effective CPAP level. Similarly, Series (17) found that treatment with fixed CPAP using a pressure identified by unattended APAP titration reduced the AHI to < 10/hour in 38/40 subjects.

Studies have also compared the CPAP pressure chosen by attended manual titration and APAP titration. Lloberes et al. (18) compared a partially attended APAP titration with a manual CPAP titration on another night. In 15 of 20 patients the difference between the APAP pressure (taken as P95) and the CPAP chosen by manual titration was equal to or less than 1 cm H_2O. Stradling et al. (19) used a randomized parallel-group design and found the APAP and manual titration pressures to be very similar in two well-matched groups of OSA patients (APAP: 8.2 ± 2.1, manual CPAP titration: 8.7 ± 2.1 cm H_2O). The selection of the effective pressure on the APAP night was performed after visualization of raw data. The pressure effective "most" of the time during APAP titration was chosen.

Fletcher et al. (20) studied the feasibility of using ambulatory monitoring for diagnosis followed by ambulatory APAP titration/treatment as therapy for a large group with OSA. Exclusion criteria included a suspicion of other sleep disorders (narcolepsy, restless legs syndrome), complicating medical illnesses, acute decompensation requiring hospitalization, or a prior diagnosis of OSA. Of the 45 patients that underwent APAP titration, it was deemed adequate in 35 (78%).

Based on a literature search pre-2002 the Standards of Practice Committee of the American Academy of Sleep Medicine did not recommend the routine use of unattended APAP for the choice of a fixed CPAP prescription pressure (1). Since this literature review, further evidence of the ability of APAP devices to function in the unattended auto-titration mode has been published. In a large multicenter study, Masa et al. (21) randomized patients newly diagnosed with OSA to one of the three treatment arms using a parallel-group design. The study groups included: (*i*) standard attended titration with polysomnography, (*ii*) auto-titration at home, or (*iii*) use of a level of CPAP chosen by a prediction formula (22) followed by pressure adjustment based on spouse observations. The randomization was performed after a 20-minute trial of CPAP during the day. Of note, 23% of the original study population was excluded because of severe nasal congestion, prior palate surgery, refusal to participate, psychiatric incapacity, alcohol addiction, inability to place the CPAP mask, and absence of a partner at home. In the auto-titrating arm patients were seen after one night of auto-titration. The CPAP prescription pressure was chosen as the 90th percentile pressure. If the patient slept poorly (patient report) or the machine information revealed high leak, the auto-titration was repeated on a second or third night. About 5% of patients in the auto-adjusting arm were considered titration failures. One night of titration was successful in 98 of 119 patients. In the predicted formula group, CPAP was chosen based on neck size, body mass index, and the AHI (22). Pressure was increased for observed apnea or snoring by fixed protocol. The patients were treated with CPAP in all three groups and adherence and outcomes measures were compared between the groups. There was no difference in the improvement in the Epworth sleepiness scale (subjective sleepiness), adherence (objective hours per night), drop out rates, or quality-of-life measures. The mean CPAP levels in all three groups were similar (around 9 cm H_2O). The mean nightly use was approximately five hours. This large study suggests that ambulatory APAP titration is as effective as manual titration (provided similar methods and exclusions are used). However, the large number of excluded patients and the relatively low mean pressure may mean that this finding may not apply to all populations of OSA patients. The 20-minute CPAP trial during the day is a very appealing technique for early identification of patients likely to need attended titration or who will be unable to tolerate positive pressure at all.

In summary, there is convincing evidence that auto-titrating PAP devices can be useful for identifying an appropriate fixed CPAP level in appropriate patients. Recent studies have provided evidence that unattended as well as attended titration can be effective. However, it is likely that unattended APAP titration will not be effective in a significant proportion of OSA patients. In general, patients with a significant proportion of central apneas, those with low baseline SaO_2 values or who have difficulty applying the mask and/or operating an APAP device are probably best studied using attended manual titration with polysomnography. A brief practice trial with APAP may be useful to identify mask leak or nasal congestion problems requiring intervention before the patient takes the APAP device home. If APAP titration is performed, close review of the data is needed to ensure that the titration was adequate. Those patients not having an adequate APAP titration should be referred for a traditional CPAP titration.

Technique of Auto-Titration

As with manual attended PAP titrations with polysomnography, patient education, and mask fitting are essential for successful auto-titration. Patients must feel comfortable applying the mask interface and operating the APAP device if an unattended titration is planned. One study found a short 20-minute trial of APAP to be very useful in identifying patient problems including claustrophobia, mask leak or an inability to operate the device (21). The physician ordering the APAP titration designates the lower and upper pressure limits (for example, 4 and 20 cm H_2O). The APAP device then titrates between these limits. Depending on the type of APAP device utilized, information on applied pressure, leak, snoring, flattening, and a moving time average of the AHI is stored in the device memory. After transfer to a computer the information is available for review. It is possible to determine statistics for all or a portion of the data. Most devices allow the ability to look at one or more single nights of data in detail (pressure, leak, residual events vs. time) (Fig. 4). Periods of high leak and the frequently associated increase in pressure can be appreciated. High leak can result in many devices promptly increasing pressure until the upper pressure limit is reached. In addition to detailed time profiles, summary statistics can be displayed for a single night or multiple nights. Typically available information includes: 90th or 95th percentile pressure, median pressure, maximum pressure, maximum leak, median leak, and residual AHI.

Usually either the 90th or 95th percentile pressure is chosen for the prescription pressure. However, simply noting one number can be very misleading. The clinician must first determine if the titration duration (amount of sleep on the device) was adequate and if the residual AHI is reasonably low (AHI < 5–10/hour). Patients with suboptimal or inconclusive APAP titrations should have a repeat APAP titration or be referred for an attended lab PAP titration. High-residual AHI could be secondary to frequent central apneas, high leak, or too low maximum pressure limit. High leak could be secondary to inadequate mask seal or mouth leak if a nasal mask is being utilized. Patients with a high AHI and leak may undergo a repeat APAP titration after mask adjustment or change to a full-face mask (or addition of a chin strap) as indicated. A persistently high-residual AHI despite repeated attempts at APAP titration would be an indication of the need for a traditional manual PAP titration.

In Figure 4 an example of an ideal titration is shown. Leak is relatively low as is the residual AHI. The lower and upper pressure limits in this example were 4 and 15 cm H_2O. A prescription pressure of 10 cm H_2O was chosen based on the 95th percentile pressure of 9.4 cm H_2O. Figure 5 shows a less ideal titration. Here there is a

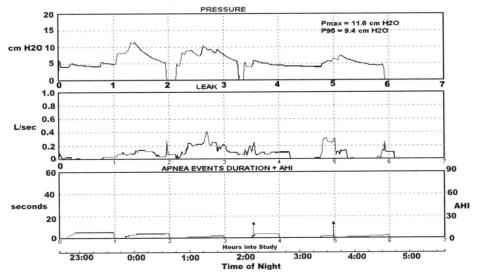

FIGURE 4 This is a single night profile of pressure, leak, and residual apnea-hypopnea index (AHI) of an ideal titration. The leak and residual AHI are low. The 95th percentile pressure was 9.4 cm H_2O. The patient was treated with a prescription pressure of 10 cm H_2O. *Source*: From Ref. 42.

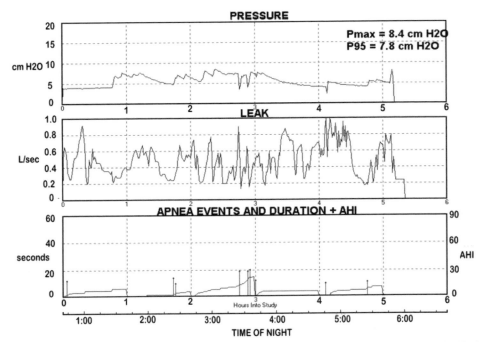

FIGURE 5 This is a single night profile of pressure, leak and residual apnea-hypopnea index (AHI) of a fair titration. The leak is higher than ideal (> 0.4 L/s) at times. However, the residual AHI remained low. The 95th percentile pressure was 7.8 cm H_2O. The prescription pressure was chosen to be 8 cm H_2O.

high leak but the residual AHI remains low. In Figure 6 an unacceptable auto-titration is shown. Very high leak is obvious and the machine pressure climbed to the upper pressure limit and stayed there for most of the night. In Table 2 examples of results for two patients undergoing auto-titration are illustrated. In patient one the statistics from five days of monitoring showed a low-residual AHI. In patient two, the results of a single night showed a very high residual apnea index. The latter patient underwent an attended titration and was found to have a significant number of central apneas.

A number of portable monitoring units can interface with selected APAP devices. For example, airflow, respiratory effort, oxygen saturation, body position, and delivered pressure can be recorded for clinician analysis (23). This is especially helpful if one night of APAP titration is utilized. For example, absence of supine sleep could result in a lower than typically needed prescription pressure. This is also a reason that it is often helpful to have the patient use the APAP device for several nights. Average statistics over a week may more accurately represent a typical night's pressure requirements. Information from pulse oximetry during the APAP titration can identify the need for the addition of supplemental oxygen.

CHRONIC TREATMENT WITH AUTO-POSITIVE AIRWAY PRESSURE (AUTO-ADJUSTING POSITIVE AIRWAY PRESSURE)

When originally developed one anticipated advantage of APAP devices was that delivery of the lowest effective pressure in any circumstance (sleep stage, body position) would

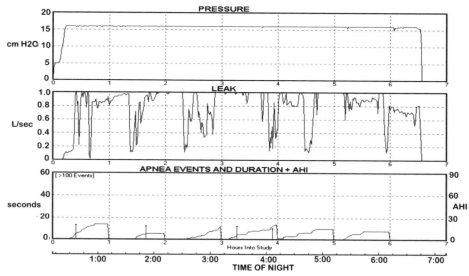

FIGURE 6 This is a single night profile of pressure, leak and residual apnea–hypopnea index (AHI) of an unacceptable auto-positive airway pressure titration. The leak is very high. The pressure increased to the upper limit (16 cm H_2O) and remained there for most of the night. The AHI was also elevated. This titration would need to be repeated with a better mask seal or use of a full-face mask if mouth leak was believed to be present.

improve acceptance and adherence to positive pressure treatment. This was based on the premise that a lower mean nightly pressure would improve patient tolerance to PAP treatment. Alternatively, chronic treatment with an auto-adjusting device would obviate the need for an attended or unattended PAP titration.

Auto-Positive Airway Pressure Vs. Continuous Positive Airway Pressure Treatment

A number of studies have examined the hypothesis that chronic treatment with auto-adjusting PAP would increase the adherence. Some studies did find higher adherence with APAP compared to fixed CPAP treatment (24–27). However, several other studies did not confirm this result (10,28–32). A meta-analysis (Fig. 7) by Ayas

TABLE 2 Auto-Positive Airway Pressure Statistics

	Patient 1	Patient 2
Days	5	1
P_{max}	8.2	10
P95	7.8	8
AI (/hr)	2	15
HI (/hr)	3	5
AHI (/hr)	5	20
Median leak (L/s)	0.2	0.4

Note: Patient 2 had a high residual AHI.
Abbreviations: AI, apnea index; HI, hypopnea index; AHI, apnea-hypopnea index.

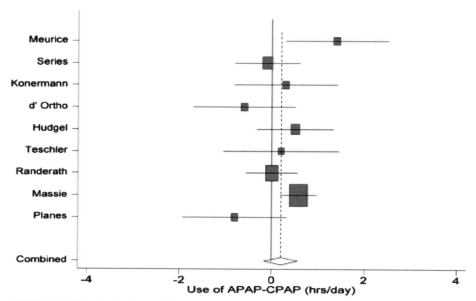

FIGURE 7 Effects of auto-positive airway pressure (APAP) versus continuous positive airway pressure (CPAP) on adherence. A positive score indicated a better adherence to APAP than CPAP. The X axis is the nightly adherence with APAP minus adherence with CPAP. Y axis: studies reporting adherence ordered by publication year. The bottom diamond represents the pooled effect, with the dashed line drawn though the mean of this estimate. The composite data are consistent with no increase in adherence on APAP versus CPAP treatment. *Source*: From Ref. 33.

et al. (32) concluded that there was no significant increase in adherence with APAP treatment compared to fixed CPAP in these studies. In evaluating studies of adherence several issues must be considered. First, pressure intolerance is not the major issue for many patients (34). Second, the difference in the mean pressure on APAP and an adequate fixed pressure is oft en only 1 to 2 cm (30) H_2O (Fig. 8). One would not expect such a small pressure difference to change adherence.

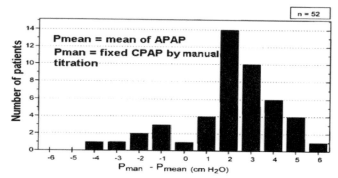

FIGURE 8 The number of patients with displayed differences between the manual effective continuous positive airway pressure (Pman) and the mean nightly pressure on auto-positive airway pressure (APAP). While a few patients had a much lower mean pressure on APAP compared to the fixed pressure (Pman), the difference was only 1 or 2 cm H_2O in most patients. *Source*: From Ref. 30.

Are there subsets of OSA patients who would adhere better to APAP than fixed CPAP? One might expect a potential advantage for APAP devices in patients with pressure intolerance, high prescription pressures, or a large variation in the required pressure during the night (postural or REM-related OSA) (35). However, Noseda et al. (36) found no evidence for increased adherence in patients with a high variability in pressure requirement. A major problem with this study is that it did not target pressure intolerant patients. Of interest, Hukins (32) found evidence of lower leak and fewer reported side effects on APAP compared to fixed CPAP treatment. Lowering the mean pressure might be expected to minimize mask leak or the tendency for mouth leak. Leak, especially mouth leak, often results in dryness that may not respond to the addition of heated humidity (37–39). Thus, chronic APAP treatment provides a useful alternative in patients with a mask or mouth leak problem that does not respond to interventions such as a change in mask type or size or an increase in the delivered humidity.

Although APAP treatment appears to have no advantage over CPAP with respect to adherence in unselected patients, several studies have demonstrated a patient preference for APAP (30,32,40). It would be useful to be able to predict which patients might prefer treatment with APAP. Marrone et al. (40) compared APAP and fixed CPAP treatment using a crossover design. Of 22 patients, 14 preferred APAP treatment. However, analysis of group characteristics found no factor that would predict a preference for APAP. Of interest is the finding that only those patients with a preference for APAP had higher adherence to APAP than CPAP. Thus, if a patient is having difficulty with CPAP, a trial of APAP is a reasonable intervention. If APAP is preferred, improved adherence is likely with this mode of treatment compared to fixed CPAP. Furthermore, information stored in the machine such as leak or residual events may help diagnose problems with treatment.

Patients with difficulty tolerating CPAP due to pressure intolerance ("cannot breathe out") are often switched to BPAP. One study compared intervention with APAP to that with BPAP in patients with difficult-to-treat sleep apnea (41). The inclusion criteria were patients requiring CPAP > 12 cm H_2O, those not tolerating CPAP, and those with central apneas that worsened on CPAP. Both APAP and BPAP improved subjective sleepiness with equivalent adherence. A majority of the patients preferred APAP at the end of the study. As APAP devices are considerably less expensive than BPAP devices, this study suggests that a trial of APAP treatment should be given consideration when CPAP is not well-tolerated.

Although the fact that APAP treatment does not improve adherence over fixed CPAP selected by manual titration, the equivalence of these treatments suggests another role for APAP devices. That is, patients diagnosed with OSA could be treated with chronic APAP without the need for either traditional laboratory titration or auto-titration. Any additional cost of APAP devices over CPAP would usually be less than the cost of an in-laboratory CPAP titration. In fact, one study (31) found both a cost saving and a reduction in the time needed to adjust the PAP treatment to a satisfactory level. Indeed it is a common experience that the optimal level of CPAP determined by an attended in-laboratory titration often requires alteration for patient tolerance, side effects, or control of daytime sleepiness.

Technique of Chronic Auto-Positive Airway Pressure Treatment

The physician usually orders the lower and upper limits of positive pressure. The APAP device then delivers the lowest effective pressure between these limits.

The upper and lower pressure limits could be placed as wide as possible (4–18 cm H_2O) or narrowed based on information from a previous CPAP titration or previous nights of APAP use. Some patients find starting at 4 cm H_2O uncomfortable and it may take some APAP machines several minutes to reach a pressure level that they find comfortable. In this case the lower pressure could be increased to 6–10 cm H_2O. Awakening with the feeling of insufficient pressure could be another situation in which the lower pressure limit should be increased. Bloating or evidence of excessive mouth leak might be an indication to lower the upper pressure limit. Alternatively, if the 90th percentile pressure essentially equals the upper pressure limit, then a higher upper pressure limit is likely needed (especially if the residual AHI is high).

Information on delivered pressure is not the only data stored in the APAP device that is potentially useful for tailoring treatment. High leak may indicate the need for another mask or a full-face mask (mouth leak). A high-residual AHI might indicate a need for an increase in either the lower or upper pressure. A high number of residual apneas might suggest that central apneas could be present.

REIMBURSEMENT CRITERIA AND ISSUES

Financial constraints may limit the use of APAP devices for chronic treatment of OSA at least in some circumstances. In the United States durable medical equipment (DME) providers receive the same reimbursement for supplying an APAP device as a CPAP device despite the greater cost of APAP. One option is to pass the extra cost to the patient who often pays out of pocket for the difference. Some patients may choose to buy a unit directly from a national discount provider over the Internet.

Unattended auto-titration is currently not reimbursed in the United States. For this reason, it has been most widely used in circumstances where reimbursement for the auto-titration is not an issue such as certain health maintenance organizations and the Veterans Health Care System. In the private sector, some DME providers are willing to provide an APAP loaner for a few days to weeks to determine a fixed CPAP pressure (if a CPAP will be provided by them at a pressure based on the study). In this setting, the patient is responsible for paying for the mask and other supplies should they decline CPAP treatment.

CONCLUSIONS

This chapter has presented evidence that APAP devices can be effective in the auto-titrating and auto-adjusting modes. They provide a useful titration or chronic treatment alternative for patients with sleep apnea. Success depends on proper patient selection, education, and detailed physician review of the stored information. Treatment or titration results could vary between brands of APAP devices. The devices may not work well in patients with central apneas or those with large mouth or mask leak. Careful physician evaluation of treatment efficacy is essential. For example, it is possible that a given patient may have better alertness or sleep with a slightly higher or lower pressure than the 90th or 95th percentile pressure identified by APAP titration. Familiarity with type of information provided by a given brand of device is essential to benefit from the stored information. As with any type of PAP treatment, close follow-up of objective adherence and outcome measures such as subjective sleepiness is essential.

REFERENCES

1. Berry RB, Parish JM, Hartse KM. The use of auto-titrating CPAP for treatment of adults with obstructive sleep apnea. Sleep 2002; 25:148–173.
2. Littner M, Hirshkowitz M, Davila D, et al. Standards of Practice Committee of the American Academy of Sleep Medicine Practice parameters for the use of auto-titrating continuous airway pressure devices for titrating pressures and treating adult patients with obstructive sleep apnea syndrome. An American Academy of Sleep Medicine Report. Sleep 2002; 15(25):143–147.
3. Teschler H, Berthon-Jones M. Intelligent CPAP systems: clinical experience. Thorax 1998; 53:S49–S54.
4. Pevernagie DA, Sheard JW Jr. Relations between sleep stage, posture and effective nasal CPAP levels in OSA. Sleep 1992; 15:162–167.
5. Oksenberg A, Silverberg DS, Arons E, et al. The sleep supine position has a major effect on optimal nasal continuous positive airway pressure. Chest 1999; 116:1000–1006.
6. Neill AM, Angus SM, Sajkov D, McEvoy RD. Effects of sleep posture on upper airway stability in patients with obstructive sleep apnea. Am J Respir Crit Care Med 1997; 155:199–204.
7. Farré R, Montserrat JM, Rigau J, Trepat X, Pinto P, Navajas D. Response of automatic continuous positive pressure devices to different sleep breathing patterns. Am J Respir Crit Care Med 2002; 166:469–473.
8. Abdenbi F, Chambille B, Escourrou P. Bench testing of auto-adjusting positive airway pressure devices. Eur Respir J 2004; 24:649–658.
9. Kessler R, Weitzenblum E, Chaouat A, Iamandt C, Alliotte T. Evaluation of unattended automated titration to determine therapeutic continuous positive airway pressure in patients with obstructive sleep apnea. Chest 2003; 123:704–710.
10. Senn O, Brack T, Matthews F, Russi EW, Bloch KE. Randomized short-term trial of two AutoCPAP devices versus fixed continuous positive airway pressure for treatment of sleep apnea. Am J Respir Crit Care Med 2003; 168:1506–1511.
11. Aloia MS, Stanchina M, Arnedt JT, Malhotra A, Millman RP. Treatment adherence and outcomes in flexible versus standard continuous positive airway pressure. Chest 2005; 127:2085–2093.
12. American Sleep Disorders Standard of Practice Committee, Chesson A. Chairman. Practice Parameters for the Indications for Polysomnography and Related procedures. Sleep 1997; 20:406–422.
13. Gagnadoux F, Rakotonanahary D, Martins de Araujo MT, et al. Evaluation of an auto-CPAP device for treatment of obstructive sleep apnea. Sleep 1999; 22:1095–1097.
14. Teschler H, Berthon-Jones M, Thompson AB, et al. Automated continuous positive airway pressure titration for obstructive sleep apnea syndrome. Am J Respir Crit Care Med 1996; 154:734–740.
15. Teschler H, Farhat AA, Exner V, et al. AutoSet nasal CPAP titration: Constancy of pressure, compliance, and effectiveness at 8 months follow-up. Eur Respir J 1997; 10:2073–2078.
16. Berkani M, Lofaso F, Chouaid C, et al. Eur Respir J 1998; 12:759–763.
17. Series F. Accuracy of unattended home CPAP titration in the treatment of obstructive sleep apnea. Am J Respir Crit Care Med 2000; 162:94–97.
18. Lloberes P, Ballester E, Montserrat JM, et al. Comparison of manual and automatic CPAP titration in patients with sleep apnea/hypopnea syndrome. Am J Respir Crit Care Med 1996; 154:1755–1758.
19. Stradling J, Barbour C, Pitson DJ, Davies RJO. Automatic nasal continuous positive airway pressure titration in the laboratory: patient outcomes. Thorax 1997; 52:72–75.
20. Fletcher EC, Stich J, Yang KL. Unattended home diagnosis and treatment of obstructive sleep apnea without polysomnography. Arch Fam Med 2000; 9:168–174.
21. Masa JF, Jimenez A, Duran J, et al. Alternative methods of titrating continuous positive airway pressure. Am J Respir Crit Care Med 2004; 170:1218–1224.
22. Miljeteig H, Hoffstein V. Determinants of continuous positive airway pressure for treatment of obstructive sleep apnea. Am Rev Respir Dis 1993; 147:1526–1530.
23. Marrone O, Insalaco, Salvaggio A, Bonsignore G. Role of different nocturnal monitorings in the evaluation of CPAP titration by autoCPAP devices. Respir Med 2005; 99:313–320.
24. Konermann M, Sanner BM, Vyleta M, et al. Use of conventional and self-adjusting nasal continuous positive airway pressure for treatment of severe obstructive sleep apnea syndrome. Chest 1998; 113:714–718.

25. Meurice JC, Marc I, Series F. Efficacy of auto-CPAP in the treatment of obstructive sleep apnea/hypopnea syndrome. Am J Respir Crit Care Med 1996; 153:794–798.

26. Hudgel DW, Fung C. A long-term randomized, cross-over comparison of auto-titrating and standard nasal continuous airway pressure. Sleep 2000; 23:645–648.

27. Massie CA, McArdle N, Hart RW, et al. Comparison between automatic and fixed positive airway pressure therapy in the home. Am J Respir Crit Care Med 2003; 167:20–23.

28. d'Ortho PM, Grillier-Lanoir V, Levy P, et al. Constant vs automatic continuous positive airway pressure therapy. Chest 2000; 118:1010–1017.

29. Teschler H, Wessendorf TE, Farhat AA, et al. Two months auto-adjusting versus conventional nCPAP for obstructive sleep apnoea syndrome. Eur Respir J 2000; 15:990–995.

30. Randerath WJ, Schraeder, Galetke W, Feldmeyer F, Rühle K-H. Autoadjusting CPAP based on impedance efficacy, compliance, and acceptance. Am J Respir Crit Care Med 2001; 163:652–657.

31. Planès C, d'Ortho M, Foucher A, et al. Efficacy and cost of home-initiated auto-nCPAP versus conventional nCPAP. Sleep 2003; 26:156–160.

32. Hukins C. Comparative study of autotitrating and fixed-pressure CPAP in the home: a randomized, single-blind crossover trial. Sleep 2004; 27:1512–1517.

33. Ayas NT, Patel SR, Malhotra A, et al. Auto-titrating versus standard continuous positive airway pressure for the treatment of obstructive sleep apnea: results of a meta-analysis: Sleep 2004; 27:249–253.

34. Rolfe I, Olson LG, Sanders NA. Long-term acceptance of continuous positive airway pressure in obstructive sleep apnea. Am Rev Respir Dis 1991; 144:1130–1133.

35. Series F, Marc I. Importance of sleep stage and body position dependence of sleep apnea in determining benefits to auto-CPAP therapy. Eur Respir J 2001; 18:170–175.

36. Noseda A, Kekmpenaers C, Kerkhofs M, Braun S, Linkowski P, Jann E. Constant vs auto-continuous positive airway pressure in patients with sleep apnea hypopnea syndrome with a high variability in pressure requirement. Chest 2004; 126:31–37.

37. Martins de Araujo MT, Vieira SB, Vasquez EC, Fleury B. Heated humidification or face mask to prevent upper airway dryness during continuous positive airway pressure therapy. Chest 2000; 117:142–147.

38. Richards GN, Cistulli PA, Ungar RG, Berthon-Jones M, Sullivan CE. Mouth leak with nasal continuous positive airway pressure increases nasal airway resistance. Am J Respir Crit Care Med 1996; 154:182–186.

39. Massie CA, Hart RW, Peralez K, Richards G. Effects of humidification on nasal symptoms and compliance in sleep apnea patients using continuous positive airway pressure. Chest 1999; 116:403–408.

40. Marrone O, Resta O, Salvaggio A, Giliberti T, Stefan A, Insalaco G. Preference for fixed or automatic CPAP in patients with obstructive sleep apnea. Sleep Med 2004; 5:247–251.

41. Randerath W, Galetke W, Ruehle KH. Auto-adjusting CPAP based on impedance versus bilevel pressure in difficult to treat sleep apnea syndrome: a prospective randomized crossover study. Med Sci Monit 2003; 9:CR353–358.

42. Berry, RB. Sleep Medicine Pearls. Philadelphia: Hanley and Belfus, 2003.

9 Critical Factors in Positive Pressure Therapy

Scott M. Leibowitz
The Sleep Disorders Center of Cardiac Disease Specialists,
Atlanta, Georgia, U.S.A.

Mark S. Aloia
Butler Hospital, Providence, Rhode Island, U.S.A.

INTRODUCTION

Obstructive sleep apnea (OSA) is a condition of cyclical or repetitive obstructions of the upper airway during sleep, with micro-arousals occurring at the termination of a respiratory event (1,2). In adults, micro-arousal activity has been postulated to disrupt the normal restorative processes of sleep and has been demonstrated to produce sleepiness and/or daytime performance deficits when induced by various sensory stimuli in normal subjects (3,4). In addition to nonrestorative sleep, OSA has been found to have a strong association with cardiovascular disease (5), including hypertension (6), congestive heart failure (7), cardiac arrhythmias (8), coronary artery disease (9), and stroke (10).

There are several different modalities that have been found to be effective for the treatment of OSA. The first-line treatment however, has become the use of positive airway pressure (PAP) therapy, especially continuous positive airway pressure (CPAP) therapy (11). The first reported use of nasal CPAP for OSA in adults was by Sullivan et al. (12) in 1981. The therapeutic mechanism of successful treatment is the creation of a "pneumatic splint" by an effective positive pressure applied to the pharynx, providing immediate relief from obstruction (13), thus allowing sleep continuity and preservation of sleep architecture (14,15).

BENEFITS OF CONTINUOUS POSITIVE PRESSURE THERAPY

Studies have shown that positive pressure therapy, if successfully implemented, can have significant impact on a variety of parameters of health and daily living. A number of studies have shown that PAP therapy significantly improves subjective and objective measures of daytime sleepiness (16,17), improves quality of life (18–20), and has a positive impact on neurocognitive function in patients with OSA (18,19).

Further studies have shown that significant reductions in adverse cardiovascular disease outcomes may be obtained with successful treatment of OSA (5,10). CPAP reduces blood pressure in hypertensive patients (21,22), reverses hemodynamic changes in the cerebral circulation (23), and may reduce pulmonary pressures in OSA patients (24). Moreover, CPAP has been shown to prevent OSA-associated bradyarrhythmias (25,26), decrease recurrence of atrial fibrillation after cardioversion (27), and abolish ventricular arrhythmias (28,29). Furthermore, patients with congestive heart failure (CHF) and OSA have shown a marked improvement in left ventricular ejection fraction and functional class after initiation of CPAP therapy (30,31).

In addition, CPAP produces many other sustained benefits that may have significant impact on long-term health outcomes, in particular, those processes that appear to contribute to the pathogenesis of cardiovascular disease. These benefits include decreased platelet activity and aggregation during sleep in OSA patients (32), a decrease in factor VII coagulant activity (VII:C) (32,33), decreased fibrinogen levels (34), increased levels of circulating nitric oxide (35,36), decreased overall sympathetic nervous system output (37,38), improved insulin sensitivity and glucose intolerance (39), reduced C-reactive protein (CRP) and interleukin-6 levels (40), and reduced serum leptin levels (41,42).

INDICATIONS TO TREAT WITH POSITIVE AIRWAY PRESSURE

All of these data suggest that CPAP should exert a favorable effect on patients with OSA, and in particular, patients with OSA and cardiovascular disease. However, unequivocal data showing long-term benefits with cardiovascular endpoints are still lacking. So, in turn, the question of which patients with OSA that will derive benefit from treatment remains somewhat controversial. Practice parameters developed by the American Academy of Sleep Medicine and published in 2006 describe the indications for PAP therapy; the main indications are described in this section (43).

In North America, OSA is remarkably prevalent in the general population, with studies showing an estimated 20% of adults with mild to asymptomatic disease and at least 5% of adults with significant disease (44). The prevalence has been estimated to be as high as 30% to 50% in some at-risk patient populations (27,45,46).

Obstructive Sleep Apnea

According to Medicare guidelines, revised in 2002, CPAP is indicated for patients with an apnea–hypopnea index (AHI) > 15 events/hour (moderate severity), regardless of symptoms; and for patients with an AHI > 5 and ≤ 14 (mild severity) with excessive daytime somnolence, impaired cognition, mood disorders, insomnia; or with the comorbidities of hypertension, ischemic heart disease, or stroke (47). However, the Medicare list of acceptable ICD-9 (International Classification of Diseases, ninth revision) codes that support medical necessity which justify the use of polysomnography to screen for and/or diagnose sleep-related breathing disorders includes only diagnoses of sleep disturbances or of hypersomnolence, disregarding comorbidities (48).

It is important to note, however, that in the seminal Wisconsin Cohort Study, it was found that only 15.5% of males and 22.6% of females with documented obstructive sleep-related respiratory events (i.e., AHI), at a rate of five events per hour or more, reported sleepiness on all three subjective measures assessed (49). Additionally, the Wisconsin Cohort Study showed a dose–response association between sleep-disordered breathing at baseline and the presence of hypertension four years later that was independent of other known risk factors, even in the presence of only mild OSA [odds ratio (OR) = 2.03; 1.2–3.17].

Based upon these data, it is prudent to screen patients with diagnostic polysomnography at risk for or previously diagnosed with primary hypertension in the presence of other associated risk factors that increase the suspicion of OSA, including witnessed apneas, snoring, obesity, large neck circumference, and a small posterior airway space, with or without overt sleep complaints. If OSA is detected, even of mild severity, then treatment with PAP therapy is warranted. Accordingly, current

Medicare guidelines support the treatment of patients with mild OSA and cardiovascular comorbidities. However, based upon current Medicare guidelines, the current indication for diagnostic polysomnography precludes the routine screening of these patients without overt sleep complaints.

Upper Airway Resistance Syndrome (See Also Chapter 18)
Another controversial area is the utility of PAP therapy in patients with upper airway resistance syndrome (UARS). This disorder is generally considered to be present in patients with severe snoring accompanied by respiratory effort-related arousals during sleep and excessive daytime sleepiness (50). Typically, overt apneas and/or hypopneas are absent, thus the patient fails to meet criteria for the diagnosis of OSA. Despite Medicare's failure to acknowledge this disease as noteworthy enough to warrant treatment, it is an important disease to acknowledge and in clinically symptomatic patients, may warrant treatment with either PAP, surgery, or more conservative approaches such as oral appliances, weight loss, or positional therapy.

Central Sleep Apnea (See Also Chapter 19)
Central sleep apnea (CSA) is a sleep-related breathing disorder that requires careful consideration when evaluating treatment options. The etiology of CSA may impact treatment decision algorithms and must be closely evaluated before determining the appropriate modality of therapy. Patients with alveolar hypoventilation or idiopathic CSA will likely benefit from PAP therapy, especially in patients with waking hypercapnea with worsening hypoxemia during sleep, as well as patients complaining of excessive daytime sleepiness. Frequently, patients who have been diagnosed with idiopathic CSA will in fact have secondary causes of central events, including unrecognized upper airway obstruction causing nasopharyngeal or non-nasal pharyngeal reflexive central events (51,52). PAP clearly has a role in treating these patients; whereas patients with true idiopathic CSA prove to be somewhat more difficult to appropriately treat. While adequate ventilation may be accomplished with a pressure- or volume-cycled ventilators (53) no definitive modality, including supplemental nocturnal oxygen (54), acetazolamide (55), and other medications (56), have proven to be consistently effective for treatment in these patients.

Another important subset of CSA patients consists of patients with Cheyne-Stokes respiration (CSA-CSR). This pattern of respiration is characterized by a crescendo–decrescendo respiratory pattern, with periods of hyperventilation followed by periods of central apneas. CSR with CSA has been reported to have prevalence rates between 33% and 45% in patients with congestive heart failure (CHF) (7,57,58). Importantly, increased mortality has been found in patients who develop CSA-CSR during sleep (59). Like idiopathic CSA, no reliable treatment modality has been found to be wholly effective in patients with CSA-CSR. While some patients with CHF seem to show improvement of CSA-CSR through optimization of cardiac function, this modality is only effective in a minority of patients (60). While CPAP has been shown to improve cardiac function and reduce adrenergic tone when used chronically (61,62), previous studies have shown improvement in survival and delays in time to transplantation (63,64). A multicenter trial of CPAP and CSA-CSR in CHF patients failed to show any significant improvement in number of hospitalizations, quality of life, or significant difference in death and heart transplantation in the CPAP-treated group (64). It is important to note that although adherence with CPAP was fairly high in this trial, hours of use in the treatment group was between 3.5 and 4 hours/night and the average AHI after treatment was 19 events per hour. Despite many shortcomings of this study, the results demonstrate the complexities and barriers in finding the optimal treatment modality of CSA-CSR.

As evidenced in previous studies, adherence with PAP therapy in patients with CSA-CSR seems equal in importance to elimination of respiratory events as a barrier to effective treatment. More recently, alternative PAP delivery mechanisms have shown promise as an effective modality for treatment of CSA-CSR; namely, timed bilevel PAP (BPAP) and/or adaptive servo-ventilation (ASV) (VPAP Adapt SV; ResMed, North Ryde, Australia). Studies have indicated that CSA-CSR is more effectively treated with bilevel PAP and ASV and equally as important, patients preferred both these modalities over CPAP; however, more data are required before the routine use of these modalities in treatment for this disease (65–67).

Pulmonary Arterial Hypertension
In 1998, the World Health Organization conference on pulmonary arterial hypertension (PAH) recognized sleep-disordered breathing as a secondary cause of PAH (68). While severe OSA and hypoxemia are more commonly associated with PAH, mild PAH is also common in patients with OSA (69–71). Patients who have been diagnosed with pulmonary hypertension should be evaluated for a sleep-related breathing disorder as a part of the initial diagnostic assessment and should be treated with PAP if OSA is present.

Chronic Obstructive Pulmonary Disease (See Also Chapter 20)
There are no data to suggest that OSA occurs with greater frequency in patients with chronic obstructive pulmonary disease (COPD), the so-called "overlap syndrome." While patients with COPD have a significant degree of nocturnal hypoxemia, in particular during rapid eye movement (REM) sleep there is no evidence to suggest that this nocturnal hypoxemia occurs due to airway obstruction. It appears rather to be caused by a combination of hypoventilation (72), ventilation–perfusion mismatch (73), and a decrease in functional residual capacity. Noninvasive positive pressure ventilation (NIPPV) has been found to reduce intubations, complications, and mortality rate in patients with acute hypercapnea due to a COPD exacerbation (74); however, it is still unclear whether patients with chronic, severe hypercapnea will derive significant survival benefit from prolonged NIPPV (75).

Restrictive Lung Disease
Restrictive lung disease is another category of pulmonary disorders that may require nocturnal PAP therapy. Lung restriction is most commonly seen in obesity, kyphoscoliosis, neuromuscular disease, interstitial lung disease, and pregnancy. PAP therapy should be used unequivocally in these patients if they have coexisting OSA. However, in the absence of OSA, PAP therapy must be considered on a case-by-case manner, depending upon the disease process being considered.

Obese patients without OSA but with obesity hypoventilation syndrome (OHS) may benefit from nocturnal PAP therapy; CPAP, BPAP, or volume cycled NIPPV. BPAP or volume cycled NIPPV allow for increased ventilatory assistance compared to PAP therapy with CPAP. Initiation of PAP therapy should be performed in an attended setting as these patients may, at times, be medically unstable, and/or require supplemental oxygen in addition to positive pressure therapy; however, oxygen therapy alone is insufficient in these patients. NIPPV has been shown to improve long-term outcomes in patients with OHS (76).

Patients with kyphoscoliosis should be considered for PAP therapy in the absence of OSA if there are complaints of daytime sleepiness or sleep disruption and/or evidence of hypoventilation, Cheyne-Stokes respirations, or central apneas, all of which may be seen in these patients (77,78). Again, initiation of PAP therapy should be performed in a supervised setting due to the likelihood of the need to titrate supplemental oxygen in addition to NIPPV as well as the possibility of acute respiratory failure developing in these patients. Acute respiratory failure due to PAP therapy may occur in these patients with its initiation due to the increased work of breathing, which may result from an increased functional residual capacity coupled with extreme chest wall stiffness. Once evidence of hypoventilation is observed, BPAP or volume cycled NIPPV will be required to adequately ventilate these patients at night and may stave off invasive ventilation for some time (79–81).

Patients with progressive neuromuscular disorders will manifest the beginnings of chronic respiratory failure with nocturnal hypoventilation. In these cases, NIPPV should appropriately be started at night with a formal, supervised titration. Stable neuromuscular disorders with partial ventilatory function, including the sequelae of poliomyelitis, tuberculosis, Duchenne muscular dystrophy (DMD), or high-level spinal cord injuries, may successfully be ventilated at night, which may, in turn improve clinical and physiologic daytime function and may, like patients with respiratory failure due to kyphoscoliosis, stave off continuous NIPPV and/or invasive ventilation (82,83).

Interstitial lung disease (ILD) is a broad group of restrictive pulmonary disorders of more than 100 different etiologies. Patients with ILD often manifest disordered sleep due to difficulties with nocturnal breathing, especially in patients with baseline $SaO_2 < 90\%$ (84). Additionally, nocturnal hypoxemia is fairly common in this group of patients and is likely due to episodic or persistent hypoventilation relative to waking ventilation, and may be more severe in REM sleep (85). PAP therapy is only indicated in patients with coexisting OSA and although no definitive clinical trials have validated its use, nocturnal oxygen in appropriate individuals is likely the treatment of choice (86).

TITRATION TECHNIQUES

The current standard of care dictates CPAP therapy be commenced and titrated under direct supervision by a trained technician. Direct supervision allows for immediate assessment of various sleep-related disturbances, direct determination of the optimal CPAP pressure, and identification of significant sleep-related comorbidities, including but not limited to nocturnal seizures, cardiac arrhythmias, parasomnia activity, and nocturnal myoclonus. Furthermore, direct supervision allows for appropriate evaluation of persistent hypoxemia with PAP therapy in the absence of overt respiratory events, which may in turn require additional titration of supplemental oxygen. To date, there is little evidence regarding the safety and efficacy of CPAP titrations performed outside of a medically-supervised setting. In fact, current evidence suggests that patients have a greater likelihood of being compliant with therapy if initial introduction to CPAP is performed in a setting where education and support by a sleep professional are a part of the initial experience, and longitudinal support and positive reinforcement are offered as an ongoing part of patient care (87–89). Auto-titrating devices have called into question the current standard; however, current evidence does not support the use of these devices for CPAP initiation and further studies are needed.

The primary goal of the PAP titration study is three-fold: introduction of and acclimation to PAP therapy, determination of optimal mask interface type and fit, and determination of the optimal pressure that will normalize sleep-disordered breathing and correct hypoxemia. Introduction of PAP therapy is a critical step in helping towards long-term adherence. Data have suggested that patients who have difficulties on the first night of therapy have less likelihood of long-term adherence and are three times more likely to use their machines for less than four hours per night than those without first night problems (90).

Before the initiation of the PAP titration, extensive education about the pathophysiology of OSA, the consequences of untreated OSA, as well as PAP therapy should be given to the patient. Videotapes and supplemental reading are additional tools that may help patient adherence. Intensive patient education has been shown to improve the likelihood of adherence in various studies (see section: Improving Adherence) (88,89). Special care should be given by the supervising technician to ensure optimal mask fit in order to improve comfort and reduce the potential for mask leak. In some cases, a chinstrap or a full-face mask may be required to eliminate mouth breathing, which should be assessed once the titration study has begun (91). Mouth breathing has been shown to adversely effect CPAP adherence and should be addressed during the initial titration night (92).

When determining a titration algorithm, it is essential to understand that elimination of apneas, hypopneas, and oxygen desaturations is the first objective, but not the endpoint of the titration. Rather, the endpoint of the titration should be elimination of snoring and respiratory-related arousals in all positions and all stages of sleep (50,93). Persistent inspiratory airflow limitation is evidenced by a flattened airflow pressure tracing and can best be demonstrated with titrations that are performed with nasal pressure-flow transducers, as opposed to thermistors or other indirect measures of airflow (94). Although esophageal pressure monitoring is the most accurate means of assessing increased respiratory effort due to flow limitation, this modality is often poorly tolerated which may in turn limit its routine use in CPAP titration studies. When inspiratory airflow limitation is associated with spontaneous arousals, it is likely due to UARS and a further increase in airway pressure is indicated (95). An uncontrolled CPAP titration patient series has been reported, which suggests that careful monitoring of esophageal pressures, and/or CPAP airflow signals, generally demonstrates continued evidence of airflow resistance until CPAP pressures have been increased to 2 cm H_2O, on average, above that needed to eliminate apneas and hypopneas (96). Surprisingly, it has been demonstrated that patients undergoing CPAP titration may display increased pressure requirements during titration from lower CPAP pressures upward, as compared to pressures required during downward titration from higher pressures (97). Accordingly, in some patients, it is appropriate during a titration study to titrate pressures upward until elimination of respiratory events has been achieved and a normal airflow pattern is attained; and then titrate downward to the return of obstructive events. This method is of particular use in patients who have difficulty tolerating PAP therapy due to high pressure requirements.

When performing a titration, it is important to note sleep stage and body position once optimal pressure is assumed as evidence that suggests that higher pressure requirements may be needed in the supine position (98) and in REM sleep (99). Once an optimal pressure has been attained, in addition to resolution of sleep-related breathing events, sleep continuity should theoretically improve, with a decrease in the number of spontaneous arousals and arousals associated with respiratory events. Commonly, slow-wave sleep rebound or REM sleep rebound will be seen with improved sleep continuity and this finding can be used as an indication that an effective pressure level is imminent (100). It has been shown that increased tidal volumes can induce central apneas in the setting of normocapnia due to neuro-chemical inhibition and possibly, baroreceptor activity (101). This finding has led to the practice of decreasing CPAP pressures when the emergence of central apneas is witnessed during an upward titration. However, it is important to continue to explore upward pressures with the appearance of central apneas, as there are several mechanisms that have been shown to elicit central apneas, including upper airway obstruction (51,52), which may be indicative of subtherapeutic pressures.

There is considerable debate regarding the use of bilevel ventilation as a strategy to improve adherence to PAP therapy in patients requiring high pressures to treat sleep-related breathing disorders. Studies using dynamic upper airway imaging have confirmed that expiratory collapse of the upper airway occurs, and does so in a more passive manner than does inspiratory airway collapse (102). This finding seems to be explained by the active, negative intraluminal pressures generated during inspiration, which are absent with the more passive expiration. As a result, it has been shown that lower expiratory pressures are required to maintain airway patency than with inspiration (103). The efficacy of using bilevel ventilation as a standard treatment modality in all patients with OSA is questionable; however, clinicians tend to consider unacceptably high CPAP pressures, as deemed by intolerance of the pressure by the patient during the study, as an indication to change to bilevel mode of ventilation. Although not studied systematically, clinicians generally feel that patients with lung disease, chest-wall disease, and/or neuromuscular disease may be most appropriate for bilevel mode of delivery of breath. There is at least one study that has suggested that bilevel PAP increases the incidence of CSA-CSR and non-CSR CSA in certain patients (104), which further reinforces the need for more studies in this area.

While CPAP therapy has been the standard of care for many years, there is a surprising lack of data validating standardized titration methods. In particular, details on the transition from CPAP therapy to bilevel therapy are lacking. In patients with OSA intolerant of CPAP, there exist primarily three different techniques employed: (*i*) an inspiratory pressure is chosen equal to the CPAP pressure where obstructive events were eliminated; (*ii*) an expiratory pressure is chosen equal to the CPAP pressure where obstructive events were eliminated; (*iii*) bilevel is initiated from a low starting pressure, beginning with baseline pressure settings and titrating upwards. Regardless of the technique followed, it is generally thought that a 4 to 5 cm H_2O difference should be preserved in order to maintain airway patency during expiration. Commonly, expiratory pressure increases are performed in the setting of persistent or reappearing apneas, while inspiratory pressure increases are made in the setting of snoring, flow limitation, or hypopneas, maintaining a 4 cm difference between the two.

The use of BPAP in patients with OHS should be initiated in a similar fashion; however, if hypoxemia persists after resolution of respiratory events, in particular during REM sleep, the addition of supplemental oxygen in these patients is appropriate. Special consideration is needed when using BPAP in patients with CSA not responsive to CPAP, especially patients with CSA-CSR in the absence of OSA. These patients will often need a "timed mode" of inspiration as the bilevel unit will not be triggered due to lack of inspiratory effort. As previously stated, these patients are extremely difficult to treat and a definitive modality of therapy has yet to be determined. In light of this fact, ASV ventilation has been developed in the hope of creating a more effective means of treating CSA-CSR and improving adherence. ASV ventilation provides positive expiratory airway pressure and inspiratory pressure support that is servo-controlled based on the detection of CSR, with a backup respiratory rate. Initial studies show great promise for this device as means of effectively controlling CSA-CSR (65–67); however, further data are needed before this modality becomes the standard of care.

Another area of debate is the use of the "split-night" study as means to diagnose and treat OSA in a single night. This strategy has been devised in an effort to decrease the financial burden of two separate studies as well as to minimize the inconvenience to the patient. There are data to suggest that this is a reasonable approach (105), however, these nonrandomized studies were biased toward patients with more severe disease (106,107). There seem to be certain patients who are best suited for the "split-night" protocol; however, data are lacking to justify the routine use of these studies in the absence of insurance mandate or appropriate patient selection.

The use of "daytime" titrations is another method that has been proposed to derive optimal pressure settings. Again, limited efficacy and adherence data call this technique into question (105) though initial nonrandomized cohort studies do show some comparable results to overnight titrations (108,109).

Many factors may contribute to the therapeutic efficacy of PAP therapy over time. In the absence of significant clinical changes, a pressure level chosen during a single night's titration is generally effective on longitudinal nights (110). However, significant weight gain (111), heavy alcohol use (112), and nasal congestion are all factors that can alter the efficacy of CPAP therapy. If a patient who initially responded to treatment begins to complain of recurrent symptoms, consider these contributing factors as a potential cause. It is imperative for the clinician to consider all causes of "residual hypersomnolence" in the treated OSA patient, and far and away the most common cause of sleepiness in Western society is insufficient sleep. Additionally though, CPAP nonadherence, coexisting sleep fragmenting disorders, and chronic medical or psychiatric conditions may also play a role in the complaint of sleepiness or fatigue in the treated OSA patient.

SIDE EFFECTS AND LIMITATIONS

Side effects from CPAP therapy tend to be minor though can often be a significant barrier between long-term adherence (113) and tend to be related either due to problems with the interface or due to positive pressure. Common complaints include nasal congestion, rhinorrhea, skin abrasion, difficulty with exhalation, chest discomfort, dry mouth, claustrophobia, conjunctivitis due to air leak, and/or aerophagia (114). Reports document up to 10% of all CPAP users complaining of some degree of persistent nasal congestion at six months after initiation of CPAP therapy (115). This finding is likely related to reduced humidification of the inspired air causing release of inflammatory mediators (116). Extremely rare are reports of serious complications including pulmonary barotrauma, pneumocephalus (subsequent to base of skull fracture), tympanic membrane rupture, massive epistaxis, subcutaneous emphysema, decreased cardiac output at high pressure, and increased intraocular pressure, which have been reported in association with the use of nasal CPAP (114,117–119). Most side effects or problems can be resolved (Table 1) with careful attention to interface options with appropriate selection of mask type and fit, careful and methodological assessment of patient symptoms, and careful monitoring of patients at risk for serious complications, such as those with bullous lung disease.

Although CPAP is the definitive treatment for sleep-related breathing disorders, there are still limitations to this therapy. The most obvious limitation is the ability of certain individuals to tolerate PAP. As will be discussed later in this chapter, adherence to CPAP therapy is the greatest obstacle for the clinician to contend with, and this is largely dictated by the patient's ability to tolerate CPAP. Additionally, certain patients require such high pressures to definitively treat their disease that mask leak is largely unavoidable, making tolerance all the more difficult to achieve. Patients with severe nasal obstruction often will not tolerate a traditional nasal mask interface and require a full-face mask, which anecdotally is less tolerated than a nasal mask. Alternatively, nasal surgery may allow for better tolerance of PAP therapy through decreased nasal resistance (120). Other issues that arise which may in turn limit an individual's adherence with therapy include lifestyle inconvenience, such as that encountered when trying to travel with a CPAP device. Fortunately, airport

TABLE 1 Common CPAP Problems and Solutions

Problem	Solutions
Aerophagia	Reduce CPAP pressure; consider BPAP or APAP
Air leakage through mouth	Add chinstrap or switch to full-face mask
Condensation of water in CPAP hose	Add insulated sleeve around hose
Claustrophobia	Switch to different mask or try nasal interface; desensitization (i.e., wearing device for progressively longer periods)
Dry mouth and/or nose	Add humidification and apply saline drops in nose; add chinstrap or switch to full-face mask
Eye irritation	Refit or adjust mask; apply saline drops in eyes; add eye mask
Inadvertently removing mask during sleep	Adjust alarm setting on machine; apply surgical tape at edge of mask and skin, since removal of tape may awaken patient and prevent removal of mask; consider PAP re-titration
Mask discomfort	Switch to different mask
Mask leak	Refit or adjust mask
Nasal congestion	Add heated humidification; add nasal saline, decongestant, antihistamine, and/or nasal steroid; switch to full-face mask; correct possible anatomic defect in nose or sinuses
Noisy device	Place device under bed or away from patient (may need extension hose), but avoid covering air intake port to device; switch to another device
Pressure intolerance	Consider PAP re-titration; instruct patient on ramp feature of device; switch to APAP, BPAP, or flexible PAP
Skin breakdown from mask at bridge of nose	Refit mask or switch to different mask; try nasal interface

Abbreviations: APAP, automatic positive airway pressure; BPAP, bilevel positive airway pressure; CPAP, continuous positive airway pressure; PAP, positive airway pressure.
Source: Courtesy of C. Kushida.

security personnel have become increasingly informed about CPAP and usually make allowances for individuals traveling with these devices.

Another potential limitation of CPAP therapy is its application in the pediatric patient population. While tonsillectomy and adenoidectomy is the mainstay of treatment for pediatric OSA, a small but significant portion of pediatric patients with OSA will have persistent sleep-disordered breathing postoperatively, indicating a craniofacial etiology for their disease (121,122). CPAP is thus indicated for treatment until such time that surgical intervention can be performed to correct the skeletal abnormality predicating the disease. Surprisingly, CPAP is relatively well-tolerated in a large percentage of these patients, with studies indicating up to 80% adherence (123,124); however, attaining adherence in pediatric patients intolerant of CPAP is fairly difficult.

Interestingly, while adherence with PAP therapy is clearly an issue, the question of how much nightly usage constitutes "adherence" is not well understood and often debated. An interesting notion that has likely fueled this debate is one that suggests that there exists a residual benefit from CPAP when used only a few hours a night, which seems to reinforce this idea of 4.5 hours/night of use to be adequate. A study by Hers et al. (125) found that in 24 patients with newly-diagnosed OSA, after being titrated to normalization of their sleep and breathing during the first half of the night, a partial improvement of OSA severity and mean oxygen severity occurred during the second half of the night without treatment. Sleep architecture was notably more fragmented during the second half of the study night without therapy. It is possible that this carryover effect is what is responsible for subjective benefits reported by patients who are only partially compliant with treatment. The topic of adherence is discussed in more detail later in this chapter.

PERIOPERATIVE MANAGEMENT

Patients undergoing any surgical procedure are susceptible to postoperative complications due to respiratory compromise. Patients with OSA are at obvious risk for a postoperative complication due to the perioperative use of narcotics and benzodiazepines, which are known to blunt the respiratory response to hypercapnea and to hypoxia as well as exacerbate upper airway obstruction (126). Unfortunately, many patients undergoing surgical procedures are not appropriately screened for OSA and may be put at risk for postoperative complications, in particular patients having outpatient surgical procedures who are sent home to a completely unmonitored environment.

There are few studies looking directly at the risk of postoperative complications associated with OSA, however, the American Society of Anesthesiologists (ASA) have recognized the risk of postoperative complications associated with patients who have undiagnosed OSA and thereby published practice guidelines outlining recommendations of how to identify and treat patients at risk. The ASA practice parameters suggest that preoperatively, anesthesiologists should work with surgeons to develop a protocol whereby patients in whom the possibility of OSA is suspected on clinical grounds are evaluated long enough before the day of surgery to allow preparation of a perioperative management plan. The recommendations go on to include preoperative preparation where preoperative initiation of CPAP should be considered, particularly if OSA is severe. As previously stated, because of their propensity for airway collapse and sleep deprivation, patients with OSA are especially susceptible to the respiratory depressant and airway effects of sedatives, narcotics, and inhaled anesthetics. Therefore, in selecting intraoperative medications, the ASA practice parameters suggest that the potential for postoperative respiratory compromise should be considered. Regional analgesic (pain relief) techniques should be considered to reduce or eliminate the requirement for systemic opioids (narcotics) in patients at increased perioperative risk from OSA. Finally, the practice parameters go on to recommend that before patients at increased perioperative risk from OSA are scheduled for surgery, a determination should be made regarding whether a given surgical procedure is most appropriately performed on an inpatient or outpatient basis. In addition, specific criteria should be met for discharging the patient after surgery to an unmonitored setting, such as the home (127).

ADHERENCE

Despite its demonstrated efficacy for treating OSA (128–130), there is some concern that CPAP adherence consistently falls below expectations. Some studies have demonstrated that the majority of patients who are prescribed CPAP either discontinue it completely or fail to use it at recommended levels (i.e., all night every night) (131,132). A review of the past 50 years of adherence to medical treatments concluded that the poorest adherence was associated with the treatment of sleep disorders (133). The majority of these studies involved treatment with CPAP. Using liberal definitions of adherence, 65% of patients were adherent with CPAP therapy compared to an overall average of 75% for all medical disorders. The continual report of low adherence may lead providers to accept less than optimal adherence, recognizing that they are limited in an attempt to try to achieve higher rates. This point is further exacerbated by the fact that few studies to date have identified the level of adherence needed to remedy some of the more common sequelae of the disorder. Moreover, there is no field standard for adherence, leading some to report adequate adherence in participants that would be characterized as suboptimal or poor by others' standards. There have been some studies and meeting presentations that suggest necessary levels of adherence to reduce the risk of cardiovascular disease and remedy functional problems (134,135). These studies generally point to use of six or more hours a night, levels less frequently reached in naturalistic studies. Perhaps the initial step to improving adherence lies in better understanding adherence as a dependent measure and what factors influence adherence over time.

Adherence as a Dependent Variable

Adherence can be a complex dependent variable. Adherence researchers have long understood that adherence is generally not normally distributed and is often resistant to attempts at modification (136). A normal distribution is assumed in linear-based statistics employed in most studies. It is true that some of these statistics are robust to violations of this assumption, but some investigators have chosen to categorize adherence into two groups (adherent or not) for this very reason. Categorization also provides a more heuristic way of describing the data. The problem with categorizing adherence is that there are no set a priori categories used by most investigators. Many use four hours a night as a cutoff for adherent CPAP use. This four-hour cutoff is most likely a result of continued report of four hours per night as the arithmetic average adherence attained in many studies. However, there is no clinical evidence to date that suggests a particular advantage to four hours per night. Similarly, Kribbs et al. (132) used two separate definitions based on intuition.

Minimal use was described as four hours per night over 70% of the nights; while optimal use was described as seven hours per night over 70% of the nights. Although appealing, these definitions again have no clinical or scientific data to support them. Even more importantly, there is evidence that adherence may be better considered in several categories rather than either adequate or poor adherence, allowing for individual differences to emerge in the approach to using CPAP. There are reports claiming to identify a critical cutoff for adherence based on clinical outcomes. One study suggested that adherence of at least six hours per night demonstrated an advantage over adherence of less than an hour a night in long-term cardiovascular morbidity and mortality (134). This six-hour cutoff has also been reported at meetings as beneficial to remedy functional outcomes associated with OSA (135). In sum, adherence with CPAP therapy is a complex variable and its complexity must be considered in statistical analyses. Despite this complexity, there is no agreed upon definition of a cutoff for adequate adherence to date.

Predictors of Adherence

Studies of CPAP nonadherence have found that the most consistent indicator of continued CPAP use is perceived improvement in sleepiness (136). In some studies, CPAP adherers have been found to be more educated and have greater daytime somnolence, while nonadherers have less severe disease and concurrent medical problems (131,132). Side effects of CPAP therapy, although often cited as a primary reason for discontinuing treatment (137,138), produce only minimal adherence improvements when treated (139). Factors such as type of mask (139), titration method (auto vs. standard) (128–140), and delivery method of PAP (CPAP vs. bilevel ventilation) (141) do not reliably produce improvements in adherence or in OSA-related symptoms. Perhaps the strongest effects on predicting adherence have been demonstrated by measures of behavioral attitudes toward CPAP use. In a seminal study, Stepnowsky et al. (142) examined the predictive utility of behavioral attitudes based on psychological theories of behavior change principles. These theories have been applied to studies of behavior change for several years and have only relatively recently been employed in adherence studies. These investigators found that these self-report measures, taken only one week after the beginning of CPAP, predicted approximately 20% to 30% of the variance in one-month adherence. Predictive utility increased when the measures were taken concurrently to measuring adherence (30–40% of the variance). Aloia et al. (143) followed this study with another study that examined the efficacy of these measures over longer follow-up periods. These investigators found that these measures predicted 20% of the variance in six-month use when taken at one week and 40% of the variance when taken concurrently with measuring adherence (at three months). Together, these studies suggest that theories of behavior change principles effectively apply to the conceptualization of why individuals do or do not adhere to CPAP. Moreover, these measures can serve as gateways into discussions with patients about their attitudes toward use rather than confronting them directly with poor adherence.

Improving Adherence

Several investigators have attempted to take various approaches to remedying the problem of CPAP adherence. Common approaches can fall into one of two categories: technological interventions or behavioral interventions. The success of these will be briefly summarized here. A more thorough review of these methods and their relative success or failure can be obtained through one of two comprehensive reviews (144,145).

Recent technological advances in the delivery of airflow have occurred, aiming to improve patient comfort, adherence, and effectiveness for reducing apneas and inspiratory flow limitation. Many of these advances, such as auto-titrating PAP (APAP), have been designed to adjust PAP throughout the night, keeping the pressure elevated when upper airway collapsing forces are high and lowering pressure when the likelihood of airway collapse is low (146). Other devices, including bilevel devices, deliver different set pressures during exhalation (lower pressure) and inhalation (higher pressure) in an attempt to improve comfort (103). Despite these advances, previous studies suggest that these different flow delivery devices do not substantially improve treatment adherence over traditional CPAP (103,147). In a Cochrane Review conducted in 2004 (145), investigators also found little evidence of a strong advantage of auto devices over fixed devices, though they are careful to mention that these devices may have utility for a subset of patient who are as yet unidentified. They also state that the limited advantage provided bilevel ventilation may be outweighed by the cost of the device. The most recent technological advancement has come in the form of flexible pressure delivery. This type of device alternates airway pressure between exhalation and inhalation on a breath-by-breath basis. Airway pressure is reduced during early exhalation in proportion to the patient's expiratory flow rate. Pressure is then increased again toward the end of exhalation when airway collapse is most likely (102). Adherence to flexible pressure technology was compared to fixed CPAP in one controlled, nonrandomized study (148). Flexible pressure was demonstrated to show an advantage of 1.7 hours a night by three months, but differences were not demonstrated on clinical outcome variables. Finally, heated humidification has also resulted in mixed findings, with a one hour a night advantage demonstrated in one study (138), while another demonstrated no advantage (149). Despite the mixed and sometimes unimpressive findings associated with technological advancements, investigators and clinicians agree that improvements in the comfort of the method of flow delivery might serve as one important target in attempting to improve patient adherence.

Several studies have applied educational and behaviorally-based interventions to the problem of CPAP adherence [for review see Engleman and Wild (144) and Haniffa et al. (145)]. Three studies have evaluated the efficacy of simple education on adherence, reasoning that increased knowledge about OSA risks and the consequences of nonadherence would result in greater use (150–152). Some improvement in adherence over short follow-up periods resulted. Two additional studies examined the efficacy of more intensive interventions for adherence compared to standard care (153,154). Findings from these studies were equivocal. Finally, one previous study reported enhanced PAP use in a small sample of participants who received systematic desensitization and sensory awareness training for CPAP-related claustrophobia (155). Collectively, these findings suggest that interventions that focus on enhancing knowledge, increasing patient–therapist interaction, or removing only one potential barrier to PAP use produce nightly improvements ranging from 0 to 2.5 hours. Some of these studies have been limited by small sample sizes, the absence of control groups, and the inclusion of programs that would present practical and fiscal barriers for most sleep clinics to implement. Nonetheless, a Cochrane report concluded that: "There is some evidence that psychological/educational interventions improve CPAP usage." (145). Aloia et al. (155) proposed applying a therapy to PAP adherence that stems from psychological theories of behavior change, which have been found to predict CPAP adherence robustly in previous studies (143,144,156). This motivational enhancement therapy (MET) employs motivational interviewing techniques to the problem of poor adherence to treatment. Early results from this therapy suggest that brief therapies in general can reduce CPAP discontinuation rates compared to standard care. The MET therapy performed best under the condition of flexible delivery of PAP, though differences were not statistically significant (157).

In summary, several studies have demonstrated small to modest effects of both technological and behavioral interventions on adherence to CPAP. The single best approach, however, has not yet been identified. This may be because there is no single best approach. It may be that patients who are strong users of treatment early on need very little if any intervention to ensure their continued use; while those struggling early on may need both technological advantages coupled with therapeutic interventions targeting behavior change. This stepped-care approach to adherence has not yet been tested but may indeed be the most efficacious manner by which to approach the problem of nonadherence.

CONCLUSIONS

OSA is a markedly prevalent disease affecting a large percentage of the general population. Despite the limitations of CPAP, it is wholly effective in treating OSA when used and tolerated with few side effects and thus, has become the mainstay of treatment. Use of CPAP, however, may pose many challenges for both the clinician and the patient. When therapy is implemented, there are many important considerations for both parties to ensure a successful outcome. Certain individuals and situations require special care to ensure optimal therapy and compliance. Ultimately, treatment with PAP therapy can provide tremendous benefits for patients with OSA and a comprehensive approach by clinicians as well as longitudinal support are critical pieces of the treatment plan.

REFERENCES

1. Guilleminault C, Tilkian A, Dement WC. The sleep apnea syndromes. Ann Rev Med 1976; 27:465–484.
2. Bassiri AG, Guilleminault C. Clinical features of evaluation of obstructive sleep apnea–hypopnea syndrome. In: Kryger MH, Roth T, Dement WC, eds. Principles and Practices of Sleep Medicine. 3rd ed. Philadelphia, PA: Saunders, 2000:868–878.
3. Philip P, Stoohs R, Guilleminault C. Sleep fragmentation in normals. Sleep 1994; 17:242–247.
4. Chugh DK, Weaver TE, Dinges DF. Neurobehavioral consequences of arousals. Sleep 1996; 19(suppl):S198–S201.
5. Peker Y, Hedner J, Norum J, Kraiczi H, Carlson J. Increased incidence of cardiovascular disease in middle-aged men with obstructive sleep apnea: a 7-year follow-up. Am J Respir Crit Care Med 2002; 166:159–165.
6. Peppard PE, Young T, Palta M, Skatrud J. Prospective study of the association between sleep-disordered breathing and hypertension. N Engl J Med 2000; 342:1378–1384.
7. Javaheri S, Parker TJ, Wexler L, et al. Occult sleep-disordered breathing in stable congestive heart failure. Ann Int Med 1995; 122:487–492.
8. Gami AS, Pressman G, Caples SM, et al. Association of atrial fibrillation and obstructive sleep apnea. Circulation 2004; 110:364–367.
9. Peker Y, Kraiczi H, Hedner J, Loth S, Hohansson A, Bende M. An independent association between obstructive sleep apnoea and coronary artery disease. Eur Respir J 1999; 14:179–184.

10. Marin JM, Santiago JC, Vicente E, Agusti AGN. Long-term cardiovascular outcomes in men with obstructive sleep apnoea–hypopnoea with or without treatment with continuous positive airway pressure: an observational study. Lancet 2005; 365:1046–1053.
11. Strollo PJ, Roberts RM. Obstructive sleep apnea. N Engl J Med 1996; 334:99–104.
12. Sullivan CE, Issa FG, Berthon-Jones M, Eves L. Reversal of obstructive sleep apnoea by continuous positive airway pressure applied through the nares. Lancet 1981; 1:862–865.
13. Abbey NC, Cooper KR, Kwentus JA. Benefit of nasal CPAP in obstructive sleep apnea is due to positive pharyngeal pressure. Sleep 1989; 12:420–422.
14. Loredo JS, Anocli-Israel S, Dimsdale JE. Effect of continuous positive airway pressure vs placebo continuous positive airway pressure on sleep quality in obstructive sleep apnea. Chest 1999; 116:1545–1549.
15. McArdle N, Douglas NJ. Effect of continuous positive airway pressure on sleep architecture in the sleep apnea-hypopnea syndrome: a randomized controlled trial. Am J Respir Crit Care Med 2001; 164:1459–1463.
16. Patel SR, White DP, Malhotra A, Stanchina ML, Ayas NT. Continuous positive airway pressure therapy for treating sleepiness in a diverse population with obstructive sleep apnea: results of a meta-analysis. Arch Intern Med 2003; 163:565–571.
17. Morisson F, Decary A, Petit D, Lavigne G, Malo J, Montplaisir J. Daytime sleepiness and EEG spectral analysis in apneic patients before and after treatment with continuous positive airway pressure. Chest 2001; 119:45–52.
18. Engelman HM, Kingshott RN, Wraith PK, Mackay TW, Deary IJ, Douglas NJ. Randomized placebo-controlled crossover trial of continuous positive airway pressure for mild sleep Apnea/Hypopnea syndrome. Am J Respir Crit Care Med 1999; 159: 461–467.
19. Engleman HM, Martin SE, Deary IJ, Douglas NJ. Effect of continuous positive airway pressure treatment on daytime function in sleep apnoea/hypopnea syndrome. Lancet 1994; 343:572–575.
20. Engleman HM, Martin SE, Deary IJ, Douglas NJ. Effect of CPAP therapy on daytime function in patients with mild sleep apnoea/hypopnoea syndrome. Thorax 1997; 52:114–119.
21. Suzuki M, Otsuka K, Guilleminault C. Long-term nasal continuous positive airway pressure administration can normalize hypertension in obstructive sleep apnea patients. Sleep 1993; 16:545–549.
22. Dimsdale JE, Loredo JS, Profant T, et al. Effect of nasal continuous positive airway pressure on blood pressure: a placebo trial. Hypertension 2000; 35:144–147.
23. Diomedi M, Placidi F, Cupini LM, et al. Cerebral hemodynamic changes in sleep apnea syndrome and effect of continuous positive airway pressure treatment. Neurology 1998; 51:1051–1056.
24. Alchanatis M, Tourkohoriti G, Kakouros S, et al. Daytime pulmonary hypertension in patients with obstructive sleep apnea: the effect of continuous positive airway pressure on pulmonary hemodynamics. Respiration 2001; 68:566–572.
25. Becker H, Brandenburg U, Peter JH, et al. Reversal of sinus arrest and atrioventricular conduction block in patients with sleep apnea during nasal continuous positive airway pressure. Am J Respir Crit Care Med 1995; 151:2215–2218.
26. Stegman SS, Burroughs JM, Henthorn RW. Asymptomatic bradyarrhythmias as a marker for sleep apnea: appropriate recognition and treatment may reduce the need for pacemaker therapy. Pacing Clin Electrophysiol 1996; 19:899–904.
27. Kanagala R, Murali NS, Friedman PA, et al. Obstructive sleep apnea and the recurrence of atrial fibrillation. Circulation 2003; 107:2589–2594.
28. Harbison J, O'Reilly P, McNicholas WT. Cardiac rhythm disturbances in the obstructive sleep apnea syndrome: effects of nasal continuous positive airway pressure therapy. Chest 2000; 118:591–595.
29. Javaheri S. Effects of continuous positive airway pressure on sleep apnea and ventricular irritability in patients with heart failure. Circulation 2000; 169:156–162.
30. Malone S, Liu PP, Holloway R, et al. Obstructive sleep apnoea in patients with dilated cardiomyopathy: effects of continuous positive airway pressure. Lancet 1991; 338:1480–1484.
31. Kaneko Y, Floras JS, Usui K, et al. Cardiovascular effects of continuous positive airway pressure in patients with heart failure and obstructive sleep apnea. N Engl J Med 2003; 348:1233–1241.

32. Sanner BM, Konermann M, Tepel M, et al. Platelet function in patients with obstructive sleep apnea in ischemic stroke. Am J Respir Crit Care Med 2000; 22:21–27.
33. Chin K, Kita H, Noguchi T, et al. Improvement of factor VII clotting activity following long-term NCPAP treatment in obstructive sleep apnoea syndrome. QJM 1998; 91:627–633.
34. Chin K, Ohi M, Kita H, et al. Effects of NCPAP therapy on fibrinogen levels in obstructive sleep apnea syndrome. Am J Respir Crit Care Med 1996; 153:1972–1976.
35. Ohike Y, Kozaki K, Iijima K, et al. Amelioration of vascular endothelial dysfunction in obstructive sleep apnea syndrome by nasal continuous positive airway pressure—possible involvement of nitric oxide and symmetric NG, NG-dimethylarginine. Circ J 2005; 32(11 suppl):S548–S553.
36. Zhang XL, Yin KS, Mao H, Wang H, Yang Y. Effect of continuous positive airway pressure treatment on vascular endothelial function in patients with obstructive sleep apnea hypopnea syndrome and coronary artery disease. Chin Med J 2004; 117:844–847.
37. Narkiewicz K, de Borne PJH, Cooley RL, Dyken ME, Somers VK. Sympathetic activity in obese subjects with and without obstructive sleep apnea. Circulation 1998; 98:772–776.
38. Usui K, Bradley TD, Spaak J, et al. Inhibition of awake sympathetic nerve activity of heart failure patients with obstructive sleep apnea by nocturnal continuous positive airway pressure. J Am Coll Cardiol 2005; 45:2008–2011.
39. Harsch IA, Pour Schahin S, Radespiel-Troger M, et al. Continuous positive airway pressure treatment rapidly improves insulin sensitivity in patients with obstructive sleep apnea syndrome. Am J Respir Crit Care Med 2004; 169:156–162.
40. Yokoe T, Minoguchi K, Matsuo H, et al. Elevated levels of C-reactive protein and interleukin-6 in patients with obstructive sleep apnea syndrome are decreased by nasal continuous positive airway pressure. Circulation 2003; 107:1129–1134.
41. Ip MS, Lam KS, Ho C, Tsang KW, Lam W. Serum leptin and vascular risk factors in obstructive sleep apnea. Chest 2000; 118:569–571.
42. Chin K, Shinizu K, Nakamura T, et al. Changes in intra-abdominal visceral fat and serum leptin levels in patients with obstructive sleep apnea syndrome following nasal continuous positive airway pressure therapy. Circulation 1999; 100:706–712.
43. Kushida CA, Littner MR, Hirshkowitz M, et al. Practice parameters for the use of continuous and bilevel positive airway pressure devices to treat adult patients with sleep-related breathing disorders. Sleep 2006; 29:375–380.
44. Young T, Peppard PE, Gottlieb DJ. Epidemiology of obstructive sleep apnea: a population health perspective. Am J Respir Crit Care Med 2002; 165:1217–1239.
45. Javaheri S. Sleep disorders in systolic heart failure: a prospective study of 100 male patients. The final report. Int J Cardiol 2006; 106:21–28.
46. Schafer H, Koehler U, Ewig S, et al. Obstructive sleep apnea as a risk marker in coronary artery disease. Cardiology 1999; 92:79–84.
47. Centers for Medicare and Medicaid Services Manual. Section 60–17. Revised April 1, 2002.
48. Centers for Medicare and Medicaid Services. Empire Medicaid Services: Local coverage determination. Last review March 9, 2006. www.empiremedicare.com/newypolicy/policy/|8201_final.htm.
49. Young T, Palta M, Dempsey J, Skatrud J, Weber S, Badr S. The occurrence of sleep-disordered breathing among middle-aged adults. N Engl J Med 1993; 328(17):1230–1235.
50. Guilleminault C, Stoohs R, Clark A, et al. A cause of excessive daytime sleepiness: the upper airway resistance syndrome. Chest 1993; 104:781–787.
51. Suratt PM, Turner BL, Withoit SC. Effect of intranasal obstruction on breathing during sleep. Chest 1986; 90:324–329.
52. Issa F, Sullivan C. Reversal of central sleep apnea using nasal CPAP. Chest 1986; 90:165–171.
53. Guilleminualt C, Stoohs R, Shnieder H, et al. Central alveolar hypoventilation and sleep: treatment by intermittent positive pressure ventilation through nasal mask in an adult. Chest 1989; 96:1210–1212.
54. McNicholas W, Carter J, Rutherford R, et al. Beneficial effect of oxygen in primary alveolar hypoventilation with central sleep apnea. Am Rev Respir Dis 1982; 125:773–775.

55. White D, Zwillich C, Pickett C, et al. Central sleep apnea: improvement with acetazolamide therapy. Arch Intern Med 1982; 142:1816–1819.
56. Guilleminault C, van den Hoed J, Mitler M. Clinical overview of the sleep apnea syndromes. In: Guilleminault C, Dement W, eds. Sleep Apnea Syndromes. New York: Alan R Liss, 1978:1–11.
57. Sin DD, Fitzgeral F, Parker JD, et al. Risk factors for central and obstructive sleep apnea in 450 men and women with congestive heart failure. Am J Respir Crit Care Med 1999; 160:1101–1106.
58. Lofaso F, Verschueren P, Rande JL, Harf A, Goldenberg F. Prevalence of sleep-disordered breathing in patients on a heart transplant waiting list. Chest 1994; 106:1689–1694.
59. Hanly PJ, Zuberi-Khokar NS. Increased mortality associated with Cheyne-Stokes respiration in patients with congestive heart failure. Am J Respir Crit Care Med 1996; 153:272–276.
60. Tremel F, Pepin J, Veale D, et al. High prevalence and persistence of sleep apnoea in patients referred for acute left ventricular failure and medically treated over 2 months. Eur Heart J 1999; 20:1201–1209.
61. Naughton MT, Lie PP, Bernard DC, et al. Treatment of congestive heart failure and Cheyne-Stokes respiration during sleep by continuous positive airway pressure. Am J Respir Crit Care Med 1995; 151:92–97.
62. Kaye DM, Mansfield D, Aggarwal A, et al. Acute effects of continuous positive airway pressure on cardiac sympathetic tone in congestive heart failure. Circulation 2001; 103:2336–2338.
63. Sn DD, Logan AG, Fitgerald FS, et al. Effects of continuous positive airway pressure on cardiovascular outcomes in heart failure patients with and without Cheyne-Stokes respiration. Circulation 2000; 102:61–66.
64. Bradley TD, Logan AG, Kimoff RJ, et al. Continuous positive airway pressure for central sleep apnea and heart failure. N Engl J Med 2005; 353:2025–2033.
65. Pepperell JC, Maskell NA, Jones DR, et al. A randomized controlled trial of adaptive ventilation for Cheyne-Stokes Breathing in heart failure. Am J Respir Crit Care Med 2003; 168:1109–1114.
66. Teschler H, Dohring J, Wang YM, Berthon-Jones M. Adaptive pressure support servo-ventilation: a novel treatment for Cheyne-Stokes breathing in heart failure. Am J Respir Crit Care Med 2003; 168:1109–1114.
67. Philippe C, Stoica-Herman, Drouot X, et al. Compliance with and effectiveness of adaptive servo-ventilation versus continuous positive airway pressure in the treatment of Cheyne-Stokes respiration in heart failure over a six month period. Heart 2006; 92:337–342.
68. Rich S, ed. Primary pulmonary hypertension: executive summary from the World Symposium on Primary Pulmonary Hypertension. Geneva, World Health Organization, 1998.
69. Sanner BM, Doberauer C, Konermann M, et al. Pulmonary hypertension in patients with obstructive sleep apnea syndrome. Arch Intern Med 1997; 157:2483–2487.
70. Chaouat A, Weitzenblum E, Krieger J, et al. Pulmonary hemodynamics in the obstructive sleep apnea syndrome. Chest 1996; 109:380–386.
71. Laks L, Lehrhaft B, Grunstein RR, et al. Pulmonary hypertension in obstructive sleep apnea. Eur Respir J 1995; 8:537–541.
72. Catterall JR, Douglas NJ, Calverley PM, et al. Transient hypoxemia during sleep in chronic obstructive pulmonary disease is not a sleep apnea syndrome. Am Rev Respir Dis 1983; 128:24–29.
73. Catterall JR, Calverley PM, MacNee W, et al. Mechanism of transient nocturnal hypoxemia in hypoxic chronic bronchitis and emphysema. J Appl Physiol 1985; 59:1698–1703.
74. Lighttowler JV, Wedzicha JA, Elliot MW, Ramm FS. Non-invasive pressure ventilation to treat respiratory failure from exacerbations of chronic obstructive pulmonary disease: Cochrane systematic review and meta-analysis. Br Med J 2003; 326:185–187.
75. Meecham Jones DJ, Paul EA, Jones PW, Wedzicha JA. Nasal pressure support ventilation plus oxygen compared with oxygen therapy alone in hypercapnic COPD. Am J Respir Crit Care Med 1995; 152:538–544.

76. Perez de Llano LA, Golpe R, Ortiz Piquer M, et al. Short-term and long-term effects of nasal intermittent positive pressure ventilation in patients with obesity-hypoventilation syndrome. Chest 2005; 128:587–594.

77. Mezon BL, West P, Israels J, et al. Sleep breathing abnormalities in kyphoscoliosis. Am Rev Respir Dis 1980; 122:617.

78. Guilleminault C, Kurland G, Winkle R, et al. Severe kyphoscoliosis, breathing, and sleep: The "Quasimodo" syndrome during sleep. Chest 1981; 79:6.

79. Hill NS, Eveloff SE, Carlisle CC, et al. Efficacy of nocturnal nasal ventilation in patients with restrictive thoracic disease. Am Rev Respir Dis 1992; 145:365–371.

80. Buyse B, Meersseman W, Demedts M. Treatment of chronic respiratory failure in kyphoscoliosis: oxygen or ventilation? Eur Respir J 2003; 22:525–528.

81. Masa JF. Noninvasive positive pressure ventilation and not oxygen may prevent overt ventilatory failure in patients with chest wall disease. Chest 1997; 112:201–213.

82. Ward S, Chatwin M, Heather S, Simonds AK. Randomised controlled trial of non-invasive ventilation (NIV) for nocturnal hypoventilation in neuromuscular and chest wall disease patients with daytime normocapnia. Thorax 2005; 60:1019–1024.

83. Konagaya M, Sakai M, Wakayama T, et al. Effect of intermittent positive pressure ventilation on lifespan and causes of death in Duchenne muscular dystrophy. Rinsho Shinkeigaku 2005; 45:643–646.

84. Perez-Padilla R, West P, Lertzman M, et al. Breathing during sleep in patients with interstitial lung disease. Am Rev Respir Dis 1985; 132:224–229.

85. Tatsumi K, Kimuar H, Kunitomo F, et al. Arterial oxygen desaturation during sleep in interstitial pulmonary disease: correlation with chemical control of breathing during wakefulness. Chest 1989; 95:962–967.

86. Crockett AJ, Cranston JM, Antic N. Domiciliary oxygen for interstitial lung disease. Cochrane Database Syst Rev 2001; (3):CD002883.

87. Means MK, Edinger JD, Husain AM. CPAP compliance in sleep apnea patients with and without laboratory CPAP titration. Sleep Breath 2004; 8:7–14.

88. Zozula R, Rosen R. Compliance with continuous positive airway pressure therapy: assessing and improving treatment outcomes. Curr Opin Pulm Med 2001; 7:391–398.

89. Hoy CJ, Vennelle M, Kingshott RN, et al. Can intensive support improve continuous positive airway pressure use in patients with the sleep apnea/hypopnea syndrome? Am J Respir Crit Care Med 1999; 159:1096–1100.

90. Lewis KE, Seale L, Bartle IE, et al. Early predictors of CPAP use for the treatment of obstructive sleep apnea. Sleep 2004; 27:134–138.

91. Bachour A, Hurmerinta K, Maasilta P. Mouth closing device (chinstrap) reduces mouth leak during nasal CPAP. Sleep Med 2004; 5:261–267.

92. Bachour A, Maasilta P. Mouth breathing comprises adherence to nasal continuous positive airway pressure. Chest 2004; 126:1248–1254.

93. Montserrat JM, Ballester E, Olivi H, et al. Time-course of stepwise CPAP titration: behavior of respiratory and neurological variables. Am J Respir Crit Care Med 1995; 152:1854–1859.

94. Hosselet JJ, Norman RG, Ayappa I, et al. Detection of flow limitation with a nasal cannula/pressure transducer system. Am J Respir Crit Care Med 1998; 157:1461–1467.

95. Meurice JC, Paquereau J, Denjean A, et al. Influence of correction of flow limitation on continuous positive airway pressure efficiency in sleep apnoea/hyponoea syndrome. Eur Respir J 1998:1121–1127.

96. Miles LE, Crichton DA, Vishnevskaya Z. Sustained inspiratory airflow limitation: a preferred measure of partial upper airway obstruction. J Sleep Res 2000; 11(suppl 1):156.

97. Bureau MP, Series F. Comparison of two in-laboratory titration methods to determine effective pressure levels in patients with obstructive sleep apnoea. Thorax 2000; 55:741–745.

98. Pevernagie DA, Shepard JW Jr. Relations between sleep stage, posture and effective nasal CPAP levels in OSAHS. Sleep 1992; 15:162–167.

99. Marrone O, Insalaco G, Bonsignore MR, et al. Sleep structure correlates of continuous positive airway pressure variations during application of an autotitrating continuous positive airway pressure machine in patients with obstructive sleep apnea syndrome. Chest 2002; 121:759–767.

100. Issa FG, Sullivan CE. The immediate effects of nasal continuous positive airway pressure treatment on sleep pattern in patients with obstructive sleep apnea syndrome. Electroencephalogr Clin Neurophysiol 1986; 63:10–17.
101. Leevers AM, Simon PM, Dempsey JA. Apnea after normocapnic mechanical ventilation during NREM sleep. J Appl Physiol 1994; 77:2079–2085.
102. Schwab RJ, Gefter WB, Hoffman EA, et al. Dynamic upper airway imaging during awake respiration in normal subjects and patients with sleep disordered breathing. Am Rev Respir Dis 1985; 131:401–408.
103. Sanders MH, Kern N. Obstructive sleep apnea treated by independently adjusted inspiratory and expiratory positive airway pressures via nasal mask: physiologic and clinical implications. Chest 1990; 98:317–324.
104. Johnson KG, Johnson DC. Bilevel positive airway pressure worsens central apneas during sleep. Chest 2005; 128:2141–2150.
105. Gay P, Weaver T, Loube D, Iber C. Evaluation of positive airway pressure treatment for sleep related breathing disorders in adults: a review by the positive airway pressure task force of the Standards of Practice Committee of the American Academy of Sleep Medicine. Sleep 2006; 29:381–401.
106. Fleury B, Rakotonanahary D, Tehindrazanarivedlo AD, et al. Long term compliance to continuous positive airway pressure therapy (nCPAP) set up during a split-night polysomnography. Sleep 1994; 17:512–515.
107. Sanders MH, Kern NB, Costantino JP, et al. Adequacy of prescribing positive airway pressure therapy by mask for sleep apnea on the basis of a partial-night trial. Am Rev Respir Dis 1993; 147:1169–1174.
108. Rosenthal L, Nykamp K, Guido P, et al. Daytime CPAP titration: a viable alternative for patients with severe obstructive sleep apnea. Chest 1998; 114:1056–1060.
109. Rudkowski JC, Verschelden P, Kimoff RJ. Efficacy of daytime continuous positive airway pressure titration in severe obstructive sleep apnoea. Eur Respir J 2001; 18:535–541.
110. Jokic R, Klimaszewski A, Sridhar G, et al. Continuous positive airway pressure requirement during the first month of treatment in patients with severe obstructive sleep apnea. Chest 1998; 114:1061–1069.
111. Miljeteigh H, Hoffstein V. Continuous positive airway pressure for treatment of obstructive sleep apnea. Am Rev Respir Dis 1993; 147:1526–1530.
112. Berry RB, Desa MM, Lights RW. Effect of ethanol on the efficacy of nasal continuous positive airway pressure as a treatment for obstructive sleep apnea. Chest 1991; 99:339–343.
113. Engleman HM, Asgari-Jirhandeh N, McLeod AL, et al. Self-reported use of CPAP and benefits of CPAP therapy: a patient survey. Chest 1996; 109:1470–1476.
114. Strollo PJ Jr, Sanders MH, Atwood CW. Positive pressure therapy. Clin Chest Med 1998; 19:55–68.
115. Pepin JL, Leger P, Veale D, et al. Side effects of nasal continuous positive airway pressure in sleep apnea syndrome: study of 193 patients in two French sleep centers. Chest 1995; 107:375–381.
116. Richards GN, Cistulli PA, Ungar RG, et al. Mouth leak with continuous positive airway pressure increases nasal airway resistance. Am J Respir Crit Care Med 1996; 154:182–186.
117. Herrejon SA, Inchaurraga AI, Gonzalez M. Spontaneous pneumothorax associated with the use of nighttime BiPAP with a nasal mask. Arch Bronceneumol 1998; 34:512.
118. Alvarez-Sala R, Diaz S, Prados C, et al. Increase of intraocular pressure during nasal continuous positive pressure in a patient with sleep apnea syndrome. Chest 1992; 101:1477.
119. Jarjour NN, Wilson P. Pneumocephalus associated with nasal continuous positive airway pressure in a patient with sleep apnea syndrome. Chest 1989; 96:1425–1426.
120. Nowak C, Bourgin P, Portier F, et al. Nasal obstruction and compliance to nasal positive airway pressure. Ann Otolaryngol Chir Cervicofac 2003; 120:161–166.
121. Brouillette RT, Fernback SK, Hunt CE. Obstructive sleep apnea in infants and children. J Pediatric 1982; 100:31–40.
122. Suen JS, Arnold JE, Brooks LJ. Adenotonsillectomy for treatment of obstructive sleep apnea in children. Arch Otolaryngol Head Neck Surg 1995; 121:525–530.

123. O'Donnell AR, Bjornson CL, Bohn SG, Kirk VG. Compliance rates in children using noninvasive continuous positive airway pressure. Sleep 2006; 29:651–658.
124. Marcus CL, Ward SL, Mallory GB, et al. Use of nasal continuous positive airway pressure as treatment of childhood obstructive sleep apnea. J Pediatr 1995; 127:88–94.
125. Hers V, Liistro G, Dury M, et al. Residual effect of nCPAP applied for part of the night in patients with obstructive sleep apnoea. Eur Respir J 1997; 10:973–976.
126. Gupta RM, Parvizi J, Hanssen AD, Gay PC. Postoperative complications in patients with obstructive sleep apnea syndrome undergoing hip or knee replacement: a case control study. Mayo Clin Proc 2001; 76:897–905.
127. Gross JB, Bachenberg KL, Benumof JL, et al. Practice guidelines for the perioperative management of patients with obstructive sleep apnea: a report by the American Society of Anesthesiologists Task Force on Perioperative Management of patients with obstructive sleep apnea. Anesthesiology 2006; 104:1081–1093.
128. Montserrat JM, Ferrer M, Hernandez L, et al. Effectiveness of CPAP treatment in daytime function in sleep apnea syndrome. A randomized controlled study with an optimized placebo. Am J Respir Crit Care Med 2001; 164:608–613.
129. Engleman HM, McDonald JP, Graham D, et al. Randomized crossover trial of two treatments for sleep apnea/hypopnea syndrome: continuous positive airway pressure and mandibular repositioning splint. Am J Respir Crit Care Med 2002; 166:855–859.
130. Redline S, Adams N, Strauss ME, et al. Improvement of mild sleep-disordered breathing with CPAP compared with conservative therapy. Am J Respir Crit Care Med 1998; 157:858–865.
131. McArdle N, Devereux G, Heidarnejad H, et al. Long-term use of CPAP therapy for sleep apnea/hypopnea syndrome. Am J Respir Crit Care Med 1999; 159:1108–1114.
132. Kribbs NB, Pack AI, Kline LR, et al. Objective measurement of patterns of nasal CPAP use by patients with obstructive sleep apnea. Am Rev Respir Dis 1993; 147:887–895.
133. DiMatteo MR. Variation in patients' adherence to medical recommendations: a quantitative review of 50 years of research. Medical Care 2004; 42(3):200–209.
134. Campos-Rodriguez F, Pena-Grinan N, Reyes-Nunez N, et al. Mortality in obstructive sleep apnea–hypopnea patients treated with positive airway pressure. Chest 2005; 128:624–633.
135. Weaver TE. How much is enough CPAP? Sleep Med 2003; 4:S52.
136. Burke LE, Ockene IS. Compliance in healthcare and research. Armonk, NY: Futura Publishing Co., 2001.
137. Engleman HM, Martin SE, Douglas NJ. Compliance with CPAP therapy in patients with sleep apnoea/hypopnoea syndrome. Thorax 1994; 49:263–266.
138. Massie C, Hart R, Peralez K, et al. Effects of humidification on nasal symptoms and compliance in sleep apnea patients using continuous positive airway pressure. Chest 1999; 116:403–408.
139. Mortimore IL, Whittle AT, Douglas NJ. Comparison of nose and face mask CPAP therapy for sleep apnoea. Thorax 1998; 53:290–292.
140. Hudgel DW, Fung C. A long-term randomized, cross-over comparison of auto-titrating and standard nasal continuous positive airway pressure. Sleep 2000; 23:645–648.
141. Reeves-Hoche MK, Hudgel DW, Meck R, et al. Continuous versus bilevel positive airway pressure for obstructive sleep apnea. Am J Respir Crit Care Med 1995; 151:443–449.
142. Stepnowsky CJ Jr, Marler MR, Ancoli-Israel S. Determinants of nasal CPAP compliance. Sleep Med 2002; 3:239–247.
143. Aloia MS, Arnedt JT, Stepnowsky CJ Jr, et al. Predicting treatment adherence in obstructive sleep apnea using principles of behavior change. J Clin Sleep Med 2005; 1:247–254.
144. Engleman H, Wild MR. Improving CPAP use by patients with the sleep apnoea/hypopnoea syndrome (SAHS). Sleep Med Rev 2003; 7:81–99.
145. Haniffa M, Lasserson TJ, Smith I. Interventions to improve compliance with continuous positive airway pressure for obstructive sleep apnoea (Review). Cochrane Database Syst Rev Wiley, October 18, 2004; CD003531:1–58.

146. Teschler H, Berthon-Jones M, Thompson AB, et al. Automated continuous positive airway pressure titration for obstructive sleep apnea syndrome. Am J Respir Crit Care Med 1996; 154:734–740.

147. Ayas NT, Patel SR, Malhotra A, et al. Auto-titrating versus standard continuous positive airway pressure for the treatment of obstructive sleep apnea: results of a meta-analysis. Sleep 2004; 27:249–253.

148. Aloia MS, Stanchina ML, Arnedt JT, et al. Treatment adherence and outcomes in flexible versus continuous positive airway pressure therapy. Chest 2005; 127:2085–2093.

149. Worsnop C, Miseski S, Rochford P. Humidification of continuous positive airway pressure treatment in sleep apnoea reduces nasal symptoms. Proceedings of the Thoracic Society of Australia and New Zealand, Adelaide, 2003:178.

150. Fletcher EC, Luckett RA. The effect of positive reinforcement on hourly compliance in nasal continuous positive airway pressure users with obstructive sleep apnea. Am Rev Respir Dis 1991; 143:936–941.

151. Likar LL, Panciera TM, Erickson AD, et al. Group education sessions and compliance with nasal CPAP therapy. Chest 1997; 111:1273–1277.

152. Chervin RD, Theut S, Bassetti C, et al. Compliance with nasal CPAP can be improved by simple interventions. Sleep 1997; 20:284–289.

153. Hoy CJ, Vennelle M, Kingshott RN, et al. Can intensive support improve continuous positive airway pressure use in patients with the sleep apnea/hypopnea syndrome? Am J Respir Crit Care Med 1999; 159:1096–1871.

154. Hui DSC, Chan JKW, Choy DKL, et al. Effects of augmented continuous positive airway pressure education and support on compliance and outcome in a Chinese population. Chest 2000; 117:1410–1416.

155. Aloia MS, Arnedt JT, Riggs RL, et al. Clinical management of poor adherence to CPAP: motivational enhancement. Behav Sleep Med 2004; 2:205–222.

156. Stepnowsky CJ Jr, Ancoli-Israel S. CPAP adherence is associated with the decisional balance index [Abstract]. Sleep 2000; 23:A287–A288.

157. Aloia MS, Smith K, Arnedt JT, et al. Brief behavioral therapies reduce early PAP discontinuation rates in SAS: preliminary findings. Behav Sleep Med. In press.

10 Noninvasive Positive Ventilation

Dominique Robert
University Claude Bernard and Edouard Herriot Hospital,
Lyon, France

Laurent Argaud
Emergency and Intensive Care Department, Edouard Herriot Hospital,
Lyon, France

INTRODUCTION

In the early 1960s and 1970s limited experience with the long-term use of mechanical ventilation at home was acquired to replace or complement the ventilatory function after acute poliomyelitis and other neuromuscular or even lung diseases. Depending on the medical centers the three main methods for delivering mechanical tidal volume were used: intermittent negative pressure ventilation with iron lung or chest shell (1–3), intermittent positive pressure ventilation (IPPV) via a tracheostomy (3,4) or via a mouthpiece (5,6). In the early 1980s in spite of obvious clinical positive results, clinicians were reluctant to use these techniques, considering them as much too invasive (tracheostomy) or cumbersome and of limited efficacy (negative pressure) (7). It is now recognized, after the explosive experience of nasal continuous positive airway pressure (CPAP) to treat obstructive apnea (8), that IPPV could also be comfortably and efficiently delivered, noninvasively [noninvasive positive pressure ventilation (NIPPV)] through facial interfaces. Positive pressure is applied to the airway during inspiration at higher value than during expiration. Thus, NIPPV brings a part or even the whole tidal volume. Depending on the underlying diseases either IPPV is continuously mandatory to avoid death in case of complete or quasi-complete paralysis or is used nightly, producing enough improvement to allow free time during the daytime for spontaneous breathing. This chapter will address the use of NIPPV (to the exclusion of CPAP) in the different diseases for which it is currently proposed: principally in diseases responsible for chronic hypoventilation and incidentally in others such as obstructive sleep apnea (OSA) or problems of central drive (Cheyne-Stokes breathing, Ondine's curse). NIPPV, which is now a predominant technique, allows a progressive generalization for long-term home ventilation (9).

METHODS OF NONINVASIVE POSITIVE PRESSURE VENTILATION AND THEIR USES

Interfaces

The need to select an appropriate and properly fitted interface cannot be overemphasized due to its impact on the quality of ventilation (10–12). The aim to reach is a compromise between different objectives: minimize leaks, improve comfort, and to implement the mask easily. There are now a wide variety of different factory-made masks of different designs, shapes, sizes, and materials. It is usually possible to find a mask that suits most individuals. This explains that the initial practice of an individually made interface is now seldom needed even if it remains probably the best interface (10–15). There are currently four different types of interfaces: nasal mask, facial mask covering the nose and the mouth, nasal pillows, and mouthpieces. Nasal masks are predominantly used (10,16). Mouthpieces are now essentially indicated in the case of daytime ventilation (17,18). This may afford an excellent interface to adjunct daytime ventilation in neuromuscular patients who are unable to maintain acceptable diurnal arterial blood gases without frequent intermittent periods of assistance. The mouthpiece is positioned close to the patient's mouth where it is intermittently captured to take a few assisted breaths from the ventilator and subsequently released. An advantage is to clear the face from a face-attached interface. Thus, the patient needing assistance night and day may use a combination of interfaces.

Ventilator and Mode for Noninvasive Positive Pressure Ventilation

Ventilators use one of two basic methods: volume-preset and pressure-preset (10). With volume-preset, the ventilator always delivers the tidal volume which is set by the clinician, regardless of the patient's pulmonary system mechanics (compliance, resistance, and active inspiration). However, leaks at the skin–mask interface or through the mouth when using a nasal mask, reduce the volume received by the patient. Conversely, with pressure-preset, changes in pulmonary mechanics directly influence the flow and the delivered tidal volume (lower or higher) since the ventilator delivers the set pressure all along inspiration. Then leaks augment the flow and tend to maintain the tidal volume (19,20). It is important to understand that NIPPV is dominated both by rapid variations of nonintentional leaks and of the geometry and the resistance of the upper airway (21). Obviously, leaks and airway resistance partly interact. Facing these continuous changes the respective advantages and drawbacks of volume- and pressure-preset modes, which are opposite, make a predictable effect difficult. The way to begin and end inspiration is either initiated by the ventilator or in response to a patient effort to do so, allowing one to define the main modes: (i) control (ii) assist-control (iii) assist or spontaneous (possible only with pressure-preset). Most of the home ventilators function uniquely in volume or in pressure preset but modern ones may deliver inspiration according to the two modes. Besides the classical circuitry including two valves (on the inspiratory and expiratory limbs) alternatively closing and opening, bilevel positive airway pressure (BPAP) ventilators are simpler and therefore lend themselves to home mechanical ventilation (22). Inspiratory and expiratory pressures are alternatively established in a single circuit incorporating an intentional, calibrated leak located close to the patient or even on the mask. The theoretical disadvantage with such a circuit is the risk of a variable CO_2 rebreathing. Concern about the risk of CO_2 rebreathing is not definitively documented (23–25) even if the trend is to consider it as negligible (26–28) provided positive expiratory pressure is applied in order to eliminate CO_2 through the intentional leak (at least 2–4 cm H_2O). Depending on the ventilator, all the different modes and refined settings and even closed-loop modes usually applied in the intensive care unit, are more or less available. Some ventilators may analyze ventilation in an on-going manner, keep it in an internal memory and provide the data for further assessment. The general objective is to provide many possible capabilities in order to have enough tools to adapt and optimize patient–machine synchronization. While conceptually attractive, sufficient studies have not been performed to document or refute the advantages of such complexity in the context of noninvasive home ventilation.

Choice of the Ventilator and Mode

Many clinicians currently prefer a pressure-preset ventilator in assist mode as the first choice with the view to offer the better synchronization (9). In fact, in the studies comparing volume- and pressure-preset ventilators no clear differences in the correction of hypoventilation in short-term studies (29–37) and in long-term outcomes (38–40) are shown. This is understandable since during NIPPV, leaks and resistance changes alternate very quickly and when the pressure target does well, the volume target does not do well, and conversely. However, it is important to remain flexible by trying alternative approaches if problems occur with one or the other type of ventilator. Besides, it should be noted that batteries are unavailable or they offer a short autonomy for BPAP ventilators and this would limit security and mobility of neuromuscular patients with hypoventilation and then drive the preference to the volume ventilator.

CRITERIA TO DISCUSS NONINVASIVE POSITIVE PRESSURE VENTILATION
Signs and Symptoms of Hypoventilation

The presence of clinical symptoms and/or physiologic markers of hypoventilation are useful in identifying clinical severity as it relates to therapeutic decision-making with regard to initiation of nocturnal NIPPV. In the course of a typical progressive disease, two successive steps occur more or less rapidly: (*i*) nocturnal hypoventilation reversible during wake associated with none or a few clinical symptoms; and (*ii*) nocturnal and daylight hypoventilation associated with clinical symptoms, which show a low respiratory reserve and should be considered an unstable state with increased susceptibility to life-threatening acute ventilatory failure that may be triggered by what may otherwise be trivial additional factors (41,42). A sleep study continuously recording CO_2 (end-tidal $EtCO_2$ or transcutaneous $TcCO_2$) and/or oxygen saturation (SpO_2) is required to document nocturnal hypoventilation, which may occur throughout all sleep stages but in some cases exclusively during rapid eye movement (REM) sleep. Daytime hypoventilation is defined by an abnormally elevated partial pressure of arterial carbon dioxide ($PaCO_2$), a high-serum bicarbonate level and a relatively normal pH with associated reduction of partial pressure of arterial oxygen (PaO_2). Chronic daytime hypoventilation is an important indicator invariably associated with sleep-related hypoventilation. Thus, in the presence of diurnal hypoventilation, the reason for overnight recording is only to rule out obstructive or central apnea. Clinical symptoms indicating consequences of hypoventilation (Table 1) must be carefully evaluated since even when modest, they are important for the appreciation of disease severity and prognosis and to indicate NIPPV. Pulmonary function tests help define and quantify the ventilatory–respiratory disease but have low predictive values for chronic sleep-related hypoventilation in individual patients except in those with neuromuscular disease. Indeed, in Duchenne muscular dystrophy, hypoventilation appears only during REM sleep, all night, or during the daytime when supine inspiratory vital capacity is < 40%, < 25%, and < 12%, respectively (41). Similarly a peak cough flow < 160 L/min, related to expiratory muscle deficit, means an increased risk of accumulation of secretions that may worsen hypoventilation and trigger acute failure (18,43–46). It is crucial to notice that isolated reduced PaO_2 does not mean hypoventilation but only a mismatching of ventilation and perfusion adequately compensated or even overcompensated (low $PaCO_2$), which will not require support by mechanical ventilation but only by supplemental oxygen.

TABLE 1 Clinical Features Frequently Associated with Alveolar Hypoventilation

Shortness of breath during activities of daily living in the absence of paralysis
Orthopnea in patients with disordered diaphragmatic dysfunction
Poor sleep quality: insomnia, nightmares, and frequent arousals
Nocturnal or early morning headaches
Daytime fatigue, drowsiness and sleepiness, loss of energy
Decrease in intellectual performance
Loss of appetite and weight loss
Appearance of recurrent complications: respiratory infections
Clinical signs of cor pulmonale

Diseases That May Potentially Be Treated with Noninvasive Positive Pressure Ventilation

The principal diseases which may be addressed using NIPPV therapy are shown in Table 2. Except for those due to respiratory control or upper airway abnormalities, all may become severe enough to cause alveolar hypoventilation during sleep and daytime and eventually may impair quality of life and threaten life. In neuromuscular disorders it is important to consider the progressiveness according to each type of disease and the individual concerned.

Survival with Noninvasive Positive Pressure Ventilation in Different Diseases

NIPPV efficacy in terms of survival compared to control treatment is major information that one needs to adequately discuss NIPPV. Besides a few randomized control trials (47–50), information comes from retrospective series compared to the usual prognosis (14,40,51–58). In order to extend the analysis it is also possible to take into

TABLE 2 Main Diseases That Can Benefit from Noninvasive Positive Pressure Ventilation, Classified According to the Cause and Progressiveness of the Respiratory Impairment

Parietal disorders: (PFT abnormal: ↓ VC, ↓ FEV1, → FEV1/VC, ↓ RV, ↓ TLC)[a]	
Chest wall:	
Kyphoscoliosis	No worsening
Sequels of tuberculosis	Slow worsening
Obesity hypoventilation syndrome	Depends on obesity
Neuromuscular disorders:	
Spinal muscular atrophy	No worsening
Acid maltase deficit	Slow worsening (>15 years)
Duchenne muscular dystrophy	Intermediate worsening (5–15 yrs)
Myotonic myopathy	Intermediate worsening (5–15 yrs)
Amyotrophic lateral sclerosis	Rapid Worsening (0–3 yrs)
Lung diseases: (PFT abnormal: → or ↓ VC, ↓ FEV1, ↓ FEV1/VC, ↑ RV, ↑ TLC)[a]	
COPD	Continuous worsening
Bronchiectasis, Cystic fibrosis	Continuous worsening
Predominant ventilatory control abnormalities: (PFT normal)	
Ondine's curse	Improvement (?)
Cheyne-Stokes breathing	Depends on heart failure
Upper airway abnormalities: (PFT normal)	
Pierre Robin	No worsening
Obstructive sleep apnea	No worsening

[a]Symbols indicate actual compared to theoretical values: ↓ or ↑, decrease or increase; →, normal.
Abbreviations: COPD, chronic obstructive pulmonary disease; FEV1, forced expiratory volume in one second; PFT, pulmonary function test; RV, residual volume; TLC, total lung capacity; VC, vital capacity.

account the results obtained either with negative pressure ventilation (59) or with tracheostomy (4,60). Their conclusions are informative enough and generally accepted by the medical community even if these conclusions are refutable in terms of evidence-based medicine. In neuromuscular disease, NIPPV always increases survival. Approximate median prolongations of life depend on the age when starting NIPPV and the comorbidities (including extended paralysis): very long (> 20 years) in the sequelae of poliomyelitis; long (10 years) in spinal muscular atrophy (SMA) type 2 and 3, Duchenne muscular dystrophy, acid maltase deficiency; short in myotonic dystrophy (4 years); and very short in amyotrophic lateral sclerosis (ALS) (one year). In chest-wall abnormalities NIPPV also prolongs life: in kyphosis (15 years) and in the sequelae of tuberculosis (seven years). In lung diseases no data support a positive effect on survival: in chronic obstructive pulmonary disease (COPD) patients for whom randomized trials are negative (48,49,59) or in cystic fibrosis or bronchiectasis patients for whom data are too scarce.

Circumstances and Indications for Noninvasive Positive Pressure Ventilation

In clinical practice, NIPPV is initiated either electively or in the context of acute ventilatory failure initially treated invasively with translaryngeal intubation or noninvasively with facial interfaces (61). In the latter circumstances, the long-term necessity for NIPPV should be re-evaluated after weeks or months during follow-up since the indications for NIPPV may change as the clinical conditions improve or not. In cases of chronic and stable awake hypoventilation, the cornerstone to foresee use of NIPPV is an advanced severity with clinical symptoms of hypoventilation plus a balance of several other issues: (*i*) the main primary process explaining the hypoventilation: mechanical or lung deficit; (*ii*) the natural rate of progression appreciated as a few years or dozens of years; (*iii*) the clinical severity at the time of decision-making: actual symptoms and history of acute–subacute failure in the previous months; and (*iv*) the patient's willingness, including the family and social environment, to undertake this therapy. Indications are outlined in Table 3. NIPPV is strongly indicated in patients with chest-wall and neuromuscular disorders in the presence of clinical symptoms attributable to diurnal hypoventilation (18,62–67). There are no validated values above which NIPPV is definitely indicated; however,

TABLE 3 Typical Indications for Nocturnal Noninvasive Positive Pressure Ventilation According to Disease Process and Severity

Diseases	Symptoms Day $CO_2\uparrow^a$	Symptoms Night $CO_2\uparrow^a$	No symptoms Day $CO_2\uparrow^a$	Usual daily duration of NIPPV (hrs)
Scoliosis	Yes	Yes	Perhaps	<12
Tuberculosis	Yes	Yes	Perhaps	<12
Neuromuscular stable or slow	Yes	Perhaps	Perhaps	18–24
Neuromuscular intermediate	Yes	Perhaps	Perhaps	18–24
Neuromuscular rapid	Yes	Yes	Yes	24
COPD	Perhaps	No	No	12
Bronchiectasis, Cystic fibrosis	Perhaps	No	No	18–24
Obesity-hypoventilation	Perhaps	Perhaps	No	<12

[a]$\uparrow$, increase.
Abbreviations: COPD, chronic obstructive pulmonary disease; NIPPV, noninvasive positive pressure ventilation.

many clinicians consider treatment in scoliosis and sequelae of tuberculosis with awake $PaCO_2 > 50–55$ mmHg and a $PaO_2 < 60$ mmHg, and in neuromuscular disease, a $PaCO_2$ around 45–50 mmHg and a $PaO_2 < 70$ mmHg. In case of clear clinical symptoms less severe values may be considered as an indication to start NIPPV (65). Conversely, in COPD and probably in other lung diseases diurnal hypoventilation do not support the unequivocal utility of NIPPV (68,69). Nevertheless, this question remains open since the clinical trials are underpowered and secondary parameters like some components of the quality of life or hospitalization days, may have improved. Some observational series suggest better results (70–73). Presently, we may admit NIPPV as an option in COPD patients with symptoms of hypoventilation contributing to recurrence of acute–subacute failure, provided that long-term oxygen and drug therapy have already been optimally adjusted. During early stages with only isolated nocturnal hypoventilation, NIPPV is not mandatory but could be optional in kyphoscoliosis (74,75) and in neuromuscular diseases (75). In the latter, when worsening is both inevitable and rapid (e.g., ALS), NIPPV is valuable at an early stage provided that this is an acceptable therapeutic option for the patient.

Other particular diseases may also deserve considerations related to NIPPV use even if clinical experience remains nonconclusive. Obesity hypoventilation syndrome is dominated by morbid obesity impeding ventilation, frequent obstructive apnea and more or less reversible decreased reactivity of the respiratory centers (76). In acute–subacute as in chronic situations, NIPPV has been shown to reverse hypoventilation (77–80). But, considering the high prevalence of obstructive apnea, CPAP is also a simpler and efficient treatment. Cheyne-Stokes breathing with central and obstructive apnea in the context of severe cardiac insufficiency has been shown to negatively worsen the clinical situation and survival (81–83). Conventional NIPPV or a new modality such as adaptive servo-ventilation has been shown to alleviate apnea and improve cardiac function (84–89). Nevertheless, no conclusion about the utility of nocturnal NIPPV in terms of survival and main outcomes is available. Even more, a large study comparing O_2 and CPAP, which also alleviates apnea and improves cardiac function does not prove the clinical superiority of CPAP in term of survival even if apneas are significantly diminished (90). Pure obstructive apneas in the context of OSA could be suppressed with NIPPV. Some authors have proposed NIPPV as a second-line treatment in the case of CPAP failure. Such a possibility is not supported with enough conclusive study to be recommended (91–93). Ondine's curse, in children, is characterized by the lack of metabolic response of the respiratory centers during sleep and is responsible for severe nocturnal hypoventilation. The usual treatment is tracheostomy and nocturnal ventilation. Some clinical experience suggests that, after years, tracheostomy might be converted in some cases to nocturnal NIPPV. Obviously such options must remain in the hand of specialized teams (94).

MANAGEMENT OF NONINVASIVE POSITIVE PRESSURE VENTILATION
Initiation and Settings in the Case of Nocturnal Ventilation
The main goal of NIPPV, used at best uniquely during the night, includes the provision of improvement in arterial blood gases nearly up to normal values without discomfort and sleep disruption. The objective in case of a residual muscle ability to breathe is to provide enough improvement to allow comfortable time off the ventilator. Even if there is no absolute recommendation it is good general practice to proceed in three steps. The first step consists of selecting and adjusting the ventilator settings while the patient is awake, insuring physiological adequacy,

and patient comfort for at least one or two hours. One study, done on awake cystic fibrosis patients, found that clinical observation is as efficient as the use of physiological measurement including esophageal pressure in setting the ventilator parameters (95). Another study in patients with COPD and neuromuscular disease has shown that using physiological measurement does not improve ventilation during the day but improves ventilation and sleep quality during the night (96,97). In the second step, the clinician should judge adequacy when sleeping during a nap and/or nocturnal use. To complete this step, different options according to the resources available in each center could be used. Arterial blood gas measurements would seem ideal; however, one or few samples during the night do not represent the rapid changes observed during several continuous hours of sleep, and the invasiveness of sampling have led most clinicians to noninvasively monitor different parameters. Ideally, a complete polysomnogram recording SpO_2 and $PtcCO_2$ or $PEtCO_2$, airflow, tidal volume, airway pressure, rib cage and abdomen excursion, and sleep staging permits a complete assessment (98). When resources are not available to perform these detailed recordings, fewer measurements during overnight recordings remain informative. However, the minimal requirement is to overnight record SpO_2 in room air assessing that the normalization of SpO_2 goes with the normalization, or at least the improvement of $PaCO_2$. In addition, data related to patient tolerance, comfort, sleep quality, and well-being should be obtained. The third step consists in looking for reduction of $PaCO_2$ and augmentation of PaO_2, without dyspnoea, during the day in free ventilation after several NIPPV nights to confirm that the settings are adequate. This also gives information about the necessity or not to add daylight hours of NIPPV (at first during the nap and more when necessary). If the results are not satisfactory, alterations must be made to the settings and possibly the mask and the ventilator, and their effects checked again. In most cases, a few days are necessary to succeed.

If one uses assist pressure-preset ventilation, 10 cm H_2O of inspiratory pressure support is a suggested starting point. If necessary, the pressure level is progressively increased to achieve evidence of improvement. Pressure support higher than 20 cm H_2O is rarely necessary. Nevertheless, one observational series reports good results in COPD patients ventilated with higher (28 cm H_2O) pressure (73). In COPD, the addition of an expiratory positive pressure [positive end-expiratory pressure (PEEP) or expiratory positive airway pressure], also necessary to decrease the rebreathing with BPAP ventilators, should conceptually improve patient triggering when intrinsic PEEP exists. But, there is no long-term study proving its clinical usefulness (99,100). Depending on the ventilator capabilities and observations made of how patient and ventilator do together, more subtle settings concerning triggers, initial flow, and inspiratory time limit could be tried. A backup frequency set close to the spontaneous frequency of the patient during sleep is a reasonable substitute to avoid central apnea induced by transitory but repeated hyperventilation overpassing the apnea threshold (101).

When employing a volume-preset ventilator, the initial suggested settings may be established by adjusting the frequency of ventilator-delivered breaths so that it approximates the patient's spontaneous breathing frequency during sleep, an inspiratory time/total breathing cycle time between 0.33 and 0.5 and a relatively high tidal volume of around 10 to 15 mL/kg to insure sufficient tidal volume in case of leaks (19).

Supplemental O_2 should be added into the ventilator circuit in those patients requiring oxygen while awake due to lung parenchyma diseases (e.g., COPD, cystic fibrosis, bronchiectasis). In the absence of parenchymal disease it is only after trying to optimize all technical parameters that residual desaturation may justify additional O_2 bled into the ventilator circuit during sleep (102,103).

Continuous Noninvasive Positive Pressure Ventilation
In neuromuscular (to a lesser degree in end-stage lung diseases) the ventilator dependency may be total when starting NIPPV or may progressively increase following the gradual worsening of the disease. In the case of continuous need for ventilation, NIPPV could be used provided that the following techniques are adapted: alternate interfaces night and day, and assisted coughing available (18,104–106). Only a very well-trained team may take in charge of such an approach in patients who are completely informed and conscious of the constraints and dangers. Such application has been reported by different teams in stable neuro-muscular patients, such as those with a sequelae of poliomyelitis, high-level spinal cord injury or Duchenne muscular dystrophy (1,17,107). Alternatively, a tracheos-tomy may be performed to facilitate ventilatory assistance and secretion removal. There is no clear answer as to whether and beyond what duration a quite totally ventilator-dependent patient is better or more safely ventilated by tracheostomy or NIPPV (65,108–111). This debate will probably continue and, in the end, the decision to indicate or to convert to tracheostomy is highly dependent on the phi-losophy and capabilities of the clinical team as well as that of the patient and his/her family environmental preferences. It is essential that discussion of such issues be started as early as possible in the patient's course, well before the imperative arises. Besides, swallowing dysfunction, responsible for frequent and massive aspirations and pneumonia, observed during the course of ALS (frequent and due to bulbar origin) or of Duchenne muscular dystrophy (seldom and due to muscle weakness), is an imperative indication for tracheostomy to prolong survival, but it also raises major difficulties to communicate and to have enough personal interactions (locked-in state) (110,112). From this point of view, NIPPV, which may be easily stopped, could be a reasonable maximal option in case of rapidly devas-tating diseases like ALS, and can be considered both by the patient and medical team as a limitation of care or a palliative approach (113,114). This was confirmed since NIPPV in ALS patients with bulbar symptoms do not survive longer than controls (50).

Follow-up
Clinical follow-up and daytime arterial blood gas (ABG) measurements (or their surrogates) should be conducted regularly (two times per year for example). When possible, recordings during sleep on NIPPV, identical to those used for initiating NIPPV are useful. At any time, when there are unsatisfactory results like recurrence of clinical symptoms or hypoventilation on ABG, inadequate NIPPV must be sus-pected and objective evaluation during sleep must be undertaken. At the very least, overnight oximetry must be done. When NIPPV is determined to be suboptimal, a change in ventilator modality or setting and a review of the mask fitting may be indicated. Increasing the total duration of NIPPV use per day should also be considered, particularly when the underlying disease has progressed. Masks have to be regularly checked and changed or adapted as needed.

Management of Complications
Air Leaks During Noninvasive Positive Pressure Ventilation
To some degree, leaks are present when using nasal NIPPV during sleep in all patients. The major potential adverse effects of such leaks are reduced efficiency of ventilation and sleep fragmentation (115–118). A variety of measures, more or less

efficacious, have been suggested to address problematic leaks. These include: preventing neck flexion, reclining in a semi-recumbent position, discouraging the mouth from opening by use of a chin strap (117) or a cervical collar, switching to pressure-preset mode (19), decreasing the peak inspiratory pressure, increasing the delivered volume (20), optimizing the interface (12,16), and possibly switching to nasal pillows or a full-face mask (119). The effectiveness of these measures must be confirmed during sleep recordings.

Nasal Dryness, Congestion, and Rhinitis
With reference to the CPAP literature, the side effects of nasal dryness, congestion, and rhinitis are related to a defect of humidification promoted by air leaks (120). For patients with nasal and mouth dryness, a cold passover or a heated humidifier (the latter is more effective) (121) can be used. Heat/moisture exchangers are not well adapted to the case of leaks since the "dry" flow from the ventilator is higher than the "dampened" flow returning from the patient. In a large series, a minority of patients needed humidifiers (10).

Aerophagia
Aerophagia, or swallowing air, is frequently reported by patients, but rarely intolerable (122). Minor clinical signs are: eructation, flatulence, and abdominal discomfort. Aerophagia is usually dependent on the level of inspiratory pressure and is more commonly seen when using volume and/or mouthpiece ventilation and in the care of patients with neuromuscular disease. The incidence decreases if the peak inspiratory pressure is kept below 25 cm H_2O pressure.

NONINVASIVE POSITIVE PRESSURE VENTILATION EFFECTS (OTHER THAN SURVIVAL) AND RELATED MECHANISMS
During Ventilatory Assistance
As expected, when under NIPPV, ventilation and gas exchange are improved in all types of disease (38,70,74,123–127), even if significant episodes of transient hypoventilation, related to mouth leaks, may appear (115–118). Duration of sleep is augmented without clear changes in its quality (115,116,128). Respiratory muscles are normally put at rest but there are many exceptions due to air leaks and patient-ventilator asynchrony (129–131).

After Ventilation
When spontaneous ventilation exists and in the absence of major lung disease, gas exchange remains improved. It may persist for hours and even days before reappearance of hypoventilation (132,133). The improvement reported in many studies is important in chest-wall and neuromuscular diseases but inconsistent in COPD (123,125,134,135). Certainly, it explains improvements in clinical symptoms such as general well-being, appetite, exercise capability, headaches, ankle edema, and resurgence of acute failure, as well as decreasing hospitalization, increasing quality of life (136–138) and finally improving survival.

Three main explanations have been proposed: (*i*) improved respiratory muscle strength; (*ii*) resetting of the chemoreceptors; and (*iii*) decrease of the ventilatory load. The first hypothesis suggests that ventilatory assistance rests the respiratory muscles reversing fatigue. Indeed, inspiratory force [PI_{max} (maximum inspiratory pressure) or P_{es} (esophageal pressure) during sniff nasal pressure testing] have been found significantly augmented in four studies (56,139–141), very close in one (142) and stable in one (143). One study in which a nonvolitional objective measure using bilateral anterolateral phrenic nerve magnetic stimulation was assessed and found to be negative for improvement (142). One study in which respiratory muscle endurance was measured showed significant improvement (139). The second hypothesis suggests that, in response to chronic hypercapnia and hypoxia, the chemoreceptors commanding the respiratory centers change their set point, which perpetuates hypoventilation rather than attempting to generate nonsustainable ventilatory muscle efforts (144–147). The resumption of better ventilation during NIPPV would reset the centers to more normal values. The three studies that have looked at the hypercapnic ventilatory response have actually found significant improvement (140,142,143). It is interesting to consider that even a few hours of NIPPV during daytime can have the same effect (72,148) indicating that the determining factor is to resume hypoventilation for a relatively short daily duration. The third hypothesis suggests that an improvement of respiratory chest-wall and/or lung compliance, under the effects of positive pressure ventilation, would reduce the ventilatory load and increase the efficiency of the muscles. In the studies done on scoliosis, vital capacity significantly increased (56,139–141); while in the other two hypothesis, including also neuromuscular patients, the vital capacity remained unchanged. In one study, chest-wall and lung compliance did not change even though there was a nonsignificant trend toward an increase (142). In the three studies, periodic hyper-insufflation using higher inspiratory pressure during a few minutes in scoliosis (149,150) and ALS (151) patients, revealed an increase in compliance. It seems probable that, even if the mechanisms which explain the efficacy of NIPPV are imperfectly understood, it is likely that several factors, even if not individually significant, change and interact together to improve alveolar ventilation. The minimum mandatory duration of assistance is not clearly known. However, a relationship between a decrease of $PaCO_2$ and the pressure to ventilate has been found (141). Finally, one study reports a significant improvement of pulmonary arterial hypertension, which obviously favors clinical improvement (152).

In COPD patients, the absence of clinical results compared to scoliosis and neuromuscular disease, even if resetting of the respiratory centers has been shown (125,153), could be explained by the relatively low impairment of respiratory muscles and the importance of the lesions of the lung itself and its progressiveness.

CONCLUSIONS

Chronic ventilatory support using NIPPV improves and stabilizes the clinical course of many patients with chronic ventilatory failure. The results appear to be good in patients with restrictive disorders and poor in COPD. Among the neuromuscular disorders results are better in the slowly progressive ones. The benefit of NIPPV is reflected by the improvements in survival, blood gas composition, and clinical stability. Due to its relative simplicity and its noninvasive nature, NIPPV permits long-term mechanical ventilation to be an acceptable option to patients who otherwise would not have been treated if tracheostomy were the only alternative. In this way, nocturnal NIPPV represents a huge advance.

REFERENCES

1. Splaingard ML, Frates RC Jr, Harrison GM, et al. Home positive-pressure ventilation. Twenty years' experience. Chest 1983; 84:376–382.

2. Baydur A, Layne E, Aral H, et al. Long term non-invasive ventilation in the community for patients with musculoskeletal disorders: 46 year experience and review [see comments]. Thorax 2000; 55:4–11.
3. Duiverman ML, Bladder G, Meinesz AF, et al. Home mechanical ventilatory support in patients with restrictive ventilatory disorders: a 48-year experience. Respir Med 2006; 100:56–65.
4. Robert D, Gerard M, Leger P, et al. Permanent mechanical ventilation at home via a tracheotomy in chronic respiratory insufficiency. Rev Fr Mal Respir 1983; 11:923–936.
5. Bach JR, Alba AS, Bohatiuk G, et al. Mouth intermittent positive pressure ventilation in the management of postpolio respiratory insufficiency. Chest 1987; 91:859–864.
6. Baydur A, Gilgoff I, Prentice W, et al. Decline in respiratory function and experience with long-term assisted ventilation in advanced Duchenne's muscular dystrophy. Chest 1990; 97:884–889.
7. Hill NS. Clinical applications of body ventilators. Chest 1986; 90:897–905.
8. Sullivan CE, Issa FG, Berthon-Jones M, et al. Reversal of obstructive sleep apnea by continuous positive airway pressure applied the nares. Lancet 1981; 1:862–865.
9. Lloyd-Owen SJ, Donaldson GC, Ambrosino N, et al. Patterns of home mechanical ventilation use in Europe: results from the Eurovent survey. Eur Respir J 2005; 25:1025–1031.
10. Schonhofer B, Sortor-Leger S. Equipment needs for noninvasive mechanical ventilation. Eur Respir J 2002; 20:1029–1036.
11. Hill NS. Saving face: better interfaces for noninvasive ventilation. Intensive Care Med 2002; 28:227–229.
12. Elliott MW. The interface: crucial for successful noninvasive ventilation. Eur Respir J 2004; 23:7–8.
13. Leger P, Jennequin J, Gerard M, et al. Home positive pressure ventilation via nasal mask for patients with neuromuscular weakness or restrictive lung or chest-wall disease. Respiratory Care 1989; 34:73–77.
14. Leger P, Bedicam JM, Cornette A, et al. Nasal intermittent positive pressure ventilation. Long-term follow-up in patients with severe chronic respiratory insufficiency. Chest 1994; 105:100–105.
15. Fauroux B, Lavis JF, Nicot F, et al. Facial side effects during noninvasive positive pressure ventilation in children. Intensive Care Med 2005; 31:965–969.
16. Leger SS, Leger P. The art of interface. Tools for administering noninvasive ventilation. Med Klin 1999; 94:35–39.
17. Bach JR, Alba AS, Saporito LR. Intermittent positive pressure ventilation via the mouth as an alternative to tracheostomy for 257 ventilators users. Chest 1993; 103:174–182.
18. Finder JD, Birnkrant D, Carl J, et al. Respiratory care of the patient with Duchenne muscular dystrophy: ATS consensus statement. Am J Respir Crit Care Med 2004; 170:456–465.
19. Mehta S, McCool FD, Hill NS. Leak compensation in positive pressure ventilators: a lung model study. Eur Respir J 2001; 17:259–267.
20. Tuggey JM, Elliott MW. Titration of non-invasive positive pressure ventilation in chronic respiratory failure. Respir Med 2006; 100:1262–1269.
21. Jounieaux V, Aubert G, Dury M, et al. Effects of nasal positive-pressure hyperventilation on the glottis in normal sleeping subjects. J Appl Physiol 1995; 79:186–193.
22. Strumpf DA, Carlisle CC, Millman RP, et al. An evaluation of the respironics BiPAP bi-level CPAP device for delivery of assisted ventilation. Respir Care 1990; 35:415–422.
23. Ferguson GT, Gilmartin M. CO_2 rebreathing during BiPAP ventilatory assistance. Am J Respir Crit Care Med 1995; 151:1126–1135.
24. Lofaso F, Brochard L, Touchard D, et al. Evaluation of carbon dioxyde rebreathing during pressure support ventilation with airway management system (BiPAP) devices. Chest 1995; 108:772–778.
25. Schettino GP, Chatmongkolchart S, Hess DR, et al. Position of exhalation port and mask design affect CO_2 rebreathing during noninvasive positive pressure ventilation. Crit Care Med 2003; 31:2178–2182.
26. Hill NS, Carlisle C, Kramer NR. Effect of a nonrebreathing exhalation valve on long-term nasal ventilation using a bilevel device. Chest 2002; 122:84–91.
27. Hill N. What mask for noninvasive ventilation: is deadspace an issue? Crit Care Med 2003; 31:2247–2248.
28. Saatci E, Miller DM, Stell IM, et al. Dynamic dead space in face masks used with non-invasive ventilators: a lung model study. Eur Respir J 2004; 23:129–135.

29. Restrick LJ, Fox NC, Braid G, et al. Comparison of nasal pressure support ventilation with nasal intermittent positive pressure ventilation in patients with nocturnal hypoventilation. Eur Respir J 1993; 6:364–370.
30. Meecham Jones DJ, Wedzichia JA. Comparison of pressure and volume preset nasal ventilator systems in stable chronic respiratory failure. Eur Respir J 1993; 6:1060–1064.
31. Cinnella G, Conti G, Lofaso F, et al. Effects of assisted ventilation on the work of breathing: volume-controlled versus pressure-controlled ventilation. Am J Respir Crit Care Med 1996; 153:1025–1033.
32. Girault C, Richard JC, Chevron V, et al. Comparative physiologic effects of noninvasive assist-control and pressure support ventilation in acute hypercapnic respiratory failure [see comments]. Chest 1997; 111:1639–1648.
33. Tejeda M, Boix JH, Alvarez F, et al. Comparison of pressure support ventilation and assist-control ventilation in the treatment of respiratory failure. Chest 1997; 111:1322–1325.
34. Lien TC, Wang JH, Huang SH, et al. Comparison of bilevel positive airway pressure and volume ventilation via nasal or facial masks in patients with severe, stable COPD. Chung Hua I Hsueh Tsa Chih (Taipei) 2000; 63:542–551.
35. Laserna E, Barrot E, Beiztegui A, et al. Non-invasive ventilation in kyphoscoliosis. A comparison of a volumetric ventilator and a BIPAP support pressure device. Arch Bronconeumol 2003; 39:13–18.
36. Tuggey JM, Elliott MW. Randomised crossover study of pressure and volume noninvasive ventilation in chest wall deformity. Thorax 2005; 60:859–864.
37. Windisch W, Storre JH, Sorichter S, et al. Comparison of volume- and pressure-limited NPPV at night: a prospective randomized cross-over trial. Respir Med 2005; 99:52–59.
38. Schonhofer B, Sonneborn M, Haidl P, et al. Comparison of two different modes for non-invasive mechanical ventilation in chronic respiratory failure: volume versus pressure controlled device. Eur Respir J 1997; 10:184–191.
39. Smith IE, Laroche CM, Jamieson SA, et al. Kyphosis secondary to tuberculosis osteomyelitis as a cause of ventilatory failure. Clinical features, mechanisms, and management. Chest 1996; 110:1105–1110.
40. Janssens JP, Derivaz S, Breitenstein E, et al. Changing patterns in long-term noninvasive ventilation: a 7-year prospective study in the Geneva Lake area. Chest 2003; 123:67–79.
41. Ragette R, Mellies U, Schwake C, et al. Patterns and predictors of sleep disordered breathing in primary myopathies. Thorax 2002; 57:724–728.
42. Lo Coco D, Marchese S, Corrao S, et al. Development of chronic hypoventilation in amyotrophic lateral sclerosis patients. Respir Med 2006; 100:1028–1036.
43. Bach JR. Mechanical insufflation, exsufflation. Comparison of peak expiratory flows with manually assisted and unassisted coughing techniques. Chest 1993; 104:1553–1562.
44. Bach JR. Update and perspective on noninvasive respiratory muscle aids. Part 2: the expiratory aids. Chest 1994; 105:1538–1544.
45. Bach JR, Saporito LR. Criteria for extubation and tracheostomy tube removal for patients with ventilatory failure. A different approach to weaning. Chest 1996; 110:1566–1571.
46. Chaudri MB, Liu C, Hubbard R, et al. Relationship between supramaximal flow during cough and mortality in motor neurone disease. Eur Respir J 2002; 19:434–438.
47. Pinto AC, Evangelista T, Carvalho M, et al. Respiratory assistance with a non-invasive ventilator (BIPAP) in MND/ALS patients: survival rates in a controlled trial. J Neurol Sci 1995; 129(suppl):19–26.
48. Clini E, Sturani C, Rossi A, et al. The Italian multicentre study on noninvasive ventilation in chronic obstructive pulmonary disease patients. Eur Respir J 2002; 20:529–538.
49. Casanova C, Celli BR, Tost L, et al. Long-term controlled trial of nocturnal nasal positive pressure ventilation in patients with severe COPD. Chest 2000; 118:1582–1590.
50. Bourke SC, Tomlinson M, Williams TL, et al. Effects of non-invasive ventilation on survival and quality of life in patients with amyotrophic lateral sclerosis: a randomised controlled trial. Lancet Neurol 2006; 5:140–147.
51. Jackson M, Smith I, King M, et al. Long term non-invasive domiciliary assisted ventilation for respiratory failure following thoracoplasty. Thorax 1994; 49:915–919.
52. Simonds AK, Elliott MW. Outcome of domiciliary nasal intermittent positive pressure ventilation in restrictive and obstructive disorders. Thorax 1995; 50:604–609.
53. Aboussouan LS, Khan SU, Meeker DP, et al. Effect of noninvasive positive-pressure ventilation on survival in amyotrophic lateral sclerosis. Ann Intern Med 1997; 127:450–453.

54. Kleopa KA, Sherman M, Neal B, et al. BIPAP improves survival and rate of pulmonary function decline in patients with ALS. J Neurol Sci 1999; 164:82–88.
55. Nugent AM, Smith IE, Shneerson JM. Domiciliary-assisted ventilation in patients with myotonic dystrophy. Chest 2002; 121:459–464.
56. Gonzalez C, Ferris G, Diaz J, et al. Kyphoscoliotic ventilatory insufficiency: effects of long-term intermittent positive-pressure ventilation. Chest 2003; 124:857–862.
57. Chu CM, Yu WC, Tam CM, et al. Home mechanical ventilation in Hong Kong. Eur Respir J 2004; 23:136–141.
58. Farrero E, Prats E, Povedano M, et al. Survival in amyotrophic lateral sclerosis with home mechanical ventilation: the impact of systematic respiratory assessment and bulbar involvement. Chest 2005; 127:2132–2138.
59. Shapiro SH, Ernst P, Gray-Donald K, et al. Effect of negative pressure ventilation in severe chronic obstructive pulmonary disease [see comments]. Lancet 1992; 340:1425–1429.
60. Muir JF, Girault C, Cardinaud JP, et al. Survival and long-term follow-up of tracheostomized patients with COPD treated by home mechanical ventilation. A multicenter French study in 259 patients. French Cooperative Study Group. Chest 1994; 106:201–209.
61. Keenan SP, Sinuff T, Cook DJ, et al. Which patients with acute exacerbation of chronic obstructive pulmonary disease benefit from noninvasive positive-pressure ventilation? A systematic review of the literature. Ann Intern Med 2003; 138:861–870.
62. Robert D, Willig TN, Paulus J, et al. Long-term nasal ventilation in neuromuscular disorders: report of a consensus conference. Eur Respir J 1993; 6:599–606.
63. Make BJ, Hill NS, Goldberg AI, et al. Mechanical ventilation beyond the intensive care unit. Report of a consensus conference of the American College of Chest Physicians. Chest 1998; 113:S289–S344.
64. Clinical indications for noninvasive positive pressure ventilation in chronic respiratory failure due to restrictive lung disease, COPD, and nocturnal hypoventilation—a consensus conference report. Chest 1999; 116:521–534.
65. Shneerson JM, Simonds AK. Noninvasive ventilation for chest wall and neuromuscular disorders. Eur Respir J 2002; 20:480–487.
66. Norregaard O. Noninvasive ventilation in children. Eur Respir J 2002; 20:1332–1342.
67. Simonds AK, Ward S, Heather S, et al. Outcome of paediatric domiciliary mask ventilation in neuromuscular and skeletal disease. Eur Respir J 2000; 16:476–481.
68. Wijkstra PJ, Lacasse Y, Guyatt GH, et al. Nocturnal non-invasive positive pressure ventilation for stable chronic obstructive pulmonary disease. Cochrane Database Syst Rev 2002:CD002878.
69. Wijkstra PJ, Lacasse Y, Guyatt GH, et al. A meta-analysis of nocturnal noninvasive positive pressure ventilation in patients with stable COPD. Chest 2003; 124:337–343.
70. Sivasothy P, Smith IE, Shneerson JM. Mask intermittent positive pressure ventilation in chronic hypercapnic respiratory failure due to chronic obstructive pulmonary disease. Eur Respir J 1998; 11:34–40.
71. Nava S, Fanfulla F, Frigerio P, et al. Physiologic evaluation of 4 weeks of nocturnal nasal positive pressure ventilation in stable hypercapnic patients with chronic obstructive pulmonary disease. Respiration 2001; 68:573–583.
72. Diaz O, Begin P, Andresen M, et al. Physiological and clinical effects of diurnal noninvasive ventilation in hypercapnic COPD. Eur Respir J 2005; 26:1016–1023.
73. Windisch W, Kostic S, Dreher M, et al. Outcome of patients with stable COPD receiving controlled noninvasive positive pressure ventilation aimed at a maximal reduction of Pa(CO2). Chest 2005; 128:657–662.
74. Masa JF, Celli BR, Riesco JA, et al. Noninvasive positive pressure ventilation and not oxygen may prevent overt ventilatory failure in patients with chest wall diseases. Chest 1997; 112:207–213.
75. Ward S, Chatwin M, Heather S, et al. Randomised controlled trial of non-invasive ventilation (NIV) for nocturnal hypoventilation in neuromuscular and chest wall disease patients with daytime normocapnia. Thorax 2005; 60:1019–1024.
76. Olson AL, Zwillich C. The obesity hypoventilation syndrome. Am J Med 2005; 118:948–956.
77. Sullivan CE, Berthon-Jones M, Issa FG. Remission of severe obesity-hypoventilation syndrome after short-term treatment during sleep with nasal continuous positive airway pressure. Am Rev Respir Dis 1983; 128:177–181.

78. Masa JF, Celli BR, Riesco JA, et al. The obesity hypoventilation syndrome can be treated with noninvasive mechanical ventilation. Chest 2001; 119:1102–1107.

79. de Lucas-Ramos P, de Miguel-Diez J, Santacruz-Siminiani A, et al. Benefits at 1 year of nocturnal intermittent positive pressure ventilation in patients with obesity-hypoventilation syndrome. Respir Med 2004; 98:961–967.

80. Perez de Llano LA, Golpe R, Ortiz Piquer M, et al. Short-term and long-term effects of nasal intermittent positive pressure ventilation in patients with obesity-hypoventilation syndrome. Chest 2005; 128:587–594.

81. Bradley TD, Floras JS. Sleep apnea and heart failure. Part II: central sleep apnea. Circulation 2003; 107:1822–1826.

82. Bradley TD, Floras JS. Sleep apnea and heart failure. Part I: obstructive sleep apnea. Circulation 2003; 107:1671–1678.

83. Pepin JL, Chouri-Pontarollo N, Tamisier R, et al. Cheyne-Stokes respiration with central sleep apnoea in chronic heart failure: proposals for a diagnostic and therapeutic strategy. Sleep Med Rev 2006; 10:33–47.

84. Willson GN, Wilcox I, Piper AJ, et al. Noninvasive pressure preset ventilation for the treatment of Cheyne-Stokes respiration during sleep. Eur Respir J 2001; 17:1250–1257.

85. Kohnlein T, Welte T, Tan LB, et al. Assisted ventilation for heart failure patients with Cheyne-Stokes respiration. Eur Respir J 2002; 20:934–941.

86. Teschler H, Dohring J, Wang YM, et al. Adaptive pressure support servo-ventilation: a novel treatment for Cheyne-Stokes respiration in heart failure. Am J Respir Crit Care Med 2001; 164:614–619.

87. Pepperell JC, Maskell NA, Jones DR, et al. A randomized controlled trial of adaptive ventilation for Cheyne-Stokes breathing in heart failure. Am J Respir Crit Care Med 2003; 168:1109–1114.

88. Philippe C, Stoica-Herman M, Drouot X, et al. Compliance with and effectiveness of adaptive servo-ventilation versus continuous positive airway pressure in the treatment of Cheyne-Stokes respiration in heart failure over a six month period. Heart 2006; 92:337–342.

89. Arzt M, Bradley TD. Treatment of sleep apnea in heart failure. Am J Respir Crit Care Med 2006; 173:1300–1308.

90. Bradley TD, Logan AG, Kimoff RJ, et al. Continuous positive airway pressure for central sleep apnea and heart failure. N Engl J Med 2005; 353:2025–2033.

91. Resta O, Guido P, Picca V, et al. Prescription of nCPAP and nBIPAP in obstructive sleep apnea syndrome: Italian experience in 105 subjects. A prospective two centre study. Respir Med 1998; 92:820–827.

92. Gay PC, Herold DL, Olson EJ. A randomized, double-blind clinical trial comparing continuous positive airway pressure with a novel bilevel pressure system for treatment of obstructive sleep apnea syndrome. Sleep 2003; 26:864–869.

93. Han F, Chen E, Wei H, et al. Treatment effects on carbon dioxide retention in patients with obstructive sleep apnea–hypopnea syndrome. Chest 2001; 119:1814–1819.

94. Trang H, Dehan M, Beaufils F, et al. The French Congenital Central Hypoventilation Syndrome Registry: general data, phenotype, and genotype. Chest 2005; 127:72–79.

95. Fauroux B, Nicot F, Essouri S, et al. Setting of noninvasive pressure support in young patients with cystic fibrosis. Eur Respir J 2004; 24:624–630.

96. Vitacca M, Nava S, Confalonieri M, et al. The appropriate setting of noninvasive pressure support ventilation in stable COPD patients. Chest 2000; 118:1286–1293.

97. Fanfulla F, Delmastro M, Berardinelli A, et al. Effects of different ventilator settings on sleep and inspiratory effort in patients with neuromuscular disease. Am J Respir Crit Care Med 2005; 172:619–624.

98. Lofaso F, Quera-Salva MA. Polysomnography for the management of progressive neuromuscular disorders. Eur Respir J 2002; 19:989–990.

99. Nava S, Ambrosino N, Rubini F, et al. Effect of nasal pressure support ventilation and external PEEP on diaphragmatic activity in patients with severe stable COPD. Chest 1993; 103:143–150.

100. Appendini L, Patessio A, Zanaboni S, et al. Physiologic effects of positive end expiratory pressure and mask pressure support during exacerbation of chronic obstructive pulmonary disease. Am J Respir Crit Care Med 1994; 149:1069–1076.

101. Johnson KG, Johnson DC. Bilevel positive airway pressure worsens central apneas during sleep. Chest 2005; 128:2141–2150.

102. Thys F, Liistro G, Dozin O, et al. Determinants of Fi, O2 with oxygen supplementation during noninvasive two-level positive pressure ventilation. Eur Respir J 2002; 19:653–657.

103. Schwartz AR, Kacmarek RM, Hess DR. Factors affecting oxygen delivery with bi-level positive airway pressure. Respir Care 2004; 49:270–275.

104. Bach JR. Amyotrophic lateral sclerosis: predictors for prolongation of life by noninvasive respiratory aids. Arch Phys Med Rehabil 1995; 76:828–832.

105. Tzeng AC, Bach JR. Prevention of pulmonary morbidity for patients with neuromuscular disease. Chest 2000; 118:1390–1396.

106. Dohna-Schwake C, Ragette R, Teschler H, et al. Predictors of severe chest infections in pediatric neuromuscular disorders. Neuromuscul Disord 2006; 16:325–328.

107. Curran FJ, Colbert AP. Ventilator management in Duchenne muscular dystrophy and postpoliomyelitis syndrome: twelve years' experience. Arch Phys Med Rehabil 1989; 70:180–185.

108. Bach JR. Indications for tracheostomy and decannulation of tracheostomized ventilator users. Monaldi Arch Chest Dis 1995; 50:223–227.

109. Bach JR, Bianchi C, Aufiero E. Oximetry and indications for tracheotomy for amyotrophic lateral sclerosis. Chest 2004; 126:1502–1507.

110. Hayashi H, Oppenheimer E. ALS patients on TPPV totally locked-in state, neurologic findings and clinical implications. Neurology 2003; 61:135–137.

111. Cazzolli PA, Oppenheimer EA. Home mechanical ventilation for amyotrophic lateral sclerosis: nasal compared to tracheostomy-intermittent positive pressure ventilation. J Neurol Sci 1996; 139(suppl):123–128.

112. Tsara V, Serasli E, Voutsas V, et al. Burden and coping strategies in families of patients under noninvasive home mechanical ventilation. Respiration 2006; 73:61–67.

113. Polkey MI, Lyall RA, Davidson AC, et al. Ethical and clinical issues in the use of home non-invasive mechanical ventilation for the palliation of breathlessness in motor neurone disease. Thorax 1999; 54:367–371.

114. Simonds AK. Ethics and decision making in end stage lung disease. Thorax 2003; 58:272–277.

115. Bach JR, Robert D, Leger P, et al. Sleep fragmentation in kyphoscoliotic individuals with alveolar hypoventilation treated by NIPPV. Chest 1995; 107:1552–1558.

116. Meyer TJ, Pressman MR, Benditt J, et al. Air leaking through the mouth during nocturnal nasal ventilation: effect on sleep quality. Sleep 1997; 20:561–569.

117. Teschler H, Stampa J, Ragette R, et al. Effect of mouth leak on effectiveness of nasal bilevel ventilatory assistance and sleep architecture. Eur Respir J 1999; 14:1251–1257.

118. Gonzalez J, Sharshar T, Hart N, et al. Air leaks during mechanical ventilation as a cause of persistent hypercapnia in neuromuscular disorders. Intensive Care Med 2003; 29:596–602.

119. Mehta S, Hill NS. Noninvasive ventilation. Am J Respir Crit Care Med 2001; 163:540–577.

120. Richards GN, Cistulli PA, Ungar RG, et al. Mouth leak with nasal continuous positive airway pressure increases nasal airway resistance. Am J Respir Crit Care Med 1996; 154:182–186.

121. Randerath WJ, Meier J, Genger H, et al. Efficiency of cold passover and heated humidification under continuous positive airway pressure. Eur Respir J 2002; 20:183–186.

122. Hill NS. Complications of noninvasive ventilation. Respir Care 2000; 45:480–481.

123. Strumpf DA, Millman RP, Carlisle CC, et al. Nocturnal positive-pressure ventilation via nasal mask in patients with severe chronic obstructive pulmonary disease. Am Rev Respir Dis 1991; 144:1234–1239.

124. Elliott MW. Noninvasive ventilation in chronic ventilatory failure due to chronic obstructive pulmonary disease. Eur Respir J 2002; 20:511–514.

125. Meecham Jones DJ, Paul EA, Jones PW, et al. Nasal pressure support ventilation plus oxygen compared with oxygen therapy alone in hypercapnic COPD. Am J Respir Crit Care Med 1995; 152:538–544.

126. Barbé F, Quera-Salva MA, de Lattre J, et al. Long-term effects of nasal intermittent positive-pressure ventilation on pulmonary function and sleep architecture in patients with neuromuscular diseases. Chest 1996; 110:1179–1183.

127. Benhamou D, Muir JF, Raspaud C, et al. Long-term efficiency of home nasal mask ventilation in patients with diffuse bronchiectasis and severe chronic respiratory failure. Chest 1997; 112:1259–1266.
128. Schonhofer B, Kohler D. Effect of non-invasive mechanical ventilation on sleep and nocturnal ventilation in patients with chronic respiratory failure. Thorax 2000; 55:308–313.
129. Brochard L. Noninvasive pressure support ventilation: physiological and clinical results in patients with COPD and acute respiratory failure. Monaldi Arch Chest Dis 1997; 52:64–67.
130. Carrey Z, Gottfried SB, Levy RD. Ventilatory muscle support in respiratory failure with nasal positive pressure ventilation. Chest 1990; 97:150–158.
131. L'Her E, Deye N, Lellouche F, et al. Physiologic effects of noninvasive ventilation during acute lung injury. Am J Respir Crit Care Med 2005; 172:1112–1118.
132. Jimenez JFM, de Cos Escuin JS, Vicente CD, et al. Nasal intermittent positive pressure ventilation. Analysis of its withdrawal. Chest 1995; 107:383–388.
133. Karakurt S, Fanfulla F, Nava S. Is it safe for patients with chronic hypercapnic respiratory failure undergoing home noninvasive ventilation to discontinue ventilation briefly? Chest 2001; 119:1379–1386.
134. Gay PC, Hubmayr RD, Stroetz RW. Efficacy of nocturnal nasal ventilation in stable, severe chronic obstructive pulmonary disease during a 3-month controlled trial. Mayo Clin Proc 1996; 71:533–542.
135. Lin CC. Comparison between nocturnal nasal positive pressure ventilation combined with oxygen therapy and oxygen monotherapy in patients with severe COPD. Am J Respir Crit Care Med 1996; 154:353–358.
136. Windisch W, Freidel K, Matthys H, et al. Health-related quality of life (HRQL) in patients receiving home mechanical ventilation. Pneumologie 2002; 56:610–620.
137. Markstrom A, Sundell K, Lysdahl M, et al. Quality-of-life evaluation of patients with neuromuscular and skeletal diseases treated with noninvasive and invasive home mechanical ventilation. Chest 2002; 122:1695–1700.
138. Domenech-Clar R, Nauffal-Manzur D, Perpina-Tordera M, et al. Home mechanical ventilation for restrictive thoracic diseases: effects on patient quality-of-life and hospitalizations. Respir Med 2003; 97:1320–1327.
139. Schonhofer B, Wallstein S, Wiese C, et al. Noninvasive mechanical ventilation improves endurance performance in patients with chronic respiratory failure due to thoracic restriction. Chest 2001; 119:1371–1378.
140. Dellborg C, Olofson J, Hamnegard CH, et al. Ventilatory response to CO2 re-breathing before and after nocturnal nasal intermittent positive pressure ventilation in patients with chronic alveolar hypoventilation. Respir Med 2000; 94:1154–1160.
141. Budweiser S, Heinemann F, Fischer W, et al. Impact of ventilation parameters and duration of ventilator use on non-invasive home ventilation in restrictive thoracic disorders. Respiration 2006; 73:488–494.
142. Nickol AH, Hart N, Hopkinson NS, et al. Mechanisms of improvement of respiratory failure in patients with restrictive thoracic disease treated with non-invasive ventilation. Thorax 2005; 60:754–760.
143. Annane D, Quera-Salva MA, Lofaso F, et al. Mechanisms underlying effects of nocturnal ventilation on daytime blood gases in neuromuscular diseases. Eur Respir J 1999; 13:157–162.
144. Elliott MW, Mulvey DA, Moxham J, et al. Domiciliary nocturnal nasal intermittent positive pressure ventilation in COPD: mechanisms underlying changes in arterial blood gas tensions. Eur Respir J 1991; 4:1044–1052.
145. Fernandez E, Weinert P, Meltzer E, et al. Sustained improvement in gas exchange after negative pressure ventilation for 8 hours per day on 2 successive days in chronic airflow limitation. Am Rev Respir Dis 1991; 144:390–394.
146. Hill NS, Eveloff SE, Carlisle C, et al. Efficacy of nocturnal nasal ventilation in patients with restrictive thoracic disease. Am Rev Respir Dis 1992; 145:365–371.
147. Annane D, Chevrolet JC, Chevret S, et al. Nocturnal mechanical ventilation for chronic hypoventilation in patients with neuromuscular and chest wall disorders. Cochrane Database Syst Rev 2000:CD001941.

148. Schonhofer B, Geibel M, Sonneborn M, et al. Daytime mechanical ventilation in chronic respiratory insufficiency. Eur Respir J 1997; 10:2840–2846.
149. Bergowsky EH. State of the art: respiratory failure in disorders of the thoracic cage. Am Rev Respir J 1979; 119:643–669.
150. Simonds AK, Parker RA, Branthwaite MA. The effect of intermittent positive-pressure hyperinflation in restrictive chest wall disease. Respiration 1989; 55:136–143.
151. Lechtzin N, Shade D, Clawson L, et al. Supramaximal inflation improves lung compliance in subjects with amyotrophic lateral sclerosis. Chest 2006; 129:1322–1329.
152. Schonhofer B, Barchfeld T, Wenzel M, et al. Long term effects of non-invasive mechanical ventilation on pulmonary haemodynamics in patients with chronic respiratory failure. Thorax 2001; 56:524–528.
153. Elliott MW. Non-invasive ventilation—mechanisms of benefit. Med Klin (Munich) 1999; 94:2–6.

11 Upper Airway Surgery in the Adult

Donald M. Sesso
Department of Otolaryngology/Head and Neck Surgery, Stanford University Medical Center, Palo Alto, California, U.S.A.

Nelson B. Powell and Robert W. Riley
Department of Otolaryngology/Head and Neck Surgery, Stanford University Medical Center and Division of Sleep Medicine, Department of Behavioral Sciences, Stanford School of Medicine, Palo Alto, California, U.S.A.

Jerome E. Hester
Department of Otolaryngology/Head and Neck Surgery, Stanford University Medical Center, Palo Alto, California, U.S.A.

INTRODUCTION

Sleep-disordered breathing (SDB) is a collective term, which encompasses snoring, upper airway resistance syndrome (UARS), obstructive sleep apnea-hypopnea syndrome, and obstructive sleep apnea (OSA). These terms describe a partial or complete obstruction of the upper airway during sleep. Patency of the pharyngeal airway is maintained by two opposing forces: negative intraluminal pressure and the activity of the upper airway musculature. Anatomical or central neural abnormalities can disrupt this delicate balance with resultant compromise of the upper airway. This reduction of airway caliber may cause sleep fragmentation and subsequent behavioral derangements, such as excessive daytime sleepiness (EDS) (1–3). Thus, medical and surgical therapy attempt to alleviate this obstruction and increase airway patency.

Surgical management was the first therapeutic modality employed to treat SDB. Kuhlo (4) described placement of a tracheotomy tube in an attempt to bypass upper airway obstruction in Pickwickian patients. Although effective, tracheotomy is not readily accepted by most patients and does not address the specific sites of pharyngeal collapse. These regions include the nasal cavity/nasopharynx, oropharynx, and hypopharynx. Often, multilevel obstruction is present. Consequently, the surgical armamentarium has evolved to create techniques, which correct the specific anatomical sites of obstruction. The objective of surgical intervention is to eliminate SDB. To achieve this goal, it is necessary to alleviate all levels of obstruction in an organized and safe protocol. Ultimately, it is the obligation of the surgeon to counsel the patient regarding all surgical techniques, risks, complications, and alternative medical therapies.

Medical management is often considered the primary treatment of SDB, however, there are exceptions. Treatment may consist of weight loss, avoidance of alcohol, and sedating medications and manipulation of body position during sleep (5–9). Currently, continuous positive airway pressure (CPAP) or bilevel positive airway pressure devices are the preferred methods of treatment and the standard to which other modalities are compared. The efficacy of CPAP has clearly been demonstrated

(10,11). Yet, a subset of patients struggle to comply with or accept CPAP therapy (12,13). Consequently, patients who are unwilling or unable to comply with medical treatment may be candidates for surgery.

RATIONALE FOR SURGICAL TREATMENT OF SLEEP-DISORDERED BREATHING

The rationale for surgical treatment of the upper airway is to alleviate or minimize the pathophysiologic and neurobehavioral derangements associated with upper airway obstruction. The goal is to achieve outcomes that are equivalent to those of medical management. Ideally, this would include an improved quality of life with a reduction in cardiopulmonary and neurologic morbidity (14–17).

SURGICAL INDICATIONS

Indications for surgery are defined in Table 1. All patients require a comprehensive evaluation to determine if they meet the criteria for surgery. Polysomnography as well as a history and physical examination are essential to make this determination. The subgroup of patients whose apnea-hypopnea index (AHI) is less than 20 may still be candidates for surgery. Surgery is considered appropriate if these patients have associated EDS, which results in altered daytime performance or comorbidities as recognized by the Center for Medicare and Medicaid Services (including stroke and ischemic heart disease). For those patients whose EDS is not explained by the severity of their sleep apnea or resolved with CPAP therapy, consideration may be given to obtaining a multiple sleep latency test or the maintenance of wakefulness test to determine other etiologies of sleepiness (18,19). In these patients, surgery is unlikely to be beneficial. Other factors exist, which could predict poor surgical outcomes and consequently, render a patient to be unsuitable for surgery. These factors are listed in Table 2.

PREOPERATIVE EVALUATION

Proper screening and selection of patients for surgery is paramount to achieve successful outcomes and to minimize postoperative complications. The preoperative evaluation requires a comprehensive medical history, head and neck examination, polysomnography, fiberoptic nasopharyngolaryngoscopy, and lateral cephalometric analysis. A thorough review of this data can determine the extent of SDB severity,

TABLE 1 Surgical Indications

Apnea-hypopnea index $\geq 20^a$ events per hour of sleep
Oxygen desaturation nadir < 90%
Esophageal pressure (P_{es}) more negative than −10 cm H_2O
Cardiovascular derangements (arrhythmia, hypertension)
Neurobehavioral symptoms (excessive daytime sleepiness)
Failure of medical management
Anatomical sites of obstruction (nose, palate, tongue base)

[a]Surgery may be indicated with an AHI < 20 if accompanied by excessive daytime fatigue.
Source: From Ref. 18.

TABLE 2   Poor Surgical Candidates

Severe pulmonary disease
Unstable cardiovascular disease
Morbid obesity
Alcohol or drug abuse
Psychiatric instability
Unrealistic expectations

Source: From Ref. 18.

uncover comorbidities, and assist in risk management. Furthermore, this systematic approach will identify probable anatomic sites of obstruction. Armed with this information, a safe, site-specific surgical protocol can be presented to the patient.

In addition, a surgeon must listen to the concerns and expectations of their patients. Often, these may differ than those of the physician. Thus, educating a patient about SDB and expected outcomes of surgery should be undertaken prior to any intervention.

PHYSICAL EXAMINATION (SEE ALSO CHAPTER 1)

A complete physical exam with vital signs, weight and neck circumference should be performed on every patient. Included in this evaluation is a detailed head and neck examination. Specific attention is focused in the regions that have been well described as potential sites of upper airway obstruction, such as the nose, palate, and base of tongue (20–25). Nasal obstruction can occur as a result of alar collapse, septal deviation, and turbinate hypertrophy or sinonasal masses. These can be identified on anterior rhinoscopy. The oral cavity should be examined for dental occlusion, periodontal disease and any lesions, including torus mandibulae or torus palatinus. Examination of the oropharyngeal and hypopharyngeal regions includes a description of the tonsils, palate, lateral pharyngeal walls, and tongue base. A variety of grading systems, such as Mallampati's, have been developed to establish a standard of describing the degree of obstruction caused by these structures (26,27). However, it was Fujita who first proposed a classification system to define the levels of upper airway obstruction in OSA patients (28,29). Laryngeal anatomy can be evaluated by indirect laryngoscopy or fiberoptic exam (see Fiberoptic Nasopharyngolaryngoscopy section).

POLYSOMNOGRAM (SEE ALSO CHAPTER 3)

A polysomnogram (PSG) is a vital part of the preoperative evaluation. The study must be carefully reviewed by the surgeon, with particular attention focused on the AHI and oxygen desaturation nadir. These data will guide appropriate surgical treatment, as well as preoperative and postoperative management. As with any intervention, a postoperative PSG is needed to assess a patient's response to surgery. Failure to obtain this study may result in an inadequately treated patient.

FIBEROPTIC NASOPHARYNGOLARYNGOSCOPY

Obstruction of the nasal airway, pharynx, and larynx can all be visualized during fiberoptic exam. In particular, the larynx can be more closely observed for such

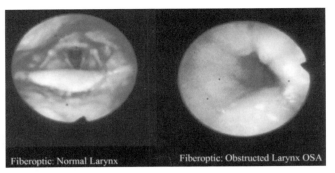

FIGURE 1 (*See color insert.*) Fiberoptic laryngoscopy. Note that the entire vocal folds of the normal larynx can be visualized (*left*). Müller's maneuver results in velopharyngeal and hypopharyngeal collapse with airway obstruction. Vocal folds are obscured by soft tissue in this abnormal exam (*right*). *Abbreviation*: OSA, obstructive sleep apnea.

abnormalities as an omega-shaped epiglottis, vocal fold paralysis or obstructing lesions. Evaluation of the posterior airway space (PAs) is required to determine if obstruction occurs at the palate and/or tongue base. Furthermore, the posterior airway space is examined at rest as well as during provocative maneuvers. One such technique, Müller's maneuver, has been evaluated by Sher et al. (30) to identify potential sites of obstruction and to predict surgical success. This test involves inspiration against a closed oral and nasal airway, while keeping the glottis open. Photo documentation of findings may prove useful for surgical planning and patient education (Fig. 1).

Fiberoptic examination is not only important to evaluate the upper airway for obstruction but aids in determining ease of intubation. These data can be invaluable to both the surgeon and anesthesiologist, as they determine the best method to intubate a patient.

CEPHALOMETRIC ANALYSIS

The lateral cephalogram is the most cost-effective radiographic study of the bony facial skeleton and soft tissues of the upper airway. Using these landmarks, Riley et al. (31) were first to describe anthropomorphic measurements, which can be performed to ascertain skeletal facial abnormalities. Magnetic resonance imaging (MRI) and computed tomography (CT) scanning have proven to be effective in radiographic studies; however, these tools are often reserved for investigational studies due to expense and time (32–34). Although not as detailed as CT scan or MRI, the cephalogram allows measurement of the length of the soft palate, skeletal proportions, posterior airway space, and hyoid position. Studies have shown the cephalogram to be valid in assessing obstruction, and in fact, it compares favorably to three-dimensional volumetric computed tomographic scans of the upper airway (35). As with other tests, this modality may underestimate the degree of obstruction, due to the fact that the study is not performed while the patient is sleeping.

SURGICAL TREATMENT SUMMARY

The aim of surgical treatment is to alleviate upper airway obstruction and its associated neurobehavioral symptoms and morbidities. No longer is a 50% reduction in the

TABLE 3   Powell-Riley Definition of Surgical Responders

Apnea-hypopnea index < 20 events per hour of sleep[a]
Oxygen desaturation nadir ≥ 90%
Excessive daytime sleepiness alleviated
Response equivalent to CPAP on full-night titration

[a]A reduction of the apnea-hypopnea index by 50% or more is considered a cure if
the preoperative apnea-hypopnea index is less than 20.
Abbreviation: CPAP, continuous-positive airway pressure.
Source: From Ref. 18.

AHI deemed acceptable (Table 3). Rather, the objective is to treat to cure (normalization of respiratory events and elimination of hypoxemia). This goal can only be accomplished if a careful and systematic evaluation is performed on every patient. Since obstruction may occur at multiple levels, it may be necessary to treat more than one site. Failure to recognize or treat all anatomical levels will lead to persistent obstruction. Thus, the surgeon must be committed to treating the entire upper airway.

Once a surgical plan has been developed, this must be communicated to the patient and our medical colleagues. Successful treatment of a SDB patient typically requires a multidisciplinary team. This team will assist in the preoperative and postoperative course to minimize risk and potential complications. Prior to surgical treatment, a review of treatment options and risks must be discussed with the patient. Only after the patient fully understands the process and has consented to surgery can the treatment plan proceed.

The surgeon has a variety of procedures available within his or her armamentarium to treat SDB. Selecting the appropriate surgery for a patient can be challenging. However, we have created a two-phase surgical protocol (Powell-Riley surgical protocol) as a logically directed plan to treat the specific areas of upper airway obstruction (36,37). This protocol (Table 4) as well as other contemporary surgical techniques (Table 5) will be discussed in this chapter.

POWELL-RILEY TWO-PHASE SURGICAL PROTOCOL

This protocol consists of two distinct phases. The procedures included in each phase are listed in Table 4. Developed to prevent unnecessary surgery, this method is a conservative surgical approach to the SDB patient. Phase II surgery has documented success rates exceeding 90%; however, a substantial number of patients may not

TABLE 4   Powell-Riley Protocol Surgical Procedures

Phase I
Nasal surgery (septoplasty, turbinate reduction, nasal valve grafting)
Tonsillectomy
Uvulopalatopharyngoplasty or uvulopalatal flap
Mandibular osteotomy with genioglossus advancement
Hyoid myotomy and suspension
Temperature-controlled radiofrequency[a]—turbinates, palate, tongue base
Phase II
Maxillomandibular advancement osteotomy
Temperature-controlled radiofrequency[a]—tongue base

[a]Temperature-controlled radiofrequency is typically used as an adjunctive treatment.
Select patients may choose temperature-controlled radiofrequency as primary treatment.

TABLE 5 Alternative Upper Airway Surgical Techniques

Pharyngeal obstruction
Temperature-controlled radiofrequency
Pillar® palatal implant system
Laser-assisted uvulopalatoplasty
Injection snoreplasty
Hypopharyngeal obstruction
Genial bone advancement trephine system (GBAT™)
Repose™ genioglossus advancement hyoid myotomy
Temperature-controlled radiofrequency
Midline glossectomy and lingualplasty
Airway bypass surgery
Tracheotomy

---

need such extensive surgery (38,39). In fact, patients have a realistic chance to be cured by phase I surgery alone. However, it is difficult to predict surgical outcomes for an individual patient. Conservative surgery (phase I) is therefore recommended initially with the plan to perform postoperative PSG to assess response to surgery. Those patients who are incompletely treated would then be considered for phase II surgery. As with any treatment protocol, exceptions may occur. There are select cases in which phase II surgery may be the appropriate initial step, as in nonobese patients with marked mandibular deficiency and normal palates (40).

Phase I surgery is directed towards the three potential sites of upper airway obstruction (nose, palate, and tongue base). Essentially, these surgical approaches treat the soft tissue of the upper airway. Neither dental occlusion nor the facial skeleton is altered. Clinical response is determined by PSG. The PSG is obtained four to six months following surgery to allow for adequate healing. Patients who have persistent SDB are prepared for phase II surgery.

Phase II surgery refers to maxillomandibular advancement osteotomy (MMO) or bimaxillary advancement. MMO helps clear hypopharyngeal obstruction, which would be the only region incompletely treated by phase I. This is the only procedure which physically creates more room for the tongue to be advanced anteriorly, thus enlarging the posterior airway space.

SURGICAL OUTCOMES

As noted previously, simply reducing the AHI by 50% is no longer considered a cure for SDB. Rather, surgical intervention aims to attain the results obtained by CPAP therapy. Consequently, a more comprehensive criterion was established to determine surgical success or cure (Table 3).

Clinical response to phase I surgery ranges from 42% to 75% (38,41–45). Our published data have shown that approximately 60% of all patients are cured with phase I surgery (38). Factors that portend less successful outcomes are a mean respiratory disturbance index (RDI) greater than 60, oxygen desaturation below 70%, mandibular deficiency (sella nasion point B < 75°) and morbid obesity [body mass index (BMI) > 33 kg/m²]. However, it is imprudent to forego phase I surgery in these patients, since a reasonable percentage may not require more aggressive surgery (37).

Incomplete treatment by phase I surgery is primarily related to persistent hypopharyngeal obstruction. Those patients who have failed treatment or who have been incompletely treated would then be considered for phase II surgery (MMO). MMO is a more aggressive surgery, which requires more intensive operative and postoperative care. Patients must be prepared for a recovery period of four to six weeks. Although the convalescence period may be extensive, documented success rates exceed 90% (38,46–49).

SURGICAL PREPARATION

As with any surgery, ensuring that a patient is medically stable for the operative procedure can reduce postoperative complications. This evaluation includes appropriate laboratory, cardiopulmonary, and radiographic testing. In patients with existing comorbid medical conditions (diabetes, hypothyroidism, cardiovascular disease, and pulmonary disease), consultation with the appropriate medical specialist should be sought.

Furthermore, for those patients who are tolerant of CPAP, they should be encouraged to use this modality for at least two weeks prior to surgery. Preoperative CPAP can alleviate the issues associated with sleep deprivation and may reduce the risk of postobstructive pulmonary edema (50). In 1988, Powell et al. (51) recommended the use of preoperative CPAP for all patients who have an RDI greater than 40 and an oxygen desaturation of 80% or less. According to this protocol, the surgeon must consider insertion of a temporary tracheotomy for those patients with severe OSA (RDI greater than 60 and/or SaO_2 less than 70%) who are intolerant of CPAP therapy. Tracheotomy is rarely needed at our center and must be determined on a case-by-case basis.

SURGICAL PROCEDURES—PHASE I
Nasal Reconstruction
Nasal obstruction can occur due to incompetent nasal valves, septal deviations or chronically enlarged turbinates. A patent nasal airway is essential for normal respiration and sleep. Obstruction can increase airway resistance and result in mouth breathing. Opening of the mouth rotates the mandible posteriorly and inferiorly, which in turn causes the tongue to prolapse into the posterior airway space. A plethora of techniques (septoplasty, alar grafting, and turbinate reduction) exist to treat nasal obstruction. These techniques and their results have been well established in the head and neck literature. The choice of procedure depends upon surgeon preference and experience.

Nasal reconstruction can improve quality of life and may improve OSA in select patients (52,53). In addition, improvement of the nasal airway may improve a patient's tolerance of nasal CPAP (54). Rarely, however, will alleviating nasal obstruction cure OSA.

Although most treatments of the nasal cavity are well established, treatment of the turbinates is an evolving technique. Our preferred method is submucosal turbinoplasty with a radiofrequency probe. Submucosal turbinoplasty can be performed with radiofrequency or a microdebrider. Radiofrequency is rarely associated with complications such as bleeding or crusting. However, the ultimate goal of reducing submucosal erectile tissue, while preserving the ciliated, surface mucosa is the same (55,56).

Uvulopalatopharyngoplasty/Uvulopalatal Flap
Ikematsu (57) is credited with developing the uvulopalatopharyngoplasty (UPPP) for the treatment of habitual snoring. This technique was later adapted to treat SDB and snoring by Fujita et al. (29) in 1981. Since this time, multiple variations have

TABLE 6 Fujita Classification of Obstructive Regions

Type I: Palate (normal base of tongue)
Type II: Palate and base of tongue
Type III: Base of tongue (normal palate)

Source: From Ref. 28.

been developed to treat the obstructing tissues of the soft palate, lateral pharyngeal walls, and tonsils.

UPPP is an excellent technique to alleviate isolated retropalatal (Table 6) obstruction (Fujita Type I). Performed under general anesthesia, a portion of the palate, uvula, lateral pharyngeal walls, and tonsils may be removed (Fig. 2). This is conservative surgery, which an experienced surgeon can perform with ease. Results vary depending upon the skill of the surgeon, the technique selected, and the severity of disease. Unfortunately, there is often a stigma associated with UPPP due to the intensity of postoperative pain and variable cure rates.

A meta-analysis of the cure rate of UPPP was performed by Sher et al. (46) in 1996. UPPP was found to have a success rate of 39% for curing OSA. Such a high failure rate is most likely related to the fact that a large percentage of these patients had coexisting, unrecognized hypopharyngeal obstruction. Undoubtedly, UPPP can clear the palatal airway of excessive tissue and, if utilized appropriately, can improve SDB. While capable of improving select patients, UPPP is seldom credited with curing moderate or severe SDB. In fact, this procedure may be over-utilized as an isolated surgical procedure to cure SDB by those who have failed to identify tongue base obstruction. However, if UPPP is used appropriately or combined with

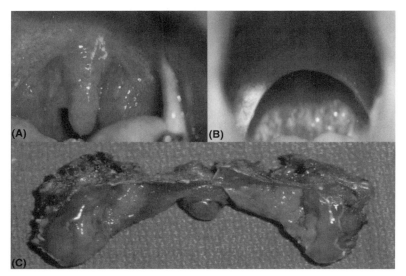

FIGURE 2 (See color insert.) Uvulopalatopharyngoplasty. (**A**) This patient demonstrates tonsillar hypertrophy, an elongated uvula and redundant tissue of the lateral pharyngeal wall resulting in a narrowed airway space. (**B**) Removal of the tonsils, lateral pharyngeal wall mucosa, and soft palate mucosa has enlarged the airway. (**C**) Excised surgical specimen.

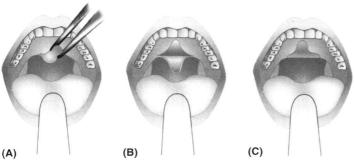

(A)   **(B)**   **(C)**

FIGURE 3 (*See color insert.*) Uvulopalatal flap technique. (**A**) The mucosal crease is identified by reflecting the uvula. This marks the superior limit of dissection. (**B**) Incision is planned on the lingual aspect of the soft palate. (**C**) Wound is closed with 3–0 Vicryl sutures. These sutures may be removed to release the flap if velopharyngeal insufficiency should occur. *Source*: From Ref. 121.

procedures aimed at other anatomical sites of obstruction the results can be much more gratifying.

The uvulopalatal flap (UPF) was introduced by Powell et al. as a modification of the UPPP in 1996 (Figs. 3 and 4). The goal was to reduce the incidence of velopharyngeal insufficiency (VPI) by using a potentially reversible flap that could be "taken down" early in the recovery period if complications arose. In addition, the UPF technique was found to have less postoperative pain on a visual analog scale, as compared to traditional UPPP. The reason for reduced pain is due to the fact that no sutures are placed on the free edge of the palate (58). The indications for performing the UPF are the same as UPPP. However, this flap is contraindicated in patients with excessively long and thick palates. In these patients, the flap created will be too bulky and could potentially eliminate a favorable outcome.

Major complications (myocardial infarction, complete airway obstruction, and severe hemorrhage) following UPPP are less than 1.5% (59). More commonly, patients complain of postoperative pain and mild palatal swelling. Voice changes, taste disturbances and dysphagia have been reported, but are typically transient. Although rare, VPI and nasopharyngeal stenosis are often the result of poor surgical technique. The temptation to maximize results by removing large portions of the palate should

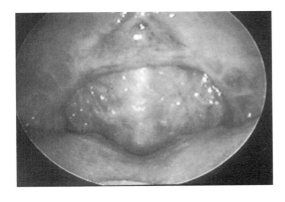

FIGURE 4 (*See color insert.*) Uvulopalatal flap (UPF). Postoperative view of a UPF.

be resisted to prevent VPI. Judicious resection of tissue and proper patient selection can aid in preventing these complications.

Mandibular Osteotomy with Genioglossus Advancement

Genioglossus advancement is indicated for patients with documented hypopharyngeal obstruction (Table 6) (Fujita Type II–III). The rationale of this surgery is to enlarge the posterior airway space by preventing prolapse of the tongue during sleep. Considered part of phase I of the Powell-Riley protocol, it may be used alone or in combination with other procedures depending upon the regions of obstruction.

This surgery is a conservative maxillofacial technique, since an osteotomy is created in the mandible without changing the dental occlusion. Thus, a limitation of this surgery is that no additional room is created for the tongue, in contrast to maxillomandibular advancement. Essentially, the genial tubercle and the attached genioglossus muscle are advanced anteriorly. The degree of advancement is dependent upon the thickness of the anterior portion of the mandible and the compliance of the genioglossus muscle. Less muscle compliance will provide a greater degree of tension. Unfortunately, there is no study to determine the compliance of the genioglossus muscle preoperatively.

Surgery can be performed under intravenous sedation or general anesthesia. Blood loss is usually negligible. A lateral cephalometric radiograph and a panoramic dental radiograph are critical in the preoperative planning. The panoramic radiograph allows the surgeon to identify the genial tubercle and to assess the root length of the mandibular canine and central incisor teeth. Sclerotic bone in the symphyseal region of the mandible aids in locating the genial tubercle. Furthermore, the film should be reviewed for evidence of periodontal disease.

Knowledge of the anatomy is vital to capture the majority of the genioglossus muscle fibers within the rectangular osteotomy and to avoid complications. As the muscle's insertion includes the genial tubercle and the lingual surface of the mandible adjacent to the tubercle, the osteotomy must be designed to encompass this region. Thus, the width of the bone fragment should be at least 14 mm and the height about 10 mm (60,61). To avoid injury to the roots of the canine teeth, the vertical osteotomies should be medial to the canine dentition. Careful planning is also required in performing the horizontal osteotomies. The surgeon must be cognizant of the roots of the incisor dentition and the inferior border of the mandible. It is recommended that the superior osteotomy be placed at least 5 mm inferior to the root apices to avoid injury (62). In addition, the inferior osteotomy should be approximately 10 mm above the inferior border of the mandible to prevent a potential fracture.

In 1986, Riley et al. (63) developed the rectangular osteotomy technique (Fig. 5) to advance the genial tubercle for patients with hypopharyngeal obstruction. This procedure is within the rubric of phase I surgery. Subsequently, they evaluated 239 patients who completed phase I surgery and underwent postoperative PSG. Most of these patients had genioglossus advancement with hyoid suspension and UPPP. The overall success rate was 61%. The data were further extrapolated to determine the correlation between disease severity and response rates. Patients with mild disease had a cure rate of 77%, while those with severe disease had a cure rate of 42% (38). Similar results were reported in other studies (43–45,64). In Sher's (46) meta-analysis of patients who only underwent UPPP, the overall responder rate

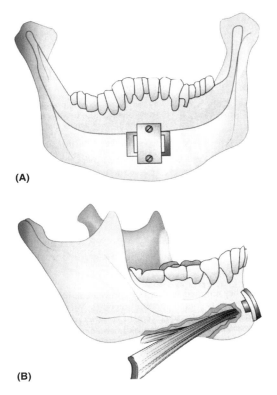

(A)

(B)

FIGURE 5 (*See color insert.*) Mandibular osteotomy with genioglossus advancement. A rectangular osteotomy is created in the anterior mandible. The genial tubercle and the attached genioglossus muscle are advanced anteriorly. The bony fragment is rotated 90° to overlap the inferior border of the mandible and secured to the mandible with a titanium screw. *Source*: From Ref. 121.

was 39%. Thus, it became evident that the addition of genioglossus advancement can substantially increase success rates for treating SDB.

Postoperative edema or hematoma is usually self-limiting. Obstruction of the airway due to edema or hematoma is the most distressing complication following surgery but it has not been observed in our series. The use of CPAP in the early postoperative period reduces edema and maintains the patency of the airway (65,66). Meticulous hemostasis and aggressive antihypertensive management are critical to prevent hematoma formation. As previously mentioned, inferior border mandible fractures can occur if the osteotomy is incorrectly designed. This complication has been essentially eliminated by performing a rectangular osteotomy, which leaves the inferior border of the mandible intact. Any technique which violates the inferior border increases the risk of a pathologic fracture. Minor complications, such as wound infection, transient anesthesia of the teeth or lower lip, and root injury requiring endodontic therapy have an incidence rate of 2%, 6%, and 1%, respectively, at our center.

Hyoid Myotomy and Suspension

The genioglossus and geniohyoid muscles as well as the middle pharyngeal constrictors insert on the hyoid bone. Consequently, the position of the hyoid complex is important in maintaining the patency of the hypopharyngeal airway.

Van de Graaff et al. (67) reported that anterior hyoid advancement improved the posterior airway space in a canine model. In 1984, Kaya (68) was the first to demonstrate this concept in human subjects. Thus, the rationale for hyoid myotomy and suspension is to alleviate hypopharyngeal obstruction by advancing the hyoid complex in an anterior direction. This procedure is considered as part of phase I surgery and may be performed as an isolated procedure or in combination with other techniques.

Currently, we rarely perform hyoid suspension simultaneously with genioglossus advancement. The added trauma to the hypopharyngeal region can be problematic for the patient to tolerate, and it may prolong recovery. Furthermore, UPPP and genioglossus advancement may have enlarged the posterior airway space, so as to eliminate the need for additional surgery. Hyoid myotomy and suspension has become an adjunctive procedure to treat tongue base obstruction for those who previously underwent genioglossus advancement.

Originally, this surgery involved suspending the hyoid to the mandible with fascia lata (63). However, this required additional incisions and dissection to harvest the fascia lata and expose the mandible. In order to reduce the extent of surgery, the technique has been modified to suspend the hyoid bone to the superior border of the thyroid cartilage (42). A single horizontal incision is made at the level of the hyoid. Both the hyoid bone and thyroid cartilage are exposed. The hyoid is advanced anteriorly and secured to the thyroid cartilage with three or four permanent sutures (Fig. 6). Either general or local anesthesia may be utilized (69).

As stated previously, the overall success rate for phase I surgery was 61%. However, the majority of patients underwent genioglossus advancement with hyoid suspension and UPPP (38). Riley and Powell (42) found that hyoid myotomy and suspension improved SDB and corrected EDS in 75% of consecutively treated patients ($n = 15$) with documented sleep apnea. Yet, these patients also had previous genioglossus advancement. Two studies have reviewed the outcomes of patients treated with hyoid suspension alone without concurrent or previous genioglossus advancement for hypopharyngeal obstruction. The success rate from these studies ranged from 17% to 78% (69,70). Our experience has indicated that hyoid suspension is not efficacious as primary treatment of hypopharyngeal obstruction, but rather may be reserved as an adjunctive therapy.

Major complications are exceedingly rare with this surgery. The potential for airway obstruction exists, but this has not been observed at our center. Seroma or hematoma formation may occur; however, the use of surgical drains has reduced this complication. Transient aspiration or dysphagia can be observed but usually

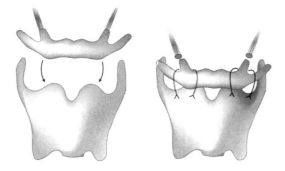

FIGURE 6 (*See color insert.*) Hyoid myotomy and suspension. The hyoid bone and thyroid cartilage are exposed via a small neck incision. The hyoid bone is advanced anteriorly and secured to the thyroid cartilage with three or four permanent sutures. *Source*: From Ref. 121.

will resolve within 10 days. If these symptoms persist, removal of the suspension sutures should alleviate this problem (71). Meticulous dissection of the suprahyoid musculature protects vital structures. Specifically, dissection should not extend lateral to the lesser cornu or superior to the upper border of the hyoid to avoid injury to the superior laryngeal nerve and hypoglossal nerve, respectively. Infection can be managed with wound care and antibiotics should it occur.

SURGICAL PROCEDURES—PHASE II
Maxillomandibular Advancement Osteotomy

MMO, also referred to as bimaxillary surgery, is considered phase II of the Powell-Riley two-phase surgical protocol. The rationale for MMO is to ameliorate refractory hypopharyngeal obstruction by advancing the mandible and maxilla forward.

Treatment of SDB by skeletal surgery was first described by Kuo et al. (72) and Bear and Priest (73). Subjective improvements in SDB were reported, but there was no postoperative PSG to support these claims. Subsequently, our group objectively documented an improvement in sleep apnea following mandibular advancement (74). Numerous studies have since reiterated these findings (49,75,76).

MMO enlarges both the hypopharyngeal and pharyngeal airway by expanding the skeletal facial framework. It is the only surgery in our protocol, which physically creates more space for the tongue in the oral cavity. In addition, it exerts further tension on the velopharyngeal and suprahyoid musculature to prevent their posterior collapse. Advancements of 10 to 15 mm are usually required to adequately clear the posterior airway space of obstruction.

Although some authors have advocated maxillomandibular advancement as primary therapy for hypopharyngeal obstruction, we usually reserve this surgery for those who are incompletely treated with phase I surgery (36,77). Our experience has demonstrated reasonable response rates with phase I treatment; thus, we attempt less invasive surgery prior to MMO surgery. For those patients inadequately treated with phase I surgery, the source of obstruction is typically the hypopharynx.

Initially, MMO was advocated for patients with maxillomandibular deficiency. However, only approximately 40% of patients with SDB have contributing craniofacial deficiency (78). Potentially creating temporomandibular joint dysfunction or compromising facial esthetics was of concern in performing MMO in patients without mandibular or maxillary deficiency, but studies have since proven that MMO is effective in these patients without resulting in these complications. In fact, skeletal facial advancement may impart a more youthful esthetic appearance (79,80).

Maxillomandibular advancement had been used for many years to treat malocclusion. The surgery has undergone several modifications for the treatment of SDB. The primary modification is a bony advancement of 10 to 15 mm, which tends to be greater than those needed to treat malocclusion. Care must be taken to preserve the descending palatine arteries of the maxilla, and, the dental occlusion should be preserved. This is accomplished by placing arch bars or orthodontic bands prior to the osteotomies. A Le Fort I maxillary osteotomy is performed above the roots of the teeth. The maxilla is down fractured and then advanced anteriorly. Stabilization of the maxilla is accomplished with rigid plate fixation. Mandibular advancement is achieved by a sagittal split osteotomy (Fig. 7). Care is taken to preserve the inferior alveolar nerves. Fixation is maintained by bi-cortical screws and mono-cortical plating. Proper alignment of the dental occlusion is needed prior to fixation.

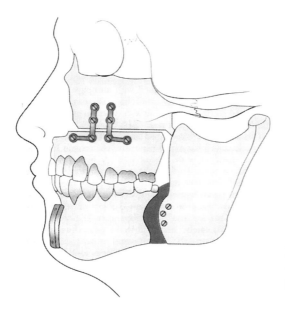

FIGURE 7 (*See color insert.*) Maxillo-mandibular advancement osteotomy (MMO). The maxilla and mandible are advanced 10 to 15 mm. A Le Fort I osteotomy and bilateral sagittal split mandibular osteotomy are performed. The advanced segments of bone are stabilized with bi-cortical screws and rigid plate fixation. Note the genioglossus advancement performed prior to MMO. *Source*: From Ref. 121.

Published data regarding the results of MMO has been well established (47,49,77,81,82). In 1992, we reported 91 patients who underwent bimaxillary surgery. The success rate of phase II therapy was 97% (38). Despite the potential for some skeletal relapse, the long-term success of MMO remains greater than 90% (83). An enlarged posterior airway space can be visualized on postoperative cephalograms (Fig. 8). Ultimately, in order for surgery to be considered efficacious, it must

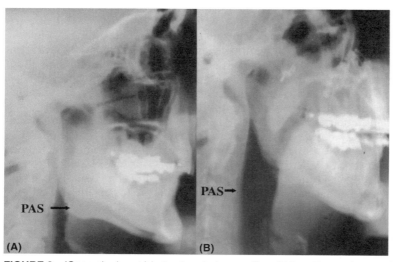

FIGURE 8 (*See color insert.*) Lateral cephalogram films. This patient underwent both phase I and phase II of the Powell-Riley protocol for sleep-disordered breathing. (**A**) Preoperative film. (**B**) Postoperative film—note the markedly widened posterior airway space (PAS).

achieve rates of cure similar to CPAP therapy. In 1990, Riley et al. (84) demonstrated no statistical difference between nasal CPAP and surgery in improving sleep architecture and SDB. Consequently, if a logical, stepwise surgical approach is used in treating SDB patients, cure rates similar to that of medical management can be offered.

As mentioned previously, loss of the airway is the most feared complication following surgery. Risk can be reduced by appropriately utilizing preoperative CPAP and controlling blood pressure (65,66). Necrosis of the palate has been observed as a result of compromised blood supply, although it is quite rare (85). Identifying and protecting the descending palatine vessels can prevent this complication. Skeletal relapse with resulting malocclusion may occur in 15% of patients. This usually does not result in recurrence of SDB, and can easily be managed with occlusal equilibration. Pain is well controlled with oral analgesics and is not as intense as palatal surgery. Perhaps the most common complaint following MMO surgery is anesthesia or paresthesias of the dentition and perioral region. This symptom is expected in the early recovery period and will resolve within 6 to 12 months for most patients.

CONTEMPORARY TREATMENT ALTERNATIVES FOR PHARYNGEAL RECONSTRUCTION
Temperature-Controlled Radiofrequency of the Palate

Radiofrequency ablation (RF) of tissue has many applications in the medical and surgical fields. It has been used to treat benign prostatic hypertrophy and Wolfe-Parkinson-White syndrome (86,87). Powell and Riley adapted this modality to treat redundant tissue of the upper airway in patients with SDB. The initial investigation trial was performed in a porcine model. Histologic assessments revealed a well-circumscribed lesion with normally healing tissue without damage to peripheral nerves. Volumetric analysis noted an initial inflammatory response, which resolved within 48 hours. A 26.3% volumetric reduction of tissue was documented on the 10th postoperative day (88). Based upon the positive studies in animal models, RF was attempted on human palates to treat snoring and SDB. Subsequent trials were then applied to the nasal turbinates and tongue base.

Temperature-controlled radiofrequency (TCRF) has several advantages as compared to traditional techniques when treating SDB. This procedure is minimally invasive and can be performed on an outpatient basis. The mucosal layer of tissue is spared, thus resulting in less pain and complications. Lower temperatures allow for more precise treatment and reduce thermal injury to adjacent tissue. TCRF heats treated tissue from 47 to 90°C. Electrocautery and laser procedures can heat tissue from 750 to 900°C. More precise control of thermal energy and limited submucosal tissue injury results in less morbidity without sacrificing efficacy.

Treatment is administered by inserting an electrode probe into the submucosal layer of the tissue to be ablated. Low frequency (465 kHz), low heat electromagnetic energy is administered to denature tissue protein. This region of necrosis is resorbed by the body with resulting volumetric reduction and stiffening of the tissue.

TCRF treatment of the palate reduced subjective snoring scores by 77% and reduced EDS (89). Multiple studies have shown TCRF of the palate improves snoring as effectively as other treatment modalities (90–92). Relapse of snoring has been noted at rates similar to those obtained by other treatment protocols (93). However, patients are more likely to undergo repeat RF treatments than more invasive procedures. While outcomes may be similar for different treatment options for snoring, the main advantage RF offers is minimal postoperative pain. Typically, ibuprofen is used for analgesia after TCRF. Narcotics are not commonly needed to alleviate pain following TCRF, while they are needed in nearly all patients who undergo UPPP or laser-assisted palatoplasty (94). Although improvement in SDB has been documented following TCRF, it is unlikely to cure palatal obstruction as primary therapy. Blumen et al. (95) demonstrated a significant reduction in RDI following TCRF of the palate in patients with mild-to-moderate disease. It is our experience that, due to the bulk of tissue which needs to be reduced, TCRF is best utilized as an adjunctive technique to treat palatal obstruction.

TCRF is well-tolerated. The incidence of postoperative complications is exceedingly low. A study of the postoperative outcomes demonstrated no major complications and less than a 1% chance of minor complications (96). Mucosal ulceration or sloughing was defined as a minor complication. Airway obstruction, hemorrhage, palatal fistula, and severe dysphagia are potential serious negative outcomes.

Pillar® Palatal Implant System

The Pillar® palatal implant (Restore Medical, Inc., St. Paul, Minnesota, U.S.) was introduced as a treatment for snoring in 2003. These implants are composed of polyethylene terephthalate (PET). This material has been used since the 1960s in other implantable medical products. PET is biocompatible and inert resulting in minimal tissue reaction to the implant. The nature of the material allows tissue ingrowth to stabilize the material. Histologic analysis of the implant system indicates that a chronic inflammatory response occurs as a result of PET implantation. Inflammation results in the formation of a fibrous capsule. This process should be complete within four weeks.

The rationale for this procedure is to stiffen the soft palate, and thus reduce palatal flutter and snoring. Implantation of the PET material imparts a degree of rigidity to the palate. Additional stiffening of the palate is achieved by fibrosis and formation of capsule in response to the inflammatory reaction (97).

The procedure is minimally invasive and can be performed in the clinic setting. A handheld applicator is used to insert the PET implants. After the palate is anesthetized, an 18 mm by 1.5 mm implant is placed in the midline above the uvula. The implants should be positioned in the muscular layer of the soft palate. Two additional implants are placed 2 mm lateral to the midline on each side. Postoperative antibiotics are given to prevent infection. Pain can usually be controlled with over-the-counter analgesics (98,99).

The Pillar Implant received FDA clearance for the treatment of snoring and mild-to-moderate OSA. Originally, this implant was studied to determine its role in eliminating snoring. The outcomes of these studies indicate that the implant system has efficacy and relapse rates similar to other treatment modalities (98,100–101). However, these studies often excluded patients with OSA and did not always obtain a PSG. More recently, Nordgård evaluated 25 patients with mild-to-moderate sleep apnea to determine if palatal implants could alleviate SDB. All patients underwent PSG before and after treatment. Inclusion in the study required an AHI of 10 to 30 and a BMI of ≤ 30. AHI was reduced from a mean of 16.2 to a mean of 12.1. The AHI was reduced to below 10 in 48% of patients at 90 days post-implant (102).

Pain and mild palatal swelling can occur postoperatively, yet they are transient. The most common complication was implant extrusion. Different rates of extrusion have been noted from 2.7% to 8.8% (98,99). The most feared negative outcome would be aspiration of an extruded implant. This has not been documented in the literature. The palate must have a length > 25 mm in order to be eligible to receive an implant. Surgeon inexperience and short palatal length may increase the incidence of implant extrusion.

Laser-Assisted Uvulopalatoplasty

Laser-assisted uvulopalatoplasty (LAUP) has been used as an office-based procedure to treat snoring and SDB. The rationale and indications for this procedure are the same as for UPPP. However, this surgery was developed as an alternative to performing UPPP in the operating room.

The technique attempts to shorten and stiffen the soft palate via a series of carbon dioxide laser incisions. A portion of the uvula is resected and vertical incisions are made lateral to the uvula. Redundant tissue of the lateral pharyngeal may be excised. Local anesthesia is used for this procedure. Walker et al. (103) demonstrated a 48% success rate; however, 21% of patients had worsening of their SDB following LAUP.

LAUP is associated with significant palatal edema, and concerns exist regarding the safety of performing this procedure in the office. Terris et al. (104) noted a four-fold increase in the apnea index and a significant narrowing of the airway at 72 hours following LAUP. These findings prompted them to discourage LAUP in patients with moderate or severe sleep apnea. Other complications, such as palatal incompetence and hemorrhage, have been reported . With the advent of less painful techniques, the popularity of LAUP has waned (105). In fact, a variety of procedures are now available with similar cure rates to treat the palate with less pain and morbidity.

Injection Snoreplasty

Palatal injection sclerotherapy (injection snoreplasty) was introduced as an inexpensive, minimally invasive office procedure that treats palatal flutter snoring. Essentially, a sclerotherapy agent is injected into the submucosal layer of the soft palate to promote fibrosis and scarring (106). Several different sclerotherapy agents have been employed to stiffen the soft palate. The two most commonly used agents are 3% sodium tetradecyl sulfate (sotradecol) and 50% ethanol (107). The average number of injections required to achieve adequate reduction in snoring was 1.2 injections per patient. Exclusion criteria for this modality include comorbid diseases that interfere with wound healing (uncontrolled diabetes, uncontrolled hypothyroidism, and periodontal disease), marked tonsillar hypertrophy, previous surgical procedures for snoring, and significant OSA. Complete cessation or a significant reduction in snoring was reported by 92% of patients or bed partners. However, the rate of snoring relapse was 18% at long-term follow-up (106,108). The success and relapse rates of injection snoreplasty are similar to those of other modalities used to treat snoring (93,109,110).

In addition, to the cost effectiveness of this technique, injection snoreplasty offers the advantage of mild pain without a significant recovery period. In fact, most patients experience no interruption in the activities of daily life. This procedure can be performed during a routine office visit. The most common reported complications are palatal swelling and superficial mucosal breakdown. These are managed with observation. Other more serious complications include mucosal ulceration, palatal fistulae, VPI and anaphylaxis to the agent. This technique has not shown to significantly reduce the RDI (106,108).

CONTEMPORARY TREATMENT ALTERNATIVES FOR
HYPOPHARYNGEAL OBSTRUCTION
Genial Bone Advancement Trephine System

The genial bone advancement trephine system (GBAT™) (Stryker Leibinger Corporation, Kalamazoo, Minnesota, U.S.) attempts to alleviate tongue base obstruction by advancing the genial tubercle. This modality is a modification of the rectangular mandibular osteotomy with genioglossus advancement. The rationale and indications for the GBAT procedure are the same as for traditional genioglossus advancement.

Identification of the genial tubercle is essential to perform the surgery. A circular osteotomy is created in the mandible with the provided trephine (12 mm or 14 mm). The bone segment with the attached genioglossus muscle is advanced and secured to the anterior mandible with a rigid plate (111). The surgeon must ensure that the mandible has sufficient size to accommodate the osteotomy without violating the apices of the tooth roots and the inferior border of the mandible.

As this technique is a simple modification of existing genioglossus advancement, one would expect similar outcomes. Miller et al. studied 35 patients who underwent the GBAT procedure with simultaneous UPPP for SDB. The RDI and apnea index were reduced by 70%. Furthermore, the lowest oxygen desaturation increased from 80% to 88% and the posterior airway space increased by 4.7 mm. Overall, the cure rate was 67% (111). Studies have demonstrated subjective improvement in SDB with the GBAT procedure (112). However, long-term objective studies have not documented the success rate of the GBAT technique when used as primary treatment for SDB.

GBAT was developed as a device which would allow a one-step osteotomy and advancement of the genial tubercle. The intention is to allow the surgeon to perform the osteotomy with greater ease and speed. While the device is effective in capturing the genial tubercle, there are significant complications (111–113). Major complications have been noted to be as high as 15% (111). These complications include exposure of the hardware, persistent infection and hematoma of the floor of the mouth requiring drainage. The potential for tooth root injury and pathologic fracture of the mandible exists. Other minor complications noted in traditional genioglossus surgery can occur with the GBAT system. However, the most worrisome complication is avulsion of the genioglossus muscle by the trephine. The circular motion of the trephine places the muscle at greater risk of avulsion as compared to the rectangular osteotomy technique.

Although the GBAT system is capable of capturing the genial tubercle and has an acceptable rate of cure, it does not offer a significant advantage versus traditional surgery. Traditional genioglossus osteotomy can be performed in a similar amount of time. Furthermore, the GBAT system lacks the tactile sensation provided by a sagittal saw, which could potentially result in trauma to the floor of the mouth and muscle avulsion. Lastly, once the genioglossus muscle is avulsed, it is exceedingly difficult to salvage the surgery.

Repose™ Genioglossus Advancement Hyoid Myotomy

The Repose™ (Influent, Inc., San Francisco, California, U.S.) genioglossus advancement hyoid myotomy suspension suture technique is a minimally invasive procedure to treat hypopharyngeal obstruction (114). The concept of the surgery is to place tension on the redundant tissues of the tongue base and/or the hyoid complex by anchoring a suture to the mandible. These sutures are passed through the base of the tongue or the hyoid bone. No tissue is removed and there is minimal dissection. Thus, the procedure can be performed quickly and with less tissue trauma.

The surgery is performed under general anesthesia. A small incision is placed in the floor of the mouth. A screw is then inserted into the lingual surface of the mandible for the tongue procedure. A suture is passed through the base of the tongue and secured to the screw anchored to the mandible. For the hyoid procedure, a screw is inserted into the inferior border of the mandible. A permanent suture attached to the screw is tunneled to the level of the hyoid bone. The suture is passed around the hyoid bone with resulting anterior displacement of the hyoid complex.

The Repose system has been evaluated as primary therapy and in combination with UPPP to treat SDB. Subjective improvements in snoring and daytime fatigue have been noted. Also, a reduction of the RDI and apnea index with improvement of oxygen saturation was observed. Unfortunately, the overall cure rate was approximately 20% in several studies (115,116).

Mild complications can be associated with this surgery. Sialadenitis (salivary gland inflammation), wound infection, trauma to the neurovascular bundle of the tongue, and dysphagia can occur. In terms of the long-term efficacy of this technique, the most important issue is whether or not the suture is able to prevent the hypopharyngeal muscles from prolapsing into the posterior airway space.

Temperature-Controlled Radiofrequency of the Tongue
TCRF applied to the tongue has been shown to improve the RDI; however, the results have varied (117,118). While RF may have a role as primary therapy for mild SDB or UARS, we consider this to be an adjunctive therapy for most patients. RF is minimally invasive and can be performed in the office. Many patients will require multiple treatments. Thus, therapy can be extended over several months. However, this protocol is intended to prevent complications associated with delivering large amounts of energy to the tongue.

Complications are extremely uncommon and are similar to those of other sites treated with RF. If performed properly, this procedure is safe and offers promising outcomes for patients.

Midline Glossectomy and Lingualplasty
Midline glossectomy (MLG) has been used for many years to treat macroglossia. However, this procedure is quite invasive and results in considerable edema of the tongue. MLG is associated with significant postoperative pain. In addition, many patients require a tracheotomy to protect their airway. As a result, patients are reluctant to undergo this surgery.

A variation of traditional glossectomy surgery is the laser glossectomy and lingualplasty described by Woodson and Fujita (119). They reported a 77% responder rate using the criteria of a postoperative RDI less than 20. Despite these encouraging results, a complication rate of 27% was noted. Other transcervical submucosal approaches have been developed to resect a portion of the tongue base (120). However, these procedures can be complicated and require extensive dissection. Typically, these surgeries require placement of a tracheotomy tube and thus meet patient resistance.

AIRWAY BYPASS SURGERY
Tracheotomy

Tracheotomy was once the only treatment available for SDB. By creating an external opening in the trachea, the obstructing tissue of the upper airway was bypassed. This provided immediate resolution of airway obstruction during sleep. However, tracheotomy is poorly accepted by patients. This prompted a search for more conservative site-specific surgical procedures. In addition, the advent of CPAP provided a nonsurgical method to prevent upper airway obstruction. The efficacy of CPAP has markedly reduced the number of patients needing tracheotomy (51).

Yet, indications still exist for the insertion of a tracheotomy tube. A tracheotomy should be inserted when there is a need to secure an airway prior to a multi-phased protocol. Furthermore, it should be considered in morbidly obese patients with severe SDB and an oxygen desaturation below 70%, especially in those who cannot tolerate CPAP. Patients with significant cardiac disease may not be able to tolerate hypoxemia following surgery; thus a tracheotomy may be warranted. A tracheotomy may be temporary if the upper airway is subsequently reconstructed to alleviate obstruction.

CONCLUSIONS

Management of a patient with SDB requires a multidisciplinary team. Patients need to be counseled regarding all medical and surgical treatments that are available. CPAP therapy is considered first-line treatment. However, a referral for a surgical evaluation should be offered to patients, especially in those struggling to tolerate nasal CPAP. The surgeon must educate a patient regarding complications and expected efficacy. Patients should have a realistic expectation of outcomes. Armed with this knowledge, a patient can make an informed decision regarding their care.

Long-term cure rates similar to nasal CPAP can be achieved with surgery (84). A systematic evaluation of each patient and a rationale stepwise surgical approach are necessary to produce these outcomes. While not all procedures have similar outcomes, new technology is evolving to offer less invasive options to patients.

REFERENCES

1. Schwab RJ, Kuna ST, Remmers JE. Anatomy and physiology of upper airway obstruction. In: Kryger MH, Roth T, Dement WC, eds. Principles and Practices of Sleep Medicine, 4th ed. Philadelphia: Elsevier Saunders, 2005:983–1000.
2. American Academy of Sleep Medicine. Sleep related breathing disorders in adults: recommendations for syndrome definition and measurement techniques in clinical research. Sleep 1999; 22:667–689.
3. Kales A, Cadieux RJ, Bixler EO, et al. Severe obstructive sleep apnea. I: Onset, clinical course, and characteristics. J Chronic Dis 1985; 38(5):419–425.
4. Kuhlo W, Doll E, Franck MD. Erfolgreiche Behandlung eines Pickwick Syndroms durch eine Dauertrachekanuele. Dtsch Med Wochenschr 1969; 94:1286–1290.
5. Harman EM, Wynne JW, Block AJ. The effect of weight loss on sleep-disordered breathing and oxygen saturation in morbidly obese men. Chest 1982; 82(3):291–294.
6. Guilleminault C. Weight loss in sleep apnea. Chest 1989; 96(3):703–704.
7. Rubinstein I, Colapinto N, Rotstein L, et al. Improvement in upper airway function after weight loss in patients with obstructive sleep apnea. Am Rev Respir Dis 1988; 138(5):1192–1195.
8. Cartwright RD, Lloyd S, Lilie J, et al. Sleep position training as treatment for sleep apnea syndrome: a preliminary study. Sleep 1985; 8(2):87–94.
9. Issa FG, Sullivan CE. Alcohol, snoring and sleep apnea. J Neurol Neurosurg Psychiatry 1982; 45(4):353–359.

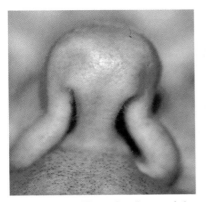

FIGURE 1.1 Bilateral collapse of the nasal rim that is frequently observed during inspiration in patients with obstructive sleep apnea-associated nasal resistance. (*See p. 11*)

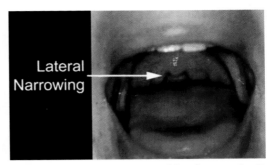

FIGURE 1.3 Lateral narrowing of the pharyngeal wall. *Source*: Photograph courtesy of Kannan Ramar, M.D.

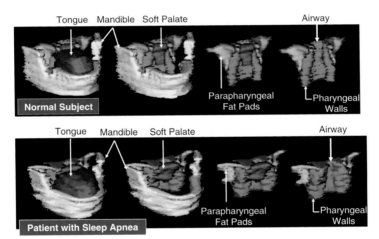

FIGURE 4.5 Volumetric reconstruction of axial magnetic resonance images in a normal subject (*top panel*) and a patient with sleep apnea (*bottom panel*). (*See p. 66*)

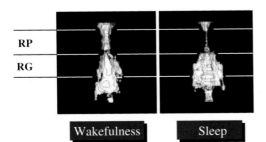

FIGURE 4.7 Volumetric state-dependent airway imaging in a normal subject using magnetic resonance imaging. (*See p. 74*)

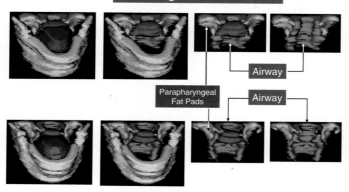

FIGURE 4.10 Upper airway soft tissue [soft palate (purple), the tongue (orange/rust), the lateral pharyngeal walls (green), parapharyngeal fat pads (yellow)] and craniofacial [mandible (gray)] magnetic resonance imaging reconstructions before and after a 17% weight loss in a normal woman. (*See p. 77*)

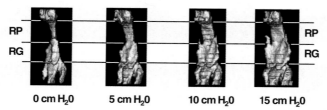

FIGURE 4.11 Volumetric magnetic resonance imaging reconstruction of the upper airway in a normal subject with progressively greater continuous positive airway pressure (CPAP) (0 to 15 cm H_2O) settings. (*See p. 78*)

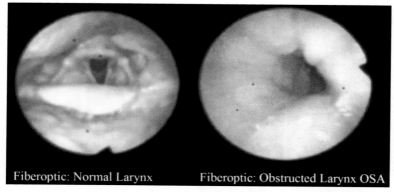

FIGURE 11.1 Fiberoptic laryngoscopy. (*See p. 194*)

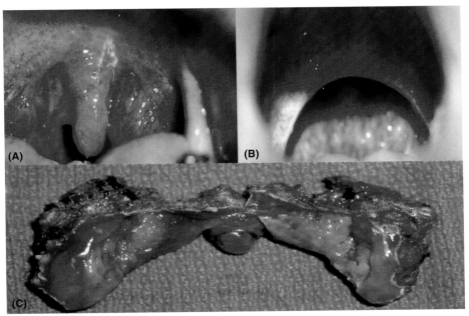

FIGURE 11.2 Uvulopalatopharyngoplasty. (*See p. 198*)

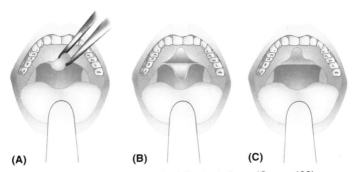

FIGURE 11.3 Uvulopalatal flap technique. (*See p. 199*)

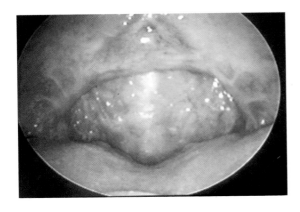

FIGURE 11.4 Uvulopalatal flap (UPF). Postoperative view of a UPF.

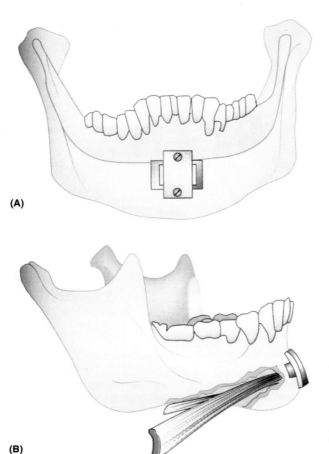

(A)

(B)

FIGURE 11.5 Mandibular osteotomy with genioglossus advancement. A rectangular osteotomy is created in the anterior mandible. The genial tubercle and the attached genioglossus muscle are advanced anteriorly. The bony fragment is rotated 90° to overlap the inferior border of the mandible and secured to the mandible with a titanium screw. *Source*: From Ref. 121.

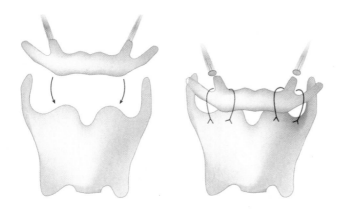

FIGURE 11.6 Hyoid myotomy and suspension. The hyoid bone and thyroid cartilage are exposed via a small neck incision. The hyoid bone is advanced anteriorly and secured to the thyroid cartilage with three or four permanent sutures. *Source*: From Ref. 121.

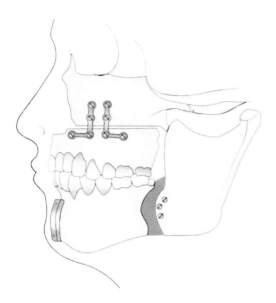

FIGURE 11.7 Maxillomandibular adv-ancement osteotomy (MMO). The maxilla and mandible are advanced 10 to 15 mm. A Le Fort I osteotomy and bilateral sagittal split mandibular osteotomy are performed. The advanced segments of bone are stabi-lized with bi-cortical screws and rigid plate fixation. Note the genioglossus advancement performed prior to MMO. *Source*: From Ref. 121.

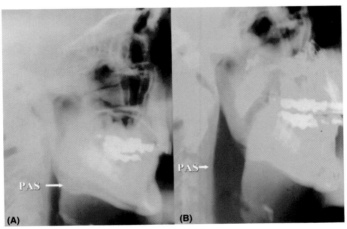

FIGURE 11.8 Lateral cephalogram films. (*See p. 204*)

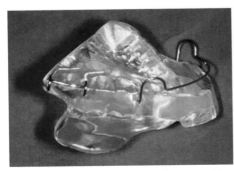

FIGURE 12.1 An example of a monobloc (one-piece) mandibular advancement splint.

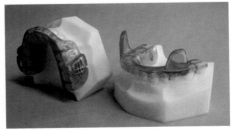

FIGURE 12.2 An example of a duobloc (two-piece) mandibular advancement splint (SomnoMed MAS™, Australia). (*See p. 218*)

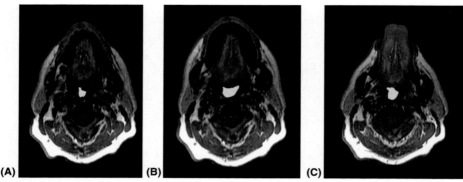

FIGURE 12.3 Axial magnetic resonance imaging scans at the retroglossal level at baseline (**A**), with a mandibular advancement splint (**B**), and with a tongue retaining device (**C**) in the same patient, taken in the awake state. (*See p. 219*)

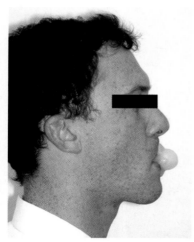

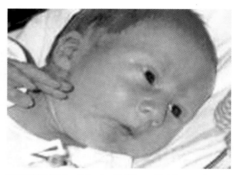

FIGURE 15.2 Infant with Pierre Robin syndrome; micrognathia, specifically mandibular hypoplasia, as depicted is characteristic of this disorder.

FIGURE 12.4 The effect of a tongue retaining device in holding the tongue out of the mouth by use of a suction cap.

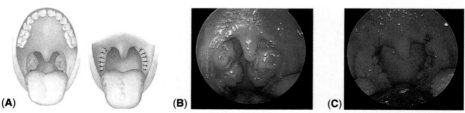

FIGURE 15.3 (**A**) Schematic diagram illustrating oral cavity before (*left*) and after (*right*) tonsillectomy. (**B**) Patient's oral cavity depicting hypertrophied tonsils. (**C**) Same patient's oral cavity following tonsillectomy.

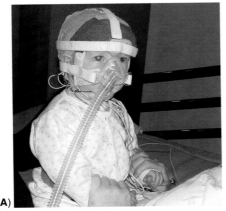 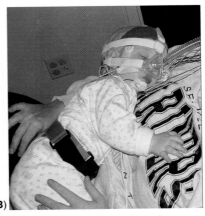

(A)   (B)

FIGURE 15.4   (**A**) Child awake and (**B**) asleep while wearing a continuous positive airway pressure mask during polysomnographic monitoring in a sleep laboratory. Note wires connected to recording electrodes that are placed on the face and on the scalp, which are hidden beneath the head wraps used to prevent dislodgement of electrodes.

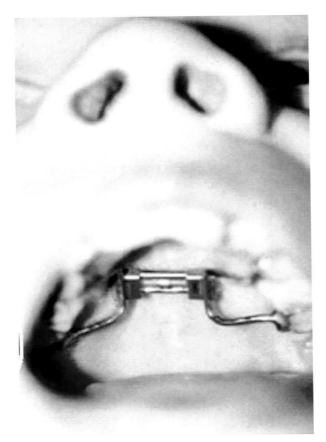

FIGURE 15.5 Maxillary osteogenic distraction device placed below the palate of a child's mouth. *Source*: Photograph courtesy of Kannan Ramar, MD.

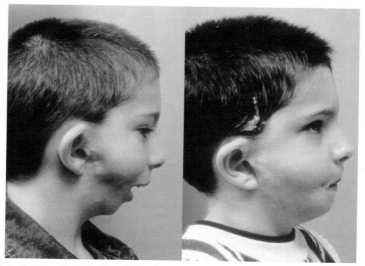

FIGURE 15.6 Profile of child's face (**A**) before and (**B**) after mandibular distraction osteogenesis.

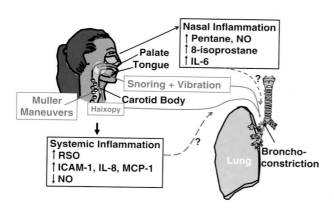

FIGURE 23.2 Potential interactions between OSA, nasal inflammation, systemic inflammation, and their possible link to asthma severity. (*See p. 392*)

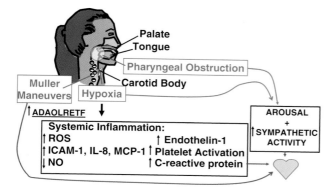

FIGURE 23.4 Potential interactions between OSA, systemic inflammation, and their possible link to cardiovascular disease. (*See p. 399*)

10. Sullivan CE, Issa FG, Berthon-Jones M, et al. Reversal of obstructive sleep apnea by continuous positive airway pressure applied through the nares. Lancet 1981; 1(8225):862–865.

11. Ballestar E, Badia JR, Hernandez L, et al. Evidence of the effectiveness of CPAP in the treatment of sleep apnea/hypopnea syndrome. Am J Respir Crit Care Med 1999; 159(5 Pt 1):495–501.

12. Sin DD, Mayers I, Man GC, et al. Long-term compliance rates of CPAP in obstructive sleep apnea: a population-based study. Chest 2002; 121(2):430–435.

13. Means MK, Edinger JD, Husain AM. CPAP compliance in sleep apnea patients with and without laboratory CPAP titration. Sleep Breath 2004; 8(1):7–14.

14. He J, Kryger M, Zorick T, et al. Mortality and apnea index in obstructive sleep apnea: experience in 385 male patients. Chest 1998; 94(1):9–14.

15. Dyugovskaya L, Lavie P, Lavie L. Increased adhesion molecules expression and production of reactive oxygen species in leukocytes of sleep apnea patients. Am J Respir Crit Care Med 2002; 165(7):934–939.

16. Dincer HE, O'Neill W. Deleterious effects of sleep-disordered breathing on the heart and vascular system. Respiration 2006; 73(1):124–130.

17. Yaggi HK, Concato J, Kernan WN, et al. Obstructive sleep apnea as a risk factor for stroke and death. N Engl J Med 2005; 353(19):2034–2041.

18. Powell NB, Riley RW, Guilleminault C. Surgical management of sleep-disordered breathing. In: Kryger MH, Roth T, Dement WC, eds. Principles and Practices of Sleep Medicine, 4th ed. Philadelphia: Elsevier Saunders, 2005:1081–1097.

19. Mickelson SA. Patient selection for surgery. In: Terris DJ, Goode RL, eds. Surgical Management of Sleep Apnea and Snoring. Boca Raton: Taylor & Francis, 2005:223–232.

20. Riley R, Guilleminault C, Powell NB, et al. Palatopharyngoplasty failure, cephalometric roentgenograms, and obstructive sleep apnea. Otolaryngol Head Neck Surg 1985; 93(2):240–244.

21. Shepard J, Gefter W, Guilleminault C, et al. Evaluation of the upper airway in patients with obstructive sleep apnea. Sleep 1991; 14(4):361–371.

22. Rivlin J, Hoffstein V, Kalbfleisch J, et al. Upper airway morphology in patients with idiopathic obstructive sleep apnea. Am Rev Respir Dis 1984; 129(3):355–360.

23. Rojewski TE, Schuller DE, Clark RW, et al. Videoendoscopic determination of the mechanism of obstruction in obstructive sleep apnea. Otolaryngol Head Neck Surg 1984; 92(2):127–131.

24. Remmers JE, DeGrott WJ, Sauerland EK, et al. Pathogenesis of upper airway occlusion during sleep. J Appl Physiol 1978; 44(6):931–938.

25. Olsen K, Kern E, Westbrook P. Sleep and breathing disturbance secondary to nasal obstruction. Otolaryngol Head Neck Surg 1981; 89(5):804–810.

26. Mallampati SR, Gatt SP, Gugino LD, et al. A clinical sign to predict difficult tracheal intubation: a prospective study. Can Anaesth Soc J 1985; 32(4):429–434.

27. Friedman M, Ibrahim H, Joseph NJ. Staging of obstructive sleep apnea/hypopnea syndrome: a guide to appropriate treatment. Laryngoscope 2004; 114(3):454–459.

28. Fujita S. Pharyngeal surgery for obstructive sleep apnea and snoring. In: Fairbanks D, Fujita S, Ikematsu T, et al, eds. Snoring and Obstructive Sleep Apnea. New York: Raven Press, 1987:101–128.

29. Fujita S, Conway W, Zorick F, et al. Surgical correction of anatomical abnormalities in obstructive sleep apnea syndrome: uvulopalatopharyngoplasty. Otolaryngol Head Neck Surg 1981; 89(6):923–934.

30. Sher AE, Thorpy MJ, Shrintzen RJ, et al. Predictive value of Müller maneuver in selection of patient for uvulopalatopharyngoplasty. Laryngoscope 1985; 9512:1483–1487.

31. Riley R, Guilleminault C, Herran J, et al. Cephalometric analyses and flow volume loops in obstructive sleep apnea patients. Sleep 1983; 6(4):303–311.

32. Ikeda K, Ogura M, Oshima T, et al. Quantitative assessment of the pharyngeal airway by dynamic magnetic resonance imaging in obstructive sleep apnea syndrome. Ann Otol Rhinol Laryngol 2001; 110(2):183–189.

33. Welch KC, Foster GD, Ritter CT, et al. A novel volumetric magnetic resonance imaging paradigm to study upper airway anatomy. Sleep 2002; 25(5):532–542.

34. Shepard JW, Stanson AW, Sheedy PF, et al. Fast-CT evaluation of the upper airway during wakefulness in patients with obstructive sleep apnea. Prog Clin Biol Res 1990; 345:273–279.

35. Riley R, Powell N, Guilleminault C. Cephalometric roentgenograms and computerized tomographic scans in obstructive sleep apnea. Sleep 1986; 9(4):514–515.

36. Riley R, Powell N, Guilleminault C, et al. Obstructive sleep apnea syndrome: a surgical protocol for dynamic upper airway reconstruction. J Oral Maxillofac Surg 1993; 51(7):742–747.
37. Powell NB, Riley RW, Robinson A. Surgical management of obstructive sleep apnea syndrome. Clin Chest Med 1998; 19(1):77–86.
38. Riley R, Powell N, Guilleminault C. Obstructive sleep apnea syndrome: a review of 306 consecutively treated surgical patients. Otolaryngol Head Neck Surg 1993; 108(2):117–125.
39. Riley RW, Powell NB. Maxillofacial surgery and obstructive sleep apnea syndrome. Otolaryngol Clin North Am 1990; 23(4):809–826.
40. Powell NB, Riley RW. A surgical protocol for sleep disordered breathing. Oral Maxillofac Surg Clin North Am 1995; 7(2):345–356.
41. Riley R, Powell N, Guilleminault C. Inferior mandibular osteotomy and hyoid myotomy suspension for obstructive sleep apnea: a review of 55 patients. J Oral Maxillomaxfac Surg 1989; 47(2):159–164.
42. Riley R, Powell N, Guilleminault C. Obstructive sleep apnea and the hyoid: a revised surgical procedure. Otolaryngol Head Neck Surg 1994; 111(6):717–721.
43. Ramirez SG, Loube DI. Inferior sagittal osteotomy with hyoid bone suspension for obese patients with sleep apnea. Arch Otolaryngol Head Neck Surg 1996; 122(9):953–957.
44. Johnson NT, Chinn J. Uvulopalatopharyngoplasty and inferior sagittal mandibular osteotomy with genioglossus advancement for treatment of obstructive sleep apnea. Chest 1994; 105(1):278–283.
45. Lee N, Givens C, Wilson J, et al. Staged surgical treatment of obstructive sleep apnea syndrome: a review of 35 patients. J Oral Maxillofac Surg 1999; 57(4):382–385.
46. Sher AE, Schechtman KB, Piccirillo JF. The efficacy of surgical modifications of the upper airway in adults with obstructive sleep apnea syndrome. Sleep 1996; 19(2):156–177.
47. Waite PD, Wooten V, Lachner J, et al. Maxillomandibular advancement surgery in 23 patients with obstructive sleep apnea syndrome. J Oral Maxillofac Surg 1989; 47(12):1256–1261.
48. Hochban W, Brandenburg U, Hermann PJ. Surgical treatment of obstructive sleep apnea by maxillomandibular advancement. Sleep 1994; 17(7):624–629.
49. Hochban W, Conradt R, Brandenburg U, et al. Surgical maxillofacial treatment of obstructive sleep apnea. Plast Reconstr Surg 1997; 99(3):619–626.
50. McConkey P. Postobstructive pulmonary oedema—a case series and review. Anaesth Intensive Care 2000; 28(1):72–76.
51. Powell N, Riley R, Guilleminault C, et al. Obstructive sleep apnea, continuous positive airway pressure, and surgery. Otolaryngol Head Neck Surg 1988; 99(4):362–369.
52. Olsen K. The role of nasal surgery in the treatment of obstructive sleep apnea. Otolaryngol Head Neck Surg 1991; 2(5):63–68.
53. Hoijer U, Ejnell H, Hedner J, et al. The effects of nasal dilatation on snoring and obstructive sleep apnea. Arch Otolaryngol Head Neck Surg 1992; 118(3):281–284.
54. Powell N, Zonato A, Weaver E, et al. Radiofrequency treatment of turbinate hypertrophy in subjects using continuous positive airway pressure: a randomized, double-blind, placebo-controlled clinical pilot trial. Laryngoscope 2001; 111(10):1783–1790.
55. Utley DS, Goode RL, Hakim I. Radiofrequency energy tissue ablation for the treatment of nasal obstruction secondary to turbinate hypertrophy. Laryngoscope 1999; 109(5): 683–686.
56. Passali D, Lauriello M, Anselmi M, et al. Treatment of hypertrophy of the inferior turbinate: long-term results in 382 patients randomly assigned to therapy. Ann Otol Rhinol Laryngol 1999; 108(6):569–575.
57. Ikematsu T. Study of snoring, fourth report: therapy [in Japanese]. Jpn Otorhinolaryngol 1964; 64:434–435.
58. Powell NB, Riley RW, Guilleminault C, et al. A reversible uvulopalatal flap for snoring and obstructive sleep. Sleep 1996; 19(17):593–599.
59. Kezirian EJ, Weaver EM, Yueh B, et al. Incidence of serious complications after uvulopalatopharyngoplasty. Laryngoscope 2004; 114(3):450–453.
60. Mintz SM, Ettinger AC, Geist JR, et al. Anatomic relationship of the genial tubercles to the dentition as determined by cross-sectional tomography. J Oral Maxillofac Surg 1995; 53(11):1324–1326.

61. Silverstein K, Costello BJ, Giannakpoulos H, et al. Genioglossus muscle attachments: an anatomic analysis and the implications for genioglossus advancement. Oral Surg Oral Med Oral Pathol Oral Radiol Endod 2000; 90(6):686–688.
62. McBride KL, Bell WH. Chin surgery. In: Bell WH, Proffit WR, White RP, eds. Surgical Correction of Dentofacial Deformities. 1st ed. Philadelphia: WB Saunders, 1980:1210–1281.
63. Riley R, Powell N, Guilleminault C. Inferior sagittal osteotomy of the mandible with hyoid myotomy-suspension: a new procedure for obstructive sleep apnea. Otolaryngol Head Neck Surg 1986; 94(5):589–593.
64. Yoa M, Utlet D, Terris D. Cephalometric parameters after multi-level pharyngeal surgery for patients with obstructive sleep apnea. Laryngoscope 1998; 108(6):789–795.
65. Riley RW, Powell NB, Guilleminault C, et al. Obstructive sleep apnea surgery: risk management and complications. Otolaryngol Head Neck Surg 1997; 117(6):648–652.
66. Li KK, Powell N, Riley R. Postoperative management of the obstructive sleep apnea patient. Oral Maxillofac Surg Clin North Am 2002; 14:401–404.
67. Van de Graaff W, Gottfried S, Mitra J, et al. Respiratory function of hyoid muscles and hyoid arch. J Appl Physiol 1984; 57(1):197–204.
68. Kaya N. Sectioning the hyoid bone as a therapeutic approach for obstructive sleep apnea. Sleep 1984; 7(1):77–78.
69. Neruntarat C. Hyoid myotomy with suspension under local anesthesia for obstructive sleep apnea syndrome. Eur Arch Otorhinolaryngol 2003; 260(5):286–290.
70. Bowden MT, Kezirian EJ, Utley D, et al. Outcomes of hyoid suspension for the treatment of obstructive sleep apnea. Arch Otolaryngol Head Neck Surg 2005; 131(5):440–445.
71. Li KK, Riley R, Powell N. Complications of obstructive sleep apnea surgery. Oral Maxilllofac Surg Clin North Am 2003; 15:297–304.
72. Kuo PC, West RA, Bloomquist DS. The effect of mandibular osteotomy in three patients with hypersomnia and sleep apnea. Oral Surg Oral Med Oral Pathol 1979; 48(5):385–392.
73. Bear SE, Priest JH. Sleep apnea syndrome: correction with surgical advancement of the mandible. J Oral Surg 1980; 38(7):543–549.
74. Powell NB, Guilleminault C, Riley RW, et al. Mandibular advancement and obstructive sleep apnea syndrome. Bull Eur Physiopathol Respir 1983; 19(6):607–610.
75. Conradt R, Hochban W, Bradenburg U, et al. Long-term follow-up after surgical treatment of obstructive sleep apnoea by maxillomandibular advancement. Eur Respir J 1997; 10(1):123–128.
76. Smatt Y, Ferri J. Retrospective study of 18 patients treated by maxillomandibular advancement with adjunctive procedures for obstructive sleep apnea syndrome. J Craniofac Surg 2005; 16(5):770–777.
77. Prinsell JR. Maxillomandibular advancement surgery in a site-specific treatment approach for obstructive sleep apnea in 50 consecutive patients. Chest 1999; 116(6):1503–1506.
78. Hochban W, Brandenburg U. Morphology of the viscerocranium in obstructive sleep apnoea syndrome—cephalometric evaluation of 400 patients. J Craniomaxillofac Surg 1994; 22(4):205–213.
79. Li KK, Riley RW, Powell NB, et al. Maxillomandibular advancement for persistent obstructive sleep apnea after phase I surgery in patients without maxillomandibular deficiency. Laryngoscope 2000; 110(10 Pt 1):1684–1688.
80. Li KK, Riley RW, Powell NB, et al. Patient's perception of the facial appearance after maxillomandibular advancement for obstructive sleep apnea syndrome. J Oral Maxillofac Surg 2001; 59(2):377–380.
81. Riley R, Powell N, Guilleminault C. Maxillofacial surgery and obstructive sleep apnea: a review of 80 patients. Otolaryngol Head Neck Surg 1989; 101(3):353–361.
82. Bettega G, Pepin J, Veale D, et al. Obstructive sleep apnea syndrome: fifty-one consecutive patients treated by maxillofacial surgery. Am J Crit Care Med 2000; 162(2 Pt 1):641–649.
83. Riley R, Powell N, Li K, et al. Surgery and obstructive sleep apnea: long-term clinical outcomes. Otolaryngol Head Neck Surg 2000; 122(3):415–421.
84. Riley RW, Powell NB, Guilleminault C. Maxillofacial surgery and nasal CPAP: a comparison of treatment for obstructive sleep apnea syndrome. Chest 1990; 98(6): 1421–1425.
85. Lanigan DT, Hey JH, West RA. Aseptic necrosis following maxillary osteotomies: report of 36 cases. J Oral Maxillofac Surg 1990; 48(2):142–156.

86. Issa M, Oesterling J. Transurethral needle ablation (TUNA): an overview of radiofrequency thermal therapy for the treatment of benign prostatic hyperplasia. Curr Opin Urol 1996; 6:20–27.
87. Jackman WM, Wang XZ, Friday KJ, et al. Catheter ablation of accessory atrioventricular pathways (Wolfe-Parkinson-White syndrome) by radiofrequency current. N Engl J Med 1991; 324(23):1605–1611.
88. Powell NB, Riley RW, Troell RJ, et al. Radiofrequency volumetric reduction of the tongue: a porcine pilot study for the treatment of obstructive sleep apnea syndrome. Chest 1997; 111(5):1348–1355.
89. Powell NB, Riley RW, Troell RJ, et al. Radiofrequency volumetric tissue reduction of the palate in subjects with sleep-disordered breathing. Chest 1998; 113(5):1163–1174.
90. Wedman J, Miljeteig H. Treatment of simple snoring using radiowaves for ablation of uvula and soft palate: a day-case surgery procedure. Laryngoscope 2002; 112(7 Pt 1):1256–1259.
91. Johnson J, Pollack G, Wagner R. Transoral radiofrequency treatment of snoring. Otolaryngol Head Neck Surg 2002; 127(3):235–237.
92. Stuck BA, Maurer JT, Hein G, et al. Radiofrequency surgery of the soft palate in the treatment of snoring: a review of the literature. Sleep 2004; 27(3):551–555.
93. Li KK, Powell NB, Riley RW, et al. Radiofrequency volumetric reduction of the palate: an extended follow-up study. Otolaryngol Head Neck Surg 2000; 122(3):410–414.
94. Troell RJ, Powell NB, Riley RW, et al. Comparison of postoperative pain between laser-assisted uvulopalatoplasty, uvulopalatopharyngoplasty, and radiofrequency volumetric tissue reduction of the palate. Otolaryngol Head Neck Surg 2000; 122(3):402–409.
95. Blumen M, Dahan S, Fleury B, et al. Radiofrequency ablation for the treatment of mild to moderate obstructive sleep apnea. Laryngoscope 2002; 112(11):2086–2092.
96. Kezirian EJ, Powell NB, Riley RW, et al. Incidence of complications in radiofrequency of the upper airway. Laryngoscope 2005; 115(7):1298–1304.
97. Friedman M, Ramakrishnan V, Bliznikas D, et al. Patient selection and efficacy of Pillar implant technique for treatment of snoring and obstructive sleep apnea/hypopnea syndrome. Otolaryngol Head Neck Surg 2006; 134(2):187–196.
98. Romanow JH, Catalano PJ. Initial U.S. pilot study: palatal implants for the treatment of snoring. Otolaryngol Head Neck Surg 2006; 134(4):551–557.
99. Nordgård S, Stene BK, Skjøstad KW, et al. Palatal implants for the treatment of snoring: long-term results. Otolaryngol Head Neck Surg 2006; 134(4):558–564.
100. Ho WK, Wei WI, Chung KF. Managing disturbing snoring with palatal implants. A pilot study. Arch Otolaryngol Head Neck Surg 2004; 130(6):753–758.
101. Nordgård S, Wormdal K, Bugten V, et al. Palatal implants: a new method for the treatment of snoring. Acta Otolaryngol 2004; 124(8):970–975.
102. Nordgård S, Stene BK, Skjøstad KW. Soft palate implants for the treatment of mild to moderate obstructive sleep apnea. Otolaryngol Head Neck Surg 2006; 134(4):565–570.
103. Walker RP, Grigg-Damberger MM, Gopalsami C, et al. Laser-assisted uvulopalatoplasty for snoring and obstructive sleep apnea: results in 170 patients. Laryngoscope 1995; 105(9 Pt 1):938–943.
104. Terris DJ, Clerk AA, Norbash AM, et al. Characterization of post-operative edema following laser-assisted uvulopalatoplasty using MRI and polysomnography: implication for the outpatient treatment of obstructive sleep apnea syndrome. Laryngoscope 1996; 106(2 Pt 1):124–128.
105. Littner M, Kushida CA, Hartse K, et al. Practice parameters for the use of laser-assisted uvulopalatoplasty: an update for 2000. Sleep 2001; 24(5):603–619.
106. Brietzke SE, Mair EA. Injection snoreplasty: how to treat snoring without all the pain and expense. Otolaryngol Head Neck Surg 2001; 124(5):503–510.
107. Brietzke SE, Mair EA. Injection snoreplasty: investigation of alternative sclerotherapy agents. Otolaryngol Head Neck Surg 2004; 130(1):47–57.
108. Brietzke SE, Mair EA. Injection snoreplasty: extended follow-up and new objective data. Otolaryngol Head Neck Surg 2003; 128(5):605–615.
109. Levin BC, Becker GD. Uvulopalatopharyngoplasty for snoring: long term results. Laryngoscope 1994; 104(9):1150–1152.
110. Wareing MJ, Callanan VP, Mitchell DB. Laser assisted uvuloplasty: six and eighteen month results. J Laryngol Otol 1998; 112(7):639–641.

111. Miller FR, Watson D, Boseley M. The role of the Genial Bone Advancement Trephine system in conjunction with uvulopalatopharyngoplasty in the multilevel management of obstructive sleep apnea. Otolaryngol Head Neck Surg 2004; 130(1):73–79.
112. Lewis MR, Ducic Y. Genioglossus muscle advancement with the genioglossus bone advancement technique for base of tongue obstruction. J Otolaryngol 2003; 32(3): 168–173.
113. Hennessee J, Miller FR. Anatomic analysis of the Genial Bone Advancement Trephine System's effectiveness at capturing the genial tubercle and its muscular attachments. Otolaryngol Head Neck Surg 2005; 133(2):229–233.
114. DeRowe A, Gunther E, Fibbi A, et al. Tongue-base suspension with a soft tissue-to-bone anchor for obstructive sleep apnea: preliminary clinical results of a new minimally invasive technique. Otolaryngol Head Neck Surg 2000; 122(1):100–103.
115. Miller FR, Watson D, Malis D. Role of the tongue base suspension suture with the Repose System bone screw in the multilevel surgical management of obstructive sleep apnea. Otolaryngol Head Neck Surg 2002; 126(4):392–398.
116. Woodson BT. A tongue suspension suture for obstructive sleep apnea and snorers. Otolaryngol Head Neck Surg 2001; 124(3):297–303.
117. Li K, Powell N, Riley R, et al. Temperature-controlled radiofrequency tongue base reduction for sleep-disordered breathing: long-term outcomes. Otolaryngol Head Neck Surg 2002; 127(3):230–234.
118. Stuck B, Maurer J, Verse T, et al. Tongue base reduction with temperature controlled radiofrequency volumetric tissue reduction for treatment of obstructive sleep apnea syndrome. Acta Otolaryngol 2002; 122(5):531–536.
119. Woodson BT, Fujita S. Clinical experience with lingualplasty as part of the treatment of severe obstructive sleep apnea. Otolaryngol Head Neck Surg 1992; 107(1):40–48.
120. Chabolle F, Wagner I, Blumen MB, et al. Tongue base reduction with hyoepiglottoplasty: a treatment for severe obstructive sleep apnea. Laryngoscope 1999; 109(8):1273–1280.
121. Troell RJ, Powell NB, Riley RW. Hypopharyngeal airway surgery for obstructive sleep apnea syndrome. Semin Respir Crit Care Med 1998; 19(2):175–183.

Oral Appliances

Peter A. Cistulli
Centre for Sleep Health & Research, Royal North Shore Hospital and The University of Sydney and Woolcock Institute of Medical Research, Sydney, Australia

M. Ali Darendeliler
Discipline of Orthodontics, Faculty of Dentistry, The University of Sydney and Department of Orthodontics, Sydney Dental Hospital, Sydney, Australia

INTRODUCTION

The last decade has seen the emergence of oral appliances in the clinical management of snoring and obstructive sleep apnea (OSA). This has been driven by the need for simple and effective treatment options for these highly prevalent disorders. The idea of using a dental prosthesis to reduce upper airway obstruction is not new. Pierre Robin (1) described such a concept in children with life-threatening upper airway obstruction related to micrognathia and glossoptosis, well before OSA was even recognized as a disorder. The use of oral appliances for the treatment of sleep-related upper airway obstruction was first reported some 25 years ago (2,3). A key milestone in the field was the systematic review conducted by the American Academy of Sleep Medicine (AASM) a decade ago (4), highlighting the inadequacy of existing evidence at that time and the need for rigorous scientific evaluation. Whilst it has taken a relatively long time for the evidence base to reach a level that supports their use in clinical practice, that time has now arrived, and it is important for clinicians involved in the management of snoring and OSA to have a sound working knowledge about this treatment modality.

In general terms, this treatment approach relies on repositioning of the mandible and/or tongue and related soft tissues in such a way that the upper airway caliber is increased and the propensity to sleep-related airway narrowing and collapse is mitigated (5). The potential advantages of such an approach, particularly relative to the current gold standard continuous positive airway pressure (CPAP), include its simplicity, portability, lack of noise and need for a power source, and potentially lower cost, all of which have a positive impact on patient acceptance.

TYPES OF ORAL APPLIANCES

Oral appliances used for OSA generally fall into one of two classes, viz. mandibular advancement splints (MAS) and tongue retaining devices (TRD). MAS induce protrusion of the mandible by anchoring a removable device to part of or the entire upper and lower dental arches, while TRD use a suction cavity to protrude the tongue out of the mouth. MAS are far more widely used in clinical practice and there is an extensive literature on their use, compared to TRD. There are many designs available, but they generally fall into either one-piece (monobloc) or two-piece (duobloc) configurations (Figs. 1 and 2). Beyond this, they can differ substantially in size, type of material, degree of customization to the patient's dentition,

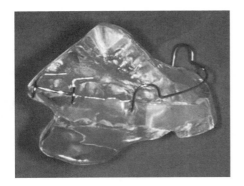

FIGURE 1 (*See color insert.*) An example of a monobloc (one-piece) mandibular advancement splint.

coupling mechanism, amount of occlusal coverage, titratability of mandibular advancement, degree of mandibular mobility permitted (vertical and lateral), and allowance for oral respiration. The impact of these design differences on clinical outcomes is largely unknown at this stage, and this suggests the need for caution in extrapolating the results of studies using one type of appliance to all types of appliances.

Two-piece splints consist of an upper and a lower removable plate with some type of intermaxillary coupling (Fig. 2). There are several modes of coupling between the upper and the lower plates, such as elastic or plastic connectors, metal pin and tube connectors, hook connectors, acrylic extensions or magnets. There has been a steady shift toward the predominant use of two-piece appliances in clinical practice because of the advantages they often confer, including titratability over time and permission of movement (vertical and/or lateral). Although prefabricated appliances are commercially available, it is considered that the best retention, comfort, and side-effect profile is achieved with custom-made oral appliances.

MECHANISMS OF ACTION

The prevailing view has been that the primary mechanism of action of MAS arises from the anterior movement of the tongue, and the consequent increase in the anteroposterior dimensions of the oropharynx. It now appears that this is an overly simplistic view, based on a growing number of studies that indicate rather more

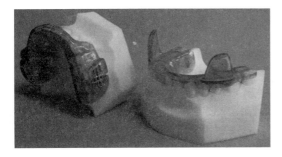

FIGURE 2 (*See color insert.*) An example of a duobloc (two-piece) mandibular advancement splint (SomnoMed MAS™, Australia), comprising separate upper and lower plates, with a unique "fin" coupling mechanism that permits the full range of mouth opening and closing, limited lateral movement, and titratable mandibular advancement.

complex anatomical changes. Such studies have used a range of imaging modalities, including computerized tomography (6), magnetic resonance imaging (MRI) (7), and nasopharyngoscopy (8). Not surprisingly, airway volume increases with mandibular advancement. Of some surprise has been the consistent observation of an increase in cross-sectional area of the velopharynx, in both the lateral and anteroposterior dimensions, and increases in the lateral dimension of the oropharynx (Fig. 3). These changes are thought to be mediated through the intricate linkages that exist between the muscles of the tongue, soft palate, lateral pharyngeal walls, and the mandibular attachments. In particular, it has been proposed that the improvement in velopharyngeal dimensions is mediated through stretching of the palatoglossal and palatopharyngeal arches (9). Notably, it appears that there is interindividual variability in the airway configurational changes that occur with mandibular advancement, and this is likely to have major relevance to the variable clinical response associated with this treatment modality.

There remains uncertainty about the extent to which oral appliance effects are mediated through neuromuscular pathways. Whilst there are some studies indicating that oral appliances stimulate genioglossus muscle activity (10,11), the clinical significance of this has not been borne out by "placebo" controlled studies using inactive oral appliances, which have shown little change in sleep-disordered breathing parameters (12,13). This suggests that the primary mechanism of action is mechanical rather than neuromuscular. The mechanical effect results in greater airway stability, evidenced by reduced upper airway closing pressure during sleep (14). In a study of anesthetized OSA patients, Kato et al. (15) found a dose-dependent reduction in closing pressure of all pharyngeal segments.

The mechanism of action of TRD is likely to be a little different compared with mandibular advancement devices. The forward movement of the tongue out of the oral cavity tends to be greater than the tongue advancement achieved with a mandibular advancement device (Fig. 4), and this may produce more favorable anatomical changes in the retroglossal region (Fig. 3). In addition, it is possible that they counteract the effect of gravity on the tongue in the supine position.

A useful conceptual model for understanding the mechanism of action of an oral appliance is to consider the upper airway as a lumen, surrounded by soft tissue, and contained within a bony box (16). According to such a model, the shape and

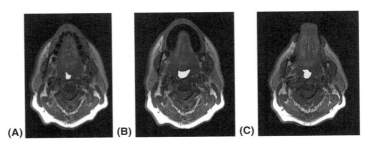

(A)   (B)   (C)

FIGURE 3   (*See color insert.*) Axial magnetic resonance imaging scans at the retroglossal level at baseline (**A**), with a mandibular advancement splint (**B**), and with a tongue retaining device (**C**) in the same patient, taken in the awake state, showing enlargement of cross-sectional area mediated by changes in both anteroposterior and lateral dimensions. Note the difference in airway changes between the two oral appliances.

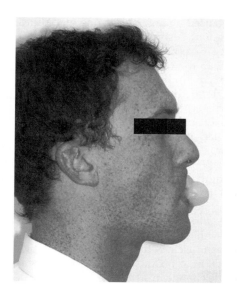

FIGURE 4 (*See color insert.*) The effect of a tongue retaining device in holding the tongue out of the mouth by use of a suction cap.

size of the airway is determined by the surrounding tissue pressure, which in turn is determined by the amount of tissue contained within the box. Hence one would predict that mandibular advancement would reduce tissue pressure by enlarging the box. This has been observed in an animal study, which found that mandibular advancement reduced tissue pressure and upper airway resistance (17). In contrast, one would hypothesize that TRD reduce the amount of tissue in the box by pulling the tongue out of the mouth, thereby reducing tissue pressure.

CLINICAL OUTCOMES

Since the systematic review of 1995 (4), there has been a substantial increase in the quantity and quality of research evaluating oral appliances (5,18). Whilst the early focus was on polysomnographic outcomes, there has been a necessary shift toward the evaluation of the impact of oral appliances on a range of important health outcomes, including daytime symptoms, neurocognitive function, and cardiovascular outcomes. The more recent studies have tended to employ rigorous randomized controlled trial methodologies and have advocated stringent, clinically relevant, definitions of treatment outcome. Comparisons with CPAP, other active and inactive oral devices, and oral tablet placebo have been published, assessing a range of important outcome measures. Despite this progress, there remain challenges in drawing definitive recommendations for clinical practice because of uncertainties about the generalizability of research findings to all types of oral appliances and patient subgroups. A contemporary systematic review, commissioned by the AASM, has formed the basis of revisions to the AASM practice parameters (19,20).

Polysomnography

The effect of oral appliances on polysomnographic outcomes has been extensively evaluated, and there is strong evidence of clinical benefit in controlling or significantly reducing the number of obstructive breathing events and arousals, and improving arterial oxygen saturation, particularly in the mild-to-moderate OSA range. The overall success rate is dependent on the definition used, with almost 70% of patients achieving a greater than 50% reduction in the apnea–hypopnea index (AHI) (19), and up to 50% achieving an AHI < 5/hour (12,13,21). Given that the aim of treatment is to resolve OSA, it is important that the more stringent definition of treatment outcome be used.

With regards to oxygen saturation parameters, studies have identified improvements in the minimum oxygen saturation, but rarely to normal levels. This is not surprising as, unlike CPAP, oral appliances do no inflate the lungs. With regards to sleep architecture and arousals, the data are less consistent, with only some studies reporting an increase in rapid eye movement sleep and reductions in the arousal index (12,13,21).

Less is known regarding the efficacy of TRD. Modest reductions in AHI (22), and improvements in minimum oxygen saturation and oxygen desaturation index (23) have been reported. Limited data suggest that supine-dependent OSA and absence of obesity are associated with a more favorable outcome (22).

Hypersomnolence
Whilst there has been a consistent observation across studies that subjective day-time sleepiness improves with oral appliances, randomized controlled trials using inactive control devices suggest that at least part of this improvement could be a placebo effect (12,13), similar to that identified with sham CPAP and oral tablet placebo (24,25). With regards to objective sleepiness there are indications of a small improvement, although more work is required in this area. In one study, the mean sleep latency on the multiple sleep latency test after four weeks of MAS treatment was significantly improved compared with an inactive control oral device, but the mean increase was relatively small (1.2 minutes) (13). Two studies compared oral appliances to CPAP over 8 to 12 weeks, using the maintenance of wakefulness test, and found no significant difference (26,27).

Neuropsychological
The few studies that have examined neurocognitive outcomes suggest an improvement with oral appliances. Comparisons have been made to inactive oral device, CPAP, and tablet placebo. An enhancement in psychomotor speed has been reported after one month of active treatment (28). The two studies comparing oral appliance to CPAP are somewhat conflicting, with one indicating no difference between treatments across a range of domains (27), and the other suggesting differential effects (26). The latter study found that oral appliance improved tension-anxiety, divided attention, and executive functioning, but CPAP was superior in improving psychomotor speed and other aspects of mood state (26). Notably, this study included a placebo arm (tablet) and found a significant placebo effect for many of the neurocognitive measures.

Cardiovascular
Given the strong association between OSA and cardiovascular morbidity and mortality, it is important to know whether oral appliance treatment has a similar beneficial cardiovascular effect compared with CPAP. To date, the only cardiovascular outcome to be assessed is blood pressure, and two randomized placebo-controlled

studies, using intention-to-treat analyses, have reported a modest reduction in 24-hour blood pressure (2–4 mmHg) with oral appliance treatment over period of one month (29) and three months (26). One study compared an oral appliance to CPAP, and found a small reduction in nocturnal diastolic blood pressure with oral appliance only (26). More recently, an uncontrolled study involving 161 subjects reported reductions in office blood pressure, with the change being significantly correlated to baseline blood pressure (30). These early studies suggest a beneficial effect of oral appliances, and additional work is required to further examine blood pressure and other cardiovascular outcomes.

Quality-of-Life

Quality-of-life is an important health outcome, and has been demonstrated to improve with CPAP treatment. The effect of oral appliance therapy remains unclear from the existing limited literature. A study published in 2004 found that three months of oral appliance treatment improved the quality-of-life as measured by the Functional Outcomes of Sleep Questionnaire mean score and Short Form 36 (SF-36) overall health score compared to placebo tablet, with a similar effect to CPAP (26). In contrast, Engleman et al. (27) reported that CPAP was superior to oral appliance treatment in improving well-being more than three months, as assessed by the SF-36 scores for health transition and mental component (27). A long-term study evaluated quality-of-life in a randomized one-year follow-up of oral appliance treatment or uvulopalatopharyngoplasty (UPPP), and found that vitality, contentment, and sleep scores improved significantly in both groups, but the surgical group demonstrated significantly greater contentment than the oral appliance group (31). Placebo-controlled studies are needed to examine the long-term impact of oral appliance treatment on quality-of-life.

Snoring

Oral appliances, unlike CPAP, have an important role in the management of habitual snoring, regardless of the presence of OSA. The majority of patients report improvement, largely based on partner reports (32). From an objective point of view, snoring frequency and intensity have been shown to reduce substantially (40–60% for snoring frequency and 3 decibels for mean intensity) compared to an inactive oral control device (12,13).

Comparison with Other Treatments

There are seven published randomized controlled trials comparing oral appliances to CPAP, and these have been the subject of published systematic reviews (33,34). It is important to note that there is significant variability amongst these studies in terms of the type of oral appliance used, the measurement techniques used for assessing treatment response (e.g., home monitoring versus in-laboratory monitoring), inclusion criteria (including severity of OSA), definitions of severity and treatment response, treatment interval, and drop-out rates, making it difficult to draw firm clinical recommendations. What is clear, is that CPAP is superior at reducing the AHI and improving oxygen saturation, but not arousal index, sleep architecture, or objective sleepiness (33,34). However, patient preference in most of the studies was in favor of oral appliance treatment. In terms of symptomatic outcomes, particularly daytime sleepiness (subjective and objective) but also neuropsychological measures, no substantial differences have been identified between CPAP and oral appliance treatments (33,34). When one considers the recent studies showing a similar reduction in blood pressure with oral appliance as that seen with CPAP, it raises the important possibility that the health effects of both treatments are of similar magnitude, as a result of the superior efficacy of CPAP being offset by its inferior adherence relative to oral appliances. This is an area that merits considerable attention, as it has major implications for clinical practice.

To date, there has only been one randomized study comparing oral appliance therapy to a surgical procedure (UPPP) in patients with mild-to-moderate OSA, over a four-year period (31). They found that both short- (one-year) and long-term (four-year) outcomes were better with oral appliance treatment (31).

Adherence

It is clear from the CPAP literature that treatment adherence in OSA patients is often not optimal. In the case of CPAP, this is partly attributable to the obtrusive nature of the treatment. Little work has been carried out to evaluate adherence to oral appliance treatment. A key problem is that there is currently no routinely available procedure for measuring objective use, which may differ considerably from partner or self-reported usage. A number of studies suggest that patients use their oral appliance on most nights and for the majority of the sleeping period, at least in the short-term (12,13,35). The only report in the literature in which objective adherence was measured used a novel intraoral monitoring device: patients used the appliance on an average of 6.8 hours per night (ranging between 5.6 and 7.5 hours) (36), which is similar to the findings of studies that used subjective measures. In the intermediate term (one year) the median use is approximately 77% of nights (19). Long-term adherence, up to five years, also seems to be acceptable amongst selected patients (37). Reasons for stopping treatment include the development of side effects, appliance wear and tear, and attenuation of the efficacy of treatment over time (37). It is likely that adherence is influenced by many factors, including appliance attributes, patient characteristics, and the quality of dental treatment and follow-up procedures. Studies are required to define the relative importance of these and other factors, so that appropriate clinical recommendations aimed at optimizing adherence can be developed. In the only comparison of MAS and TRD treatment adherence to date, Barthlen et al. (38) reported that adherence was superior with MAS (100% vs. 62%).

PREDICTION OF TREATMENT OUTCOME

Despite active research, a key unresolved issue limiting the role of oral appliances for the treatment of OSA is the inability to reliably predict treatment response. A number of studies have examined the influence of polysomnographic and anthro-pomorphic factors on oral appliance treatment outcome. In general, it is considered that a good response is more likely in mild-to-moderate OSA, although benefit in severe OSA has been reported (12,13). Cephalometric variables such as a shorter soft palate, longer maxilla, decreased distance between mandibular plane and hyoid bone, alone or in combination with other anthropomorphic and polysomnographic variables, are thought to provide some predictive power (12,39). Clinical features reported to be associated with a better outcome include younger age, lower body mass index, supine-dependent OSA (40), smaller oropharynx, smaller overjet, shorter soft palate, and smaller neck circumference (41). Whilst there is a suggestion that there is a "dose-dependent" response to mandibular advancement, namely that greater advancement is associated with greater reductions in sleep-disordered breathing (15), this has not been a consistent finding across studies. Importantly, worsening of OSA with oral appliance has been noted, and hence mandibular advancement per se will not always be of benefit.

Physiological studies indicate that retroglossal, rather than velopharyngeal, collapse during sleep is highly predictive of success (42). Upper airway imaging during wakefulness may aid in predicting treatment response. One study using MRI examined the airway response to the Müller maneuver, with and without mandibular advancement, and found that the persistence of collapse during mandibular advancement was predictive of treatment failure (7). Our own ongoing work with MRI indicates that while baseline airway and soft tissue anatomical characteristics do not differ between responders and nonresponders, the changes consequent to mandibular advancement do differ such that increases in airway volume are reasonably predictive of a favorable outcome (43). Whilst such studies are helpful in understanding fundamental mechanisms, the clinical utility of such approaches is limited and further work is required to develop simpler techniques for predicting outcome.

A relatively novel approach to the problem has been the development of single-night titration procedures using hydraulic or electronic means of incrementally advancing the mandible during sleep to determine treatment responsiveness and the required dose of advancement. Two studies have demonstrated that such an approach is feasible, and that treatment outcome can be predicted with a reasonable degree of accuracy (44,45). Further work to translate these findings into clinical practice is warranted.

ADVERSE EFFECTS

All oral appliances, regardless of design, have potential short- and long-term side effects. Most MAS are modified or similar to orthopedic appliances used routinely in the treatment of mandibular deficiencies for growth modification. Dental and bony changes associated with the use of orthopedic appliances in growing patients are well-documented, and are a desirable effect of treatment (46,47). However, MAS are largely prescribed to adult OSA patients for use during sleep only, and dental and skeletal changes would be considered undesirable. The main action of MAS is to increase the airway space by providing a stable anterior position of the mandible and advancement of the tongue, soft palate, and related tissues. This action of the MAS mediates posteriorly directed pressure on the upper dentition and anteriorly directed pressure on the lower dentition and causes immediate bite and jaw posture changes. Since there are no adaptive growth and/or major remodeling changes in adults, postural jaw modification may trigger dental and temporomandibular joint (TMJ) discomfort.

Most patients experience acute side effects during the initial phase of treatment. Excessive salivation (38–50%) and transient dental discomfort (33%), particularly of the upper and lower front teeth, for a brief time after awakening, are commonly reported with initial use and may prevent early acceptance of an oral appliance (19). TMJ discomfort (12.5–33%), dryness of the mouth (28–46%), gum irritation (20%), headaches and bruxism (12.5%) are other side effects that have been reported (12,19,48). Although these acute side effects are common, for most patients these are minor and transient, subsiding with continued use of the oral appliance.

Potential long-term adverse effects can be broken and/or loosened teeth, dislodgement of existing dental restorations, tooth mobility, periodontal complications, muscle spasms, and otalgia (49–53). These complications can often be avoided by simple recognition and appropriate early response to initial complaints. To monitor for these potential problems, it is suggested that patients with oral appliances should make periodic visits to the treating dental clinician. There are now published studies assessing long-term adverse effects out of seven years of use. Occlusal changes are predominantly characterized by a reduction in overjet and overbite, that is, backward movement of the upper front teeth, forward movement of the lower front teeth, and mandible and an increase in lower facial height (Fig. 5) (51–54). Even though the degree of overjet reduction is generally small, ranging from 0.4 mm to 3 mm (51), these changes can be clinically important. However, these changes uncommonly warrant cessation of treatment, and have to be weighed against the benefit provided by the oral appliance and the desirability of alternative treatments.

Previous studies have suggested that changes occur within the first two years of MAS use, after which they appear to stabilize (55). However, such studies have had methodological problems. More recently, a seven-year follow-up study reported progressive changes over time and also found that the magnitude of reduction in overjet was correlated with the magnitude of the initial overbite (56,57). Even though the influence of oral appliance design on side effects is not yet well-studied, the use of soft elastomeric devices, even if less durable, appears to provide some relative protection from large reductions in overjet (58). Predictably, the prevalence of side effects increases with more frequent use of the device (58). Whilst the literature suggests that the changes in the occlusion are largely temporary and revert after cessation of MAS use, permanent dental side effects requiring orthodontic treatment have been reported in a minority of cases (48). Hence it is important that patients are fully informed about these potential risks before commencing treatment. Whilst not yet investigated, it may be possible to avoid such side effects with the use of prosthetic and/or auxiliary implants as anchorage units on the upper and lower jaws. These types of anchorage units are currently successfully used to avoid unwanted effects of orthodontic forces.

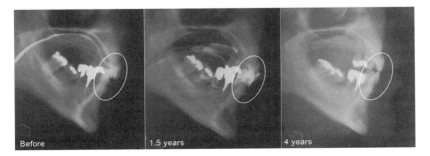

FIGURE 5 Close-up cephalometric radiographs of a 44-year-old female patient before, after 1.5 years, and after four years of mandibular advancement splint use, showing considerable reduction in overjet and overbite during that time.

CLINICAL PRACTICE ISSUES
Indications and Contraindications
According to the updated AASM practice parameters published in 2006, oral appliances are indicated in patients with mild-to-moderate OSA who prefer this form of treatment over CPAP, or who do not respond to or are unable to tolerate CPAP (20). The AASM also recommends that patients with severe OSA be considered for CPAP in preference to oral appliances whenever possible, given its greater efficacy. A major clinical limitation of oral appliance therapy, stemming from the need for titration during an acclimatization period, is in circumstances where there is an imperative to commence treatment quickly. This includes situations involving severe symptomatic OSA (e.g., concern about driving risk), with or without coexistent medical comorbidities such as ischaemic heart disease.

Not all patients are suitable candidates for the use of oral appliances. This treatment modality has no known role in treating central sleep apnea or hypoventilation states. Some case reports have shown OSA being worsened by oral appliance therapy (59,60), and this together with the known potential for a placebo reponse (12,13), highlights the need for objective assessment of treatment response. Caution is warranted in patients with TMJ problems, and it may be advisable to seek expert dental/specialist assessment prior to initiation of treatment. Insufficient number of teeth to permit adequate retention of the appliance may preclude treatment. It is commonly accepted that 10 teeth on each dental arch would represent the minimum number required (61). Less teeth will increase the partition of the pressure on each tooth and will cause more dental side effects. Similarly, the presence of periodontal disease may promote excessive tooth movement with an oral appliance. These cases may benefit from using TRD, although there is no strong evidence for this approach. In partial denture patients, the denture may become loose after the use of splints due to dental movements. All these factors tend to limit the scope of this form of therapy, and one European study has suggested that up to one-third of patients are excluded on the basis of such factors (62).

Clinical Evaluation and Management
An interdisciplinary, medical, and dental approach to diagnosis and management would appear to be conducive to good patient care. It is generally recommended that initial medical assessment and diagnosis precede the prescription and initiation of oral appliance therapy (20). Once the medical decision to proceed with oral appliance therapy has been made, it is recommended that the dental component be carried out by appropriately qualified and experienced dental practitioners (20). During the initial dental consultation the oral health status is assessed for suitability and informed consent is obtained. A lateral cephalometric X-ray may be advisable to evaluate airway continuity and dimensions as well as for baseline documentation of the position and angulation of the teeth. A regular alginate impression with buccal and palatal soft tissue features is required. The precision of the impression depends on the design of the splint. A construction bite in an initial 75% protrusive mandibular position using regular pink wax is advised, as this amount of initial activation will represent a clinically reliable start point for the acclimatization phase (12). Existence of crowns and bridges, periodontally compromised teeth, as well as inadequate under-cuts need to be identified; these areas may need reduced retention, reduced in and out shear pressure, and may require modification of the

regular appliance design. Extra clasps may be needed to increase retention in some cases. Following the insertion of the splint, patients may encounter problems fitting the splint and irritations to soft or hard tissues. These need to be corrected as soon as possible. It is common for patients to have uncomfortable sleep during the first few nights, but they usually reach an appropriate length of sleep after about a week. At the completion of titration, the patient should be re-evaluated from a medical perspective to ascertain the clinical response and to make decisions regarding the appropriateness of long-term use.

Appliance Selection

This is area requiring considerable research. Considering that there is wide variability in the reported efficacy across different studies, there is a strong suggestion that oral appliance design, in addition to dental expertise and titration procedures, has an important influence on treatment outcome.

The appropriate design of the appliance needs to take into consideration the occlusal and dental health, hard and soft tissues, the number of anchorage teeth, and the need for sagittal adjustment and/or reactivation, and this will vary on a case-by-case basis. Duobloc designs are generally preferable because of greater comfort and the ability to titrate, allowing attainment of the most comfortable and efficient position of the mandible and greater degree of lower jaw movements. MAS that permit lateral jaw movement or opening and closing whilst maintaining advancement may confer advantages in terms of reduction of the risk of complications and better patient acceptance. However, monobloc devices, whilst more rigid and bulky, are sometimes used to resolve issues related to anchorage needs, dental conditions, and the occlusal relationship.

Another important consideration is the vertical dimension of the oral appliance. Minimum vertical opening depends on the amount of overbite. Initial opening may be required before advancement of the mandible is possible, particular in cases with deep overbite (Fig. 6). However, if overbite is absent there may be no necessity to increase the vertical dimension. There are conflicting data on the effect of the degree of bite opening induced by oral appliances on treatment outcome, although most patients appear to prefer minimal interocclusal opening (21). In mouth breathing patients, splint design must have an anterior opening to permit comfortable breathing. In the case of edentulous patients wearing partial dentures, splint design should adapt to dental structures without dentures. In cases of insufficient teeth and concerns about retention there may be role for TRD.

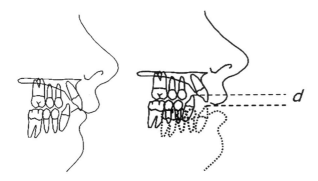

FIGURE 6 Schematic diagram showing the influence of the depth of bite on the distance (*d*) of vertical opening required in order to permit advancement of the mandible. The deeper the bite, that is, the greater the overlap between upper and lower incisors in occlusion (as per this example), the greater the amount of vertical opening required.

Titration Protocol

A period of acclimatization, over a period of weeks or months, is generally needed to initiate treatment. During this period incremental advancement of the mandible is performed according to clinical response and comfort, followed by medical reassessment to determine clinical response. This is currently a major limitation of the therapy, particularly in patients where rapid initiation of treatment is warranted. Furthermore, there is considerable interindividual variability in the degree of protrusion and time frame required to achieve a positive clinical outcome. The degree of protrusion required generally ranges between 50% and 90% of the maximum protrusion (12,35,63). The correlation between the amount of advancement and therapeutic effect is not strong. Hence, there is no basis for providing a fixed amount of advancement (e.g., 75% of maximal protrusion) to all patients, as has been proposed by some authors (64,65). The amount of advancement may be also limited by the degree of tolerance of the patient. Essentially no research has been undertaken to define the optimal procedures for this acclimatization period. It is unclear whether the advent of single-night titration procedures will enable a reduction in the duration of acclimatization required to attain an optimal result (66).

Follow-up Procedures

Once successful acclimatization is complete, and efficacy is verified, it is generally recommended that patients undergo dental review every six months for the first year, and yearly beyond that (20). This is to monitor clinical efficacy, adherence, oral health and occlusion, and device deterioration. Medical follow-up is required to assess the clinical response to treatment, usually with polysomnography or a portable monitoring device. Subsequent medical review is required to assess adherence and ongoing efficacy of the treatment. This may require periodic review with polysomnography if there is concern about attenuation of efficacy.

CONCLUSIONS

Despite the encouraging progress witnessed over the last decade, a number of key unresolved issues represent barriers to the widespread use of oral appliances in the treatment of snoring and OSA. In particular, the inability to predict treatment outcome creates uneasiness at the prospect of an unsatisfactory outcome, involving a not insubstantial investment of time and money on the part of the patient. Hence further research aimed at identifying clinical factors that predict success and failure are critical. Another important issue is the need for an acclimatization phase before maximal efficacy is achieved. Research comparing different acclimatization protocols, including the potential clinical use of single-night titration protocols, may herald the development of a more efficient process. Such an approach would hopefully assist with the individualization of treatment "dosage," that is the degree of mandibular advancement required to control OSA in the individual patient. There is an ongoing need for long-term follow-up studies, with an emphasis on both efficacy and adherence. The development of objective adherence monitors, as is available for CPAP therapy, would be an important advance. Given the likely important, but largely unstudied, influence of appliance design on treatment outcome and side effects, the field requires comparative studies to help guide clinical recommendations regarding choice of appliance.

To date, there has been little or no consideration for the potential of combining therapies in order to achieve an adeqaute clinical outcome (67). For example, the combination of weight loss and an oral appliance would be expected to produce an additive benefit, and may be useful for converting oral appliance partial responders to complete responders. In a similar vein, experimental data suggest that the combination of electical stimulation and mandibular advancement produces a synergistic effect on airway caliber (68). Another more speculative example is the combination of a pharmacological compound with mandibular advancement. Such possibilities warrant exploration, with the aim of developing "tailored" management approaches for the diverse OSA phenotypes that are evident in clinical practice (69).

REFERENCES

1. Robin P. Glossoptosis due to atresia and hypertrophy of the mandible. Am J Dis Child 1934; 48:541–547.
2. Meier-Ewert K, Schafer H, Kloss W. Proceedings of the Seventh European Congress on Sleep Research, 1984, Munich.
3. Soll BA, George PT. Treatment of obstructive sleep apnea with a nocturnal airway-patency appliance [Letter]. N Engl J Med 1985; 313:386–387.
4. American Sleep Disorders Association. Practice parameters for the treatment of snoring and obstructive sleep apnea with oral appliances. Sleep 1995; 18:511–513.
5. Cistulli PA, Gotsopoulos H, Marklund M, Lowe AA. Treatment of snoring and obstructive sleep apnea with mandibular repositioning appliances. Sleep Med Rev 2004; 8:443–457.
6. Gale DJ, Sawyer RH, Woodcock A, Stone P, Thompson R, O'Brien K. Do oral appliances enlarge the airway in patients with obstructive sleep apnoea? A prospective computerized tomographic study. Eur J Orthod 2000; 22:159–168.
7. Sanner BM, Heise M, Knoben B. MRI of the pharynx and treatment efficacy of a mandibular advancement device in obstructive sleep apnoea syndrome. Eur Respir J 2002; 20:143–150.
8. Ryan CF, Love LL, Peat D, Fleetham JA, Lowe AA. Mandibular advancement oral appliance therapy for obstructive sleep apnoea: effect on awake calibre of the velopharynx. Thorax 1999; 54:972–977.
9. Isono S, Tanaka A, Tagaito Y, et al. Pharyngeal patency in response to advancement of the mandible in obese anesthetized persons. Anesthesiology 1997; 87:1055–1062.
10. Yoshida K. Effect of a prosthetic appliance for treatment of sleep apnea syndrome on masticatory and tongue muscle activity. J Prosthet Dent 1998; 79:537–544.
11. Tsuiki S, Ono T, Kuroda T. Mandibular advancement modulates respiratory-related genioglossus electromyographic activity. Sleep Breath 2000; 4:53–58.
12. Mehta A, Qian J, Petocz P, Darendeliler MA, Cistulli PA. A randomized, controlled study of a mandibular advancement splint for obstructive sleep apnea. Am J Respir Crit Care Med 2001; 163:1457–1461.
13. Gotsopoulos H, Chen C, Qian J, Cistulli PA. Oral appliance therapy improves symptoms in obstructive sleep apnea: a randomized, controlled trial. Am J Respir Crit Care Med 2002; 166:743–748.
14. Ng AT, Gotsopoulos H, Qian J, Cistulli PA. Effect of oral appliance therapy on upper airway collapsibility in obstructive sleep apnea. Am J Respir Crit Care Med 2003; 168:238–241.
15. Kato J, Isono S, Tanaka A, et al. Dose-dependent effects of mandibular advancement on pharyngeal mechanics and nocturnal oxygenation in patients with sleep-disordered breathing. Chest 2000; 117:1065–1072.
16. Watanabe T, Isono S, Tanaka A, Tanzawa H, Nishino T. Contribution of body habitus and craniofacial characteristics to segmental closing pressures of the passive pharynx in patients with sleep-disordered breathing. Am J Respir Crit Care Med 2006; 165:260–265.
17. Kairaitis K, Stavrinou R, Parikh R, Wheatley JR, Amis TC. Mandibular advancement decreases pressures in the tissues surrounding the upper airway in rabbits. J Appl Physiol 2006; 100:349–356.
18. Ng AT, Gotsopoulos H, Darendeliler MA, Cistulli PA. Oral appliance therapy for obstructive sleep apnea. Treat Respir Dis 2005; 4:409–422.
19. Ferguson KA, Cartwright R, Rogers R, Schmidt-Nowara W. Oral appliances for snoring and obstructive sleep apnea: a review. Sleep 2006; 29:244–262.

20. Kushida CA, Morgenthaler TI, Littner MR et al. Practice parameters for the treatment of snoring and obstructive sleep apnea with oral appliances: an update for 2005. An American Academy of Sleep Medicine report. Sleep 2006; 29:240–243.

21. Pitsis AJ, Darendeliler MA, Gotsopoulos H, Petocz P, Cistulli PA. Effect of vertical dimension on efficacy of oral appliance therapy in obstructive sleep apnea. Am J Respir Crit Care Med 2002; 166:860–864.

22. Cartwright RD, Stefoski D, Calderelli D, et al. Toward a treatment logic for sleep apnea: the place of the tongue retaining device. Behav Res Ther 1988; 26:121–126.

23. Higurashi N, Kikuchi M. Miyazaki S, et al. Effectiveness of a tongue-retaining device. Psychiatry Clin Neurosci 2002; 56:331–332.

24. Engleman HM, Kingshott RN, Wraith PK, Mackay TW, Deary IJ, Douglas NJ. Randomized placebo-controlled crossover trial of continuous positive airway pressure for mild sleep apnea/hypopnea syndrome. Am J Respir Crit Care Med 1999; 159:461–467.

25. Pepperell JC, Ramdassingh-Dow S, Crosthwaite N, et al. Ambulatory blood pressure after therapeutic and subtherapeutic nasal continuous positive airway pressure for obstructive sleep apnoea: a randomised parallel trial. Lancet 2002; 359:204–210.

26. Barnes M, McEvoy RD, Banks S, et al. Efficacy of positive airway pressure and oral appliance in mild to moderate obstructive sleep apnea. Am J Respir Crit Care Med 2004; 170:656–664.

27. Engleman HM, McDonald JP, Graham D, et al. Randomized crossover trial of two treatments for sleep apnea/hypopnea syndrome: continuous positive airway pressure and mandibular repositioning splint. Am J Respir Crit Care Med 2002; 166:855–859.

28. Naismith SL, Winter VR, Hickie IB, Cistulli PA. Effect of oral appliance therapy on neurobehavioral functioning in obstructive sleep apnea: a randomized controlled trial. J Clin Sleep Med 2005; 1:374–380.

29. Gotsopoulos H, Kelly JJ, Cistulli PA. Oral appliance therapy reduces blood pressure in obstructive sleep apnea. A randomized, controlled trial. Sleep 2004; 27:934–941.

30. Yoshida K. Effect on blood pressure of oral appliance therapy for sleep apnea syndrome. Int J Prosthodont 2006; 19:61–66.

31. Walker-Engström ML, Tegelberg Å, Wilhelmsson B, Ringqvist I. 4-year follow-up of treatment with dental appliance or uvulopalatopharyngoplasty in patients with obstructive sleep apnea: a randomized study. Chest 2002; 121:739–746.

32. Schmidt-Nowara W, Lowe A, Wiegand L, Cartwright R, Perez-Guerra F, Menn S. Oral appliances for the treatment of snoring and obstructive sleep apnea: a review. Sleep 1995; 18:501–510.

33. Hoekema ASB, de Bont LG. Efficacy and co-morbidity of oral appliances in the treatment of obstructive sleep apnea–hypopnea: a systematic review. Crit Rev Oral Biol Med 2004; 15:137–155.

34. Lim J, Lasserson TJ, Fleetham J, Wright J. Oral appliances for obstructive sleep apnoea. The Cochrane Database of Systematic Reviews 2006, Issue 1. Art. No.: CD004435. DOI: 10.1002/14651858.CD004435.pub3.

35. Ferguson KA, Ono T, Lowe AA, Al-Majed S, Love LL, Fleetham JA. A short term controlled trial of an adjustable oral appliance for the treatment of mild to moderate obstructive sleep apnoea. Thorax 1997; 52:362–368.

36. Lowe AA, Sjoholm TT, Ryan CF, Fleetham JA, Ferguson KA, Remmers JE. Treatment, airway and compliance effects of a titratable oral appliance. Sleep 2000; 23:S172–S178.

37. Marklund M, Stenlund H, Franklin KA. Mandibular advancement devices in 630 men and women with obstructive sleep apnea and snoring. Chest 2004; 125:1270–1278.

38. Barthlen GM, Brown LK, Wiland MR, Sadeh JS, Patwari J, Zimmerman M. Comparison of three oral appliances for treatment of severe obstructive sleep apnea syndrome. Sleep Med 2000; 1:299–305.

39. Mayer G, Meier-Ewert K. Cephalometric predictors for orthopaedic mandibular advancement in obstructive sleep apnoea. Eur J Orthod 1995; 17:35–43.

40. Marklund M, Persson M, Franklin KA. Treatment success with a mandibular advancement device is related to supine-dependent sleep apnea. Chest 1998; 114:1630–1635.

41. Liu Y, Lowe AA. Factors related to the efficacy of an adjustable oral appliance for the treatment of obstructive sleep apnea. Chin J Dent Res 2000; 3:15–23.

42. Ng AT, Qian J, Cistulli PA. Oropharyngeal collapse predicts treatment response with oral appliance therapy in obstructive sleep apnea. Sleep 2006; 29(5):666–671.
43. Zeng B, Ng AT, Liu B, Darendeliler MA, Cistulli PA. Effect of mandibular advancement splint on awake upper airway anatomy. Proceed Am Thorac Soc 2006; 3:868 (abstract).
44. Tsai WH, Vazquez JC, Oshima T et al. Remotely controlled mandibular positioner predicts efficacy of oral appliances in sleep apnea. Am J Respir Crit Care Med 2004; 170:366–370.
45. Petelle B, Vincent G, Gagnadoux F, Rakotonanahary D, Meyer B, Fleury B. One-night mandibular advancement titration for obstructive sleep apnea syndrome: a pilot study. Am J Respir Crit Care Med 2002; 165:1150–1153.
46. Illing HM, Morris DO, Lee RT. A prospective evaluation of Bass, Bionator and Twin Block appliances. Part I—The hard tissues. Eur J Orthod 1998; 20:501–516.
47. Ruf S, Pancherz H. Long-term TMJ effects of Herbst treatment: a clinical and MRI study. Am J Orthod Dentofacial Orthop 1998; 114:475–483.
48. Fritsch KM, Iseli A, Russi EW, Bloch KE. Side effects of mandibular advancement devices for sleep apnea treatment. Am J Respir Crit Care Med 2001; 164:813–818.
49. Pantin CC, Hillman DR, Tennant M. Dental side effects of an oral device to treat snoring and obstructive sleep apnea. Sleep 1999; 22:237–240.
50. Marklund M, Sahlin C, Stenlund H, Persson M, Franklin KA. Mandibular advancement device in patients with obstructive sleep apnea: long-term effects on apnea and sleep. Chest 2001; 120:162–169.
51. Marklund M, Franklin KA, Persson M. Orthodontic side-effects of mandibular advancement devices during treatment of snoring and sleep apnoea. Eur J Orthod 2001; 23:135–144.
52. Bondemark L, Lindman R. Craniomandibular status and function in patients with habitual snoring and obstructive sleep apnoea after nocturnal treatment with a mandibular advancement splint: a 2-year follow-up. Eur J Orthod 2000; 22:53–60.
53. Rose EC, Staats R, Virchow C. Occlusal and skeletal effects of an oral appliance in the treatment of obstructive sleep apnea. Chest 2002; 122:871–877.
54. Bondemark L. Does 2 years' nocturnal treatment with a mandibular advancement splint in adult patients with snoring and OSAS cause a change in the posture of the mandible? Am J Orthod Dentofacial Orthop 1999; 116:621–628.
55. Robertson CJ. Dental and skeletal changes associated with long-term mandibular advancement. Sleep 2001; 24:531–537.
56. de Almeida FR, Lowe AA, Sung JO, Tsuiki S, Otsuka R. Long-term sequellae of oral appliance therapy in obstructive sleep apnea patients. Part 1. Cephalometric analysis. Am J Orthod Dentofacial Orthop 2006; 129:195–204.
57. de Almeida FR, Lowe AA, Otsuka R, Fastlicht S, Farbood M, Tsuiki S. Long-term sequellae of oral appliance therapy in obstructive sleep apnea patients. Part 2. Study-model analysis. Am J Orthod Dentofacial Orthop 2006; 129:205–213.
58. Marklund M. Predictors of long-term orthodontic side effects from mandibular advancement devices in patients with snoring and obstructive sleep apnea. Am J Orthod Dentofacial Orthop 2006; 129:214–221.
59. Ferguson KA, Ono T, Lowe AA, Keenan SP, Fleetham JA. A randomized crossover study of an oral appliance vs nasal-continuous positive airway pressure in the treatment of mild-moderate obstructive sleep apnea. Chest 1996; 109:1269–1275.
60. Henke E, Frantz DE, Kuna ST. An oral elastic mandibular advancement device for obstructive sleep apnea. Am J Respir Crit Care Med 2000; 161:420–425.
61. Otsuka R, de Almeida FR, Lowe AA, Ryan F. A comparison of responders and nonresponders to oral appliance therapy for the treatment of obstructive sleep apnea. Am J Orthod Dentofacial Orthop 2006; 129:222–229.
62. Petit F, Pepin J, Bettega G, et al. Mandibular advancement devices: rate of contraindications in 100 consecutive obstructive sleep apnea patients. Am J Respir Crit Care Med 2002; 166:274–278.
63. L'Estrange PR, Battagel JM, Harkness B. A method of studying adaptive changes of the oropharynx to variation in mandibular position in patients with obstructive sleep apnoea. J Oral Rehabil 1996; 23:699–711.

64. Clark GT, Arand D, Chung E, Tong D. Effect of anterior mandibular positioning on obstructive sleep apnea. Am Rev Respir Dis 1993; 147:624–629.
65. O'Sullivan RA, Hillman DR, Mateljan R, Pantin C, Finucane KE. Mandibular advancement splint: an appliance to treat snoring and obstructive sleep apnea. Am J Respir Crit Care Med 1995; 151:194–198.
66. Cistulli PA, Gotosopoulos H. Single night titration of oral appliance therapy for obstructive sleep apnea: a step forward? Am J Respir Crit Care Med 2004; 170:353–354.
67. Cistulli PA, Grunstein RR. Medical devices for the diagnosis and treatment of obstructive sleep apnea. Expert Rev Med Devices 2005; 2:749–763.
68. Oliven A, Tov N, Odeh M, Geitini L, Steinfeld U, Schwartz AR. Effect of genioglossus contraction and mandibular advancement on upper airway pressure-flow relationships in patients with obstructive sleep apnea. Am J Respir Crit Care Med 2005; 117:A87.
69. White DP. Pathogenesis of obstructive and central sleep apnea. Am J Respir Crit Care Med 2005; 172:1363–1370.

Adjunctive and Alternative Therapies

Alan T. Mulgrew, Krista Sigurdson, and Najib T. Ayas
Sleep Disorders Program and Respiratory Division, University of British Columbia, Vancouver, British Columbia, Canada

INTRODUCTION

Obstructive sleep apnea (OSA) is a common under-recognized disorder affecting approximately 4% of middle-aged males and 2% of middle-aged females (1). The disease is characterized by the repetitive collapse of the upper airway during sleep, leading to sleep fragmentation, daytime sleepiness, cognitive dysfunction, motor vehicle crashes, and cardiovascular sequelae (2–5). Positive airway pressure therapy (Chapters 6–9), oral appliances (Chapter 12), and surgery (Chapters 11 and 15) are the most commonly employed treatment modalities for this disease, and are described in detail in these other chapters. This chapter will focus on adjunctive and alternative therapies for sleep apnea. In particular, we will discuss the roles of behavioral therapies, weight loss, positional therapy, correction of other medical disorders, oxygen, and pharmaceutical agents in the treatment of sleep apnea.

BEHAVIORAL THERAPIES

All patients with OSA should be given advice concerning the avoidance of activities or agents that may worsen their disease. These include alcohol and sedative/hypnotics (benzodiazepines, narcotics, zolpidem, zopiclone, baclofen) (see also Chapter 17), as well as smoking, anabolic steroids, and sleep deprivation.

Alcohol is a gamma aminobutyric acid agonist that acts as a respiratory depressant and increases upper airway resistance; it has a greater effect on upper airway dilator muscle activity compared to the ventilatory pump muscles (such as the diaphragm), predisposing to upper airway collapse (6,7). Most studies have found that the administration of alcohol prior to bedtime leads to worsening of sleep-disordered breathing (7). Therefore, we advise our untreated patients with OSA to refrain from alcohol use at least four to five hours prior to bedtime. In contrast, moderate amounts of alcohol seem to have little effect on pressure requirements in patients treated with continuous positive airway pressure (CPAP). This was elegantly demonstrated in a study by Teschler et al. (8) who administered 1.5 mL/kg of vodka (approximately equivalent to a half bottle of wine) to 14 subjects with uncomplicated OSA; after alcohol, there was no increase in the median or 95th percentile pressure requirement (as assessed by auto-titrating CPAP). However, this study may not be applicable to patients with concomitant cardiorespiratory disease (especially if hypercapnic) or to higher doses of alcohol.

Sedative hypnotics should be used with caution in individuals with OSA, as they may exacerbate disease. Benzodiazepines decrease the arousal response to hypoxia and hypercapnia leading to increased apnea duration (9). Furthermore, Berry et al. (10) showed that even a small (0.25 mg) dose of the benzodiazepine, triazolam (Halcion®), increased the duration of apneas and worsened oxygen saturation in patients with severe OSA. Zolpidem (Ambien®), a nonbenzodiazepine sedative, does not cause increased desaturation in patients with mild-to-moderate chronic obstructive pulmonary disease; however, the effects on patients with sleep apnea are unclear, with a potential for increasing nocturnal desaturation. In one study, a significant effect of zopiclone (Imovane®) on respiratory parameters was not seen, but this study only included eight patients with upper airway resistance syndrome (8). The effects of sedatives on CPAP pressure are unclear, but there is the potential for the required pressure to be increased. We thus advise close clinical monitoring of patients with OSA treated with CPAP after prescription of sedative medications.

Baclofen (Kemstro®) is a commonly used muscle relaxant and antispasmodic drug. Finnimore et al. (11) demonstrated no significant effect of baclofen on the apnea–hypopnea index (AHI) in 10 snorers with mild sleep apnea; there was a trend for the oxygen saturation to be reduced after baclofen, but the magnitude was small. However, only one dose (25 mg) of medication was given and the effects of more substantial and frequent doses, especially chronically, are unknown.

The effects of narcotics on sleep apnea have been poorly studied. No increase in sleep-disordered breathing was found in normal subjects given small doses of oral narcotic analgesics [2–4 mg of hydromorphone (Dilaudid®, Palladone®)] (12). However, postoperative intravenous narcotic analgesia was associated with more episodes of nocturnal desaturation compared to regional analgesia with bupivacaine (Marcaine®), implying that systemic narcotics may increase sleep apnea severity (13). Chronic use of methadone (Dolophine®, Methadose®) may cause central sleep apnea and desaturation; because these central apneas do not respond well to CPAP, this may complicate therapy in patients with concomitant OSA (14).

One would expect that smoking would aggravate sleep apnea by increasing upper airway edema. Wetter et al. (15) demonstrated that current smokers had a three-fold greater risk of OSA compared to nonsmokers. However, a report from the Sleep Heart Health Study found an inverse relationship between smoking and sleep apnea (16). Nevertheless, given the multiple adverse effects of smoking on the development of cardiovascular and lung disease, we recommend that OSA patients should stop smoking.

Administration of exogenous androgens has been used in older patients to improve muscle mass and physical functioning. Male gender is a risk factor for sleep apnea, suggesting that androgens may worsen sleep-disordered breathing. Exogenous testosterone has been shown to worsen sleep-disordered breathing in hypogonadal men, predominately through nonanatomic effects (17,18). If possible, androgens in patients with OSA should be avoided; otherwise, we advise careful monitoring of OSA patients after prescription of exogenous androgens to ensure that no worsening of sleep apnea has occurred.

Finally, a single night of sleep deprivation may result in an increase in the number and length of apneas (19). This is likely because sleep deprivation results in decreases in genioglossus tone and increased collapsibility of the upper airway (9,20). Therefore, all patients with OSA should be counseled to obtain adequate amounts of nocturnal sleep.

CARDIOVASCULAR RISK FACTOR REDUCTION

Patients with OSA are at increased risk of developing cardiovascular disease (21). In part, this is related to the concomitant presence of a variety of cardiovascular risk factors. That is, these patients have a high prevalence of the following: male gender, smoking, diabetes, obesity, hypertension, and increased cholesterol (22). We recommend a low threshold for screening all patients with sleep apnea for the presence of hypercholesterolemia, hypertension, and diabetes; and initiating appropriate therapy if indicated.

WEIGHT LOSS

Approximately 70% of patients with OSA are obese. The mechanism by which obesity increases the propensity for OSA is unclear, but likely involves fat deposition around the upper airway (23,24). These deposits compromise the size of the airway lumen and may put the upper airway dilating muscles at a mechanical disadvantage. Data from the Sleep Heart Health Study (25) confirms the relationship between weight gain and the development of OSA; almost 40% of patients who started the study without sleep apnea, and who gained 10 kg during the five-year follow-up period, developed moderate OSA as defined by a respiratory disturbance index of > 15. The beneficial effects of weight loss were not as striking as the deleterious effects of weight gain, particularly in women. Nevertheless, weight loss of 10 kg or more in men had approximately five times the odds of a 15 unit or greater reduction in respiratory disturbance index compared with weight stability, suggesting that all obese patients with sleep apnea should be counseled and encouraged to lose weight.

Unfortunately, treatment of obesity is notoriously difficult among those with OSA. In one series of 216 overweight patients with OSA, 11.1% were successfully treated by weight loss alone; however, after three years, only 3% had maintained this remission (26).

In obese patients, three types of therapy have been attempted to promote weight loss: diet and exercise, pharmacological therapy, and bariatric surgery.

Diet and exercise have had limited success in the treatment of obesity. The majority of those who enroll in a typical weight loss program will continue to be obese. No consensus has been reached regarding the optimal weight reduction diet in terms of the proportion of carbohydrates and fat (27). Kansanen et al. (28) showed that weight loss with a very low calorie diet is an effective treatment for OSA having favorable effects on oxygen desaturation index, blood pressure, and baroreflex sensitivity. Maintaining weight loss is another significant barrier to the success of this treatment with the majority of patients regaining weight after a period leading to a recurrence of OSA (26,29). Cognitive behavioral therapy appears to achieve satisfactory weight loss with improvement in OSA and may be of benefit in weight loss maintenance (30).

Weight-bearing exercise for more than 20 minutes five days a week can be helpful in promoting weight loss as well as improving overall health. Additionally, the effect of exercise on OSA extends beyond its effect on patient weight. Data from the Wisconsin Cohort Study indicate that a lack of exercise was associated with increased severity of sleep-disordered breathing independent of body habitus (31). Conversely, exercise training can improve sleep apnea without improving body mass index (BMI) (32)—whether this effect is a result of stabilized muscle tone or increased respiratory drive is unclear.

Pharmacological therapy for obesity is controversial, mainly due to side effects of medications and questionable efficacy. Aminorex (Menocil®), used historically in the 1960s, was associated with an increased risk of pulmonary hypertension. More recently, dexfenfluramine (Fen-Phen®) has shown an association with cardiac valvular abnormalities as well as pulmonary vascular changes (33,34). Newer agents have been successful in achieving weight loss while avoiding significant side-effects. Orlistat (Xenical®), a lipase inhibitor is effective in maintaining weight reduction after dieting (35) and in achieving weight reduction when used as part of a weight management program (36,37). Sibutramine (Meridia®), a serotonin reuptake inhibitor has also been successful in achieving weight loss, particularly when used in combination with lifestyle modification (38). Long-term follow-up data are lacking for these agents and there is no trial data indicating effects on sleep apnea parameters. One trial has been performed, which indicates that use of sibutramine was not associated with worsening of OSA as a direct pharmacological effect (39). It is likely that trial evidence will soon be available to clarify the role of these agents in the management of OSA.

Bariatric surgery encompasses a variety of operative techniques designed to promote weight reduction. Several randomized controlled trials (40–42) and many case series have demonstrated the efficacy of these surgical techniques in the treatment of obesity and its metabolic complications. Newer laparoscopic techniques appear to reduce operative morbidity while maintaining efficacy. No randomized trials report the effects of bariatric surgery in OSA patients but a comprehensive meta-analysis outlining the impact of bariatric surgery on weight loss and on four obesity comorbidities (including OSA) was published in 2004 (43). Comorbidity outcomes were separated according to total resolution or resolution/improvement of the condition. The percentage of patients in the total population ($n = 1195$) whose OSA resolved was 85.7% [95% confidence interval (CI), 79.2–92.2%]. The percentage of patients in the total population ($n = 726$) whose OSA resolved or improved was 83.6% (95% CI, 71.8–95.4%). Evidence for changes in OSA was predominantly available for gastric bypass patients. This was particularly so for the AHI, which decreased by 33.85 per hour (95% CI, 17.5–50.2 per hour). We currently would consider bariatric surgery for morbidly obese individuals (BMI > 40 kg/m²) who have failed conservative measures at weight loss.

POSITIONAL THERAPY

The upper airway is influenced by body position due to the effects of gravity on pharyngeal structures and lung volumes (44). In particular, the pharyngeal airway is less collapsible in the lateral position than in the supine position (45), and consequently, AHI is often less in the lateral position (46). Positional sleep apnea is defined as: a total AHI > 5 events/hour, a 50% reduction in the AHI between the supine and nonsupine postures, and an AHI that normalizes in the nonsupine posture. In a large series of patients referred for overnight polysomnography (PSG) to rule out OSA, Mador et al. (47) found a high prevalence (49.5%) of positional sleep apnea in patients with mild disease (AHI 5–15), which decreased to 19.4% in patients with moderate disease (AHI, 15–30) and only 6.5% in severe patients (AHI > 30).

Positional therapy could be considered, if positional sleep apnea can be documented by PSG [including a period of rapid eye movement (REM) sleep in the lateral position]. This consists of using methods to prevent individuals from sleeping in the supine posture; selected patients may have an efficacy similar to CPAP (48).

Techniques used include sewing a tennis ball onto the back of the pajama top, attaching a pillow to the sleeper's back with a belt, or wearing a knapsack to bed. Gravity-activated alarms may also be useful in keeping subjects in the lateral position during sleep (49). Simple elevation of the upper body does not reduce sleep apnea indices but does stabilize the airway and may allow therapeutic levels of CPAP to be substantially reduced (45). Once positional therapy is prescribed, careful follow-up of symptoms is necessary to ensure adequate therapy.

CORRECTION OF OTHER MEDICAL DISORDERS

Treatment of hypothyroidism, acromegaly, and nasal congestion may improve the severity of OSA. OSA is common in patients with hypothyroidism, and it is believed that hypothyroidism predisposes to the development of OSA (50). The mechanism for this association may include weight gain, tongue enlargement, muscle dysfunction, and changes in respiratory drive. In patients with sleep apnea, the prevalence of undiagnosed hypothyroidism has been reported in the range of 3.1% to 11.5% (51,52). Whether all patients with OSA should be screened for hypothyroidism is controversial (53). Nevertheless, treatment of hypothyroidism may lead to an improvement of OSA (54), and is likely to improve symptoms of daytime fatigue and promote weight loss (55). Treatment of hypothyroidism masquerading as OSA—so called "secondary sleep apnea" may result in resolution of symptoms (56). Having a low threshold for testing thyroid function in patients with OSA is recommended.

Acromegaly is a rare disease characterized by hypersecretion of growth hormone and is associated with an increased prevalence (60–70%) of both obstructive and central sleep apnea (57,58). Sleep apnea likely results from structural abnormalities induced by growth hormone leading to upper airway narrowing, and increased respiratory drive leading to breathing instability due to increased gain of the respiratory controller (59). Treatment with octreotide (Sandostatin®) may lead to improvement of sleep-disordered breathing (60,61). Consequently, appropriate testing for acromegaly should be performed in patients with suggestive clinical findings.

Nasal pathology is associated with OSA (62). This may be related to increased negative pressure in the pharynx during inspiration due to the increased nasal resistance or interference with reflexes designed to protect the patency of the upper airway (63). In patients with concomitant OSA and seasonal allergic rhinitis, use of nasal steroids has been associated with improvement in AHI and nasal airflow resistance (64). Studies looking at the effects of other nasal decongestants have shown limited success in alleviating OSA (65). A study using an external nasal dilator in patients with mild OSA demonstrated a small increase in nocturnal oxygen saturation, but no change in AHI or sleep architecture (66). Surgical repair of nasal pathology has resulted in dramatic improvements of sleep apnea in a small case series (67) though the majority does not seem to derive benefit (68). Regardless, one should examine OSA patients for symptoms and signs of nasal pathology and consider surgical or medical treatment if abnormalities are found. Treatment of nasal pathology may also increase tolerance with CPAP therapy.

OXYGEN

Use of supplemental oxygen in patients with OSA results in substantial improvements in nocturnal desaturation and cardiac bradyarrhythmias; however, because the underlying pathophysiology is not changed, only modest reductions in the AHI are seen (69). Variable effects on hypersomnolence are seen with oxygen therapy with some studies showing improvement (70) and others showing no change (71,72). Hence, oxygen cannot be considered a first-line treatment for OSA, but may be considered as a temporizing measure if significant hypoxemia is present and CPAP or other therapies cannot be tolerated (73). Furthermore, oxygen should be considered in patients with substantial desaturation despite adequate CPAP therapy. These patients often have concomitant pulmonary pathology (e.g., emphysema).

Transtracheal delivery of oxygen is another mode of oxygen delivery that has showed promise. Delivery of oxygen below the level of obstruction appears to be a more effective strategy for stabilizing respiration. Two studies have shown improvement in AHI and subjective symptoms in patients treated with transtracheal oxygen (74,75). Data are quite limited; however, the relative invasiveness of this procedure limits its use to patients with severe desaturation in whom alternative measures have been unsuccessful.

PHARMACOLOGIC THERAPY OF OBSTRUCTIVE SLEEP APNEA
Drugs that Increase Respiratory Drive (See Also Chapter 17)
Patients with OSA have compromised upper airway anatomy making the airway more vulnerable to collapse (76–80). During wakefulness, reflex mechanisms lead to increased upper airway dilator muscle activity keeping the collapsible part of the upper airway open (79,81). However, with sleep onset, these reflex mechanisms are lost resulting in a fall in upper airway dilator muscle activity, and upper airway collapse in those anatomically susceptible (82). A variety of respiratory stimulants have been used to increase upper airway muscle activity during sleep in an attempt to treat patients with sleep apnea. Thus far, the results have been disappointing and no drug can currently be recommended.

The prevalence of sleep apnea increases after menopause, suggesting that female hormones may play a protective effect on sleep-disordered breathing (83). Medroxyprogesterone (Cycrin®, Provera®) is a respiratory stimulant and has been used to treat OSA by increasing central neural drive to the pharyngeal muscles. Strohl et al. (84) demonstrated improvement in 4/9 patients with OSA in an uncontrolled study; of note, three of the four subjects who improved were hypercapnic suggesting that they may have had an element of obesity-hypoventilation syndrome in addition to OSA. Subsequent studies, however, have not been as impressive, with mild to no improvement of OSA after treatment with progesterone (85,86), even in postmenopausal women (87). Furthermore, the combined use of estrogen and progesterone does not appear to be effective (88).

At this time, progesterone cannot be considered an effective treatment for OSA, though it may play an adjunctive role in patients with the obesity-hypoventilation syndrome by its effects on central respiratory drive. However, the potential procoagulant effects of progesterone should be considered, especially given the high doses required and their increased risk of thromboembolic and cardiovascular disease (89).

Protriptyline (Vivactil®), a tricyclic antidepressant, has also been proposed as a treatment of OSA (90). Overall, protriptyline may modestly decrease the AHI and degree of oxygen desaturation. Though protriptyline may increase genioglossus tone (perhaps through its anticholinergic effect), the predominant mechanism is likely through its suppression of REM sleep (the stage of sleep during which OSA is usually the most severe). This drug has a variety of side effects including urinary retention, dry mouth, and impotence. Therefore, although this drug may be a reasonable option in patients with mild, predominately REM-associated OSA, the drug is often poorly tolerated due to the myriad of adverse side effects.

Other respiratory stimulants such as nicotine, theophylline (Theolair®, Uniphyl®), acetazolamide (Diamox®), naloxone (Narcan®), almitrine, and bromocriptine (Parlodel®) are also not useful in treating OSA (91–93). Serotonergic drugs are described in more detail subsequently.

Serotonin and Sleep Apnea (See Also Chapter 17)

Serotonin is thought to be a key neurotransmitter involved in the modulation of upper airway tone. The hypoglossal nerve, which supplies the genioglossus muscle, is depolarized by serotonin. During sleep (especially REM sleep), there is a reduction in serotonergic output to the hypoglossal nucleus—suggesting that augmentation of serotonin around the nucleus may increase upper airway tone and improve sleep-disordered breathing. Although animal studies have shown increased genioglossus muscle activity when serotonin activity is augmented on brainstem preparations, the data that this therapy is likely to benefit human patients with OSA are limited (94–96).

Because serotonin does not cross the blood–brain barrier, selective serotonin reuptake inhibitors (SSRIs) have been used to counter the reduction in upper airway muscle activity (which occurs at sleep onset in OSA patients). Sunderram et al. (97) administered paroxetine (Paxil®, Pexeva®) to 11 normal subjects and measured genioglossus electromyography under varying conditions (CPAP, hypercapnia, room air); the use of paroxetine resulted in a significant increase in genioglossus activity suggesting that the drug may be helpful. However, the results in patients with OSA have been disappointing. Berry et al. (98) administered a single dose 40 mg dose of paroxetine to eight men with severe OSA; although peak genioglossus activity increased, there was no effect on the severity of sleep apnea (75 events/hour vs. 74 events/hour for drug vs. placebo, respectively). Kraiczi et al. (99) performed a placebo-controlled crossover trial of paroxetine (20 mg/day) and placebo in 20 patients with OSA. After treatment, there was a significant difference in AHI in the paroxetine versus the placebo group (36 vs. 30 events per hour) but the overall magnitude was small. There was no significant difference in symptoms.

SSRIs cannot presently be recommended as a treatment option for OSA, especially given their potential toxicities (i.e., insomnia, REM suppression, worsened periodic limb movements, increased appetite, serotonin syndrome, and hypomania). One possibility is that the amount of serotonergic input into the hypoglossal nucleus during sleep may be insufficient for the effectiveness of reuptake inhibitors. As such, direct serotonin agonists (or antagonists acting at autoregulatory presynaptic receptors) may be more effective in treating patients with sleep apnea, and we await future studies in this area (100).

Etanercept (Enbrel®)

OSA is thought to activate systemic inflammation. Tumor necrosis factor (TNF) is a proinflammatory cytokine that is increased in patients with OSA (101). Because this molecule is also somnogenic, it has been hypothesized that some of the sleepiness in patients with OSA may be related to levels of this cytokine. Similarly, antagonists of TNF may improve daytime sleepiness. This hypothesis was tested in a crossover

trial published by Vgontzas et al. (102). These investigators administered etanercept, a molecule that binds to TNF and which has been used in the treatment of
rheumatoid arthritis, to eight patients with OSA. Use of etanercept resulted in an
improvement of objective sleepiness (multiple sleep latency test reduced by three
minutes) and a reduction in AHI of eight events per hour compared to placebo.
From a mechanistic standpoint, this study was interesting as it suggests that treatment of inflammation may improve symptoms in OSA patients. Limitations of this
study included the small sample size and the nonrandom order of the interventions
(i.e., all patients received placebo first). In addition, anti-TNF therapies are costly
and are associated with substantial side effects including life-threatening infections,
making this therapy impractical at the current time (103).

Modafinil (Provigil®) (See Also Chapter 17)

Modafinil is a novel wake-promoting agent with an unclear mechanism of action.
A number of studies have demonstrated that this drug is effective in treating
patients with residual sleepiness after OSA therapy. For instance, Black and
Hirshkowitz (104) published in 2005 a 12-week randomized multicenter trial of
OSA patients with residual hypersomnolence despite use of CPAP (i.e., Epworth
sleepiness scale score ≥ 10). A total of 309 patients were randomized to either
placebo, 200 mg modafinil per day, or 400 mg modafinil per day. Patients on
modafinil had significant improvements in objective daytime sleepiness (as measured by the maintenance of wakefulness test) and the Epworth sleepiness scale
score. Adherence was similar in all three groups. The drug was reasonably well-
tolerated; however, six patients had to withdraw because of headaches, five for
chest pain, and four for dizziness. Although the manuscript was written by the
authors, the data were analyzed by the sponsoring company. These data are consistent with a previous report (105) and suggest that modafinil improves residual
daytime sleepiness in patients using CPAP.

However, it must be stressed that modafinil does not treat sleep apnea, it only
treats the symptom of sleepiness. In CPAP-treated patients with sleep apnea who
complain of residual daytime sleepiness, attention should be initially directed
towards verifying adherence and effectiveness of therapy and excluding other
causes of hypersomnolence (e.g., limb movements of sleep, narcolepsy, depression,
medications, inadequate daily sleep, systemic illness). Of concern, one small study
suggests that CPAP adherence may be reduced with modafinil because of symptom
improvement (106). Even though this was not demonstrated in the large trial referenced in the previous paragraph, adherence may be worse in patients not followed
closely as part of a clinical trial. Also, the long-term consequences of chronic use of
modafinil are unclear, especially with respect to the cardiovascular system.
Nevertheless, modafinil may be a useful adjunct in the treatment of patients with
substantial sleepiness despite adherence with CPAP, and after a search for other
causes of sleepiness is unfruitful. Careful monitoring of CPAP adherence and side
effects after prescription is recommended.

CONCLUSIONS

The various adjunctive and alternative therapies discussed in this chapter are summarized in Table 1. In general, pharmacologic therapies as sole treatment of OSA have
not been successful and/or have substantial side effects and are not recommended.

TABLE 1 Summary of Alternative/Adjunctive Treatments of Obstructive Sleep Apnea

Treatment	Advantages	Disadvantages	Comments
Behavioral (i.e., avoid smoking, sleep deprivation, sedatives, alcohol; maintain nasal patency)	May have other health benefits	Will rarely eliminate OSA	Advised in everyone with OSA
Weight loss	May have other health benefits	Low success rate	Advised in all obese OSA patients
Positional therapy	Low cost	Effective in only a minority of cases	Consider as an alternative in patients with positional OSA
Correction of other medical disorders (hypothyroidism, acromegaly, severe nasal obstruction)	Treatment of these disorders may improve or eliminate OSA Secondary health benefits	These are rare causes of OSA Treatment does not usually eliminate OSA	Consider these diseases in the evaluation of all OSA patients
Oxygen	Convenient Improves oxygenation	Does not eliminate upper airway obstruction and sleep fragmentation	Not recommended as primary therapy Useful as adjunctive therapy in patients who desaturate despite CPAP
Pharmacologic therapy for OSA	Convenient	Inconsistent efficacy Side effects	Not presently recommended for OSA
Etanercept	May reduce sleepiness	Cost Potentially severe side effects Paucity of data	Not recommended
Modafinil	Convenient Reduces symptoms	Long-term effects unclear May reduce CPAP adherence Side effects Cost	Consider in selected patients with persistent sleepiness despite CPAP

Abbreviations: CPAP, continuous positive airway pressure; OSA, obstructive sleep apnea.

Adjunctive therapies that may be helpful include: the aggressive treatment of obesity, the maintenance of nasal patency, the avoidance of androgens, the avoidance of sedatives (including alcohol), and the treatment of underlying disorders such as hypothyroidism and acromegaly. Modafinil may play a limited role in patients persistently sleepy despite adherence with CPAP therapy. Further work to better define the basic neurophysiology of sleep apnea may lead to novel pharmacologic therapies that may effectively treat our patients.

ACKNOWLEDGMENTS

Dr. Ayas is supported by a Scholar Award from the Michael Smith Foundation for Health Research, a New Investigator Award from the CIHR/BC Lung Association, and a Departmental Scholar Award from the University of British Columbia. Dr. Mulgrew is supported by a BC Lung Fellowship and by the CIHR/HSFC IMPACT training program.

REFERENCES

1. Young T, Palta M, Dempsey J, Skatrud J, Weber S, Badr S. The occurrence of sleep-disordered breathing among middle-aged adults. N Engl J Med 1993; 328(17): 1230–1235.
2. Epstein LJ, Weiss W. Clinical consequences of obstructive sleep apnea. Semin Respir Crit Care Med 1998; 19:123–132.
3. Teran-Santos J, Jimenez-Gomez A, Cordero-Guevara J. The association between sleep apnea and the risk of traffic accidents. Cooperative Group Burgos-Santander. N Engl J Med 1999; 340(11):847–851.
4. Ayas NT, Epstein LJ. Oral appliances in the treatment of obstructive sleep apnea and snoring. Curr Opin Pulm Med 1998; 4(6):355–360.
5. Sajkov D, Wang T, Saunders NA, Bune AJ, Neill AM, Douglas Mcevoy R. Daytime pulmonary hemodynamics in patients with obstructive sleep apnea without lung disease. Am J Respir Crit Care Med 1999; 159(5 Pt 1):1518–1526.
6. Krol RC, Knuth SL, Bartlett D. Selective reduction of genioglossal muscle activity by alcohol in normal human subjects. Am Rev Respir Dis 1984; 129(2):247–250.
7. Issa FG, Sullivan CE. Alcohol, snoring and sleep apnea. J Neurol Neurosurg Psychiatry 1982; 45(4):353–359.
8. Teschler H, Berthon-Jones M, Wessendorf T, Meyer HJ, Konietzko N. Influence of moderate alcohol consumption on obstructive sleep apnoea with and without AutoSet nasal CPAP therapy. Eur Respir J 1996; 9(11):2371–2377.
9. Leiter JC, Knuth SL, Bartlett D Jr. The effect of sleep deprivation on activity of the genioglossus muscle. Am Rev Respir Dis 1985; 132(6):1242–1245.
10. Berry RB, Kouchi K, Bower J, Prosise G, Light RW. Triazolam in patients with obstructive sleep apnea. Am J Respir Crit Care Med 1995; 151(2 Pt 1):450–454.
11. Finnimore AJ, Roebuck M, Sajkov D, McEvoy RD. The effects of the GABA agonist, baclofen, on sleep and breathing. Eur Respir J 1995; 8(2):230–234.
12. Robinson RW, Zwillich CW, Bixler EO, Cadieux RJ, Kales A, White DP. Effects of oral narcotics on sleep-disordered breathing in healthy adults. Chest 1987; 91(2):197–203.
13. Catley DM, Thornton C, Jordan C, Lehane JR, Royston D, Jones JG. Pronounced, episodic oxygen desaturation in the postoperative period: its association with ventilatory pattern and analgesic regimen. Anesthesiology 1985; 63(1):20–28.
14. Wang D, Teichtahl H, Drummer O, et al. Central sleep apnea in stable methadone maintenance treatment patients. Chest 2005; 128(3):1348–1356.
15. Wetter DW, Young TB, Bidwell TR, Badr MS, Palta M. Smoking as a risk factor for sleep-disordered breathing. Arch Intern Med 1994; 154(19):2219–2224.
16. Newman AB, Nieto FJ, Guidry U, et al. Relation of sleep-disordered breathing to cardiovascular disease risk factors: the Sleep Heart Health Study. Am J Epidemiol 2001; 154(1):50–59.

17. Liu PY, Yee B, Wishart SM, et al. The short-term effects of high-dose testosterone on sleep, breathing, and function in older men. J Clin Endocrinol Metab 2003; 88(8):3605–3613.
18. Schneider BK, Pickett CK, Zwillich CW, et al. Influence of testosterone on breathing during sleep. J Appl Physiol 1986; 61(2):618–623.
19. Guilleminault C, Rosekind M. The arousal threshold: sleep deprivation, sleep fragmentation, and obstructive sleep apnea syndrome. Bull Eur Physiopathol Respir 1981; 17(3):341–349.
20. Series F, Roy N, Marc I. Effects of sleep deprivation and sleep fragmentation on upper airway collapsibility in normal subjects. Am J Respir Crit Care Med 1994; 150(2):481–485.
21. Marin JM, Carrizo SJ, Vicente E, Agusti AG. Long-term cardiovascular outcomes in men with obstructive sleep apnoea–hypopnoea with or without treatment with continuous positive airway pressure: an observational study. Lancet 2005; 365(9464):1046–1053.
22. Kiely JL, McNicholas WT. Cardiovascular risk factors in patients with obstructive sleep apnoea syndrome. Eur Respir J 2000; 16(1):128–133.
23. Mortimore IL, Marshall I, Wraith PK, Sellar RJ, Douglas NJ. Neck and total body fat deposition in nonobese and obese patients with sleep apnea compared with that in control subjects. Am J Respir Crit Care Med 1998; 157(1):280–283.
24. Horner RL, Mohiaddin RH, Lowell DG, et al. Sites and sizes of fat deposits around the pharynx in obese patients with obstructive sleep apnoea and weight matched controls. Eur Respir J 1989; 2(7):613–622.
25. Newman AB, Foster G, Givelber R, Nieto FJ, Redline S, Young T. Progression and regression of sleep-disordered breathing with changes in weight: the Sleep Heart Health Study. Arch Intern Med 2005; 165(20):2408–2413.
26. Sampol G, Munoz X, Sagales MT, et al. Long-term efficacy of dietary weight loss in sleep apnoea/hypopnoea syndrome. Eur Respir J 1998; 12(5):1156–1159.
27. Strychar I. Diet in the management of weight loss. CMAJ 2006; 174(1):56–63.
28. Kansanen M, Vanninen E, Tuunainen A, et al. The effect of a very low-calorie diet-induced weight loss on the severity of obstructive sleep apnoea and autonomic nervous function in obese patients with obstructive sleep apnoea syndrome. Clin Physiol 1998; 18(4):377–385.
29. Wooley SC, Garner DM. Obesity treatment: the high cost of false hope. J Am Diet Assoc 1991; 91(10):1248–1251.
30. Kajaste S, Brander PE, Telakivi T, Partinen M, Mustajoki P. A cognitive-behavioral weight reduction program in the treatment of obstructive sleep apnea syndrome with or without initial nasal CPAP: a randomized study. Sleep Med 2004; 5(2):125–131.
31. Peppard PE, Young T. Exercise and sleep-disordered breathing: an association independent of body habitus. Sleep 2004; 27(3):480–484.
32. Netzer N, Lormes W, Giebelhaus V, et al. Physical training of patients with sleep apnea. Pneumologie 1997; 51(suppl):779–782.
33. Connolly HM, Crary JL, McGoon MD, et al. Valvular heart disease associated with fenfluramine-phentermine. N Engl J Med 1997; 337(9):581–588.
34. Abenhaim L, Moride Y, Brenot F, et al. Appetite-suppressant drugs and the risk of primary pulmonary hypertension. International Primary Pulmonary Hypertension Study Group. N Engl J Med 1996; 335(9):609–616.
35. Hill JO, Hauptman J, Anderson JW, et al. Orlistat, a lipase inhibitor, for weight maintenance after conventional dieting: a 1-year study. Am J Clin Nutr 1999; 69(6):1108–1116.
36. Chanoine JP, Hampl S, Jensen C, Boldrin M, Hauptman J. Effect of orlistat on weight and body composition in obese adolescents: a randomized controlled trial. JAMA 2005; 293(23):2873–2883.
37. Davidson MH, Hauptman J, DiGirolamo M, et al. Weight control and risk factor reduction in obese subjects treated for 2 years with orlistat: a randomized controlled trial. JAMA 1999; 281(3):235–242.
38. Wadden TA, Berkowitz RI, Womble LG, et al. Randomized trial of lifestyle modification and pharmacotherapy for obesity. N Engl J Med 2005; 353(20):2111–2120.
39. Martinez D, Basile BR. Sibutramine does not worsen sleep apnea syndrome: a randomized double-blind placebo-controlled study. Sleep Med 2005; 6(5):467–470.

40. Lujan JA, Frutos MD, Hernandez Q et al. Laparoscopic versus open gastric bypass in the treatment of morbid obesity: a randomized prospective study. Ann Surg 2004; 239(4):433–437.
41. Lee WJ, Huang MT, Yu PJ, Wang W, Chen TC. Laparoscopic vertical banded gastroplasty and laparoscopic gastric bypass: a comparison. Obes Surg 2004; 14(5):626–634.
42. Hall JC, Watts JM, O'Brien PE, et al. Gastric surgery for morbid obesity. The Adelaide Study. Ann Surg 1990; 211(4):419–427.
43. Buchwald H, Avidor Y, Braunwald E, et al. Bariatric surgery: a systematic review and meta-analysis. JAMA 2004; 292(14):1724–1737.
44. Pevernagie DA, Stanson AW, Sheedy PF II, Daniels BK, Shepard JW Jr. Effects of body position on the upper airway of patients with obstructive sleep apnea. Am J Respir Crit Care Med 1995; 152(1):179–185.
45. Neill AM, Angus SM, Sajkov D, McEvoy RD. Effects of sleep posture on upper airway stability in patients with obstructive sleep apnea. Am J Respir Crit Care Med 1997; 155(1):199–204.
46. Oksenberg A, Silverberg DS, Arons E, Radwan H. Positional vs nonpositional obstructive sleep apnea patients: anthropomorphic, nocturnal polysomnographic, and multiple sleep latency test data. Chest 1997; 112(3):629–639.
47. Mador MJ, Kufel TJ, Magalang UJ, Rajesh SK, Watwe V, Grant BJ. Prevalence of positional sleep apnea in patients undergoing polysomnography. Chest 2005; 128(4): 2130–2137.
48. Jokic R, Klimaszewski A, Crossley M, Sridhar G, Fitzpatrick MF. Positional treatment vs continuous positive airway pressure in patients with positional obstructive sleep apnea syndrome. Chest 1999; 115(3):771–781.
49. Cartwright RD, Lloyd S, Lilie J, Kravitz H. Sleep position training as treatment for sleep apnea syndrome: a preliminary study. Sleep 1985; 8(2):87–94.
50. Winkelman JW, Goldman H, Piscatelli N, Lukas SE, Dorsey CM, Cunningham S. Are thyroid function tests necessary in patients with suspected sleep apnea? Sleep 1996; 19(10):790–793.
51. Lin CC, Tsan KW, Chen PJ. The relationship between sleep apnea syndrome and hypothyroidism. Chest 1992; 102(6):1663–1667.
52. Resta O, Pannacciulli N, Di Gioia G, Stefano A, Barbaro MP, De Pergola G. High prevalence of previously unknown subclinical hypothyroidism in obese patients referred to a sleep clinic for sleep disordered breathing. Nutr Metab Cardiovasc Dis 2004; 14(5): 248–253.
53. Mickelson SA, Lian T, Rosenthal L. Thyroid testing and thyroid hormone replacement in patients with sleep disordered breathing. Ear Nose Throat J 1999; 78(10):768–771, 774–775.
54. Rajagopal KR, Abbrecht PH, Derderian SS, et al. Obstructive sleep apnea in hypothyroidism. Ann Intern Med 1984; 101(4):491–494.
55. Resta O, Carratu P, Carpagnano GE, et al. Influence of subclinical hypothyroidism and T4 treatment on the prevalence and severity of obstructive sleep apnoea syndrome (OSAS). J Endocrinol Invest 2005; 28(10):893–898.
56. Skjodt NM, Atkar R, Easton PA. Screening for hypothyroidism in sleep apnea. Am J Respir Crit Care Med 1999; 160(2):732–735.
57. Grunstein RR, Ho KY, Sullivan CE. Sleep apnea in acromegaly. Ann Intern Med 1991; 115(7):527–532.
58. Fatti LM, Scacchi M, Pincelli AI, Lavezzi E, Cavagnini F. Prevalence and pathogenesis of sleep apnea and lung disease in acromegaly. Pituitary 2001; 4(4):259–262.
59. Wellman A, Jordan AS, Malhotra A, et al. Ventilatory control and airway anatomy in obstructive sleep apnea. Am J Respir Crit Care Med 2004; 170(11):1225–1232.
60. Grunstein RR, Ho KK, Sullivan CE. Effect of octreotide, a somatostatin analog, on sleep apnea in patients with acromegaly. Ann Intern Med 1994; 121(7):478–483.
61. Herrmann BL, Wessendorf TE, Ajaj W, Kahlke S, Teschler H, Mann K. Effects of octreotide on sleep apnoea and tongue volume (magnetic resonance imaging) in patients with acromegaly. Eur J Endocrinol 2004; 151(3):309–315.
62. McNicholas WT, Tarlo S, Cole P, et al. Obstructive apneas during sleep in patients with seasonal allergic rhinitis. Am Rev Respir Dis 1982; 126(4):625–628.

63. Horner RL, Innes JA, Holden HB, Guz A. Afferent pathway(s) for pharyngeal dilator reflex to negative pressure in man: a study using upper airway anaesthesia. J Physiol 1991; 436:31–44.
64. Kiely JL, Nolan P, McNicholas WT. Intranasal corticosteroid therapy for obstructive sleep apnoea in patients with co-existing rhinitis. Thorax 2004; 59(1):50–55.
65. McLean HA, Urton AM, Driver HS, et al. Effect of treating severe nasal obstruction on the severity of obstructive sleep apnoea. Eur Respir J 2005; 25(3):521–527.
66. Bahammam AS, Tate R, Manfreda J, Kryger MH. Upper airway resistance syndrome: effect of nasal dilation, sleep stage, and sleep position. Sleep 1999; 22(5):592–598.
67. Heimer D, Scharf SM, Lieberman A, Lavie P. Sleep apnea syndrome treated by repair of deviated nasal septum. Chest 1983; 84(2):184–185.
68. Series F, St. Pierre S, Carrier G. Effects of surgical correction of nasal obstruction in the treatment of obstructive sleep apnea. Am Rev Respir Dis 1992; 146:1261–1265.
69. Smith PL, Haponik EF, Bleecker ER. The effects of oxygen in patients with sleep apnea. Am Rev Respir Dis 1984; 130(6):958–963.
70. Landsberg R, Friedman M, Ascher-Landsberg J. Treatment of hypoxemia in obstructive sleep apnea. Am J Rhinol 2001; 15(5):311–313.
71. Phillips BA, Schmitt FA, Berry DT, Lamb DG, Amin M, Cook YR. Treatment of obstructive sleep apnea. A preliminary report comparing nasal CPAP to nasal oxygen in patients with mild OSA. Chest 1990; 98(2):325–330.
72. Staniforth AD, Kinnear WJ, Starling R, Hetmanski DJ, Cowley AJ. Effect of oxygen on sleep quality, cognitive function and sympathetic activity in patients with chronic heart failure and Cheyne-Stokes respiration. Eur Heart J 1998; 19(6):922–928.
73. Fletcher EC, Munafo DA. Role of nocturnal oxygen therapy in obstructive sleep apnea. When should it be used? Chest 1990; 98(6):1497–1504.
74. Chauncey JB, Aldrich MS. Preliminary findings in the treatment of obstructive sleep apnea with transtracheal oxygen. Sleep 1990; 13(2):167–174.
75. Farney RJ, Walker JM, Elmer JC, Viscomi VA, Ord RJ. Transtracheal oxygen, nasal CPAP and nasal oxygen in five patients with obstructive sleep apnea. Chest 1992; 101(5):1228–1235.
76. Haponik EF, Smith PL, Bohlman ME, Allen RP, Goldman SM, Bleecker ER. Computerized tomography in obstructive sleep apnea. Correlation of airway size with physiology during sleep and wakefulness. Am Rev Respir Dis 1983; 127(2):221–226.
77. Schwab RJ, Gupta KB, Gefter WB, Metzger LJ, Hoffman EA, Pack AI. Upper airway and soft tissue anatomy in normal subjects and patients with sleep-disordered breathing. Significance of the lateral pharyngeal walls. Am J Respir Crit Care Med 1995; 152(5 Pt 1):1673–1689.
78. Isono S, Remmers JE, Tanaka A, Sho Y, Sato J, Nishino T. Anatomy of pharynx in patients with obstructive sleep apnea and in normal subjects. J Appl Physiol 1997; 82(4):1319–1326.
79. Malhotra A, Fogel R, Edwards JK, Shea SA, White DP. Neuromuscular compensatory mechanisms in obstructive sleep apnea: role of upper airway receptor mechanisms. Sleep 1999; 22:S259.
80. Malhotra A, Fogel R, Kikinis R, Shea S, White DP. The influence of aging and gender on upper airway structure and function. Am J Respir Crit Care Med 1999; 159:A170.
81. Mezzanotte WS, Tangel DJ, White DP. Waking genioglossal electromyogram in sleep apnea patients versus normal controls (a neuromuscular compensatory mechanism). J Clin Invest 1992; 89(5):1571–1579.
82. White DP. Sleep-related breathing disorder. 2. Pathophysiology of obstructive sleep apnoea. Thorax 1995; 50(7):797–804.
83. Young T, Finn L, Austin D, Peterson A. Menopausal status and sleep-disordered breathing in the Wisconsin Sleep Cohort Study. Am J Respir Crit Care Med 2003; 167(9): 1181–1185.
84. Strohl KP, Hensley MJ, Saunders NA, Scharf SM, Brown R, Ingram RH Jr. Progesterone administration and progressive sleep apneas. JAMA 1981; 245(12):1230–1232.
85. Rajagopal KR, Abbrecht PH, Jabbari B. Effects of medroxyprogesterone acetate in obstructive sleep apnea. Chest 1986; 90(6):815–821.
86. Cook WR, Benich JJ, Wooten SA. Indices of severity of obstructive sleep apnea syndrome do not change during medroxyprogesterone acetate therapy. Chest 1989; 96(2): 262–266.

87. Saaresranta T, Polo-Kantola P, Rauhala E, Polo O. Medroxyprogesterone in postmeno-pausal females with partial upper airway obstruction during sleep. Eur Respir J 2001; 18(6):989–995.
88. Cistulli PA, Barnes DJ, Grunstein RR, Sullivan CE. Effect of short-term hormone replace-ment in the treatment of obstructive sleep apnoea in postmenopausal women. Thorax 1994; 49(7):699–702.
89. Herkert O, Kuhl H, Sandow J, Busse R, Schini-Kerth VB. Sex steroids used in hormonal treatment increase vascular procoagulant activity by inducing thrombin receptor (PAR-1) expression: role of the glucocorticoid receptor. Circulation 2001; 104(23):2826–2831.
90. Brownell LG, West P, Sweatman P, Acres JC, Kryger MH. Protriptyline in obstructive sleep apnea: a double-blind trial. N Engl J Med 1982; 307(17):1037–1042.
91. Guilleminault C, Hayes B. Naloxone, theophylline, bromocriptine, and obstructive sleep apnea. Negative results. Bull Eur Physiopathol Respir 1983; 19(6):632–634.
92. Espinoza H, Antic R, Thornton AT, McEvoy RD. The effects of aminophylline on sleep and sleep-disordered breathing in patients with obstructive sleep apnea syndrome. Am Rev Respir Dis 1987; 136(1):80–84.
93. Tojima H, Kunitomo F, Kimura H, Tatsumi K, Kuriyama T, Honda Y. Effects of aceta-zolamide in patients with the sleep apnoea syndrome. Thorax 1988; 43(2):113–119.
94. Horner RL. Motor control of the pharyngeal musculature and implications for the pathogenesis of obstructive sleep apnea. Sleep 1996; 19(10):827–853.
95. Kubin L, Tojima H, Davies RO, Pack AI. Serotonergic excitatory drive to hypoglossal motoneurons in the decerebrate cat. Neurosci Lett 1992; 139(2):243–248.
96. Kubin L, Tojima H, Reignier C, Pack AI, Davies RO. Interaction of serotonergic excita-tory drive to hypoglossal motoneurons with carbachol-induced, REM sleep-like atonia. Sleep 1996; 19(3):187–195.
97. Sunderram J, Parisi RA, Strobel RJ. Serotonergic stimulation of the genioglossus and the response to nasal continuous positive airway pressure. Am J Respir Crit Care Med 2000; 162(3 Pt 1):925–929.
98. Berry RB, Yamaura EM, Gill K, Reist C. Acute effects of paroxetine on genioglossus activity in obstructive sleep apnea. Sleep 1999; 22(8):1087–1092.
99. Kraiczi H, Hedner J, Dahlof P, Ejnell H, Carlson J. Effect of serotonin uptake inhibition on breathing during sleep and daytime symptoms in obstructive sleep apnea. Sleep 1999; 22(1):61–67.
100. Veasey SC. Serotonin agonists and antagonists in obstructive sleep apnea: therapeutic potential. Am J Respir Med 2003; 2(1):21–29.
101. Vgontzas AN, Papanicolaou DA, Bixler EO, et al. Sleep apnea and daytime sleepiness and fatigue: relation to visceral obesity, insulin resistance, and hypercytokinemia. J Clin Endocrinol Metab 2000; 85(3):1151–1158.
102. Vgontzas AN, Zoumakis E, Lin HM, Bixler EO, Trakada G, Chrousos GP. Marked decrease in sleepiness in patients with sleep apnea by etanercept, a tumor necrosis factor-alpha antagonist. J Clin Endocrinol Metab 2004; 89(9):4409–4413.
103. Listing J, Strangfeld A, Kary S, et al. Infections in patients with rheumatoid arthritis treated with biologic agents. Arthritis Rheum 2005; 52(11):3403–3412.
104. Black JE, Hirshkowitz M. Modafinil for treatment of residual excessive sleepiness in nasal continuous positive airway pressure-treated obstructive sleep apnea/hypopnea syndrome. Sleep 2005; 28(4):464–471.
105. Pack AI, Black JE, Schwartz JR, Matheson JK. Modafinil as adjunct therapy for daytime sleepiness in obstructive sleep apnea. Am J Respir Crit Care Med 2001; 164(9): 1675–1681.
106. Kingshott RN, Vennelle M, Coleman EL, Engleman HM, Mackay TW, Douglas NJ. Randomized, double-blind, placebo-controlled crossover trial of modafinil in the treat-ment of residual excessive daytime sleepiness in the sleep apnea/hypopnea syndrome. Am J Respir Crit Care Med 2001;163(4):918–923.

14 Gender Differences in Obstructive Sleep Apnea

Vidya Krishnan and Nancy A. Collop
Division of Pulmonary/Critical Care Medicine, Johns Hopkins University, Baltimore, Maryland, U.S.A.

INTRODUCTION

Obstructive sleep apnea (OSA), the clinical entity characterized by repetitive partial and/or complete collapse of the upper airway during sleep and symptoms of excessive daytime sleepiness, has been historically described as a disease of males. Charles Dickens is often credited with the first description of OSA. He described a character, fat boy Joe, who suffered from the classic symptoms of snoring, excessive daytime sleepiness, obesity, and "dropsy." Nearly 170 years later, our interest in the pathophysiology and clinical sequelae of OSA has heightened, partly due to the identified associations of the syndrome with cardiovascular disease (1–4), motor vehicle accidents, and decreased quality of life (5). Early clinical research in the field of OSA identified the disease as a male-predominant disorder, with estimated male:female ratio for disease prevalence from 10:1 to 60:1 (6). However, these prevalence estimates are based on clinical studies that often had a referral bias of more men than women. In contemporary epidemiologic studies, the reported male:female prevalence ratios are in the order of 3:1 to 2:1, suggesting that OSA is not as rare in women as previously thought. In addition, women with OSA have clinical presentations, therapeutic considerations and prognoses that differ from men, making an accurate diagnosis and initiation of therapy a challenge and a priority. This chapter focuses on the elements of OSA, including epidemiology, risk factors, and treatment, which contribute to gender differences, as well as gender-specific conditions that may affect the clinical expression of OSA.

EPIDEMIOLOGY

OSA is the most common disease among the collection of sleep-related breathing disorders, estimated to affect up to 5% of the general United States adult population (5). Prevalence estimates from different studies are often difficult to compare, due to conflicting disease definitions. In a large U.S. community-based study, the prevalence of OSA, defined by an apnea–hypopnea index (AHI) of at least five obstructive events per hour, was found to be nearly three times higher in men than in women in an American middle-aged adult population (24% vs. 9%), and the combination of an AHI of at least five obstructive events per hour and daytime hypersomnolence is twice as common in men than in women (4% vs. 2%) (7).

Women tend to have fewer completely obstructive (apneic) events than partially obstructive (hypopneic) events, with shorter mean and maximum duration of respiratory events than in age-matched men (8). Patients with the upper airway resistance syndrome (UARS), often considered a milder form of disease than OSA on the spectrum of obstructive sleep-disordered breathing, are more likely to be women than men (9). In middle-aged men and women with OSA and similar apnea–hypopnea indices, women have a higher body mass index (BMI) (8,10,11), but with increasing age, the male predominance of OSA lessens and influence of BMI on OSA also lessens. By 50 years of age, the incidence rates of OSA by gender are similar (12).

Men are more likely to be diagnosed with supine position-dependent OSA compared to women (13), implying an anatomic component to their predisposition to developing OSA. Women are, however, more likely to experience obstructive events predominantly during rapid eye movement (REM) sleep, making apnea and hypopnea frequencies during REM between genders comparable (13,14). Perhaps, the reduced skeletal muscle tone during REM sleep nullifies any protective effect of the premenopausal state in women, and the mechanism for the protective effect involves the upper airway dilator muscle tone.

Epidemiologic studies throughout the world report similar rates of OSA in men and women as the aforementioned studies (15–17), suggesting that gender differences in the syndrome prevalence may result from genetic, rather than environmental determinants.

The difference in OSA prevalence is magnified in the clinical setting. In a large retrospective study of men and women with OSA, matched by age, BMI, AHI, and Epworth sleepiness scale score, women were more likely to present with initial symptoms of insomnia and have concomitant depression and hypothyroidism. They were less likely to have witnessed apneic events than men (18). We hypothesize that several reasons may explain this magnified gender difference in the clinic population. First, men are more likely to be recognized with classic OSA symptoms of daytime sleepiness, snoring, and witnessed apneas, and referred appropriately for management, whereas women often experience symptoms of insomnia, chronic fatigue or depression, which may not be recognized as attributable to OSA, and therefore resulting in a delay in diagnosis and treatment. Second, more severe cases of OSA are likelier to be referred for sleep evaluation, and the gender difference in prevalence of OSA may be magnified with greater severity of disease (2,19). Finally, women are also less likely than men to be accompanied to clinic by a bed partner, whose complementary sleep history is often important in identifying sleep symptoms, such as nocturnal snoring and witnessed apneas, and in portraying an accurate picture of the degree of clinical sleep disturbance. Differences in prevalence of disease by gender in the community and clinical settings have been examined including cardiovascular disease, end-stage renal disease, and acquired immunodeficiency syndrome (AIDS), and are sometimes attributed to barriers in attaining healthcare. Referral bias due to differences in time to presentation by gender, should be examined in every study of clinical populations, and considered in the interpretation of their results.

FACTORS THAT CONTRIBUTE TO OBSTRUCTIVE SLEEP APNEA

The reasons for gender differences in OSA may be traced to differences in the individual factors that contribute to OSA (Table 1). The pathophysiology of upper airway collapse during sleep is multifactorial, and differences in these factors between genders will elucidate the varied presentations.

TABLE 1 Factors Responsible for Obstructive Sleep Apnea with Potential
Gender Differences

Anatomic	Physiologic	Other
Upper airway anatomy	Local neuromuscular reflexes	Alcohol, tobacco, or drug use
Upper airway compliance	Central ventilatory control	
Body habitus	Hormonal effects	
	Arousal response	

Physical Factors
Upper Airway Anatomy
Upper airway caliber, a major determinant of OSA, is determined by parapharyngeal adiposity, craniofacial dimensions that affect mandibular size, and size of the surrounding tissues (lateral pharyngeal walls and tongue) (20). In normal men and women, although no gender difference in the distribution of fat in the neck is observed, total neck soft tissue volume is greater in men than in women (21). Using magnetic resonance imaging, soft tissue composition of the neck differs by gender, with men having larger soft palates and upper tongue volume than women (21). Both men and women with OSA are more likely to have craniofacial differences, as determined by cephalometry, compared to their normal counterparts (e.g., a lower set hyoid bone, smaller mandible or maxilla, a more retrognathic mandible) (22,23). While some studies suggest a difference by gender in the prevalence of craniofacial abnormalities, others have not.

Despite these multiple factors that would possibly predict smaller pharyngeal airway size in men, upper airway diameter is greater in men than in women in both normal (16) and OSA patients (24) during wakefulness. However, upper airway size appears to be a more important predictor of clinical severity of OSA in men than in women (24), suggesting that cross-sectional pharyngeal area alone does not explain the observed gender differences in predisposition to OSA.

The length of the pharynx, from the hard palate to the epiglottis, has been shown to be longer in men than in women (25), which can result in greater predisposition to collapse. In addition, the dynamic properties of the upper airway anatomy may contribute to the gender differences in OSA. Men have more narrowing of the oropharyngeal space in the supine position, as compared to women (26), and with mandibular movement during wakefulness (27). These upper airway characteristics support an increased tendency for upper airway collapse in men.

Upper Airway Compliance
Upper airway compliance, or collapsibility, is determined by many factors such as tonic and phasic upper airway muscle activation, biomechanical properties (e.g., connective tissue composition, surface tension), and response of the upper airway to positional stresses. Perhaps more important than the differences in static upper airway properties between men and women, differences in upper airway compliance predicts a divergence in the propensity for upper airway collapse by gender.

Upper airway imaging techniques have demonstrated an increased upper airway compliance (and subsequent increase in upper airway collapsibility) in proportion to the neck circumference (28), which tends to be higher in men than in women. Neck circumference alone, however, may only be a surrogate for the underlying soft tissue and muscle composition in the neck.

Local upper airway dilator muscle activation in response to upper airway obstruction can protect the patency of the upper airway (see section: Neuromuscular Reflexes) Little is known about the biomechanical properties of the upper airway in patients with OSA, particularly with regards to gender differences.

Body Habitus

Obesity is the strongest risk factor for OSA (7,29), with even small changes in weight resulting in clinically significant changes in upper airway collapsibility and severity of upper airway obstruction (29). The effect of obesity on obstructive apneic and hypopneic events is proposed to be mass loading of the upper airway by adiposity surrounding the pharynx, causing upper airway collapse. Therefore, the distribution of total body fat and not just overall BMI, is relevant to the risk of OSA. Women are more likely to be obese (BMI ≥ 30 kg/m^2) than men (30), but differences in fat distribution may be one reason why women have lower rates of OSA. When comparing men and women with comparable BMI and waist circumferences, men exhibited greater upper body obesity, as measured by smaller hip circumferences and greater subscapular skin fold thickness (31). The finding that women with a comparable severity of OSA as men have a greater BMI (7), may be explained by differences in distribution of body weight by gender.

Physiologic Factors

Neuromuscular Reflexes

Upper airway neuromuscular reflexes are a primary protective response to upper airway obstruction. Stretch mechanoreceptors in the pharynx and lung and chemoreceptors (responsive to O_2 and CO_2) are recognized sensors for these reflexes to protect the patency of the upper airway by activating pharyngeal dilator muscles, such as the tensor palatini and genioglossus muscles.

In patients with OSA, upper airway dilator muscles exhibit higher activation during wake (32,33). The decrease of pharyngeal muscle activation that occurs with sleep onset in these patients results in upper airway obstruction (34). Studies examining gender differences in upper airway neuromuscular reflexes with inspiratory flow limitation (IFL) are limited, but genioglossal and tensor palatini activity response to upper airway resistance loading do not appear to differ by gender (25). Similarly, genioglossus activity and diaphragmatic response to hypoxia are not different by gender (35). While these studies were performed in healthy men and women, it is unclear whether gender differences in neuromuscular reflexes exist in patients with OSA.

Local pharyngeal trauma due to repetitive upper airway collapse, resulting in diminished neuromuscular reflexes, is another proposed pathophysiology for development of apneas and hypopneas (36). Neuromuscular reflexes are physiologic compensatory mechanisms to protect the patency of the upper airway in the setting of upper airway collapse. While current studies have not explored possible gender differences in the susceptibility to local pharyngeal trauma, if one were to exist, this may explain the gender difference in the clinical manifestation of upper airway obstruction, since UARS occurs equally in men and women, whereas OSA is two to three times more common in men than women (36). The difference between these two entities may be due to gender differences in predisposition to lose neuro-muscular reflexes with repetitive upper airway trauma or the severity of upper airway collapse.

Central Ventilatory Control
Patients with IFL may mount an increased ventilatory response to meet the increased ventilatory demand. An exaggerated response to IFL, however, may result in venti-latory instability. Ventilatory instability can result in fluctuations in upper airway muscle activity, and subsequently result in upper airway obstruction, as well as sleep disruption. The physiologic mechanisms that preserve ventilation are another factor responsible for the spectrum of clinical expressions of IFL, with some mani-festing only simple snoring and others developing full-blown OSA.

Differential responses of ventilatory drive to various stimuli may also explain gender differences in the prevalence of OSA. In normal adults, men have a greater ventilatory response to hypoxia and hypercarbia during wake than women (37–39). During sleep, ventilatory response to hypoxia is similar in men and women (38), resulting in a greater reduction in ventilation in men compared to women in the wake-sleep transition and a stimulus for ventilatory instability in men during sleep. Also, gender differences exist in the apnea threshold, the level of arterial carbon dioxide below which an apnea is induced. Women have a lower apnea threshold during non-rapid eye movement (NREM) sleep than men (40), which can also pre-dispose men to greater ventilatory instability during sleep. With obesity, women exhibit augmented chemosensitivity and ventilatory response to hypoxia and hypercarbia, whereas men do not (41). This ventilatory response in women may protect them from the development of apneas and hypopneas, and may explain the higher prevalence of obesity hypoventilation syndrome in women than in men. With IFL, men have less ventilatory response than women, despite comparable degrees of minute ventilation (25). In particular, women respond to even mild degrees of IFL with a marked increase in respiratory rate, whereas men have this tachypneic response only with near-apneic inspiratory flow reduction (42).

Hormonal Effects
Many circulating hormones may directly or indirectly affect the clinical manifesta-tion of OSA, although the mechanisms and effects of these hormones are still under investigation. Sex-related hormones (e.g., estrogen, progesterone, testosterone) and other hormones, such as leptin, are implicated in changes in upper airway resis-tance and ventilatory drive (Table 2).

Estrogen and progesterone have been implicated in the gender differences in OSA. In a clinical cohort of 53 women, those with OSA had significantly lower levels of 17-hydroxyprogesterone, progesterone, and estradiol than those without OSA (43), highlighting an association between female sex hormones and OSA. Whether this relationship is a cause or an effect of the disease is unclear. Progesterone levels are directly related to ventilation and ventilatory chemoresponsiveness to hypoxia and hypercarbia (44,45). In addition, indirect evidence exists to support the effect of progesterone on upper airway dilator muscle activity. Tonic and phasic genioglos-sus activity appears to have a weak positive correlation with progesterone levels in healthy women (46).

Testosterone seems to precipitate or worsen OSA. Exogenous administration of testosterone hormone for treatment of hypogonadism in men has been associated with an increase in AHI from 6.4 to 15.4 events per hour (47). In women, the effects

TABLE 2 Hormones That Influence the Manifestation of Obstructive Sleep Apnea

Hormone	Source	Potential effects on OSA
Estrogen	Ovaries (women)	Increases upper airway resistance via mucosal edema, hyperemia, and hypersecretion
Progesterone	Ovaries (women)	Increases ventilatory drive Increases chemosensitivity to hypoxia and hypercarbia Increases tone of upper airway dilator muscles
Testosterone	Testes (men) adrenal glands	Increases obstructive apneas (unknown mechanism)
Leptin	Adipocytes (subcutaneous > visceral)	Stimulates ventilation Affects other circulating hormones Body weight control
Thyroxine	Thyroid	Increases obstructive apneas in thyroxine deficiency (unknown mechanism)
Growth hormone	Anterior pituitary gland	Increases obstructive apneas in growth hormone excess (unknown mechanism)
Cortisol	Adrenal glands	Increases REM density Increases central obesity

Abbreviations: OSA, obstructive sleep apnea; REM, rapid eye movement.

of testosterone are likely to predispose to OSA as well. Exogenous testosterone administration to one female was reported to precipitate clinically significant OSA (48). Additionally, women with polycystic ovarian syndrome, which is characterized by ovarian failure, obesity, and androgen excess, have a higher AHI than healthy women controls (22.5 vs. 6.7 events/hour) (49).

Leptin is a hormone recently identified to be associated with obesity and ventilatory control. Produced by subcutaneous adipocytes and to a lesser degree visceral adipocytes, leptin acts directly on the hypothalamus to reduce appetite and increase energy consumption (50). It also may have indirect effects on levels of reproductive hormones (51). Leptin has been shown to stimulate breathing, which in the face of increased work of breathing with obesity, may serve to preserve ventilation (29). Circulating levels of leptin are higher in women than men, which may be related to the distribution of adiposity and the higher relative contribution of subcutaneous fat versus visceral fat to leptin synthesis. In animal models, leptin has been shown to have a greater role in ventilatory control in obese female than in obese male mice during wake and NREM sleep (52). Thus, differences in leptin levels and function between men and women may explain the gender differences in ventilatory compensation to upper airway obstruction.

Arousal from Sleep

Arousal from sleep may be related to numerous factors. It has been suggested that women are more likely to experience an arousal from sleep with IFL, and subsequently do not meet the definition of OSA, because sleep is disrupted.

Arousals from sleep are primarily triggered by increased inspiratory effort. In both normal and OSA patients, arousals are best predicted by increased inspiratory effort and seems to occur consistently at a set threshold level (approximately −15 cm H_2O) (53–57).

Ventilatory responses subsequent to arousals have been shown to vary by gender, with increased minute ventilation during the first breath after arousal in men compared to women (58). The significance of these responses to arousal is still in question, but may contribute to subsequent ventilatory and upper airway instability.

Effects of Alcohol and Tobacco Use

Lifestyle choices also contribute to the development of OSA. Alcohol use results in upper airway relaxation and decreased arousal response to apneas, both of which result in exacerbation of apnea in patients with OSA and precipitation of OSA in patients at risk. However, healthy women and nonobese men do not develop apneas with even moderate ethanol ingestion (59,60).

While smoking has been implicated in increased upper airway resistance via upper airway inflammation, edema, and mucous secretion (61,62), an association between smoking and OSA has not been conclusively established. Nonetheless, alcohol and tobacco use and dependence, as determined by nationwide survey studies, do not differ significantly between men and women (63), and cannot explain the gender differences observed in the prevalence of OSA. Also, as stated previously, women with OSA are more likely to present with atypical symptoms, such as insomnia. Medications targeted at this primary complaint, such as sedatives, may exacerbate the underlying disease by promoting upper airway relaxation and increasing the threshold for arousal; however, there are no data supporting such a hypothesis.

GENDER-SPECIFIC CONDITIONS
Puberty

In prepubertal children, boys and girls have similar rates of OSA (64,65). OSA in children is usually due to anatomic upper airway obstruction from tonsillar hypertrophy, although with the rising epidemic of obesity, increased body weight is also associated with development of OSA in children. The divergence in prevalence of OSA occurs only after puberty (66), supporting the role of the sex hormones estrogen, progesterone, and testosterone in modifying the risk of developing OSA. After menarche, upper airway dilator muscle activity fluctuates over the monthly cycle (46), potentially affecting upper airway patency. In healthy women, upper airway resistance is increased in the follicular phase of the menstrual cycle, compared to the luteal phase, during wake and stage 2 NREM sleep (67).

Pregnancy

Obstructive sleep-disordered breathing is relatively uncommon in otherwise healthy young women of reproductive age. However, biochemical and physical changes associated with pregnancy have opposing effects on the risk for OSA, which alter the risk of OSA in an individual. A study published in 2005 showed that symptoms consistent with OSA (snoring, excessive daytime sleepiness) occur in 10% of pregnant women, and increase during the course of the pregnancy, particularly in women with higher baseline BMI and greater increases in neck circumference (68).

Pregnancy is associated with increased levels of several hormones. Estrogen and placental growth hormone levels, which are increased during pregnancy, cause alterations in the upper airway, including mucosal edema, hyperemia, and hypersecretion, each of which can independently increase upper airway resistance (69,70). Progesterone has dueling effects on sleep-disordered breathing during pregnancy, with a strong sedating effect resulting in increased total sleep time, while increasing the drive for ventilation, which can be protective in the setting of IFL. Cortisol levels are also increased during pregnancy, and are associated with changes in sleep architecture, such as increased REM density and decreased REM latency.

Physical changes during pregnancy, including abdominal distension, fetal movement, bladder distention, urinary frequency, backache, and heartburn, all contribute to increased sleep fragmentation and decreased REM sleep. Weight gain may precipitate or worsen pre-existing sleep apnea. Conversely, increased minute ventilation, preference for the lateral sleep position, and decreased REM sleep time during pregnancy can decrease the risk for OSA (71).

Treatment of OSA with continuous positive airway pressure (CPAP) (see section: Treatment of Obstructive Sleep Apnea) seems to be safe and effective in pregnant women with prepartum-diagnosed OSA. Adherence to therapy is particularly important in this subset of patients because of the risks to the fetus of intermittent hypoxia, sleep fragmentation, and heightened intrathoracic pressure swings with upper airway obstruction. There is indirect evidence that sleep-disordered breathing may be a culprit in pregnancy-related complications, including respiratory distress, hypertension, or preeclampsia. CPAP therapy has been shown to be potentially helpful in relieving preeclampsia in pregnant women who have sleep-disordered breathing (72,73).

Menopause

Menopause is associated with the rapid cessation of ovarian endocrine function, resulting in a reduction of endogenous estrogen and progesterone levels. The prevalence and clinical severity of OSA in women increases dramatically after menopause, with postmenopausal women having nearly double the rate of OSA of that observed in premenopausal women, even when accounting for neck circumference and BMI (74,75). This finding may be a function of heightened disease sensitivity to age in females, changes in upper airway anatomy, and physiology due to hormonal effects, or differences in fat distribution between men and women.

With menopause, there is a change in body habitus and overall fat distribution in females. In one study of 133 obese females (BMI ≥ 30 kg/m^2), postmenopausal women exhibited larger neck circumference and higher waist-to-hip circumference ratios, suggesting changes in fat distribution after menopause (76). Interestingly, postmenopausal women continued to have higher rates of OSA even after accounting for neck circumference and BMI (74,75), implying the increased risk of OSA observed after menopause in women is not completely explained by changes in fat distribution and overall body weight.

Differences in airway function may explain the differences in OSA predisposition between pre- and postmenopausal women. During the waking state, upper airway dilator activity is less in postmenopausal women than in premenopausal women during the luteal phase, when estrogen and progesterone levels are greatest (46). If this observation persists during sleep, then postmenopausal women may have a greater predisposition to upper airway collapse than premenopausal women.

Studies of the effect of hormone replacement therapy (HRT) on OSA risk in postmenopausal women, which can distinguish between hormonal and age effects, report conflicting results. Unopposed estrogen therapy has minimal to no significant effect on OSA severity (74,77), whereas combination of estrogen and progesterone is more effective in reducing apnea and hypopneas, by 50% to 80% (78,79). A large cross-sectional study also showed rates of OSA similar in postmenopausal women on HRT and premenopausal women (0.6% vs. 0.5%, respectively) (74). Other investigators have shown no reduction in overall clinical severity of OSA with either estrogen alone or estrogen plus progesterone, but have shown a modest reduction in apneas during REM (from 58 to 47 events/hour) (80). It is possible that the effect of HRT on OSA may require longer duration of therapy to show a protective effect, as these longitudinal studies were often only two to three months in duration. However, the potential negative effects of HRT preclude the recommendation of HRT for the treatment of OSA in postmenopausal women (81). Progesterone hormone therapy in males with OSA has not proven effective (82,83), suggesting that progesterone alone does not relieve OSA, but the progesterone-deficient state is what may predispose to the development of OSA.

Clinical studies comparing women with natural menopause and women with surgically induced menopause may also be helpful in elucidating the hormone and age effects of menopause on the risk of OSA, but currently these studies have not been published.

TREATMENT OF OBSTRUCTIVE SLEEP APNEA

Treatment considerations for OSA should be tailored to individual patients, and gender differences in treatment options should be factored into this decision. Young et al. (84) demonstrated a significant mortality difference in women diagnosed with OSA, as compared to men, despite comparable disease severity and treatment options. Further work with prospective studies is needed in this area.

Continuous Positive Airway Pressure and Adherence to Therapy

Nasal CPAP is the therapy of choice for OSA. While CPAP therapy is effective for resolving upper airway obstruction, adherence to therapy is overall poor, from 46% to 89% depending on the definition of adherence (85–87). Results of studies to determine the role of gender in predicting adherence to CPAP are conflicting, with men more likely to be adherent to therapy in some (88,89), while women are more likely in others (90). Measures to improve adherence, including warm air, humidification, and education, may improve CPAP adherence (91,92), although differential effects of these interventions by gender have not been investigated.

Oral Appliance Therapy

Oral appliances (OA) are an accepted therapy for OSA in patients with mild to moderate disease. OA typically come in two forms—mandibular advancement devices and tongue retention devices, both of which increase posterior pharyngeal space and relieve upper airway obstruction. Most research has been performed on mandibular advancement devices. In one large prospective study, women with OSA were more likely to have treatment success with OA than men, particularly those with milder forms of OSA (93). Men with OSA treated with OA were more likely to have treatment success when they had predominantly supine-dependent OSA and were more likely to develop treatment failure with even small changes in their BMI. Patients with a higher degree of upper airway collapse (as signified by a greater apnea/hypopnea ratio), as is more commonly seen in men, have decreased treatment benefit with OA (94,95).

Upper Airway Surgery

Upper airway surgery for treatment of OSA includes uvulopalatopharyngoplasty, laser-assisted uvuloplasty, nasal septoplasty, oromaxillofacial surgery, radiofrequency volume tissue reduction, and tracheostomy. Overall, there is controversy as to whether upper airway surgery is an effective treatment for OSA. However, in patients with identifiable upper airway abnormalities, surgical treatments may resolve upper airway obstruction and resolve OSA. There are sparse data regarding potential gender differences in the outcome of upper airway surgery for the treatment of OSA.

Weight Loss

Women with OSA appear to be heavier than their male counterparts. However, in a large community-based study, weight loss was found to be a more effective treatment strategy in men compared to women (96). Perhaps this difference may be explained by gender differences in the distribution of body fat. Men are more likely to gain and lose weight in their upper body, which appears more directly related to upper airway resistance loading.

Bariatric surgery, including gastric bypass, jejunoileal bypass, and gastroplasty, is often recommended for treatment of morbid obesity, particularly when associated with other medical complications. It has been shown to effectively decrease AHI and treat OSA (97). Nearly 80% of patients who undergo bariatric surgery are female. Men are reported to have a higher risk of postoperative mortality (98), and therefore may not be good candidates for this method of weight loss.

CONCLUSIONS

Although OSA is more common in men than women, the prevalence and impact of the disease is certainly significant in women. Variations in presenting symptoms, such as insomnia and depression, often result in misdiagnoses and delay of appropriate treatment. Differences in upper airway collapsibility, ventilatory response to upper airway obstruction, and hormonal effects are the most likely reasons for these differences in OSA by gender. The increased mortality observed in women with OSA compared to men is most concerning, and therefore therapeutic issues related to gender, such as decreased adherence to CPAP therapy and increased efficacy of oral appliance therapy in women, should be factored into the management strategy for treatment of OSA.

REFERENCES

1. Nieto FJ, Young TB, Lind BK, et al. Association of sleep-disordered breathing, sleep apnea, and hypertension in a large community-based study. Sleep Heart Health Study. JAMA 2000; 283(14):1829–1836.
2. Shahar E, Whitney CW, Redline S, et al. Sleep-disordered breathing and cardiovascular disease: cross-sectional results of the Sleep Heart Health Study. Am J Respir Crit Care Med 2001; 163(1):19–25.
3. Newman AB, Nieto FJ, Guidry U, et al. Relation of sleep-disordered breathing to cardiovascular disease risk factors: the Sleep Heart Health Study. Am J Epidemiol 2001; 154(1):50–59.

4. Peker Y, Hedner J, Norum J, et al. Increased incidence of cardiovascular disease in middle-aged men with obstructive sleep apnea: a 7-year follow-up. Am J Respir Crit Care Med 2002; 166(2):159–165.
5. Young T, Peppard PE, Gottlieb DJ. Epidemiology of obstructive sleep apnea: a population health perspective. Am J Respir Crit Care Med 2002; 165(9):1217–1239.
6. Chaudhary BA, Speir WA Jr. Sleep apnea syndromes. South Med J 1982; 75(1):39–45.
7. Young T, Palta M, Dempsey J, et al. The occurrence of sleep-disordered breathing among middle-aged adults. N Engl J Med 1993; 328(17):1230–1235.
8. Leech JA, Onal E, Dulberg C, et al. A comparison of men and women with occlusive sleep apnea syndrome. Chest 1988; 94(5):983–988.
9. Exar EN, Collop NA. The upper airway resistance syndrome. Chest 1999; 115(4): 1127–1139.
10. Guilleminault C, Quera-Salva MA, Partinen M, et al. Women and the obstructive sleep apnea syndrome. Chest 1988; 93(1):104–109.
11. Redline S, Kump K, Tishler PV, et al. Gender differences in sleep disordered breathing in a community-based sample. Am J Respir Crit Care Med 1994; 149(3 Pt 1):722–726.
12. Tishler PV, Larkin EK, Schluchter MD, et al. Incidence of sleep-disordered breathing in an urban adult population: the relative importance of risk factors in the development of sleep-disordered breathing. JAMA 2003; 289(17):2230–2237.
13. O'Connor C, Thornley KS, Hanly PJ. Gender differences in the polysomnographic features of obstructive sleep apnea. Am J Respir Crit Care Med 2000; 161(5):1465–1472.
14. Ware JC, McBrayer RH, Scott JA. Influence of sex and age on duration and frequency of sleep apnea events. Sleep 2000; 23(2):165–170.
15. Strohl KP, Redline S. Recognition of obstructive sleep apnea. Am J Respir Crit Care Med 1996; 154(2 Pt 1):279–289.
16. Brooks LJ, Strohl KP. Size and mechanical properties of the pharynx in healthy men and women. Am Rev Respir Dis 1992; 146(6):1394–1397.
17. Quintana-Gallego E, Carmona-Bernal C, Capote F, et al. Gender differences in obstructive sleep apnea syndrome: a clinical study of 1166 patients. Respir Med 2004; 98(10): 984–989.
18. Shepertycky MR, Banno K, Kryger MH. Differences between men and women in the clinical presentation of patients diagnosed with obstructive sleep apnea syndrome. Sleep 2005; 28(3):309–314.
19. Duran J, Esnaola S, Rubio R, et al. Obstructive sleep apnea–hypopnea and related clinical features in a population-based sample of subjects aged 30 to 70 yr. Am J Respir Crit Care Med 2001; 163(3 Pt 1):685–689.
20. Schwab RJ. Genetic determinants of upper airway structures that predispose to obstructive sleep apnea. Respir Physiol Neurobiol 2005; 147(2–3):289–298.
21. Whittle AT, Marshall I, Mortimore IL, et al. Neck soft tissue and fat distribution: comparison between normal men and women by magnetic resonance imaging. Thorax 1999; 54(4):323–328.
22. Ferguson KA, Ono T, Lowe AA, et al. The relationship between obesity and craniofacial structure in obstructive sleep apnea. Chest 1995; 108(2):375–381.
23. Riha RL, Brander P, Vennelle M, et al. A cephalometric comparison of patients with the sleep apnea/hypopnea syndrome and their siblings. Sleep 2005; 28(3):315–320.
24. Mohsenin V. Gender differences in the expression of sleep-disordered breathing: role of upper airway dimensions. Chest 2001; 120(5):1442–1447.
25. Pillar G, Malhotra A, Fogel R, et al. Airway mechanics and ventilation in response to resistive loading during sleep: influence of gender. Am J Respir Crit Care Med 2000; 162(5):1627–1632.
26. Martin SE, Mathur R, Marshall I, et al. The effect of age, sex, obesity and posture on upper airway size. Eur Respir J 1997; 10(9):2087–2090.
27. Mohsenin V. Effects of gender on upper airway collapsibility and severity of obstructive sleep apnea. Sleep Med 2003; 4(6):523–529.
28. Rowley JA, Sanders CS, Zahn BR, et al. Gender differences in upper airway compliance during NREM sleep: role of neck circumference. J Appl Physiol 2002; 92(6):2535–2541.
29. O'Donnell CP, Tankersley CG, Polotsky VP, et al. Leptin, obesity, and respiratory function. Respir Physiol 2000; 119(2–3):163–170.

30. Trinder J, Kay A, Kleiman J, et al. Gender differences in airway resistance during sleep. J Appl Physiol 1997; 83(6):1986–1997.
31. Millman RP, Carlisle CC, McGarvey ST, et al. Body fat distribution and sleep apnea severity in women. Chest 1995; 107(2):362–366.
32. Fogel RB, Malhotra A, Pillar G, et al. Genioglossal activation in patients with obstructive sleep apnea versus control subjects. Mechanisms of muscle control. Am J Respir Crit Care Med 2001; 164(11):2025–2030.
33. Mezzanote WS, Tangel DJ, White DP. Waking genioglossal EMG in sleep apnea patients vs. normal controls (neuromuscular compensatory mechanisms). J Clin Invest 1992; 89:1571–1579.
34. Mezzanote WS, Tangel DJ, White DP. Influence of sleep onset on upper-airway muscle activity in apnea patients vs. normal controls. Am J Respir Crit Care Med 1996; 153: 1880–1887.
35. Jordan AS, Catcheside PG, O'Donoghue FJ, et al. Genioglossus muscle activity at rest and in response to brief hypoxia in healthy men and women. J Appl Physiol 2002; 92(1):410–417.
36. Bao G, Guilleminault C. Upper airway resistance syndrome—one decade later. Curr Opin Pulm Med 2004; 10(6):461–467.
37. White DP, Douglas NJ, Pickett CK, et al. Sexual influence on the control of breathing. J Appl Physiol 1983; 54(4):874–879.
38. White DP, Douglas NJ, Pickett CK, et al. Hypoxic ventilatory response during sleep in normal premenopausal women. Am Rev Respir Dis 1982; 126(3):530–533.
39. White DP, Schneider BK, Santen RJ, et al. Influence of testosterone on ventilation and chemosensitivity in male subjects. J Appl Physiol 1985; 59(5):1452–1457.
40. Zhou XS, Shahabuddin S, Zahn BR, et al. Effect of gender on the development of hypocapnic apnea/hypopnea during NREM sleep. J Appl Physiol 2000; 89(1):192–199.
41. Kunitomo F, Kimura H, Tatsumi K, et al. Sex differences in awake ventilatory drive and abnormal breathing during sleep in eucapnic obesity. Chest 1988; 93(5):968–976.
42. Krishnan V, Pichard L, Patil S, et al. Gender differences in ventilatory response to inspiratory flow limitation during non-rapid eye movement (NREM) sleep. Proceed Am Thoracic Soc 2006; 3:A197.
43. Netzer NC, Eliasson AH, Strohl KP. Women with sleep apnea have lower levels of sex hormones. Sleep Breath 2003; 7(1):25–29.
44. Zwillich CW, Natalino MR, Sutton FD, et al. Effects of progesterone on chemosensitivity in normal men. J Lab Clin Med 1978; 92(2):262–269.
45. Regensteiner JG, Woodard WD, Hagerman DD, et al. Combined effects of female hormones and metabolic rate on ventilatory drives in women. J Appl Physiol 1989; 66(2): 808–813.
46. Popovic RM, White DP. Upper airway muscle activity in normal women: influence of hormonal status. J Appl Physiol 1998; 84(3):1055–1062.
47. Schneider BK, Pickett CK, Zwillich CW, et al. Influence of testosterone on breathing during sleep. J Appl Physiol 1986; 61(2):618–623.
48. Johnson MW, Anch AM, Remmers JE. Induction of the obstructive sleep apnea syndrome in a woman by exogenous androgen administration. Am Rev Respir Dis 1984; 129(6): 1023–1025.
49. Fogel RB, Malhotra A, Pillar G, et al. Increased prevalence of obstructive sleep apnea syndrome in obese women with polycystic ovary syndrome. J Clin Endocrinol Metab 2001; 86(3):1175–1180.
50. Considine RV, Sinha MK, Heiman ML, et al. Serum immunoreactive-leptin concentrations in normal-weight and obese humans. N Engl J Med 1996; 334(5):292–295.
51. Thomas T, Burguera B, Melton LJ III, et al. Relationship of serum leptin levels with body composition and sex steroid and insulin levels in men and women. Metabolism 2000; 49(10):1278–1284.
52. Polotsky VY, Wilson JA, Smaldone MC, et al. Female gender exacerbates respiratory depression in leptin-deficient obesity. Am J Respir Crit Care Med 2001; 164(8 Pt 1): 1470–1475.
53. Berry RB, Gleeson K. Respiratory arousal from sleep: mechanisms and significance. Sleep 1997; 20(8):654–675.

54. Gleeson K, Zwillich C, White DP. Arousal from sleep in response to ventilatory stimuli occurs at a similar degree of ventilatory effort irrespective of the stimulus. Am Rev Respir Dis 1989; 142:295–300.
55. Berry RB, Light RW. Effect of hyperoxia on the arousal response to airway occlusion during sleep in normal subjects. Am Rev Respir Dis 1992; 146(2):330–334.
56. Vincken W, Guilleminault C, Silvestri L, et al. Inspiratory muscle activity as a trigger causing the airways to open in obstructive sleep apnea. Am Rev Respir Dis 1987; 135(2):372–377.
57. Berry RB, Mahutte CK, Light RW. Effect of hypercapnia on the arousal response to airway occlusion during sleep in normal subjects. J Appl Physiol 1993; 74(5):2269–2275.
58. Jordan AS, McEvoy RD, Edwards JK, et al. The influence of gender and upper airway resistance on the ventilatory response to arousal in obstructive sleep apnoea in humans. J Physiol 2004; 558(Pt 3):993–1004.
59. Block AJ. Alcohol ingestion does not cause sleep-disordered breathing in premenopausal women. Alcohol Clin Exp Res 1984; 8(4):397–398.
60. Block AJ, Hellard DW, Slayton PC. Minimal effect of alcohol ingestion on breathing during the sleep of postmenopausal women. Chest 1985; 88(2):181–184.
61. Htoo A, Talwar A, Feinsilver SH, et al. Smoking and sleep disorders. Med Clin North Am 2004; 88(6):1575–1591, xii.
62. Benninger MS. The impact of cigarette smoking and environmental tobacco smoke on nasal and sinus disease: a review of the literature. Am J Rhinol 1999; 13(6):435–438.
63. Anthony JC, Echeagaray-Wagner F. Epidemiologic analysis of alcohol and tobacco use. Alcohol Res Health 2000; 24(4):201–208.
64. Teculescu DB, Caillier I, Perrin P, et al. Snoring in French preschool children. Pediatr Pulmonol 1992; 13(4):239–244.
65. Gaultier C. Sleep-related breathing disorders. 6. Obstructive sleep apnoea syndrome in infants and children: established facts and unsettled issues. Thorax 1995; 50(11):1204–1210.
66. Fuentes-Pradera MA, Sanchez-Armengol A, Capote-Gil F, et al. Effects of sex on sleep-disordered breathing in adolescents. Eur Respir J 2004; 23(2):250–254.
67. Driver HS, McLean H, Kumar DV, et al. The influence of the menstrual cycle on upper airway resistance and breathing during sleep. Sleep 2005; 28(4):449–456.
68. Pien GW, Fife D, Pack AI, et al. Changes in symptoms of sleep-disordered breathing during pregnancy. Sleep 2005; 28(10):1299–1305.
69. Mabry RL. Rhinitis of pregnancy. South Med J 1986; 79(8):965–971.
70. Ellegard EK. Clinical and pathogenetic characteristics of pregnancy rhinitis. Clin Rev Allergy Immunol 2004; 26(3):149–159.
71. Pien GW, Schwab RJ. Sleep disorders during pregnancy. Sleep 2004; 27(7):1405–1417.
72. Edwards N, Blyton DM, Kirjavainen T, et al. Nasal continuous positive airway pressure reduces sleep-induced blood pressure increments in preeclampsia. Am J Respir Crit Care Med 2000; 162(1):252–257.
73. Connolly G, Razak AR, Hayanga A, et al. Inspiratory flow limitation during sleep in pre-eclampsia: comparison with normal pregnant and nonpregnant women. Eur Respir J 2001; 18(4):672–676.
74. Bixler EO, Vgontzas AN, Lin HM, et al. Prevalence of sleep-disordered breathing in women: effects of gender. Am J Respir Crit Care Med 2001; 163(3 Pt 1):608–613.
75. Dancey DR, Hanly PJ, Soong C, et al. Impact of menopause on the prevalence and severity of sleep apnea. Chest 2001; 120(1):151–155.
76. Resta O, Bonfitto P, Sabato R, et al. Prevalence of obstructive sleep apnoea in a sample of obese women: effect of menopause. Diabetes Nutr Metab 2004; 17(5):296–303.
77. Polo-Kantola P, Rauhala E, Helenius H, et al. Breathing during sleep in menopause: a randomized, controlled, crossover trial with estrogen therapy. Obstet Gynecol 2003; 102(1):68–75.
78. Keefe DL, Watson R, Naftolin F. Hormone replacement therapy may alleviate sleep apnea in menopausal women: a pilot study. Menopause 1999; 6(3):196–200.
79. Pickett CK, Regensteiner JG, Woodard WD, et al. Progestin and estrogen reduce sleep-disordered breathing in postmenopausal women. J Appl Physiol 1989; 66(4):1656–1661.

80. Cistulli PA, Barnes DJ, Grunstein RR, et al. Effect of short-term hormone replacement in the treatment of obstructive sleep apnoea in postmenopausal women. Thorax 1994; 49(7):699–702.

81. Collop NA, Adkins D, Phillips BA. Gender differences in sleep and sleep-disordered breathing. Clin Chest Med 2004; 25(2):257–268.

82. Cook WR, Benich JJ, Wooten SA. Indices of severity of obstructive sleep apnea syndrome do not change during medroxyprogesterone acetate therapy. Chest 1989; 96(2):262–266.

83. Rajagopal KR, Abbrecht PH, Jabbari B. Effects of medroxyprogesterone acetate in obstructive sleep apnea. Chest 1986; 90(6):815–821.

84. Young T, Finn L. Epidemiological insights into the public health burden of sleep disordered breathing: sex differences in survival among sleep clinic patients. Thorax 1998; 53(suppl 3):S16–S19.

85. Hoffstein V, Viner S, Mateika S, et al. Treatment of obstructive sleep apnea with nasal continuous positive airway pressure. Patient compliance, perception of benefits, and side effects. Am Rev Respir Dis 1992; 145(4 Pt 1):841–845.

86. Krieger J, Kurtz D, Petiau C, et al. Long-term compliance with CPAP therapy in obstructive sleep apnea patients and in snorers. Sleep 1996; 19(9 suppl):S136–S143.

87. Meurice JC, Dore P, Paquereau J, et al. Predictive factors of long-term compliance with nasal continuous positive airway pressure treatment in sleep apnea syndrome. Chest 1994; 105(2):429–433.

88. McArdle N, Devereux G, Heidarnejad H, et al. Long-term use of CPAP therapy for sleep apnea/hypopnea syndrome. Am J Respir Crit Care Med 1999; 159(4 Pt 1):1108–1114.

89. Pelletier-Fleury N, Rakotonanahary D, Fleury B. The age and other factors in the evaluation of compliance with nasal continuous positive airway pressure for obstructive sleep apnea syndrome. A Cox's proportional hazard analysis. Sleep Med 2001; 2(3):225–232.

90. Sin DD, Mayers I, Man GC, et al. Long-term compliance rates to continuous positive airway pressure in obstructive sleep apnea: a population-based study. Chest 2002; 121(2):430–435.

91. Massie CA, Hart RW, Peralez K, et al. Effects of humidification on nasal symptoms and compliance in sleep apnea patients using continuous positive airway pressure. Chest 1999; 116(2):403–408.

92. Likar LL, Panciera TM, Erickson AD, et al. Group education sessions and compliance with nasal CPAP therapy. Chest 1997; 111(5):1273–1277.

93. Marklund M, Stenlund H, Franklin KA. Mandibular advancement devices in 630 men and women with obstructive sleep apnea and snoring: tolerability and predictors of treatment success. Chest 2004; 125(4):1270–1278.

94. Schmidt-Nowara W, Lowe A, Wiegand L, et al. Oral appliances for the treatment of snoring and obstructive sleep apnea: a review. Sleep 1995; 18(6):501–510.

95. Engleman HM, McDonald JP, Graham D, et al. Randomized crossover trial of two treatments for sleep apnea/hypopnea syndrome: continuous positive airway pressure and mandibular repositioning splint. Am J Respir Crit Care Med 2002; 166(6):855–859.

96. Newman AB, Foster G, Givelber R, et al. Progression and regression of sleep-disordered breathing with changes in weight: the sleep heart health study. Arch Intern Med 2005; 165(20):2408–2413.

97. Rasheid S, Banasiak M, Gallagher SF, et al. Gastric bypass is an effective treatment for obstructive sleep apnea in patients with clinically significant obesity. Obes Surg 2003; 13(1):58–61.

98. Livingston EH, Huerta S, Arthur D, et al. Male gender is a predictor of morbidity and age a predictor of mortality for patients undergoing gastric bypass surgery. Ann Surg 2002; 236(5):576–582.

15   Obstructive Sleep Apnea in Children

Rafael Pelayo
Stanford University Center of Excellence for Sleep Disorders, Stanford, California, U.S.A.

Kasey K. Li
Sleep Apnea Surgery Center, East Palo Alto, California, U.S.A.

INTRODUCTION

Pediatric sleep medicine has evolved into a major field of study (1). One of the most important conditions in this field is sleep-related breathing disorders (SRBD), which comprise a spectrum of disease ranging from simple snoring to potentially life-threatening obstructive sleep apnea (OSA). This clinical spectrum can occur at any age. Many clinicians learn that OSA emerged from the study of Pickwickian syndrome. However, it is important to point out that in Charles Dickens' first novel, *The Posthumous Papers of the Pickwick Club*, the classic description of snoring with arousals and excessive daytime sleepiness was not of Mr. Pickwick (although he probably did have OSA) but instead it was the boy, Joe, who constantly falls asleep in any situation at any time of day. The first medical description in English of children with abnormal breathing in sleep is attributed to William Osler (2) in his 1892 textbook. Osler wrote a dramatic description of the condition: "Chronic enlargement of the tonsillar tissue is an affection of great importance, and may influence in an extraordinary way the mental and bodily development of children. At night the child's sleep is greatly disturbed, the respirations are loud and snoring, and there is sometimes prolonged pauses, followed by deep, noisy inspiration. The child may wake up in a paroxysm of shortness of breath.... In long-standing cases the child is very stupid-looking, responds slowly to questions, and may be sullen and cross."

In the modern medical literature, Guilleminault (3) reported the first series of children with OSA in 1976. That report describes the essential clinical features of this condition. Eight children, 5 to 14 years of age, were diagnosed using nocturnal polysomnograms. Guilleminault wrote that excessive daytime sleepiness, decrease in school performance, abnormal daytime behavior, enuresis, morning headache, abnormal weight, and progressive development of hypertension should suggest the possibility of a sleep apnea syndrome when any of these symptoms is associated with loud snoring interrupted by pauses during sleep. Surgery was advocated to eliminate the symptoms.

More recently, there has been a realization that patients may be symptomatic in the absence of frank apneas (4,5). This has led to use of the term "sleep-disordered breathing (SDB)" to better describe the clinical spectrum, which includes OSA, upper airway resistance syndrome (UARS), and sleep hypopnea syndrome.

The management of pediatric sleep disorders may appear to some clinicians as time consuming and impractical but it can be a very rewarding experience. Sleep disorders in children are relatively common and readily treatable. However, as the modern practice of sleep medicine has grown many sleep clinicians have a background in adult pulmonary medicine and may feel uncomfortable or hesitant caring for small children. On the other hand, for most pediatricians sleep medicine does not play a large role in their training curriculum or postgraduate education (6). Since most clinicians reading this text predominately treat adults it is important to first review the broader concepts of pediatric sleep medicine before focusing on SRBD. The reader should keep in mind that most sleep disorders have familial patterns. Adults with sleep disorders may have children with sleep disorders. Children with sleep disorders may have parents with sleep disorders. *If you are not providing care to the children in your community then who is?* From the outset of the modern history of clinical sleep medicine the treatment of children was an integral part of the comprehensive care provided at the Stanford University Sleep Disorders Clinic (3) and young children were among the clinic's first patients. Unfortunately, our general pediatric colleagues are unlikely to have adequate expertise for the comprehensive care of these disorders. For this reason the American Board of Sleep Medicine has always included pediatrics as a required area of study. All sleep medicine experts are strongly encouraged to include the care of children to their clinical skills.

Current knowledge of sleep disorders in children has not been incorporated into most medical training programs. This reality is hard to reconcile with the high prevalence of sleep disorders in children. Sleep problems represent one of the most frequent complaints of parents (7,8). Persistent problems contribute to maternal depression, parenting stress, and subsequent child behavior problems (9). The 1993 National Commission on Sleep Disorders concluded that 25% of parents had some concerns of about their children's sleep (10). One survey estimated that 38% of children had experienced parasomnias such as sleepwalking or sleep terrors, 14% had excessive daytime sleepiness, and 11% had SDB (11).

When a very young child or infant is brought for an evaluation of a possible sleep problem, a common question of the parents or caretakers is whether the problem is due to a behavioral or physical cause. A quick way to attempt to answer the question is to find out if the problem is present only when the child sleeps separate from the parent/care provider or is present regardless of where or with whom the child sleeps. If the problem disappears when the child sleeps with a parent but reappears when the child sleeps alone, a behavioral cause may be more likely. On the other hand, if the problem is always present whenever the child sleeps then a physical cause may be more likely. However, this should only be used as a part of an initial diagnostic algorithm. Often, the sleep problem is neither purely behavioral nor purely physical, but rather represents a combination of these factors.

Another common question asked about a child's sleep is: *"how much time does my child need to sleep?"* The focus should not be solely on the time or quantity but ultimately the overall quality of the sleep need to be considered. To determine if an older child is getting enough sleep the first question that needs to be answered is: *"does the child awaken spontaneously feeling refreshed?"* One of the authors (RP) recalls a three-year-old boy that said: "Doctor, sleeping makes me tired." This child realized that despite being told many times that he needed to sleep to have energy in the morning he felt worse when he woke up than when he went to bed. He turned out to have OSA secondary to adenotonsillar hypertrophy. This case illustrates the importance of not focusing only on the total sleep time but the overall sleep quality.

When a child has trouble sleeping, parents will often turn to a variety of paperback advice books on the market. The quality of advice offered is quite variable and conflicting. Clinicians should be aware of the advice put forth by the more popular books since parents may quote or have specific questions about the material as it applies to their child. Also parents are unlikely to seek a clinician's opinion if the advice book has solved the problem, so the questions that do arise are sometimes the result of frustration or confusion about what the parents have read. Often these books do not provide any long-term longitudinal data about the amount of time that a normal child spends sleeping at different ages.

NORMAL SLEEP IN CHILDREN

The basic principles of normal sleep are the same for children and adults. Normal sleep can be simply described as the ability to fall asleep easily, sleep through the night, and wake up feeling refreshed.

Long-term longitudinal data have been published by Iglowstein et al. (12) to illustrate the developmental course and age-specific variability of sleep patterns. As part of the Zurich Longitudinal Studies, they followed 493 children for 16 years. The study used structured sleep-related questionnaires at 1, 3, 6, 9, 12, 18, and 24 months after birth and then at annual intervals until 16 years of age. Total sleep duration decreased from an average of 14.2 hours [standard deviation (SD)=1.9 hours] at six months of age to an average of 8.1 hours (SD=0.8 hours) at 16 years of age. Total sleep duration decreased across the studied cohorts (1974–1993) because bedtime became later, but wake time remained essentially unchanged. Between 1.5 years and 4 years of age, there was a prominent decline in napping habits. At 1.5 years of age 96.4% of children had naps; by four years of age only 35.4% napped.

This is consistent with a prior study of napping patterns by Weissbluth (13). Napping patterns were monitored in a cohort of 172 children followed from six months to seven years of age. There were no differences in the number of naps at six months of age or the pattern of napping based on gender, birth order, and whether naps disappeared spontaneously or were stopped by the parents. Total daytime sleep remained a stable individual characteristic between 6 and 18 months of age. A pattern of two naps per day was well-established by 9 to 12 months of age and one afternoon nap by 15 to 24 months. The duration of naps from two to six years was two hours. During the third and fourth year, napping occurred in the majority of children, but at decreasing rates. A minority of children was napping by five to six years and naps usually disappeared by age seven. If a child continues to nap by the age of seven years, it is possible that a sleep disorder may be present. Naps may not be called naps but rather reported as falling asleep while riding home from school.

However, napping behavior must be put into a cultural and possibly racial context. It would be less concerning if napping or "siestas" are part of the child's cultural environment. A more recent survey of napping patterns reported remarkable racial differences in reported napping and night-time sleep patterns beginning as early as age three and extending to at least eight years of age (14). In this study a more gradual age-related decline in napping was found for black children. At age 8, 39.1% of black children were reported to nap, compared with only 4.9% of white children. Black children also napped significantly more days per week, had shorter average nocturnal sleep durations, and slept significantly less on weekday nights than on weekend nights. Despite differences in sleep distribution, total weekly sleep duration (diurnal and nocturnal) was nearly identical for the two racial groups at each year of age.

The information on sleep and napping patterns is usually obtained from parental report. A study from Brown University combined parental sleep diaries with objective information from actigraphy (15). This study consisted of 169 normal children from 12 months to 60 months of age. This cross-sectional sample of children wore actigraphs for one week while their mothers kept concurrent diaries. Bedtimes and sleep start times were earliest, and time in bed and sleep period times were longest for 12-month-old children. Rise time, sleep end time, and nocturnal sleep minutes did not differ across age groups. Actigraphic estimates indicated that children aged one to five years slept an average of 8.7 hours at night. Actigraph-based nocturnal wake minutes and wake bouts were higher than maternal diary reports for all age groups. Daytime naps decreased across age groups and accounted for most of the difference in 24-hour total sleep over age groups. Children in families with lower socioeconomic status had later rise times, longer time in bed, more nocturnal wake minutes and bouts, and more night-to-night variability in bedtime and sleep period time. Not surprisingly, this study reported children with longer naps slept less at night.

In adults and most children, rapid eye movement (REM) periods occur in cycles of approximately 90 minutes throughout the night. REM latencies may be longer in younger children (16). New data suggest that the length of the REM/non-REM (NREM) cycle fluctuates with age (17). At the end of every REM cycle there is usually an arousal or brief awakening. In infants REM cycles are shorter (approximately 40–60 minutes). Parents may be concerned that their infant seems to "wake up every hour." These brief awakenings may be part of the child's normal rhythm but an overly attentive parent may inadvertently reinforce and prolonged the awakenings. On the other hand, it is possible that the child's awakenings are due to a condition that is exacerbated by REM sleep such as OSA. The percent of the total sleep time spent in REM decreases from birth when it may take up 50% of the total sleep time to approximately 20% at three years of age. It remains at this percent throughout adulthood.

Delta or slow-wave sleep represents our deepest sleep as measured by the arousal threshold (amount of stimulation needed to wake up the sleeper). Delta sleep has homeostatic properties: it increases in duration and intensity in response to sleep deprivation. The amount of delta sleep is at least 10% of the total sleep time in children and decreases after adolescence. It clusters in the first third of the night. During delta sleep it is extremely difficult to arouse children. If aroused, they often appear disoriented and cognitively slowed. Parasomnias such as sleepwalking and sleep terrors usually emerge from slow-wave sleep and in children commonly occur in the first third of the night.

GENERAL PRINCIPLES

Sleep disorders should be considered whenever a child is being evaluated for a behavioral problem. Insufficient quality or quantity of sleep may be associated with learning difficulties and attention problems (8,18–23). When a child does not sleep well it can disrupt the entire household and lead to significant stress for the family (24–26). Unrecognized and under-treated sleep disturbances may carry over into adulthood (27).

In pediatrics, a medical history usually starts with the history of the pregnancy and delivery. However, an adequate history of a child's sleep disorder should begin with a history of the sleep patterns of the parents/caretakers before they were ever parents. For example, if an infant sleeps continuously for seven hours at night and the mother was in the habit of sleeping 6.5 hours before the pregnancy she might be pleased with the way the child is sleeping. However, if the mother usually slept for eight or nine hours she might complain that the child is not sleeping enough at night. If a parent had a history of occasional insomnia before the infant was born, the parent might be overly sensitized to interruptions of sleep by the infant, whereas another parent might find the disruption more tolerable. A parent who has a history of snoring or mild OSA might be less able to tolerate what would otherwise be considered normal or expected interruptions of sleep by a child.

The child and family's cultural background must be taken into account when evaluating a complaint of poor sleep. Also the influence of other family members or caretakers, such as grandparents, in shaping the family's views should be considered. The parents need to agree about their expectations of the child's sleep, especially if the parents come from different cultural backgrounds. The individual parent (mother or father) may view the infant's sleep pattern from quite different perspectives.

In any evaluation, it is crucial to keep in mind the interaction between the physiological need for sleep and the psychology of sleep. All of us sleep best when we go to sleep feeling safe and comfortable. We learn to feel this way by forming associations with our sleeping environment and these associations are formed starting from infancy. Infant and children, like adults, may develop maladaptive associations that result in sleep difficulties. When evaluating school-age children for a sleep problem it is important to ask the child directly if he or she is scared of the dark or of being alone. The parents may minimize these concerns and the children may be too embarrassed to volunteer the information.

It is not uncommon in a clinical situation to have two or more sleep disorders interacting in the same patient. A child may have an awakening due to difficulty breathing from sleep apnea, but then be unable to return to sleep because he or she has not learned to settle back down without the parents' intervention.

PHARMACOLOGICAL GUIDELINES

There is relatively little information available on the pharmacological management of sleep disorders in children. Most pharmacological guidelines were developed for sleep disorders in adults and must be empirically extrapolated to children. The medications are typically neither Food and Drug Administration (FDA)-approved for the specific sleep disorder nor for the pediatric age range. The physician is often forced to prescribe medications as an "off label" indication. This may result in frustrating insurance reimbursement delays or denials for the family (28). These reimbursement problems may affect the availability of a specific medication, the family's adherence with the medication or force the physician to prescribe a less desirable alternative medication (29). The medication may not be available commercially in an easily administered format. Very young children may not be able to swallow pills, and may require the pharmacist to compound the medication into a suspension. In addition, due to the natural aversion among both parents and physicians to use medications for pediatric sleep disorders, medications are usually prescribed as a last resort or in the most refractory situations. Fortunately, this situation may be changing as the FDA is requesting more pediatric data from newly approved drugs and we may expect more pediatric clinical drug trials in the future (30).

At times, a decision to use medication in a child may be made not necessarily to assist the child as much as to help the parents or other family members sleep better. It is not unusual that parents may finally seek help for a child's long-standing sleep problem when the parents feel they can no longer put up with interruptions to their own sleep. Further complicating the pharmacological treatment of sleep disorders in children is the general lack of specialized training in sleep disorders available to the healthcare providers who are working with these children. Failure to consider or properly apply nondrug treatments as part of the comprehensive management of the child may also lead to unsatisfactory results. These factors may result in children that are not properly managed due to either underdosing or overdosing of medication, or incorrect medication selection.

There may be an over-reliance on the effects of the medication by both the parents and healthcare provider without adequate application of behavioral techniques to help improve the child's sleep. A common scenario in clinical practice is parents' complaint of a child's paradoxical reaction to a hypnotic medication. "It made it worse" or "he became hyper" may be the parents' complaint. This may occur because the timing or the dose provided was incorrect. The parents may expect that once a medication has been finally prescribed to help their child sleep that it will "knockout" the child. It is important that the healthcare provider advising this family take into account the circadian modulation of alertness. Humans will typically experience an enhanced alertness in the evening. If a hypnotic is given during this circadian time window, the medication may not work or the child may be frightened by hypnagogic hallucinations. If a medication has been previously shown to shorten sleep latency by only 20 or 30 minutes, giving this medication two or three hours prior to the usual falling asleep time could elicit this common scenario. This same medication given at a more appropriate circadian time could be effective. Children may also be given a medication and then be allowed to play or watch television until the medication "kicks in." This may also result in frightening hypnagogic hallucinatory phenomenon.

This lack of proper management of the sleep problem may be particularly common among children with neurological or psychiatric disabilities (31–34). If the child cannot communicate what they feel is causing the sleep difficulty incorrect assumptions may be made by the family and/or healthcare provider. In cases of insomnia, this can result in an escalating cycle of progressively more sedating agents with increasing likelihood of adverse effects. Concomitant daytime sedation may occur which may interfere with the child's therapeutic program and exacerbate the child's disabilities. In some situations, the fear of putative addiction may limit the physician or the family from using pharmacotherapy adequately to improve the child's sleep.

SLEEP-RELATED BREATHING DISORDERS
Clinical Features
Although SRBD in children have many important similarities to the adult versions of these diseases, there are also marked differences in presentation, diagnosis, and management (Table 1). While awake breathing is typically silent, and the most obvious of nocturnal SRBD is snoring. Snoring indicates turbulent airflow and is not normal in children (21,35–39). The American Academy of Pediatrics (AAP) has recommended all children should be screened for snoring as part of well child care (40). *If a sleeping animal is vulnerable to be attacked by a predator, why would it make breathing noises when its guard is down?* Indeed animals in the wild do not seem to snore; only domestic animals snore. Not all snoring is due to OSA. It may be due to other forms of obstruction such as nasal allergies or a cold (41,42).

The prevalence of SDB in children was studied by Rosen et al. (43), who performed a cross-sectional study of school-aged children in a Cleveland cohort. The cohort consisted of 829 children, 8 to 11 years old, all of whom had unattended in-home overnight cardiorespiratory sleep recordings. SDB was defined by either parent-reported habitual snoring or objectively-measured OSA. Forty (5%) children

TABLE 1 Comparison of Sleep-Related Breathing Disorders in
Adults Vs. Children

	Adults	Children
Symptoms	Sleepiness, fatigue, nocturia	Behavioral problems, learning difficulty, nocturnal enuresis
Gender	More common and severe in males	No difference prior to puberty
Physical findings	Obese, large neck circumference	High-arched palate, enlarged tonsils, orthodontic problems, less likely obese, failure to thrive
Apnea duration	10 seconds	Two breaths
Diagnostic criteria	AHI $\geq$ 5	AHI $\geq$ 1
Primary treatment	Positive airway pressure	Adenotonsillectomy

Abbreviation: AHI, apnea-hypopnea index.

were classified as having OSA [median apnea–hypopnea index (AHI) = 7.1 per hour], and another 122 (15%) had primary snoring without OSA. The remaining 667 (80%) had neither snoring nor OSA. Functional outcomes were assessed with two parent ratings scales of behavior problems: the Child Behavioral Checklist and the Conners Parent Rating Scale-Revised:Long. Children with SDB had significantly higher odds of elevated problem scores in the following domains: externalizing, hyperactive, emotional lability, oppositional, aggressive, internalizing, somatic complaints, and social problems. The authors concluded that children with relatively mild SDB, ranging from primary snoring to OSA, have a higher prevalence of problem behaviors, with the strongest, most consistent associations for externalizing, hyperactive-type behaviors. An interesting finding in this study was that only 55% of the parents of children diagnosed by polysomnography with OSA reported loud snoring. If pediatricians and surgeons screen for OSA by asking the parents/ caregiver if the child snores loudly, they may miss close to half of the cases (44).

The daytime behavior is an important difference between adults and children with SDB. The abnormal daytime sleepiness may be recognized more often by schoolteachers than by parents of young children. An increase in total sleep time or an extra-long nap may be considered as normal by parents. Nonspecific behavioral difficulties are mentioned to the pediatrician such as abnormal shyness, hyperactivity, developmental delays, rebellious or aggressive behavior (45). Chervin et al. found conduct problems and hyperactivity are frequent among children referred for SDB during sleep. They surveyed parents of children aged 2 to 14 years at two general clinics between 1998 and 2000. Parents of 872 children completed the surveys. Bullying and other specific aggressive behaviors were generally two to three times more frequent among children at high risk for SDB (46). Other daytime symptoms may include speech defects, poor appetite, or swallowing difficulties (4,47). Nocturnal enuresis or bedwetting accidents should raise suspicion of possible SDB (48).

Many of these children are mouth breathing. Regular mouth breathing should always lead to suspicion of SDB (49). Children with SDB may avoid going to bed at night due to hypnagogic hallucinations. Upon awakening these children may report morning headaches, dry mouth, confusion or irritability. As mentioned, daytime sleepiness may not be obvious depending on the age. It may translate only as a complaint of daytime tiredness or may also present itself as a tendency to take naps easily anywhere.

A study from Israel found that children with SDB had lower scores on neuro-cognitive testing compared to controls but the scores improve after treatment (23). This prospective study of 39 children aged five to nine years underwent a battery of neurocognitive tests containing process-oriented intelligence scales. Children with SDB had lower scores compared with healthy children in some Kaufman Assessment Battery for Children (K-ABC) subtests and in the general scale Mental Processing Composite, indicating impaired neurocognitive function. Six to 10 months after adenotonsillectomy, the children with OSAs demonstrated significant improvement in sleep characteristics, as well as in daytime behavior. Their neurocognitive perfor-mance improved considerably, reaching the level of the control group in the sub-tests Gestalt Closure, Triangles, Word Order, and the Matrix analogies, as well as in the K-ABC general scales, Sequential and Simultaneous Processing scales, and the Mental Processing Composite scale. The authors concluded neurocognitive func-tion is impaired in otherwise healthy children with SDB. Most functions improve to the level of the control group, indicating that the impaired neurocognitive functions are mostly reversible, at least 3 to 10 months following adenotonsillectomy (23). An abrupt and persistent deterioration in grades must also raise the question of abnormal sleep and SDB (20,21,50,51).

In schools the tiredness and sleepiness may be labeled as "inattentiveness in class," "daydreaming," or "not being there" (22,52). Concerns about school perfor-mance were raised in the original description of OSA syndrome in children (3). More recently, the possible association between SDB, learning problems, and atten-tion-deficit disorder has been studied (8,18,19,21,22,52–56). A study by Gozal et al. examined the hypothesis that domains of neurobehavioral function would be selec-tively affected by SDB. They study children with reported symptoms of attention-deficit/hyperactivity disorder (ADHD) and also determined the incidence of snoring and other sleep problems in 5- to 7-year-old children in a public school system. Children with reported symptoms of ADHD and control children were ran-domly selected for an overnight polysomnographic assessment and a battery of neurocognitive tests. Frequent and loud snoring was reported for 673 children (11.7%). Similarly, 418 (7.3%) children were reported to have hyperactivity/ADHD. Children with reported symptoms of ADHD and control children were randomly selected for an overnight polysomnographic assessment and a battery of neurocog-nitive tests. Eighty-three children with parentally reported symptoms of ADHD had sleep studies together with 34 control children. After assessment with the ADHD subscale of the Conners Parent Rating Scale, 44 children were designated as having "significant" symptoms of ADHD, 27 as "mild," and 39 designated as "none" (con-trols). Overnight polysomnography indicated that OSA was present in 5% of those with significant ADHD symptoms, 26% of those with mild symptoms, and 5% of those with no symptoms. The authors concluded an unusually high prevalence of snoring was identified among a group of children designated as showing mild symptoms of ADHD based on the Conners ADHD subscale. SDB can lead to mild ADHD-like behaviors that can be readily misperceived and potentially delay the diagnosis and appropriate treatment (22).

Additional clinical signs of SDB include increased respiratory efforts with nasal flaring, suprasternal or intercostal retractions, abnormal paradoxical inward motion of the chest occurring during inspiration, and sweating during sleep. The sweating may be limited to only the nuchal region particularly in infants; it may be severe enough to necessitate changing clothes during the night. The parents may mention the child feeling warm at night or preferring to sleep without a blanket.

Parents may also observe the child stop breathing, then gasping for breath. It is surprising to note how often parents have observed abnormal breathing patterns during sleep but were never questioned about it by pediatricians during regular visits. Information regarding the sleep position is helpful. Typically, the neck is hyper-extended and the mouth is open. Another typical sleeping position is prone with the knee tucked under the chest with head turned to the side and hyperextended. Rarely, the child with SDB prefers to sleep propped up on several pillows (4).

Parasomnias may be triggered or exacerbated by SDB. Ohayon (57) has found that individuals identified with SDB have a much higher incidence of nightmares, with reports of "drowning," "being buried alive," and "choking." SDB leads to sleep fragmentation or disruption. Any condition that disrupts slow-wave sleep may lead to sleep terrors and sleepwalking in children (58). SDB should be included in the evaluation of any child with parasomnias.

A physical finding that may be overlooked in a child with SDB is a narrow and high-arched palate (4). Interestingly, the description of attention-deficit disorder in the Diagnostic and Statistical Manual of Mental Disorders (DSM-IV) mentions that minor physical anomalies such as high-arched palates may be present (59). Since both conditions may have similar daytime behavior in the same age group, a child with SDB could be misidentified as having attention-deficit disorder. The possibility of a sleep disorder being present should be considered in any child being evaluated for attention-deficit disorder. This is particularly important since treatment of SDB may improve behavior and academic performance (60,61).

Diagnostic Criteria

The diagnostic criteria used for adults with OSA cannot be used reliably in children (5,49,62,63). The diagnosis of SDB is based on the history, physical findings, and supportive data. Laboratory testing should be, ideally, tailored to the clinical question. For example, if there are concerns about excessive daytime sleepiness, a multiple sleep latency test (MSLT) may be indicated (64). The MSLT is ideally performed in subjects who are at least eight years old.

The polysomnogram in a child uses the same technology and the same type of information as recorded in adults. Airflow, respiratory effort, and pulse oximetry comprise the breathing measurements usually monitored. Breathing can be measured with different techniques, ranging from qualitative techniques such as nasal thermocouples which use the temperature difference between inhaled and exhaled air to record individual breaths, to quantitative and invasive measures such as esophageal pressure measurements. The latter technique is less tolerable than others but is particularly helpful to distinguish central from obstructive apneas. End-tidal CO_2 monitoring is another technique that can help detect transient episodes of hypoventilation. Currently, the technique that balances need for quantification with tolerability is measuring airflow using a nasal pressure cannula (65,66). This technique allows for the identification of more subtle breathing episodes but can be harder to interpret than earlier techniques, in particular when a child is mouth breathing.

This nasal pressure cannula has facilitated the measurement of an additional abnormal respiratory event, RERA, which is an acronym for respiratory event-related arousal. The term respiratory disturbance index (RDI) may now include the total number of apneas, hypopneas, and RERAs divided by the total sleep time. The RDI should be distinguished from the AHI. However, some sleep study reports may equate the RDI with the AHI if the sleep study did not measure RERAs.

The clinician needs to be aware that these terms may be used interchangeably, potentially causing confusion.

The multitude of available techniques to measure breathing makes it difficult to compare the results from different studies. Along with the absence of controlled studies, another problem with understanding pediatric SDB is that definitions for key terms vary. OSAs are defined as lasting at least 10 seconds in adults. However, since children have faster respiratory rates clinically significant apneas can occur in less time (Fig. 1). Apneas as brief as three or four seconds may have oxygen desaturations. There is no universally accepted definition of hypopneas in children. The clinician needs to know how apneas and hypopneas are defined and scored when interpreting a polysomnogram report. The most recent edition of the International Classification of Sleep Disorders (ICSD-2) defines OSA in children as having an AHI ≥ 1 (67). In adults a higher AHI of five is required. Unfortunately it is not uncommon for an adult cutoff value to be used in children (68). There is also controversy as to when the adult cutoff value should be applied; the onset of puberty or the age of 18 years is often debated.

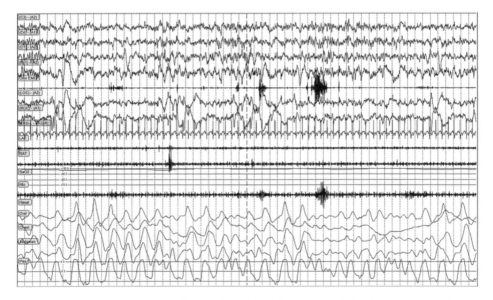

FIGURE 1   Polysomnogram of a 10-year-old girl depicting several obstructive apneas and hypopneas during a 60-second epoch of rapid eye movement (REM) sleep, accompanied by esophageal pressure "crescendos," intermittent snoring (as detected by the Chin EMG and Mic), and oxygen desaturations. Note the rapid respiration rate consistent with that of a child. *Abbreviations*: C3-A2, C4-A1, O1-A2, Fp1-A2, electroencephalogram electrodes placed centrally (C3, C4), occipitally (O1), and fronto-parietally (Fp1), and referenced to the right (A2) or left (A1) ear; Chin EMG, electromyogram recorded from chin muscles; LOC, left eye electro-oculogram; ROC, right eye electro-oculogram; EKG, electrocardiogram; LAT and RAT, electromyogram recorded from the left and right anterior tibialis muscles, respectively; SaO_2, pulse oximetry; Mic, microphone to detect snoring; Nasal, nasal pressure measured by pressure transducer; Oral, oral airflow measured by thermistor; Chest and Abdomen, impedance bands to measure thoracic and abdominal movement, respectively; P_{es}, esophageal pressure to measure transmitted intrathoracic pressure. *Source*: Courtesy of Clete A. Kushida, MD, PhD.

Controversy exists over whether a diagnosis of OSA, or the larger spectrum of SDB, should be routinely made without a formal polysomnogram. While some have suggested that this diagnosis can be made in patients using either the history and physical, or the history, physical, and an audio- or videotape, others have found an inability of clinical history alone to distinguish primary snoring from OSA in children (69). The situation is further complicated by the description of UARS in children, which may have been missed in the studies cited above. Therefore, a sleep study is the most definitive test for SDB (70,71). Currently, some otolaryngologists who treat SDB in children may make the surgical recommendation based on clinical findings of airway obstruction, sometimes reviewing an audio- or videotape (72,73). The clinicians must be aware of the potential pitfalls to this practice. Certainly there are individual cases in which a diagnostic sleep studies are not available, but ideally they should be the exception. The challenge we face in sleep medicine is providing easily-accessible and cost-effective care working within a multidisciplinary model. We do not know, for certain, how accurate clinical diagnosis is without objective testing. Until we have a better answer, the diagnostic gold standard should not be disregarded particularly in a tertiary care setting. The American Thoracic Society, American Academy of Sleep Medicine, and AAP all support the use of sleep studies (70,74,75).

SDB is not the only sleep disorder a child may have. Clinical impression may have both false negatives and positives resulting in possible misdiagnosis or unnecessary surgery. For example, without confirmatory testing, a child with symptomatic periodic limb movements might be misdiagnosed with SDB and may have unnecessary surgery. Periodic limb movements of sleep and restless legs syndrome may not be rare in children (76). These syndromes can have a vague or difficult history to elicit.

Sudden Infant Death Syndrome

Sudden infant death syndrome (SIDS) remains one of the most common causes of death among infants throughout the world. In the United States there has been a major decrease in the incidence of SIDS since the AAP released its recommendation in 1992 that infants be placed down for sleep in a nonprone position. A public health initiative was developed using the slogan "back to sleep." The recommendations also included the need to avoid redundant soft bedding and soft objects in the infant's sleeping environment. The AAP further refined its position in 2000 and no longer recognized side sleeping as a reasonable alternative to fully supine sleeping. In 2005, the AAP again provided further recommendations to decrease the incidence of SIDS. These included recommending that adults do not share a bed with infants. Instead adults should share the bedroom but sleep on a different surface. The AAP also recommended using pacifiers in the beginning of the night but replacing them in the children's mouths if they fell out during the night (77). Concerns have been raised that these newer guidelines may have the unintended consequences of disrupting the sleep of families by the infants creating an association with the need for the pacifiers in order to return to sleep during the night. Other experts have also expressed concerns that discouraging bed sharing may decrease nursing and bonding (78–81).

Sleep-Disordered Breathing in Special Populations

SDB may occur more often in special populations (82–86). Any condition or syndrome associated with craniofacial anomalies may be associated with SDB. Pierre Robin (Fig. 2), Apert's and Crouzon's are among these syndromes. Approximately

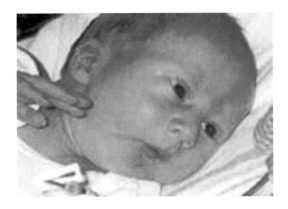

FIGURE 2 (*See color insert.*) Infant with Pierre Robin syndrome; micrognathia, specifically mandibular hypoplasia, as depicted is characteristic of this disorder.

half of all children with Down syndrome have SDB. However, symptoms of day-time sleepiness and sleep disruptions at night may be due to non-neurological factors such as maxillofacial abnormalities, large tonsils or adenoids, micrognathia, large tongues, or other abnormalities. Sleep disorders often occur in patients with neuromuscular disease because of associated weakness in respiratory muscles, which is further exacerbated by hypotonia during sleep. In disorders such as Duchenne's muscular dystrophy, daytime pulmonary function studies do not predict the degree of apneic events during sleep. Rather, these patients can have nocturnal oxygen desaturation, significant sleep fragmentation, recurrent hypoventilation, and reduced REM sleep. These patients are also at increased risk for aspiration during sleep. Diagnosis and treatment of SDB in these patients can be an important part of comprehensive management.

Treatment
Not only are the diagnostic criteria different in children than adults but also the treatment options. SDB in adults has four treatments options which may be combined. The most common treatment is continuous positive airway pressure (CPAP) to help splint open the upper airway (see also Chapter 6). When CPAP is used correctly snoring should be absent during sleep. There are several sophisticated surgical options with a wide range of success (see also Chapter 11). In adults, oral appliances, which help reposition the mandible, have improved breathing during sleep in selected patients (see also Chapter 12). As a conservative measure, adults with SDB are advised to sleep off their backs, lose weight, and avoid alcohol before sleeping (see also Chapter 13).

Unlike adults, in children surgery is the most common treatment for SDB. Adenotonsillectomy is the most common initial treatment for SDB in children (Fig. 3). This procedure can be extremely effective and result in dramatic improvements (and very grateful parents). When surgery is being entertained, as a general rule, the adenoids and tonsils should both be removed during the same surgery. It is tempting in very small children to only remove the adenoids if the tonsils do not appear overly enlarged since this allows for less postoperative pain and lower risk of adverse events such as bleeding. This practice should be discouraged since even though the tonsils do not seem enlarged the surgeon must keep in mind that they are examining a child that is awake and sitting. The relative posterior airway space

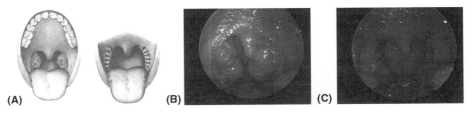

FIGURE 3 (*See color insert.*) (**A**) Schematic diagram illustrating oral cavity before (*left*) and after (*right*) tonsillectomy. (**B**) Patient's oral cavity depicting hypertrophied tonsils. (**C**) Same patient's oral cavity following tonsillectomy.

may be obstructed when the child is supine, the tongue falling back and the airway narrowing during REM sleep hypotonia. Also in a growing child the tonsils may also grow larger. If only the adenoids are removed there is the risk of having to later return for further surgery to remove the tonsils. Clinicians should be aware that there are several different techniques used to remove tonsils and this may play a role in the efficacy of treatment.

The anesthesiologist should be familiar with OSA since postoperative pulmonary complications can occur (87). Children with OSA are often thinner than expected. This is may be due to multiple factors including the greater caloric demand of breathing through a narrow airway and possible disruption of growth hormone secretion. Children after OSA surgery may unexpectedly increase their weight (88).

Surgery does not always completely cure the child's SDB. The true cure rate of this surgery for SDB is unknown (23,28,89,90). Most studies that have performed postsurgical sleep studies have used older adult definitions of sleep apnea in the children. Suen et al. designed a prospective study of 69 children aged 1 to 14 years who were referred to an otolaryngologist. Of the 69 children 35 (51%) had a RDI > 5 on polysomnography. Thirty children with a RDI > 5 underwent adenotonsillectomy. Of the 30 children 26 had follow-up polysomnography following surgery. All 26 children had a lower RDI after surgery, although four patients still had a RDI > 5. Using a RDI cut off of 5, the cure rate of surgery would be 85%. However, three children snored with postoperative RDI < 5. If those subjects were considered to have residual SDB then the cure rate of surgery would only be 73%. All patients improved with adenotonsillectomy but the true cure rate is not clear. The possibility of residual SDB should always be considered after surgery if the child is symptomatic. Suen et al. concluded history and physical findings were not useful in predicting outcome (91). Different surgical techniques may improve the success of surgery in these children (92).

Some may argue that patients with clear-cut cases of SDB may skip the postoperative sleep study. However, the adult experience teaches us that it is precisely these obviously more severe or "clear-cut" cases that will have residual disease. Adenotonsillectomy will not change the relationship of tongue size and shape to the palate. The parents may report that the child is "100% better" yet still has residual obstruction. If the child still has trouble paying attention in school, a sleep problem may be overlooked and no longer be considered a possibility. The child may end up labeled as having attention-deficit disorder because there was no postoperative sleep test done (36,93).

CPAP therapy should be considered if surgery is not a viable option for the child (94–96) (Fig. 4). CPAP uses a small air compressor attached to a mask via a

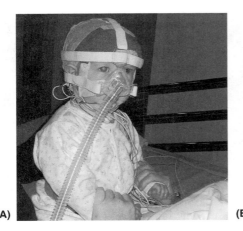 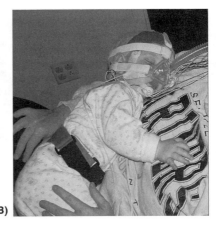

(A)   **(B)**

FIGURE 4   (*See color insert.*) (**A**) Child awake and (**B**) asleep while wearing a continuous positive airway pressure mask during polysomnographic monitoring in a sleep laboratory. Note wires connected to recording electrodes that are placed on the face and on the scalp, which are hidden beneath the head wraps used to prevent dislodgement of electrodes.

hose. The mask usually only covers the nose but masks are available that cover the nose and mouth. By forcing positive air pressure in the airway, the negative pressure of inspiration can be countered to avoid airway narrowing or collapse. CPAP is effective but can be cumbersome to use. Over time the CPAP devices have become smaller and quieter. The masks have also improved with many more styles and sizes available. In the recent past in the United States there was no CPAP mask certified for home use in children. Clinicians needed to obtain the mask from outside of the country or used the smallest available adult mask. This has now changed. CPAP has been approved for home use in children in the United States. A wider range of mask sizes and styles should now become available.

Despite these advances CPAP remains a second choice over surgery in most children (70). This is due to the advantage of having a surgical option. The main drawbacks of using CPAP are related to getting a proper-fitting CPAP mask. If the mask is not fitted correctly the air pressure may leak out causing discomfort and sleep disruption. If the mask is too tight it can cause facial abrasions or bruising. In small children the possibility of the CPAP mask interfering with growth of the maxilla should be considered. As the child grows CPAP may require adjustments both in terms of mask size and the amount of pressure delivered to the airway. In addition to a continuous pressure delivery mode, a bilevel mode [bilevel positive airway pressure, (BPAP)] is available. In this mode, the pressure on expiration is lowered from the inspiratory pressure (see also Chapter 7). This may allow the device to be more comfortable and may be preferred in patients with neuromuscular weakness. The most recent advance in positive airway pressure has been the development of machines, which can adjust the pressure required to keep the airway open on a breath-by-breath basis. These so-called "smart CPAP" or auto-positive airway pressure units (see also Chapter 8) are promising but are not part of the mainstream treatment of children at this time (94).

The treatment of residual or persistent OSA after surgery is a difficult clinical situation. CPAP has been the recommended option yet CPAP can be cumbersome.

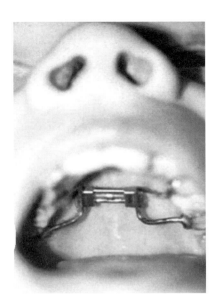

FIGURE 5 (*See color insert.*) Maxillary osteogenic distraction device placed below the palate of a child's mouth. *Source*: Photograph courtesy of Kannan Ramar, MD.

If a child has clinically significant SDB after adenotonsillectomy and CPAP is not an option or not tolerated the clinician had been forced to consider more aggressive surgery such as a tracheostomy or palliative use of supplemental oxygen. A search for better alternatives is underway. The application of more sophisticated surgical techniques with the possible use of orthodontic treatments is being pursued (97–100). In adults with persistent sleep apnea after a uvulopalatoplasty the remaining obstruction is often at the level of the base of the tongue. This may be due to a combination of retrognathia and a narrow hard palate. The most effective surgical correction at this level of obstruction is bilateral maxillo-mandibular advancement. This surgery is not advised for the growing bones of young children.

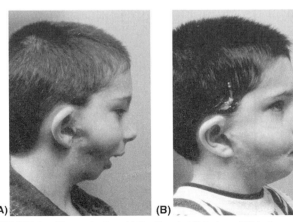

(A)   **(B)**

FIGURE 6 (*See color insert.*) Profile of child's face (**A**) before and (**B**) after mandibular distraction osteogenesis.

The base of tongue obstruction can be minimized in some children with rapid maxillary expansion (99,101). By widening the child's palate the tongue can fit into its natural position on the hard palate and be less likely to slide back into the hypopharynx (Fig. 5). This procedure is most effective when there is a significant narrow and high-arched palate. Such osteogenic distraction techniques are very promising. These techniques were traditionally reserved in children with cranio-facial anomalies to lengthen bones. These techniques are starting to be adapted for persistent SDB to bring the mandible forward and increase the posterior airway space in the pharynx (Fig. 6).

CONCLUSIONS

There are important similarities and differences between SRBD in adults and children. SDB may manifest in children with daytime behavioral problems. It is important for clinicians to be aware that snoring is unlikely to be normal in a child. Diagnostic criteria in children recognize an AHI ≥ 1 as abnormal. Unlike adults, surgery is the primary treatment for children. Residual SDB is possible after surgery. Treatment options are evolving for this situation and may involve all modalities of positive airway pressure, further surgery and/or orthodontic procedures.

REFERENCES

1. Lamberg L. Pediatric sleep medicine comes of age. JAMA 2005; 293(19):2327–2329.
2. Osler W. Chronic tonsillitis. The Principles and Practice of Medicine. New York: Appleton and Co., 1892:335–339.
3. Guilleminault C, Eldridge FL, Simmons FB, Dement WC. Sleep apnea in eight children. Pediatrics 1976; 58(1):23–30.
4. Guilleminault C, Pelayo R, Leger D, Clerk A, Bocian RC. Recognition of sleep-disordered breathing in children. Pediatrics 1996; 98(5):871–882.
5. Carroll JL. Obstructive sleep-disordered breathing in children: new controversies, new directions. Clin Chest Med 2003; 24(2):261–282.
6. Owens JA. The practice of pediatric sleep medicine: results of a community survey. Pediatrics 2001; 108(3):E51.
7. Spruyt K, O'Brien LM, Cluydts R, Verleye GB, Ferri R. Odds, prevalence and predictors of sleep problems in school-age normal children. J Sleep Res 2005; 14(2):163–176.
8. Mulvaney SA, Goodwin JL, Morgan WJ, Rosen GR, Quan SF, Kaemingk KL. Behavior problems associated with sleep disordered breathing in school-aged children—the Tucson children's assessment of sleep apnea study. J Pediatr Psychol 2006; 31(3):322–330.
9. Wake M, Morton-Allen E, Poulakis Z, Hiscock H, Gallagher S, Oberklaid F. Prevalence, stability, and outcomes of cry-fuss and sleep problems in the first 2 years of life: prospective community-based study. Pediatrics 2006; 117(3):836–842.
10. Research NCoSD. Wake up America: a national sleep alert: report of the National Commission on Sleep Disorders Research/submitted to the United States Congress and to the Secretary, U.S. Department of Health and Human Services, 1993.
11. Archbold KH, Pituch KJ, Panahi P, Chervin RD. Symptoms of sleep disturbances among children at two general pediatric clinics. J Pediatr 2002; 140(1):97–102.
12. Iglowstein I, Jenni OG, Molinari L, Largo RH. Sleep duration from infancy to adolescence: reference values and generational trends. Pediatrics 2003; 111(2):302–307.
13. Weissbluth M. Naps in children: 6 months–7 years. Sleep 1995; 18(2):82–87.
14. Crosby B, LeBourgeois MK, Harsh J. Racial differences in reported napping and nocturnal sleep in 2- to 8-year-old children. Pediatrics 2005; 115(1 suppl):225–232.
15. Acebo C, Sadeh A, Seifer R, Tzischinsky O, Hafer A, Carskadon MA. Sleep/wake patterns derived from activity monitoring and maternal report for healthy 1- to 5-year-old children. Sleep 2005; 28(12):1568–1577.

16. Ohayon MM, Carskadon MA, Guilleminault C, Vitiello MV. Meta-analysis of quantitative sleep parameters from childhood to old age in healthy individuals: developing normative sleep values across the human lifespan. Sleep 2004; 27(7):1255–1273.
17. Montgomery-Downs HE, O'Brien LM, Gulliver TE, Gozal D. Polysomnographic characteristics in normal preschool and early school-aged children. Pediatrics 2006; 117(3):741–753.
18. Mitchell RB, Kelly J. Behavior, neurocognition and quality-of-life in children with sleep-disordered breathing. Int J Pediatr Otorhinolaryngol 2006; 70(3):395–406.
19. Kurnatowski P, Putynski L, Lapienis M, Kowalska B. Neurocognitive abilities in children with adenotonsillar hypertrophy. Int J Pediatr Otorhinolaryngol 2006; 70(3):419–424.
20. O'Brien LM, Gozal D. Neurocognitive dysfunction and sleep in children: from human to rodent. Pediatr Clin North Am 2004; 51(1):187–202.
21. Kennedy JD, Blunden S, Hirte C, et al. Reduced neurocognition in children who snore. Pediatr Pulmonol 2004; 37(4):330–337.
22. O'Brien LM, Holbrook CR, Mervis CB, et al. Sleep and neurobehavioral characteristics of 5- to 7-year-old children with parentally reported symptoms of attention-deficit/hyperactivity disorder. Pediatrics 2003; 111(3):554–563.
23. Friedman BC, Hendeles-Amitai A, Kozminsky E, et al. Adenotonsillectomy improves neurocognitive function in children with obstructive sleep apnea syndrome. Sleep 2003; 26(8):999–1005.
24. Shang CY, Gau SS, Soong WT. Association between childhood sleep problems and perinatal factors, parental mental distress and behavioral problems. J Sleep Res 2006 Mar; 15(1):63–73.
25. McLearn KT, Minkovitz CS, Strobino DM, Marks E, Hou W. Maternal depressive symptoms at 2 to 4 months post partum and early parenting practices. Arch Pediatr Adolesc Med 2006; 160(3):279–284.
26. El-Sheikh M, Buckhalt JA, Mize J, Acebo C. Marital conflict and disruption of children's sleep. Child Dev 2006; 77(1):31–43.
27. Johnson EO, Roth T, Schultz L, Breslau N. Epidemiology of DSM-IV insomnia in adolescence: lifetime prevalence, chronicity, and an emergent gender difference. Pediatrics 2006; 117(2):e247–256.
28. Pelayo R, Chen W, Monzon S, Guilleminault C. Pediatric sleep pharmacology: you want to give my kid sleeping pills? Pediatr Clin North Am 2004; 51(1):117–134.
29. Owens JA, Rosen CL, Mindell JA. Medication use in the treatment of pediatric insomnia: results of a survey of community-based pediatricians. Pediatrics 2003; 111(5 Pt 1): e628–635.
30. http://www.fda.gov/cder/pediatric/.
31. Couturier JL, Speechley KN, Steele M, Norman R, Stringer B, Nicolson R. Parental perception of sleep problems in children of normal intelligence with pervasive developmental disorders: prevalence, severity, and pattern. J Am Acad Child Adolesc Psychiatry 2005; 44(8):815–822.
32. Polimeni MA, Richdale AL, Francis AJ. A survey of sleep problems in autism, Asperger's disorder and typically developing children. J Intellect Disabil Res 2005; 49(Pt 4):260–268.
33. Oyane NM, Bjorvatn B. Sleep disturbances in adolescents and young adults with autism and Asperger syndrome. Autism 2005; 9(1):83–94.
34. Weiskop S, Richdale A, Matthews J. Behavioural treatment to reduce sleep problems in children with autism or fragile X syndrome. Dev Med Child Neurol 2005; 47(2): 94–104.
35. Gozal D, O'Brien L, Row BW. Consequences of snoring and sleep disordered breathing in children. Pediatr Pulmonol Suppl 2004; 26:166–168.
36. Gozal D, O'Brien LM. Snoring and obstructive sleep apnoea in children: why should we treat? Paediatr Respir Rev 2004; 5(suppl A):S371–S376.
37. Montgomery-Downs HE, Gozal D. Snore-associated sleep fragmentation in infancy: mental development effects and contribution of secondhand cigarette smoke exposure. Pediatrics 2006; 117(3):e496–502.
38. Halbower AC, Mahone EM. Neuropsychological morbidity linked to childhood sleep-disordered breathing. Sleep Med Rev 2006; 10(2):97–107.

39. Gozal D, Kheirandish L. Oxidant stress and inflammation in the snoring child: confluent pathways to upper airway pathogenesis and end-organ morbidity. Sleep Med Rev 2006; 10(2):83–96.
40. Clinical practice guideline: diagnosis and management of childhood obstructive sleep apnea syndrome. Pediatrics 2002; 109(4):704–712.
41. Montgomery-Downs HE, O'Brien LM, Holbrook CR, Gozal D. Snoring and sleep-disordered breathing in young children: subjective and objective correlates. Sleep 2004; 27(1):87–94.
42. Tauman R, O'Brien LM, Holbrook CR, Gozal D. Sleep pressure score: a new index of sleep disruption in snoring children. Sleep 2004; 27(2):274–278.
43. Rosen CL, Storfer-Isser A, Taylor HG, Kirchner HL, Emancipator JL, Redline S. Increased behavioral morbidity in school-aged children with sleep-disordered breathing. Pediatrics 2004; 114(6):1640–1648.
44. Pelayo R, Sivan Y. Increased behavioral morbidity in school-aged children with sleep-disordered breathing. Pediatrics 2005; 116(3):797–798.
45. Ivanenko A, Crabtree VM, Gozal D. Sleep in children with psychiatric disorders. Pediatr Clin North Am 2004; 51(1):51–68.
46. Chervin RD, Dillon JE, Archbold KH, Ruzicka DL. Conduct problems and symptoms of sleep disorders in children. J Am Acad Child Adolesc Psychiatry 2003; 42(2):201–208.
47. Sterni LM, Tunkel DE. Obstructive sleep apnea in children: an update. Pediatr Clin North Am 2003; 50(2):427–443.
48. Weissbach A, Leiberman A, Tarasiuk A, Goldbart A, Tal A. Adenotonsilectomy improves enuresis in children with obstructive sleep apnea syndrome. Int J Pediatr Otorhinolaryngol 2006; 70(8):1351–1356.
49. Guilleminault C, Li K, Khramtsov A, Palombini L, Pelayo R. Breathing patterns in prepubertal children with sleep-related breathing disorders. Arch Pediatr Adolesc Med 2004; 158(2):153–161.
50. Archbold KH, Giordani B, Ruzicka DL, Chervin RD. Cognitive executive dysfunction in children with mild sleep-disordered breathing. Biol Res Nurs 2004; 5(3):168–176.
51. Chervin RD, Clarke DF, Huffman JL, et al. School performance, race, and other correlates of sleep-disordered breathing in children. Sleep Med 2003; 4(1):21–27.
52. O'Brien LM, Ivanenko A, Crabtree VM, et al. Sleep disturbances in children with attention deficit hyperactivity disorder. Pediatr Res 2003; 54(2):237–243.
53. Kirov R, Kinkelbur J, Heipke S, et al. Is there a specific polysomnographic sleep pattern in children with attention deficit/hyperactivity disorder? J Sleep Res 2004; 13(1):87–93.
54. Gottlieb DJ, Vezina RM, Chase C, et al. Symptoms of sleep-disordered breathing in 5-year-old children are associated with sleepiness and problem behaviors. Pediatrics 2003; 112(4):870–877.
55. Crabtree VM, Ivanenko A, Gozal D. Clinical and parental assessment of sleep in children with attention-deficit/hyperactivity disorder referred to a pediatric sleep medicine center. Clin Pediatr (Phila) 2003; 42(9):807–813.
56. Chervin RD, Archbold KH, Dillon JE, et al. Associations between symptoms of inattention, hyperactivity, restless legs, and periodic leg movements. Sleep 2002; 25(2): 213–218.
57. Ohayon MM, Guilleminault C, Priest RG. Night terrors, sleepwalking, and confusional arousals in the general population: their frequency and relationship to other sleep and mental disorders. J Clin Psychiatry 1999; 60(4):268–276.
58. Guilleminault C, Palombini L, Pelayo R, Chervin RD. Sleepwalking and sleep terrors in prepubertal children: what triggers them? Pediatrics 2003; 111(1):e17–25.
59. American Psychiatric Association. Diagnostic and Statistical Manual of Mental Disorders: DSM-IV. Washington: American Psychiatric Press, 1994.
60. Gozal D. Sleep-disordered breathing and school performance in children. Pediatrics 1998; 102(3 Pt 1):616–620.
61. Guilleminault C, Rosekind M. The arousal threshold: sleep deprivation, sleep fragmentation, and obstructive sleep apnea syndrome. Bull Eur Physiopathol Respir 1981; 17(3):341–349.
62. Uliel S, Tauman R, Greenfeld M, Sivan Y. Normal polysomnographic respiratory values in children and adolescents. Chest 2004; 125(3):872–878.
63. Rosen CL. Obstructive sleep apnea syndrome in children: controversies in diagnosis and treatment. Pediatr Clin North Am 2004; 51(1):153–167, vii.

64. Carskadon MA, Dement WC, Mitler MM, Roth T, Westbrook PR, Keenan S. Guidelines for the multiple sleep latency test (MSLT): a standard measure of sleepiness. Sleep 1986; 9(4):519–524.
65. Hosselet J, Ayappa I, Norman RG, Krieger AC, Rapoport DM. Classification of sleep-disordered breathing. Am J Respir Crit Care Med 2001; 163(2):398–405.
66. Ayappa I, Norman RG, Krieger AC, Rosen A, O'Malley RL, Rapoport DM. Non-invasive detection of respiratory effort-related arousals (REras) by a nasal cannula/pressure transducer system. Sleep 2000; 23(6):763–771.
67. International classification of sleep disorders. 2nd ed. Westchester, Illinois: American Academy of Sleep Medicine, 2005.
68. Chervin RD. How many children with ADHD have sleep apnea or periodic leg movements on polysomnography? Sleep 2005; 28(9):1041–1042.
69. Carroll JL, McColley SA, Marcus CL, Curtis S, Loughlin GM. Inability of clinical history to distinguish primary snoring from obstructive sleep apnea syndrome in children. Chest 1995; 108(3):610–618.
70. Farber JM. Clinical practice guideline: diagnosis and management of childhood obstructive sleep apnea syndrome. Pediatrics 2002; 110(6):1255–1257.
71. Schechter MS. Technical report: diagnosis and management of childhood obstructive sleep apnea syndrome. Pediatrics 2002; 109(4):e69.
72. Guilleminault C, Pelayo R. ...And if the polysomnogram was faulty? Pediatr Pulmonol 1998; 26(1):1–3.
73. Messner AH. Treating pediatric patients with obstructive sleep disorders: an update. Otolaryngol Clin North Am 2003; 36(3):519–530.
74. Standards and indications for cardiopulmonary sleep studies in children. American Thoracic Society. Am J Respir Crit Care Med 1996; 153(2):866–878.
75. Chesson AL Jr, Ferber RA, Fry JM, et al. The indications for polysomnography and related procedures. Sleep 1997; 20(6):423–487.
76. Allen RP, Picchietti D, Hening WA, Trenkwalder C, Walters AS, Montplaisi J. Restless legs syndrome: diagnostic criteria, special considerations, and epidemiology. A report from the restless legs syndrome diagnosis and epidemiology workshop at the National Institutes of Health. Sleep Med 2003; 4(2):101–119.
77. The changing concept of sudden infant death syndrome: diagnostic coding shifts, controversies regarding the sleeping environment, and new variables to consider in reducing risk. Pediatrics 2005; 116(5):1245–1255.
78. Pelayo R, Owens J, Mindell J, Sheldon S. Bed sharing with unimpaired parents is not an important risk for sudden infant death syndrome: to the editor. Pediatrics 2006; 117(3):993–994.
79. Gessner BD, Porter TJ. Bed sharing with unimpaired parents is not an important risk for sudden infant death syndrome. Pediatrics 2006; 117(3):990–991.
80. Eidelman AI, Gartner LM. Bed sharing with unimpaired parents is not an important risk for sudden infant death syndrome: to the editor. Pediatrics 2006; 117(3):991–992.
81. Bartick M. Bed sharing with unimpaired parents is not an important risk for sudden infant death syndrome: to the editor. Pediatrics 2006; 117(3):992–993.
82. Shott SR, Amin R, Chini B, Heubi C, Hotze S, Akers R. Obstructive sleep apnea: Should all children with Down syndrome be tested? Arch Otolaryngol Head Neck Surg 2006; 132(4):432–436.
83. Pavone M, Paglietti MG, Petrone A, Crino A, De Vincentiis GC, Cutrera R. Adenotonsillectomy for obstructive sleep apnea in children with Prader-Willi syndrome. Pediatr Pulmonol 2006; 41(1):74–79.
84. Onodera K, Niikuni N, Chigono T, Nakajima I, Sakata H, Motizuki H. Sleep disordered breathing in children with achondroplasia. Part 2. Relationship with craniofacial and airway morphology. Int J Pediatr Otorhinolaryngol 2006; 70(3):453–461.
85. Monfared A, Messner A. Death following tonsillectomy in a child with Williams syndrome. Int J Pediatr Otorhinolaryngol 2006; 70(6):1133–1135.
86. Suresh S, Wales P, Dakin C, Harris MA, Cooper DG. Sleep-related breathing disorder in Duchenne muscular dystrophy: disease spectrum in the paediatric population. J Paediatr Child Health 2005; 41(9–10):500–503.

87. Statham MM, Elluru RG, Buncher R, Kalra M. Adenotonsillectomy for obstructive sleep apnea syndrome in young children: prevalence of pulmonary complications. Arch Otolaryngol Head Neck Surg 2006; 132(5):476–480.
88. Roemmich JN, Barkley JE, D'Andrea L, et al. Increases in overweight after adenotonsillectomy in overweight children with obstructive sleep-disordered breathing are associated with decreases in motor activity and hyperactivity. Pediatrics 2006; 117(2):e200–208.
89. Rosen G. Identification and evaluation of obstructive sleep apnea prior to adenotonsillectomy in children: is there a problem? Sleep Med 2003; 4(4):273–274.
90. Tarasiuk A, Simon T, Tal A, Reuveni H. Adenotonsillectomy in children with obstructive sleep apnea syndrome reduces health care utilization. Pediatrics 2004; 113(2):351–356.
91. Suen JS, Arnold JE, Brooks LJ. Adenotonsillectomy for treatment of obstructive sleep apnea in children. Arch Otolaryngol Head Neck Surg 1995; 121(5):525–530.
92. Guilleminault C, Li K, Quo S, Inouye RN. A prospective study on the surgical outcomes of children with sleep-disordered breathing. Sleep 2004; 27(1):95–100.
93. Pelayo R, Powell N. Evaluation of obstructive sleep apnea by polysomnography prior to pediatric adenotonsillectomy. Arch Otolaryngol Head Neck Surg 1999; 125(11):1282–1283.
94. Palombini L, Pelayo R, Guilleminault C. Efficacy of automated continuous positive airway pressure in children with sleep-related breathing disorders in an attended setting. Pediatrics 2004; 113(5):e412–417.
95. Malow BA, Weatherwax KJ, Chervin RD, et al. Identification and treatment of obstructive sleep apnea in adults and children with epilepsy: a prospective pilot study. Sleep Med 2003; 4(6):509–515.
96. Marcus CL, Rosen G, Ward SL, et al. Adherence to and effectiveness of positive airway pressure therapy in children with obstructive sleep apnea. Pediatrics 2006; 117(3):e442–451.
97. Guilleminault C, Li KK. Maxillomandibular expansion for the treatment of sleep-disordered breathing: preliminary result. Laryngoscope 2004; 114(5):893–896.
98. Li KK. Surgical therapy for obstructive sleep apnea syndrome. Semin Respir Crit Care Med 2005; 26(1):80–88.
99. Pirelli P, Saponara M, Guilleminault C. Rapid maxillary expansion in children with obstructive sleep apnea syndrome. Sleep 2004; 27(4):761–766.
100. Li HY, Li KK, Chen NH, Wang PC. Modified uvulopalatopharyngoplasty: the extended uvulopalatal flap. Am J Otolaryngol 2003; 24(5):311–316.
101. Cistulli PA. Rapid maxillary expansion in obstructive sleep apnea—hope on the horizon? Sleep 2004; 27(4):606–607.

16   Obstructive Sleep Apnea in the Elderly

Lavinia Fiorentino and Sonia Ancoli-Israel
*Department of Psychiatry, University of California, San Diego and Veterans
Affairs San Diego Healthcare System, San Diego, California, U.S.A.*

INTRODUCTION

Many older adults complain of poor sleep. Foley reported that sleep disruption
becomes a common problem in aging adults, with reports of 50% of adults over the
age of 65 complaining of poor sleep (1). A variety of factors contribute to sleep disruption in the elderly, including underlying medical and psychiatric illness, medication use, circadian rhythm disturbances, and specific sleep disorders (2). One type
of sleep disorder most commonly diagnosed in the elderly, with prevalence reports
of 20% to 81%, is sleep-disordered breathing (SDB) (3–5). In general, SDB encompasses a variety of sleep-related breathing disorders ranging from benign snoring to
obstructive sleep apnea (OSA); however, the term is often used to refer to OSA.
In this chapter, we will use the terms SDB and OSA interchangeably, except when
explicitly stated otherwise.

OSA is a condition characterized by cessation of regular breathing during
sleep. Apneas refer to complete cessation of respiration and hypopneas refer to partial or reduced respiration. For the diagnosis of sleep apnea, each apneic or hypopneic event must last a minimum of 10 seconds and recur throughout the night. Each
respiratory event generally results in repeated arousals from sleep as well as nocturnal hypoxemia. The apnea index (AI) is the number of apneas per hour of sleep and
the total number of apneas plus hypopneas per hour of sleep is called the apnea–
hypopnea index (AHI) or respiratory disturbance index (RDI).

EPIDEMIOLOGY

The prevalence of SDB is higher in the elderly compared to younger adults and in
older men compared to older women. Among middle-aged adults between 30 and
60 years of age, the prevalence of SDB [defined by an AHI ≥ 5, along with the presence of excessive daytime somnolence (EDS)], has been estimated to be 4% for men
and 2% for women (6). Among older adults, as reviewed by Ancoli-Israel (3), the
prevalence of SDB (defined by different levels of AHI) was estimated to be between
19.5% to 60% for women and 28% to 62% for men. Studies that have looked at the
combined prevalence rates for men and women report prevalence rates ranging
from 5.6% to 45% (3). SDB has been reported to be more prevalent in postmenopausal compared to premenopausal women, although the reason for this remains
unclear (7).

Studies using longitudinal and cross-sectional designs have shown that
the prevalence of SDB increases or stabilizes with increasing age (4,8–10). Hoch
et al. (10) in 1990 reported that the prevalence of SDB and median AHI increased

significantly from age 60 to 90 years. The authors found an AHI ≥ 5 in 2.9% of those aged 60 to 69, 33.3% of those aged 70 to 79, and 39.5% of those aged 80 to 89 (10).

Ancoli-Israel et al. in a large study on randomly selected community-dwelling elderly between the age of 65 and 95 years reported that 24% had an AI ≥ 5 with an average AI of 13. In addition, 81% of the study participants had an AHI ≥ 5, with an average AHI of 38. Using more stringent criteria, the prevalence rates reported were 62% for an AHI ≥ 10, 44% for an AHI ≥ 20, and 24% for an AHI ≥ 40 (4). The higher rates of SDB found in this study might be the result of objective sleep record- ings rather than subjective measurements (such as self-reported snoring with observed apneas), which were used in many previous studies (11).

A study of a community-based cohort of more than 6400 individuals in the Sleep Heart Health Study reported prevalence rates of SDB by 10-year age groups (mean age 63.5 years with an age range of 40–98 years) (12). Among those between 60 and 69 years old, 32% had an AHI of 5 to 14 and 19% had an AHI ≥ 15; between 70 and 79 years old, 33% had an AHI of 5 to 14 and 21% had an AHI ≥ 15; and between 80 and 98 years old, 36% had an AHI of 5 to 14 and 20% had an AHI ≥ 15. When focusing on participants with an AHI ≥ 15, it was shown that the prevalence of SDB increased slightly for every 10-year age group except in participants between 75 and 85 years old.

Greater prevalence of SDB has been found in elderly people in nursing homes compared to those who live independently (13–15). Ancoli-Israel et al. studied 235 nursing home patients and found that 70% to 90% had an AHI ≥ 5 and 50% had an AHI ≥ 20 (14,15). Higher SDB rates were also found in patients with dementia (16,17). Hoch et al. (18) reported that more than 40% of Alzheimer's disease (AD) patients had SDB significantly higher than age-matched depressed or healthy elderly subjects. Ancoli-Israel (3) reviewed seven different studies examining the prevalence of SDB in those elderly with dementia versus without dementia and reported prevalence rates ranging from 33% to 70% in demented subjects, compared with the reported 5.6% to 45% rate found in the nondemented elderly.

RISK FACTORS

There are several known risk factors for SDB in the elderly, including increasing age, male gender, obesity, and symptomatic status (19). The most predictive physical finding of SDB in younger adults is obesity [body mass index (BMI) greater than or equal to 28 kg/m^2] (19), with approximately 40% of those with a BMI over 40 and 50% of those with a BMI over 50 having SDB (20). In the older adult, obesity is still a strong predictor of SDB (4,19,21).

Other risk factors for developing SDB include: the use of sedating medica- tions, alcohol consumption, family history, race, smoking, and upper airway config- uration (19). While few studies have explored the association between race and SDB, there is some evidence to suggest that SDB may be more severe but not more prevalent in older African-Americans compared to older Caucasians (22,23). Fiorentino et al. (24), however, found that the differences in sleep between older African-Americans and older Caucasians at risk for SDB may be better accounted for by health and socioeconomic status variables rather than by sleep variables.

CLINICAL FEATURES

The symptoms and clinical presentations of SDB in the elderly are similar to those of younger adults. Snoring and excessive daytime sleepiness (EDS) are the two principal symptoms of SDB in the elderly. The snoring is caused by airway collapse or obstruction. Snoring in patients with SDB can be extremely loud, often disrupting the bed partner's sleep, and resulting in the bed partner moving into another bedroom. Enright et al. (11) in a study of 5201 older adults (age 65 and over) reported that, for males, snoring was related to younger age, marital status, and alcohol consumption, and for women snoring was related to BMI, diabetes, and arthritis.

SDB has been identified in approximately 50% of patients that habitually snore, and snoring has been shown to be an early predictor of SDB (25). It is important to note however that not all patients who snore have SDB and not all patients with SDB snore. Also, because many elderly do not have a bed partner and live alone, this symptom may at times be difficult to identify.

One of the most salient symptoms of SDB in the elderly is EDS. This symptom is most likely a result of the recurrent night-time arousals and sleep fragmentation due to the apneas, hypopneas, and hypoxemia. EDS can have profound and detrimental effects on the quality of life of elderly patients as they may often fall asleep at inappropriate times during the day. This inadvertent napping may happen while watching television or movies, reading, attending meetings, working, driving, and during conversations. EDS is associated with occupational and social difficulties, reduced vigilance, and most important in the elderly, is correlated with cognitive deficits (26).

Morbidity and Mortality Associated with Sleep-Disordered Breathing
Cardiovascular Consequences

In younger adults, SDB has been shown to be a risk factor for hypertension (27–29). Even minimal amounts of SDB (AHI 0.1–4.9), considered by most not to be pathologic, have been shown to increase the risk of developing hypertension compared to an AHI of zero (29). A link between apnea severity and elevations in blood pressure has also been reported. A study by Lavie et al. (27) showed that each additional apneic event per hour of sleep increased the odds of hypertension by 1%, and each oxygen desaturation of 10% increased the odds by 13%.

The relationship between SDB and hypertension in older adults however is not as clear. There are studies that have reported an association between hypertension and SDB in the older adult (30,31), but more recent data from the Sleep Heart Health Study suggested that there was no association between SDB and systolic/diastolic hypertension in those aged ≥ 60 years (32). A recent study in middle-aged adults found that severe SDB was associated with pulmonary hypertension and that CPAP treatment of the SDB reduced pulmonary systolic pressure (33). Similar studies are needed in the elderly.

There is evidence of SDB being associated with cardiac arrhythmia, myocardial infarction, hypercoagulable state, and sudden death (34,35). However, the relationship between SDB and cardiovascular events in the elderly is less clear as most studies have been performed in middle-age adults. The best data come from the Sleep Heart Health Study, which produced strong evidence in support of the association between SDB and ischemic heart disease (34). Results suggested a positive association between the severity of SDB (objectively measured with polysomnography) and the risk of developing cardiovascular disease including coronary artery disease and stroke. In this study, independent of known cardiovascular risk factors, even mild to moderate SDB was associated with the development of ischemic heart disease.

Severity of SDB is an important factor in predicting myocardial infarction in cardiac patients. A study by Hung et al. (36) showed that in male cardiac patients, 66 years old or younger, severe SDB was 25 times more likely to be associated with myocardial infarction compared to mild SDB. There is also evidence that snoring by itself increases the risk of ischemic heart disease in both men and women (37).

Studies have found a high prevalence of SDB in patients with congestive heart failure (38,39). Some research suggests that SDB may exacerbate or even cause the heart failure. The Sleep Heart Health Study found that the severity of SDB was positively associated with the development of congestive heart failure and, like ischemic disease, even mild to moderate SDB was associated with its development (34).

Central sleep apnea and OSA, as well as Cheyne-Stokes respiration, are all common in patients with heart failure. Javaheri et al. (39) reported that 40% to 50% of outpatients, predominantly males, with stable, mild, medically treated congestive heart failure had SDB. In addition, AHI has been shown to be a powerful predictor of poor prognosis in this group of patients (40).

Studies suggest that there is a direct relationship between cerebrovascular conditions and SDB in adults. There are reports of patients with a cerebrovascular accident having higher prevalence of SDB compared to age- and gender-matched controls without SDB (37). The Sleep Heart Health Study found an association between the severity of SDB and the risk of developing cerebrovascular disease and reported that even mild to moderate SDB increases this risk (34). In many patients the SDB persists even after the resolution of the stroke related symptoms, strengthening the argument that the SDB precedes the development of cerebrovascular disease (37). For those patients who have suffered a stroke, the presence of SDB and its severity has been found to be an independent prognostic factor related to mortality, with a 5% increase in mortality risk for each additional unit of AHI (41). In addition, similarly to traditional risk factors for stroke such as hypertension, smoking, and hyperlipidemia, there is evidence of an independent association between self-reported snoring and stroke in the elderly (42).

The nature of the relationship between SDB and cerebrovascular disease in adults and in the elderly is still to be defined; however, as reported earlier, there is evidence that SDB might precede the development of a stroke and may in fact be a risk factor (37).

Cognitive Impairment and Dementia
There is evidence that SDB affects patients' cognitive functioning. Several studies have reported the negative effect of severe SDB (AHI $\geq$ 30) on cognitive dysfunction, with specific impairments in attentional tasks, immediate and delayed recall of verbal and visual material, executive tasks, planning and sequential thinking, and manual dexterity (26,43,44). Studies examining the relationship between milder SDB and cognition are less clear-cut, and have found that mild SDB (AHI 10–20) does not cause cognitive dysfunction in the absence of sleepiness (43). However, it is important to note that SDB might not affect all areas of cognitive functioning equally, and therefore, it is possible that in a study that only examined a small number of cognitive tasks, the findings could be (falsely) negative.

Researchers have proposed two explanatory theories for the cognitive deficits found in patients with SDB. The first is that the hypoxia caused by the SDB results in the cognitive impairments. Evidence for this theory comes from studies, which found that in patients with continuous hypoxia, there is an association between the severity of cognitive dysfunction and nocturnal oxygen saturation (45,46). In particular, as the oxygen saturation decreases, the performance on various neuropsychological testing worsens. Whether this relationship holds when the hypoxia is intermittent is unclear. An important consideration to make is that the patient's performance on cognitive tasks might vary depending on the severity of SDB and hypoxia experienced the night before the testing. This variability may in fact partially explain some of the inconsistencies reported in the literature with regards to the effects of SDB on cognitive functioning. It remains unclear whether these hypoxia-related cognitive deficits are reversible with treatment.

The second theory is that the EDS contributes to the cognitive impairment found in patients with SDB. It is well known that one of the primary symptoms of SDB is EDS, and that EDS can impair cognitive functioning including auditory verbal learning (47), executive functioning, and working memory (48). It is also possible that the cognitive deficits found in SDB patients are a product of multiple factors, which may include both hypoxia and EDS. In addition, there is evidence that many of the progressive dementias involve degenerative pathologies in brainstem regions, areas that are responsible for regulating respiration and other autonomic functions relevant to sleep maintenance (49). Therefore, because many older adults suffer from dementia, it is possible that sleep disorders such as SDB may be more likely to occur in this group of patients.

There are studies showing that the severity of the dementia is associated with the severity of the SDB (14,18). In institutionalized elderly, those patients with severe dementia [based on the Dementia Rating Scale (DRS)] had more severe SDB compared to those with mild–moderate or no dementia (14). Furthermore, there was a positive relationship between severity of the SDB and dementia, and patients with more severe SDB performing worse on the DRS. A study by Kim et al. (50) estimated that an AHI = 15 is equivalent to the decrement of psychomotor efficiency associated with an additional five years of age.

There is some speculation that SDB could actually be a cause of vascular dementia (51). Studies have shown that the hypertension, arrhythmias, decreased cardiac output, stroke volume, and cerebral perfusion associated with SDB may lead to an increased likelihood of cerebral ischemia and/or localized infarcts (52).

In our own laboratory, we have studied the relationship between SDB and cognitive impairment in patients with AD that were both institutionalized and community-dwelling (3,14,15,53). We found that SDB was highly prevalent in both populations. In addition, in the institutionalized AD patients, as AHI increased, cognitive functioning worsened, even when controlling for age (14). There is also evidence to suggest that the severity of sleep disruptions in AD parallels the decline in cognitive functioning. We are currently completing a study that examines whether treatment of SDB in patients with AD results in improvement in cognitive abilities (54,55).

The prevalence of SDB is also higher in patients with Parkinson's disease (PD) compared to age-matched controls (56,57). It is known that the majority of PD patients experience subtle changes in cognition, and that approximately 40% will progress to PD dementia (58). PD patients also commonly experience alterations in respiratory function while awake; hence, there are compelling reasons to think that patients with PD may be at risk of nocturnal hypoxemia and SDB. There is evidence that in PD patients there is a degeneration of the neurons in the reticular activating system as well as a degeneration of the pathways arising from the dorsal raphe and locus coeruleus, all of which are likely to contribute to sleep disturbances and day-time sleepiness in these patients (59). The role that SDB plays in the cognitive dys-function and eventual development of dementia experienced by the majority of PD patients is a question that still needs to be explored.

Mortality

Researchers have suggested that patients with SDB may be at increased risk of death compared to those without SDB. Bliwise et al. (60) followed a cohort of noninstitu-tionalized older subjects (mean age 66) for 12 years and found that there was a 2.7 times risk of shorter survival for those with SDB.

A polysomnographic study that reviewed death certificates of patients (mostly in their 60–70 years of age) who had died of cardiac-related death, found that those who had died from midnight to 6 A.M. had a significantly higher AHI than those who died during other time intervals during the day. This study reported that for patients with SDB, the relative risk of sudden death from cardiac causes was 2.57 from midnight to 6 A.M. (35). This is particularly telling about the possible relation-ship between SDB, heart failure and death if one considers that in general the risk of sudden death from cardiac causes is highest from 6 AM to noon and lowest from midnight to 6 A.M. (61).

The estimates of mortality in patients with SDB are high. It is possible that SDB in the elderly is one of several factors which, in combination, lead to increased mortality. There are reports of increased mortality rates in patients with heart failure who develop SDB in combination with Cheyne-Stokes breathing (62,63). Hoch et al. (64) reported that in elderly patients suffering from depression and cognitive impair-ment, SDB was associated with an excess mortality rate of 450%.

Ancoli-Israel et al. (65) found that community-dwelling elderly with greater SDB (RDI ≥ 30) had significantly shorter survival rates than those with mild–moderate or no SDB. In other studies, however, AHI was not found to be an inde-pendent predictor of mortality (65,66). These studies found that cardiovascular and pulmonary conditions, including hypertension, were independent predictors of death. Ancoli-Israel et al. reported that elderly men with congestive heart failure (CHF) had more severe SDB than those with no heart disease. Furthermore, men with both conditions, heart failure and SDB, had shortened life-spans compared to those men with only CHF, only SDB or neither (Fig. 1) (67).

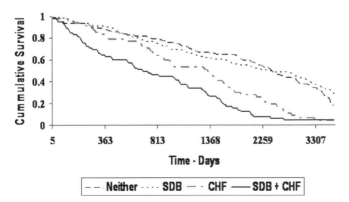

FIGURE 1 Survival curves for those with congestive heart failure (CHF), and/or sleep-disordered breathing (SDB), or neither. Those with CHF plus central sleep apnea had significantly shorter survival ($p < 0.001$) than those with just CHF or just SDB. Source: From Ref. 67.

More research is needed to clarify the exact nature of the relationship between SDB and mortality in the elderly. Furthermore, studies with older women are particularly necessary, since most studies completed have involved older men.

CLINICAL ASSESSMENT AND MANAGEMENT OF SLEEP-DISORDERED BREATHING

Presentation

As discussed earlier, EDS and snoring are the primary symptoms of SDB. The EDS manifests with high propensity to fall asleep throughout the day, sometimes inappropriately while talking to someone or even driving a car. In general, napping behavior can be intentional or inadvertent. Inadvertent napping, in particular, may be a clue that a patient has disrupted or insufficient sleep, possibly secondary to SDB. It is known that elderly patients tend to nap more frequently than younger adults, and that regular napping behavior is common in the elderly (68). Hence, it is imperative that clinicians discern whether these naps are planned or unintentional, as the latter may indicate the inability to maintain wakefulness, and thus may suggest the presence of SDB or other sleep disorder. Clinicians should also keep in mind that the EDS and the inadvertent napping may be caused by other medical conditions, such as PD, abnormal thyroid function, malignancies, depression, nocturia related to benign prostatic hypertrophy, and/or sedating medications such as long-acting hypnotics, antidepressants, antihistamines, and dopaminergics (all commonly used by the elderly).

Insomnia may also be a presenting complaint in older patients who suffer from SDB. The fragmented or restless sleep due to frequent nocturnal awakenings following the apneic events may result in a subjective complaint of difficulty sleeping, often labeled as "insomnia." In addition, SDB may present with a nocturnal confusion and/or daytime cognitive impairment, including difficulties with concentration, attention, and memory.

Diagnosis

Because EDS and snoring are common in the older population as well as being the two main clinical features of SDB, it is extremely important that clinicians do not directly assume that if an older adult has complains of snoring or EDS, that these complaints must be due to SDB, nor should they assume that snoring or EDS are normal signs of aging. A complete evaluation is always warranted.

A step-wise assessment process is suggested to accurately determine the presence of SDB in the elderly. First, a complete sleep history should be obtained, including symptoms of SDB, symptoms of other sleep disorders (e.g., restless leg syndrome), sleep-related habits and routines and, if possible, bed-partner testimonials. Secondly, the patient's medical history, including psychiatric and medical records, should be reviewed. Particular attention should be given to associated medical conditions and medications, the use of alcohol, and evidence of cognitive impairment. Lastly, if from the evidence gathered there is reason to suspect SDB, an overnight polysomnographic recording should be obtained.

The diagnosis of SDB requires an overnight polysomnogram. There may be some potential challenges in obtaining sleep studies in the elderly including difficulties with transportation, worries regarding technical equipment, understanding complicated instructions, and resistance to spending the night in an unfamiliar environment. These difficulties may be eased by offering straightforward and thorough education about the sleep recording process, anticipation of the potential difficulties implicated, and involvement of the patient's spouse or caregiver in the process. If the clinician has a high suspicion of SDB, an unattended overnight sleep study may be sufficient for diagnosis. However, it is important to note that Medicare currently reimburses only attended sleep studies.

Treatment of Sleep-Disordered Breathing in the Elderly

Treatment of SDB in the elderly is similar to treatment of SDB in younger adults. In general, several factors should be taken into account when considering SDB treatment. Age or assumed nonadherence should never alone stand as reasons to withhold treatment.

Severity and significance of the patient's symptoms should be the main guides in initiating treatment (69). Older patients with severe SDB (i.e., AHI ≥ 20) deserve a trial of treatment while in those with milder levels of SDB (i.e., AHI < 20) treatment should be considered if other conditions are present, such as hypertension, cognitive dysfunction, or EDS.

Patients should be counseled on weight loss and smoking cessation if indicated. For those with positional-related SDB, that is, with more apneic events typically occurring in the supine position, avoidance of this position and attempting to sleep on their side should be indicated and may be effective.

Some medications and substances should be avoided in older patients. In particular the long-acting, older, sedating benzodiazepines should be avoided as they are respiratory depressants and may increase the number and duration of apneas. Alcohol should be avoided because even small amounts can also exacerbate SDB.

Continuous positive airway pressure (CPAP) is the "gold standard" for the treatment of SDB (see also Chapter 6). CPAP is a device that provides continuous positive pressure via the nasal or oral airway passages, which creates an opening in the airway to permit inspiration. CPAP has been shown to be a very effective and safe treatment for SDB if used correctly (70).

Beneficial effects of CPAP in older adults with SDB have been shown in several studies. Guilleminault et al. (71) found improved nocturia, daytime somnolence, depression ratings, and quality of life scores in older males after treatment of SDB with CPAP. Another study reported that treatment of SDB with CPAP resulted in normalization of prethrombotic states in older adults, with a reported lengthening of prothrombin time and increased fibrinogen levels (72). Older adults treated for SDB with CPAP for three months showed improved cognition, particularly in the areas of attention, psychomotor speed, executive functioning, and nonverbal delayed recall (44).

As with middle aged adults, problems with CPAP adherence may occur in the elderly. However, a study that looked at CPAP adherence in demented elderly with SDB, showed that adherence was good, with the majority of patients using CPAP for about five hours a night. Depression was the only factor associated with poor adherence; age, severity of dementia, or severity of SDB did not predict nonadherence (54).

An alternative treatment for SDB patients where CPAP is not tolerated is an oral appliance (see also Chapter 12). Oral appliances should generally be reserved and considered for thinner patients with milder levels of SDB (73). Reported effectiveness ranges from 50% to 100%. However, patients with dentures are generally not candidates for this device although newer models can be fitted with dentures.

Surgical treatments are not commonly recommended in the elderly. Surgical treatments involve correcting the anatomic abnormalities most responsible for the airway obstruction. There are several possible procedures, the most common being an uvulopalatopharyngoplasty. This involves an excision of the soft palate and uvula (74), and requires general anesthesia, and is only successful in approximately 50% of cases (75). Furthermore, being 50 years old or older is associated with poorer surgical outcome (75).

When patients have trouble tolerating both CPAP and oral appliances and are poor surgical candidates, nocturnal oxygen supplementation may be considered. However, studies that have looked at the efficacy of supplemental oxygen treatment for SDB have arrived at disparate findings. It has been reported that oxygen supplementation is not as effective as CPAP in reducing apneas or improving EDS (76). However, studies have shown that providing one night of supplemental oxygen does improve the nadir oxygen saturation, but at the same time may worsen the respiratory acidosis associated with the apneas (77). There is also evidence that oxygen supplementation during sleep in patients with SDB may cause a slight increase in the mean obstructive apnea duration (77). Hence, before being prescribed oxygen for home use, patients should undergo an attended polysomnogram with oxygen supplementation to ensure that there is only a minimal increase in apnea duration if any and no worsening of cardiac arrhythmias.

CONCLUSIONS

SDB is a common condition in the elderly and is associated with complaints of EDS and snoring. The more severe cases also may present with cognitive impairments and daytime dysfunction. Although the cutoff has not yet been established, there is evidence that beyond some pathologic level of SDB, treatment is clearly beneficial. The most common treatment for SDB is CPAP, which has been shown to be both effective and acceptable in the older population.

There is a growing body of literature exploring SDB in the elderly. There is an ongoing debate in the field as to whether SDB in the elderly is a distinct pathologic condition, different than that of middle-age adults. Levy et al. (78) in a study of approximately 400 people of all ages (ranging from < 20 years to > 85 years old) reported that the severity of SDB based on AHI and oxygen saturation did not differ in those subjects 65 years of age or older when compared to those subjects < 65 years of age. However, in this study, the symptomatology and sequelae related to SDB were not reported and therefore, age differences in regards to the correlates and possible consequences of SDB were not investigated.

Some of the differences in severity found between younger and older adults might be due to correlates of older age that affect the SDB, rather than intrinsic SDB differences between the different age populations. For example, Bixler et al. (9) found that BMI is a central factor that affects SDB severity. In this study, the prevalence of SDB was higher in older men compared to younger men, however, after controlling for BMI, the severity of SDB based on number of events and oxygen saturation actually decreased with age. Furthermore, Ancoli-Israel et al. (21) in an 18-year follow-up study with more than 400 elderly patients with SDB showed that AHI did not continue to increase with age if the patient's BMI remained stable.

Controversy also exists regarding the effect of SDB on morbidity and mortality in the elderly since the research findings are at times contradictory. As discussed previously, there are several reports of increased mortality in elderly with SDB (64).

Ancoli-Israel et al. (65) found that elderly subjects with more severe SDB had signifi-cantly shorter survival, dying as soon as two years earlier, than those with mild–moderate or no SDB. On the contrary, He et al. (79) reported that an AHI ≥ 20 predicted increased mortality in SDB patients under 50 but not those over 50. Similarly, others have reported that the survival rate is reduced in middle-aged patients with SDB compared to age- and sex-matched controls, but that this pattern was not seen among older patients (80,81). Finally, Mant et al. (66) found SDB seve-rity (RDI ≥ 15) did not predict death in nondemented, independent living elderly.

Because most of the literature on SDB is based on middle-aged males, many questions about the phenomenology of SDB in other populations, including older adults in general and older women in specific, remain to be clarified. Particularly, questions that still need to be answered are whether SDB in the elderly is indeed a different disorder, and if not, the degree to which SDB might differ in younger com-pared to older adults.

ACKNOWLEDGMENTS

Supported by NIA AG08415, NCI CA112035, CBCRP 11IB-0034, CBCRP 11GB0049 M01 RR00827, and the Research Service of the VASDHS.

REFERENCES

1. Foley DJ, Monjan AA, Brown SL, Simonsick EM, Wallace RB, Blazer DG. Sleep com-plaints among elderly persons: an epidemiologic study of three communities. Sleep 1995; 18(6):425–432.
2. Ancoli-Israel S. Insomnia in the elderly: a review for the primary care practitioner. Sleep 2000; 23(suppl 1):S23–S30.
3. Ancoli-Israel S. Epidemiology of sleep disorders. In: Roth T, Roehrs TA, eds. Clinics in Geriatric Medicine. Philadelphia: W.B. Saunders Company, 1989:347–362.
4. Ancoli-Israel S, Kripke DF, Klauber MR, Mason WJ, Fell R, Kaplan O. Sleep disordered breathing in community-dwelling elderly. Sleep 1991; 14(6):486–495.
5. Redline S, Kirchner L, Quan SF, Gottlieb DJ, Kapur V, Newman A. The effects of age, sex, ethnicity, and sleep-disordered breathing on sleep architecture. Arch Intern Med 2004; 164(4):406–418.
6. Young T, Palta M, Dempsey J, Skatrud J, Weber S, Badr S. The occurrence of sleep disor-dered breathing among middle-aged adults. N Engl J Med 1993; 328:1230–1235.
7. Young T, Rabago D, Zgierska A, Austin D, Laurel F. Objective and subjective sleep qual-ity in premenopausal, perimenopausal, and postmenopausal women in the Wisconsin Sleep Cohort Study. Sleep 2003; 26(6):667–672.
8. Bliwise DL, Carskadon MA, Carey E, Dement WC. Longitudinal development of sleep-related respiratory disturbance in adult humans. J Gerontol 1984; 39:290–293.
9. Bixler EO, Vgontzas AN, Ten Have T, Tyson K, Kales A. Effects of age on sleep apnea in men. Am J Res Crit Care Med 1998; 157:144–148.
10. Hoch CC, Reynolds CFI, Monk TH, et al. Comparison of sleep-disordered breathing among healthy elderly in the seventh, eighth, and ninth decades of life. Sleep 1990; 13(6): 502–511.
11. Enright PL, Newman AB, Wahl PW, Manolio TA, Haponik EF, Boyle P. Prevalence and correlates of snoring and observed apneas in 5201 Older Adults. Sleep 1996; 19(7): 531–538.
12. Young T, Shahar E, Nieto FJ, et al. Predictors of sleep-disordered breathing in community-dwelling adults: the Sleep Heart Health Study. Arch Intern Med 2002; 162(8): 893–900.
13. Ancoli-Israel S, Parker L, Sinaee R, Fell R, Kripke DF. Sleep fragmentation in patients from a nursing home. J Gerontol 1989; 44(1):M18–M21.
14. Ancoli-Israel S, Klauber MR, Butters N, Parker L, Kripke DF. Dementia in institutional-ized elderly: relation to sleep apnea. J Am Geriatr Soc 1991; 39(3):258–263.

15. Gehrman PR, Martin JL, Shochat T, Nolan S, Corey-Bloom J, Ancoli-Israel S. Sleep disordered breathing and agitation in institutionalized adults with Alzheimer's disease. Am J Geriatr Psychiat 2003; 11(4):426–433.
16. Erkinjuntti T, Partinen M, Sulkava R, Telakivi T, Salmi T, Tilvis R. Sleep apnea in multi-infarct dementia and Alzheimer's disease. Sleep 1987; 10(5):419–425.
17. Taylor W, Phillipson EA, Moldofsky H. Cognitive function and sleep disorderd breathing in normal elderly and patients with Alzheimer's disease. In: Kuna ST, Suratt PM, Remmers JE, eds. Sleep and Respiration in Aging Adults. New York: Elsevier, 1991: 251–258.
18. Hoch CC, Reynolds CFI. Cognitive function and sleep disordered breathing in dementia: the Pittsburg experience. In: Kuna ST, Suratt PM, Remmers JE, eds. Sleep and Respiration in Aging Adults. New York: Elsevier, 1991:245–250.
19. Phillips B, Ancoli-Israel S. Sleep disorders in the elderly. Sleep Med 2001; 2(2):99–114.
20. Kripke DF, Ancoli-Israel S, Klauber MR, Wingard DL, Mason WJ, Mullaney DJ. Prevalence of sleep disordered-breathing in ages 40-64 years: a population-based survey. Sleep 1997; 20(1):65–76.
21. Ancoli-Israel S, Gehrman P, Kripke DF, et al. Long-term follow-up of sleep disordered breathing in older adults. Sleep Med 2001; 2(6):511–516.
22. Ancoli-Israel S, Klauber MR, Stepnowsky C, Estline E, Chinn A, Fell R. Sleep-disordered breathing in African-American elderly. Am J Resp Crit Care Med 1995; 152(6): 1946–1949.
23. Redline S, Tishler PV, Hans MG, Tosteson T, Strohl KP, Spry K. Racial differences in sleep-disordered breathing in African-American and Caucasians. Am J Res Crit Care Med 1997; 155(1):186–192.
24. Fiorentino L, Marler M, Stepnowsky C, Johnson SS, Ancoli-Israel S. Sleep in older African-Americans and Caucasians at risk for sleep disordered breathing. Behav Sleep Med 2006; 4(3):164–178.
25. Collop NA, Cassell DK. Snoring and sleep-disordered breathing. In: Lee-Chiong TL, Sateia MJ, Carskadon MA, eds. Sleep Medicine. Philadelphia: Hanley & Belfus, 2002:349–355.
26. Martin J, Stepnowsky C, Ancoli-Israel S. Sleep apnea in the elderly. In: McNicholas WT, Phillipson EA, eds. Breathing Disorders During Sleep. London: W.B. Saunders Company, 2002:278–287.
27. Lavie P, Herer P, Hoffstein V. Obstructive sleep apnoea syndrome as a risk factor for hypertension: population study. BMJ (Clinical Research Ed) 2000; 320(7233):479–482.
28. Nieto FJ, Young T, Lind B, et al. Association of sleep-disordered breathing, sleep apnea, and hypertension in a large community-based study. JAMA 2000; 283(14):1829–1836.
29. Peppard P, Young T, Palta M, Skatrud J. Prospective study of the association between sleep-disordered breathing and hypertension. New Eng J Med 2000; 342(19):1378–1384.
30. Berry DTR, Phillips BA, Cook YR, et al. Sleep-disordered breathing in healthy aged persons: one-year follow-up of daytime sequelae. Sleep 1989; 12(3):211–215.
31. Stoohs RA, Gingold J, Cohrs S, Harter R, Finlayson E, Guilleminault C. Sleep-disordered breathing and systemic hypertension in the older male. J Am Geriatr Soc 1996; 44(11): 1295–1300.
32. Haas DC, Foster GL, Nieto FJ, et al. Age-dependent associations between sleep-disordered breathing and hypertension: importance of discriminating between systolic/diastolic hypertension and isolated systolic hypertension in the Sleep Heart Health Study. Circulation 2005; 111:614–621.
33. Arias MA, Garcia-Rio F, Alonso-Fernandez A, Martinez I, Villamor J. Pulmonary hypertension in obstructive sleep apnoea: effects of continuous positive airway pressure. A randomized, controlled cross-over study. Eur Heart J 2006; 27(9):1106–1113.
34. Shahar E, Whitney CW, Redline S, et al. Sleep-disordered breathing and cardiovascular disease: cross sectional results of the Sleep Heart Health Study. Am J Respir Crit Care Med 2001; 163(1):19–25.
35. Gami AS, Howard DE, Olson EJ, Somers VK. Day-night pattern of sudden death in obstructive sleep apnea. New Eng J Med 2005; 352:1206–1214.
36. Hung J, Whitford EG, Parsons RW, Hillman DR. Association of sleep apnoea with myocardial infarction in men. Lancet 1990; 336:261–264.

37. Yaggi H, Mohsenin V. Obstructive sleep apnoea and stroke. lancet neurology 2004; 3: 333–342.
38. Chan J, Sanderson J, Chan JW, et al. Prevalence of sleep-disordered breathing in diastolic heart failure. Chest 1997; 111:1488–1493.
39. Javaheri S, Parker TJ, Liming JD, et al. Sleep apnea in 81 ambulatory male patients with stable heart failure types and their prevalences, consequences, and presentations. Circulation 1998; 97:2154–2159.
40. Verrier RL. Cardiovascular disorders and sleep. In: Lee-Chiong TL, Sateia MJ, Carskadon MA, eds. Sleep Medicine. Philadelphia: Hanley & Belfus, Inc., 2002:447–453.
41. Parra O, Arboix A, Montserrat JM, Quinto L, Bechich S, Garcia-Eroles L. Sleep-related breathing disorders: impact on mortality of cerebrovascular disease. Eur Respir J 2004; 24(2):267–272.
42. Jennum P, Schultz-Larsen K, Davidsen M, Christensen NJ. Snoring and risk of stroke and ischaemic heart disease in a 70 year old population. A 6-year follow-up study. Int J Epidemiol 1994; 23(6):1159–1164.
43. Redline S, Strauss ME, Adams N, et al. Neuropsychological function in mild sleep-disordered breathing. Sleep 1997; 20(2):160–167.
44. Aloia MS, Ilniczky N, Di Dio P, Perlis ML, Greenblatt DW, Giles DE. Neuropsychological changes and treatment compliance in older adults with sleep apnea. J Psychosom Res 2003; 54:71–76.
45. Bedard MA, Montplaisir J, Richer F, Malo J. Nocturnal hypoxemia as a determinant of vigilance impairment in sleep apnea syndrome. Chest 1991; 100(2):367–370.
46. Findley LJ, Barth JT, Powers DC, Wilhoit SC, Boyd DG, Suratt PM. Cognitive impairment in patients with obstructive sleep apnea and associated hypoxemia. Chest 1986; 90: 686–90.
47. Valencia-Flores M, Bliwise DL, Guilleminault C, Cilveti R, Clerk A. Cognitive function in patients with sleep apnea after acute nocturnal nasal continuous positive airway pressure (CPAP) treatment: sleepiness and hypoxemia effects. J Clin Exp Neuropsychol 1996; 18(2):197–210.
48. Durmer JS, Dinges DF. Neurocognitive consequences of sleep deprivation. Semin Neurol 2005; 25(1):117–129.
49. Prinz PN, Vitaliano PP, Vitiello MV, et al. Sleep, EEG and mental function changes in senile dementia of the Alzheimer's type. Neurobiol Aging 1982; 3:361–70.
50. Kim HC, Young T, Matthews CG, Weber SM, Woodward AR, Palta M. Sleep-disordered breathing and neuropsychological deficits. A population-based study. Am J Res Crit Care Med 1997; 156(6):1813–1819.
51. Bliwise DL. Review: sleep in normal aging and dementia. Sleep 1993; 16:40–81.
52. Bliwise DL. Cognitive function and sleep disordered breathing in aging adults. In: Kuna ST, Remmers JE, Suratt PM, eds. Sleep and Respiration in Aging Adults. New York: Elsevier, 1991:237–244.
53. Ancoli-Israel S, Klauber MR, Gillin JC, Campbell SS, Hofstetter CR. Sleep in non-institutionalized Alzheimer's disease patients. Aging Clin Exp Res 1994; 6(6):451–458.
54. Ayalon L, Ancoli-Israel S, Stepnowsky C, et al. Adherence to continuous positive airway pressure treatment in patients with Alzheimer's disease and obstructive sleep apnea. Am J Geriatr Psychiat 2006; 14(2):176–180.
55. Chong MS, Ayalon L, Marler M, et al. Continuous positive airway pressure reduces subjective daytime sleepiness in patients with mild to moderate Alzheimer's disease with sleep disordered breathing. J Am Geriatr Soc 2006; 54:777–781.
56. Maria B, Sophia S, Michalis M, et al. Sleep breathing disorders in patients with idiopathic Parkinson's disease. Respir Med 2003; 97(10):1151–1157.
57. Arnulf I, Konofal E, Merino-Andreu M et al. Parkinson's disease and sleepiness: an integral part of PD. Neurology 2002; 58(7):1019–1024.
58. Emre M. Dementia associated with Parkinson's disease. Lancet neurology 2003; 2: 229–237.
59. Schapira AH. Excessive daytime sleepiness in Parkinson's disease. Neurology 2004; 63(8 suppl 3):S24–S27.
60. Bliwise DL, Bliwise NG, Partinen M, Pursley AM, Dement WC. Sleep apnea and mortality in an aged cohort. Am J Public Health 1988; 78:544–547.

61. Cohen MC, Rohtla KM, Lavery CE, Muller JE, Mittleman MA. Meta-analysis of the morning excess of acute myocardial infarction and sudden cardiac death. Am J Cardiol 1997; 79:1512–1516.

62. Findley LJ, Zwillich CW, Ancoli-Israel S, Kripke DF, Tisi G, Moser KM. Cheyne-Stokes breathing during sleep in patients with left ventricular heart failure. South Med J 1985; 78:11–15.

63. Hanly PJ, Zuberi-Khokhar NS. Increased mortality associated with Cheyne-Stokes respiration in patients with congestive heart failure. Am J Respir Crit Care Med 1996; 153(1):272–276.

64. Hoch CC, Reynolds CFI, Houck PR, et al. Predicting mortality in mixed depression and dementia using EEG sleep variables. J Neuropsych Clin Neurosci 1989; 1(4):366–371.

65. Ancoli-Israel S, Kripke DF, Klauber MR, et al. Morbidity, mortality and sleep disordered breathing in community dwelling elderly. Sleep 1996; 19(4):277–282.

66. Mant A, King M, Saunders NA, Pond CD, Goode E, Hewitt H. Four-year follow-up of mortality and sleep-related respiratory disturbance in non-demented seniors. Sleep 1995; 18(6):433–438.

67. Ancoli-Israel S, DuHamel ER, Stepnowsky C, Engler R, Cohen-Zion M, Marler M. The relationship between congestive heart failure, sleep disordered breathing and mortality in older men. Chest 2003; 124(4):1400–1405.

68. Wauquier A, Van Sweden B, Lagaay AM, Kemp B, Kamphuisen HAC. Ambulatory monitoring of sleep-wakefulness patterns in healthy elderly males and females (>88 years): The "Senieur" protocol. J Am Geriatr Soc 1992; 40:109–114.

69. Ancoli-Israel S, Coy TV. Are breathing disturbances in elderly equivalent to sleep apnea syndrome? Sleep 1994; 17:77–83.

70. Grunstein R. Continuous postivie airway pressure treatment for obstructive sleep apnea-hypopnea syndrome. In: Kryger MH, Roth T, Dement WC, eds. Principles and Practice of Sleep Medicine. Philadelphia, PA: Elsevier, 2005:1066–1080.

71. Guilleminault C, Lin CM, Goncalves MA, Ramos E. A prospective study of nocturia and the quality of life of elderly patients with obstructive sleep apnea or sleep onset insomnia. J Psychosom Res 2004; 56:511–515.

72. Zhang X, Yin K, Wang H, Su M, Yang Y. Effect of continuous positive airway pressure treatment on elderly Chinese patients with obstructive sleep apnea in the prethrombotic state. Chin Med J 2003; 116(9):1426–1428.

73. Ferguson KA, Lowe AA. Oral Appliances for Sleep Disordered Breathing. In: Kryger MH, Roth T, Dement WC, eds. Principles and Practice of Sleep Medicine. Philadelphia, PA: Elsevier; 2005:1098–11-8.

74. Powell NB, Riley R, Guilleminault C. Surgical management of sleep disordered breathing. In: Kryger MH, Roth T, Dement WC, eds. Principls and Practice of Sleep Medicine. Philadelphia, PA: Elsevier, 2005:1081–1097.

75. Sher AE, Schechtman KB, Piccirillo JF. The efficacy of surgical modifications of the upper airway in adults with obstructive sleep apnea syndrome. Sleep 1996; 19(2):156–177.

76. Phillips BA, Schmitt FA, Berry DT, Lamb DG, Amin M, Cook YR. Treatment of obstructive sleep apnea. A preliminary report comparing nasal CPAP to nasal oxygen in patients with mild OSA. Chest 1990; 98(2):325–330.

77. Fletcher EC, Munafo D. Role of nocturnal oxygen therapy in obstructive sleep apnea: when should it be used? Chest 1990; 98(6):1497–1504.

78. Levy P, Pepin JL, Malauzat D, Emeriau JP, Leger JM. Is sleep apnea syndrome in the elderly a specific entity? Sleep 1996; 19(3):S29–S38.

79. He J, Kryger MH, Zorick FJ, Conway W, Roth T. Mortality and apnea index in obstructive sleep apnea: experience in 385 male patients. Chest 1988; 94:9–14.

80. Lavie P, Lavie L, Herer P. All-cause mortality in males with sleep apnoea syndrome: declining mortality rates with age. Eur Respir J 2005; 25(3):514–520.

81. Noda A, Okada T, Yasuma F, Sobue T, Nakashima N, Yokota M. Prognosis of the middle-aged and aged patients with obstructive sleep apnea syndrome. Psychiatry Clin Neurosci 1998; 52(1):79–85.

17 Medication Effects

Julie A. Dopheide
Schools of Pharmacy and Medicine, University of Southern California,
Los Angeles, California, U.S.A.

INTRODUCTION

Obstructive sleep apnea (OSA) is unique among neurologic conditions because there is no medication that is considered first-line treatment. Instead, pharmacotherapy is considered adjunctive (see also Chapter 13) to more established treatments such as, continuous positive airway pressure (CPAP) or bilevel positive airway pressure (BPAP), an oral appliance (1), or a surgical intervention such as uvulopalatopharyngoplasty (2,3). With this in mind, it is perhaps even more important to consider how an individual's routine medications impact OSA. Individuals with sleep apnea frequently take medications to manage coexisting conditions such as hypertension, diabetes, coronary artery disease, congestive heart failure, pain, a mood disorder, or nocturnal insomnia (2,4). Any medication with significant sedating or central nervous system depressant properties, including benzodiazepines and opioids can interfere with the mini-arousals necessary to stimulate breathing and maintain an intact airway in persons with OSA (5,6). Interestingly, the use of antihypertensive or antidepressant medication is a marker for increased risk of OSA, particularly if an individual is prescribed both antihypertensives and antidepressants and if their age is between 20 and 59 years old (7).

This chapter will review the literature regarding medications that improve OSA and medications that worsen OSA. Guidelines for the safe and effective use of medications for individuals with OSA and coexisting conditions will also be presented.

MEDICATIONS TO TREAT OBSTRUCTIVE SLEEP APNEA OR ITS SYMPTOMS
Modafinil
Clinical Trials
Modafinil (Provigil®) is the only Food and Drug Administration (FDA)-approved medication for improving daytime functioning and alertness in those who have only partially responded to CPAP. Three randomized, double-blind, placebo-controlled trials examined the efficacy of oral modafinil 200 mg to 400 mg once daily in patients with excessive daytime sleepiness associated with OSA. Two of the OSA trials were of parallel-group design ($n = 157$ and 309; treatment duration 4 and 12 weeks) and the third was a crossover trial ($n = 30$; treatment duration 2 weeks). In both parallel trials, but not in the crossover trial, modafinil (dosage of 200 mg or 400 mg) improved wakefulness as measured on the Epworth sleepiness scale, and significantly more patients were "better" with no reduction in CPAP use. Modafinil (Table 1, for more information on modafinil see also Chapter 13) improved functional status and health-related quality of life to a significantly greater extent than placebo (8–10). In the smaller, crossover trial, there was no significant between-group

TABLE 1   Medications That May Improve Obstructive Sleep Apnea

Medication	Mechanism for clinical benefit	Special considerations
Modafinil (treatment)	Decreases daytime sedation Stimulates hypocretin/orexin system Stimulates NE/DA Improves quality-of-life	200 mg in morning Nausea, headache common 3A4 inducer, 2C9 inhibitor Adjunct to PAP
SSRI (may improve)	Increases upper airway patency May decrease AHI	Paroxetine most well-studied Nausea, sexual side effects
HRT: estrogen/ progesterone (may improve)	Maintain upper airway patency Improves AHI	Weigh risk vs. benefit individually
Antihypertensive (may improve)	Variable, based on agent Adjunct to PAP, weight loss, oral appliance More studies needed	ACE inhibitors, cardioselective beta-adrenergic blockers may be safer than centrally acting agents: reserpine, clonidine, guanfacine

Abbreviations: ACE, angiotensin-converting enzyme; AHI, apnea-hypopnea index; DA, dopamine; HRT, hormone replacement therapy; NE, norepinephrine; PAP, positive airway pressure; SSRI, selective serotonin reuptake inhibitor.
Source: From Refs. 6, 10, 14, 17–19, 22.

difference in patients rated as "better" and there was a significant reduction in CPAP use (10). Modafinil did not have an adverse impact on night-time sleep as measured by polysomnography. The studies show no difference in wakefulness-enhancing effects between the 200 mg and 400 mg dose and so the FDA-approved dose is 200 mg per day (10). Modafinil has not been studied as an adjunct to OSA treatments other than CPAP.

Clinicians have expressed concern that the use of modafinil for OSA may result in patients feeling less inclined to consistently use CPAP (8). Taking modafinil without CPAP puts an individual at risk for more cardiovascular side effects and denies them the potential benefits of CPAP in lowering excessive sympathetic tone, lowering blood pressure, facilitating weight loss, and preventing the long-term development of cardiopulmonary diseases including heart failure (4,10).

Mechanism of Action

Modafinil's mechanism of action is not fully understood, but it is thought to activate orexin/hypocretin neurons in the hypothalamus, which are responsible for maintaining wakefulness (10). Its wakefulness-promoting effects may also be related to a reduction in gamma aminobutyric acid-ergic transmission and some potentiation of dopaminergic and noradrenergic function. An intact noradrenergic system is essential for the optimal wakefulness-promoting effects from modafinil, although it does not seem to have direct alpha-1 adrenergic agonist effects and it does not inhibit monoamine oxidase (10).

Pharmacokinetics

Pharmacokinetic (PK) data on modafinil were obtained from healthy male subjects. The possibility of PK variability in females or those with coexisting medical problems is largely unstudied. Modafinil is well-absorbed and it reaches peak plasma concentrations in 2.7 hours. The plasma half-life is approximately 15 to 17 hours and steady state is reached after two to four days. Modafinil is hepatically metabolized via P450 [cytochrome P (CYP)] isoenzymes to inactive metabolites (10). Modafinil impacts multiple isoenzymes and has the potential for significant drug interactions. It has been shown to induce CYP 3A/5 isoenzymes resulting in lower area under the curve (i.e., plot of drug concentration in plasma vs. time) of ethinylestradiol and triazolam (Halcion®), both substrates for CYP 3A4 (10,12). Modafinil can decrease the effectiveness of these drugs and other drugs metabolized by 3A4 including cyclosporine, verapamil (Calan®, Isoptin®, Verelan®), and lovastatin (Mevacor®, Altoprev®). Modafinil inhibits CYP 2C9 and 2C19 and therefore blood levels of phenytoin (Dilantin®, Phenytek®) and clozapine (Clozaril®) can be increased leading to possible toxicity (10,13).

Adverse Effects
The adverse events that were reported significantly more often in the modafinil group compared to placebo group in the clinical trials for OSA were headache ($p < 0.05$) and nausea ($p = 0.01$). In a 12-month extension study, the most commonly reported treatment-emergent adverse events in modafinil (dosage of 200–400 mg/day) recipients included infection, nervousness, headache, accidental injury, sinusitis, rhinitis, depression, anxiety, insomnia, and dizziness (5–11% of patients). Potential study participants were excluded if they had active clinical disease [e.g., hypertension, congestive heart failure, chronic obstructive pulmonary disease (COPD), depression] and so it is possible that adverse effects would be more common and significant in these groups of patients (10). Elevated blood pressure, increased heart rate, dizziness, nervousness, and insomnia have all been reported with regular use of modafinil (10).

Other Agents Used to Treat Obstructive Sleep Apnea
(See Also Chapter 13)
From the mid 1970s to the 1990s, prior to the FDA approval of modafinil, medications like protriptyline (Vivactil®), imipramine (Tofranil®), medroxyprogesterone (Cycrin®, Provera®), acetazolamide (Diamox®), and theophylline (Theolair®, Uniphyl®) were utilized to improve alertness and daytime functioning in those with OSA. Studies in small numbers of patients showed limited efficacy, usually improving mild to moderate symptoms only. Some studies showed no clinically significant benefit and currently these medications are infrequently used. All are included for the sake of completeness (6,14,15).

Protriptyline, a tricyclic antidepressant (TCA) with activating properties, was studied in doses of 10 to 30 mg every morning to improve wakefulness and decrease apneic episodes. Its proposed mechanism of action is two-fold: reducing rapid eye movement (REM) sleep which in turn reduces the longer oxygen desaturation periods characteristic of REM sleep, and enhancing upper airway tone. Imipramine, a less noradrenergic selective TCA, has demonstrated similar efficacy to protriptyline. Because of their REM suppressant effects, TCAs have been proposed as a reasonable option for individuals with REM-dependent OSA; however, the anticholinergic and cardiovascular side effects of TCAs outweigh the potential benefits for most individuals (6).

Medroxyprogesterone, a synthetic form of progesterone, is thought to stimulate respiratory drive and improve oxygenation and ventilation in a dose-related manner up to 60 mg/day. Four systematic studies have concluded that it is not beneficial for the majority of patients although one double-blind study showed a reduction of the apnea-hypopnea index (AHI) for a small number of patients (15). Medroxyprogesterone 20 mg three times a day can be considered for OSA patients who do not tolerate CPAP, who refuse surgical treatment, and who are candidates for progesterone therapy for other reasons (e.g., menopause in women, paraphilia in men).

Acetazolamide is a carbonic anhydrase inhibitor that results in the development of metabolic acidosis, which normally augments ventilation. This is how it works to prevent altitude sickness in mountain climbers. The administration of acetazolamide 500 mg to 1000 mg in divided doses reduced the frequency of apneas plus hypopneas in patients with OSA, but there was no decrease in awakenings from sleep and no improved breathing during sleep (14,15). Acetazolamide use is associated with many adverse effects including fatigue, drowsiness, nausea, vomiting, hyperglycemia, hyperuricemia, and electrolyte abnormalities. Due to lack of significant efficacy and poor tolerability, acetazolamide has no place in the routine treatment of OSA (14–16).

Theophylline is a ventilatory stimulant that blocks the ventilatory depressant action of adenosine. In a placebo-controlled trial of theophylline in OSA, there was a significant reduction in obstructive events during sleep (−29%), but sleep quality was significantly worsened by theophylline with more frequent arousals and daytime impairment. Other studies have shown that any potentially beneficial effect on sleep apnea was lost with time in the majority of patients. Theophylline has no place in the routine treatment of persons with sleep apnea (6).

MEDICATIONS THAT MAY IMPROVE OBSTRUCTIVE SLEEP APNEA OR ITS SYMPTOMS
Selective Serotonin Reuptake Inhibitors

An early trial of the serotonin precursor, tryptophan, showed that its use was associated with a moderate reduction of OSA. This led to investigations with selective serotonin reuptake inhibitors (SSRIs) mainly, fluoxetine (Prozac®, Sarafem®) and paroxetine (Paxil®, Pexeva®). Fluoxetine was associated with a 40% reduction of AHI with good tolerability. It is the most activating SSRI with an approximate 10% to 20% incidence of nocturnal insomnia in clinical trials for depression (Table 1).

Paroxetine, an SSRI that is less activating and more sedating than fluoxetine, has been studied in OSA patients in order to assess potential benefits on upper-airway patency during sleep. In double-blind, crossover fashion, paroxetine 20 mg was given to 20 male OSA patients (mean age of 52.1 years) for two six-week periods separated by a four-week washout period. Results showed paroxetine reduced the apnea index during NREM sleep but not during REM sleep. No significant effect on hypopnea indices was found. Paroxetine therapy enhanced serotonergic transmission and improved breathing during NREM sleep in OSA; however, there was no significant difference in daytime sleepiness or complaints as assessed on a visual analog scale (17). A separate double-blind crossover study in eight adult men with severe OSA showed that a single 40 mg dose of paroxetine augmented peak inspiratory genioglossus activity during NREM sleep but this effect was not sufficient to decrease the frequency of obstructive apnea (18). Available data show that paroxetine can increase upper-airway patency during sleep (17,18).

These results lend some support for the use of SSRIs in treating depression and anxiety disorders in individuals with OSA; however, they do not provide evidence to recommend the use of an SSRI for treating OSA alone or in place of CPAP or BPAP. In addition, longitudinal studies evaluating maintenance antidepressant use in patients with OSA are needed to confirm safety. Nevertheless, compared to TCAs, trazodone (Desyrel®), nefazodone (Serzone®), and mirtazapine (Remeron®), SSRIs are less sedating and therefore less likely to worsen sleep apnea by preventing centrally-mediated mini-arousals that stimulate breathing during an episode of apnea.

Estrogen and Progesterone

Estrogen and progesterone may exert a protective effect on the upper airway, preventing premenopausal women from developing sleep apnea (19). The role of hormone replacement therapy (HRT) in sleep-disordered breathing was examined in a cohort of 2852 women who were 50 years of age or older and participated in the Sleep Heart Health Study. The prevalence of sleep-disordered breathing (AHI of 15 or more) among hormone users was approximately half the prevalence among nonusers (19). The inverse association between hormone use and sleep-disordered breathing was evident in various subgroups and was particularly strong among women 50 to 59 years old. An earlier study showed that postmenopausal women had a significantly higher mean AHI compared with premenopausal women, and this significant difference persisted even after adjusting for body mass index and neck circumference (20). The effects of HRT on OSA should be taken into consideration when weighing the risk to benefit ratio of HRT for an individual perimenopausal or menopausal woman.

Cardiac/Cardiovascular Medications

Given that systemic hypertension occurs in nearly one-half of patients with OSA and conversely, 20% to 30% of patients with essential hypertension are found to have OSA (21), the impact of antihypertensive medication on OSA is poorly studied. Limited information indicates beta-blockers, angiotensin-converting enzyme (ACE) inhibitors, and calcium channel blockers can improve symptoms of OSA while improving blood pressure control (6). Both the ACE inhibitor cilazapril (Inhibace®, not commercially available in the U.S.) and the beta-blocker metoprolol (Lopressor®, Toprol®) reduced apnea-hypopnea frequency by approximately 30%. The alpha-2 adrenergic agonist clonidine (Catapres®) reduced REM sleep-related OSA activity in six out of eight patients, while no effects were seen on NREM sleep. Similar beneficial results on OSA symptoms were associated with the calcium channel blockers isradipine (Dynacirc®) and mibefradil (Posicor®) in separate studies (6). Amlodipine (Norvasc®) did not exacerbate sleep-disordered breathing in newly diagnosed hypertensive patients (22,23).

Although most results show that antihypertensive medication either improves OSA symptoms or has no significant effect, there is some concern that beta-adrenergic receptor blocking agents could result in excessively low heart rate during apneic episodes, particularly during REM sleep when autonomic instability peaks. Also, centrally acting antihypertensive medications like clonidine (Catapres®) or guanfacine (Tenex®) can cause sedation and fatigue, and worsening daytime functioning for individuals already sleepy secondary to OSA (6,14).

More impressive, are the results of positive airway pressure (PAP) in improving hypertension. One investigation of 540 consecutive patients (mean age 55.4 years) found a significant decrease in blood pressure and heart rate in OSA subjects effectively treated with CPAP. Results were greatest in those who had elevated blood pressure at the start of therapy and benefits occurred exclusively in those not taking blood pressure medication. Patients with a change in blood pressure medication during the study were excluded from analysis and therefore no conclusions can be made regarding PAPs efficacy in those who take blood pressure medicine (23). Clearly, more studies are needed to assess the effectiveness and safety of blood pressure medication in OSA patients. Until such studies are available, it is wise to recommend PAP with adjunctive antihypertensive medication to control blood pressure that remains high despite well-adjusted PAP. There are insufficient data to assess whether one antihypertensive medication is preferred in persons with OSA but there is some suggestion that ACE inhibitors may have the least potential for adverse effects in OSA patients (6,14).

MEDICATIONS OR SUBSTANCES THAT MAY WORSEN OBSTRUCTIVE SLEEP APNEA OR ITS SYMPTOMS (SEE ALSO CHAPTER 13)

Effective, nonpharmacologic treatment of OSA, particularly CPAP, has been shown to improve comorbid medical conditions (e.g., heart failure, hypertension) and decrease healthcare resource utilization (11,24). Effective CPAP can also improve the safety of concomitant medication that can worsen OSA such as sedative/hypnotics, anesthetics, analgesics, anticonvulsants, antihistamines, and antipsychotics (25,26). Table 2 lists medications that may be dangerous for individuals with sleep apnea, the mechanism of worsening apnea, and any special considerations for use. Even though CPAP can improve the safety of these concomitant medications, clinician monitoring with polysomnography in a sleep lab may be needed to facilitate

TABLE 2 Medications or Substances That May Worsen Obstructive Sleep Apnea

Medication	Mechanism	Special considerations
Opioids	CNS depression	Safe use with PAP is possible
	Brain fails to signal diaphragm to move and take in air	Patient counseling essential
		NSAID alternative possible
Anxiolytics, Benzodiazepines	CNS depression	High dose and long half-life agents most problematic
	Brain fails to signal diaphragm to move and take in air	Patient counseling essential
Hypnotics, Benzodiazepines, Z-hypnotics	CNS depression	High dose and long half-life agents most problematic
	Brain fails to signal diaphragm to move and take in air	Safe use with PAP is possible
Antipsychotics with high sedation	CNS depression	Older conventional agents: chlorpromazine, thioridazine
	Brain fails to signal diaphragm to move and take in air	Atypical agents: clozapine, olanzapine, quetiapine
Alcohol	Upper airway dysfunction	Additive effects with other agents
	CNS depression	Counseling on abstinence and consequences of alcohol use

Abbreviations: CNS, central nervous system; NSAID, nonsteroidal anti-inflammatory drug; PAP, positive airway pressure.
Source: From Refs. 6, 14, 26, 34.

adjustments in CPAP fit and to assess whether the concomitant medication is actually safe when used with CPAP.

Anesthetics, Opioids, and Barbiturates

Recommendations for safe perioperative care in the OSA patient include the use of CPAP preoperatively, consideration of intubation over fiberoptic bronchoscope during surgery, and the use of CPAP and regional anesthesia postoperatively rather than the continuous administration of opiates (26). Nasal CPAP can eliminate the postoperative risk of hypoxemia, which would then allow the use of adequate parenteral or oral analgesics. Analgesia has been achieved safely with intravenous morphine sulfate or meperidine hydrochloride (Demerol®) (intensive care unit) and oral oxycodone (OxyContin®, Roxicodone®), while patients were receiving CPAP during all periods of sleep after surgery. There were no significant reductions in SpO_2 regardless of the severity of OSA syndrome or obesity (26).

All opiates have the potential to worsen sleep apnea, compromise breathing, and even cause sleep apnea is some cases. Opioids depress respiration, by direct effect on brainstem respiratory centers and by reducing the ventilatory responsiveness to carbon dioxide and hypoxia. Central sleep apnea (CSA) was present in 30% of individuals on methadone maintenance therapy with the severity directly related to the blood level of methadone (27). CSA occurs in less than 1% of the general population (28). Any patient with CSA or OSA taking an opiate medication is at risk of cessation of breathing during sleep without proper nonpharmacologic treatment (e.g., PAP). Persons with sleep apnea should be counseled that any opiate, even oral acetaminophen/hydrocodone (Vicodin®), the most commonly prescribed opiate for acute pain, can be dangerous due to impairment of normal respiratory function. Alternative pain control (e.g., nonsteroidal anti-inflammatory drugs like ibuprofen) should be used in patients whose apnea is not well-controlled with PAP (6,27).

Barbiturates, such as phenobarbital, pentobarbital (Nembutal®), secobarbital (Seconal®), and mephobarbital (Mebaral®) have well-established respiratory-depressant effects and they should not be used in patients with OSA. A less potent barbiturate, butalbital, is found in headache remedies like Fiorinal®. It can also compromise respiratory function and it should be avoided in OSA patients (15).

Sedative/Hypnotics

Benzodiazepines are commonly prescribed orally to treat anxiety disorders, mood disorders, and insomnia. In addition, they are used parenterally as premedications before procedures such as endoscopy or minor surgery. The most prescribed agents include alprazolam (Xanax®, Niravam®), clonazepam (Klonopin®), diazepam (Valium®), lorazepam (Ativan®), midazolam (Versed®), and temazepam (Restoril®) (29). Benzodiazepines exert respiratory-depressant effects centrally in addition to decreasing upper airway tone. The respiratory-depressant effects of benzodiazepines range from mild to the most severe outcome, death (14).

Individuals with sleep apnea or COPD are most at risk for benzodiazepine-associated respiratory distress; however, parenteral midazolam use induced OSA and a severe reduction in SpO_2 in five of 21 patients with no history of OSA. Nasal CPAP reversed the respiratory deterioration in these patients (25). In another study of elderly patients with mild sleep apnea, seven subjects received temazepam 15 mg/night to 30 mg/night and eight subjects received placebo. There was no difference in respiratory distress between the two groups (30). In addition to the respiratory-depressant effects during sleep, benzodiazepines have the potential to cause next-day hangover and contribute to excessive daytime sleepiness and cognitive impairment already experienced by individuals with OSA (31). Because benzodiazepine-associated respiratory function worsening in OSA is difficult to predict, sleep experts recommend avoiding benzodiazepines in untreated patients with severe OSA, especially in those with daytime hypoventilation (14).

Zaleplon (Sonata®), zolpidem (Ambien®, Ambien® CR), and eszopiclone (Lunesta®) are nonbenzodiazepine hypnotics that act on the benzodiazepine receptor complex. They are selective for the alpha-1 benzodiazepine receptor and demonstrate hypnotic efficacy without significant anxiolytic, anticonvulsant, or muscle relaxant effects (31). All of these "Z-hypnotics" are FDA-approved for insomnia although eszopiclone and zolpidem controlled-release are the only agents approved for long-term treatment (32,33). Compared to n onselective benzodiazepines, Z-hypnotics are less likely to affect sleep architecture at recommended hypnotic doses (31–34).

Zolpidem is the most prescribed and most well-studied agent. Ten patients with stable COPD were given zolpidem 10 mg over eight consecutive nights in order to assess zolpidem's impact on respiratory function. Zolpidem did not impair sleep architecture or diurnal pulmonary function tests or central control of breathing (35). Other data indicate that zolpidem 20 mg induces a significant reduction of respiratory flow in healthy individuals and decreases oxygen saturation in patients with sleep apnea syndrome (34). Zaleplon and eszopiclone's impact on respiratory function has not been assessed in patients with COPD or OSA; however, since they possess the same pharmacologic activity, there is a dose-related potential for compromising respiratory function in patients treated with these agents as well.

Alcohol

Alcohol is not a medication per se, but it is included in this chapter since many individuals self-medicate with alcohol, a potentially fatal problem for those with OSA. Clearly, alcohol increases apnea frequency in people with pre-existing OSA but it can also induce obstructive apnea in people who otherwise only snore. Individuals with OSA should be counseled regarding the consequences of drinking alcohol, namely increased breathing difficulty that could be fatal (36).

CONCLUSIONS

Modafinil is the only FDA-approved medication indicated to manage excessive daytime sleepiness in patients with OSA who have only partially responded to CPAP. Each routine medication should be evaluated to determine its impact or lack of impact on an individual patient's breathing during sleep. Agents that may improve OSA include: SSRIs, antihypertensives, and estrogen/progesterone therapy in women. Medications or substances that may worsen sleep apnea include opioids, barbiturates, sedative/hypnotics, and alcohol. CPAP therapy can improve the safety of medications known to worsen sleep apnea. Clinician monitoring with polysomnography in a sleep laboratory is optimal to facilitate adjustments in CPAP fit and to assess whether the concomitant medication is actually safe when used with CPAP.

REFERENCES

1. Kushida CA, Littner MR, Hirshkowitz M, et al. Practice parameters for the use of continuous and bilevel positive airway pressure devices to treat adult patients with sleep-related breathing disorders. Sleep 2006; 29(3):375–380.

2. Caples SM, Gami AS, Somers VK. Obstructive sleep apnea. Ann Intern Med 2005; 142(3): 187–197.
3. Sundaram S, Bridgman SA, Lim J, Lasserson TJ. Surgery for obstructive sleep apnoea. Cochrane Database Syst Rev 2005; 1:1–66.
4. Shamsuzzaman ASM, Gersh BJ, Somers VK. Obstructive sleep apnea: implications for cardiac and vascular disease. JAMA 2003; 290(14):1906–1914.
5. Flemons WW. Obstructive sleep apnea. N Engl J Med 2002; 347(7):498–504.
6. Grunstein RR, Hedner J, Grote L. Treatment options for sleep apnea. Drugs 2001; 61(2):237–251.
7. Farney RJ, Lugo A, Jensen RL, et al. Simultaneous use of antidepressant and antihypertensive medications increases likelihood of diagnosis of obstructive sleep apnea syndrome. Chest 2004; 125:1279–1285.
8. Black JE, Hirshkowitz M. Modafinil for treatment of residual excessive sleepiness in nasal continuous positive airway pressure-treated obstructive sleep apnea/hypopnea syndrome. Sleep 2005; 28(4):464–471.
9. Pack AI, Black JE, Schwartz JRL, et al. Modafinil as adjunct therapy for daytime sleepiness in obstructive sleep apnea. Am J Respir Crit Care Med 2001; 164:1675–1681.
10. Keating GM, Raffin MJ. Modafinil: a review of its use in excessive sleepiness associated with obstructive sleep apnoea/hypopnoea syndrome and shift work sleep disorder. CNS Drugs 2005; 19(9):785–803.
11. Kaneko Y, Floras JS, Usui K, et al. Cardiovascular effects of continuous positive airway pressure in patients with heart failure and obstructive sleep apnea. N Engl J Med 2003; 348(13):1233–1241.
12. Robertson P Jr, Hellriegel ET, Arora S, et al. Effect of modafinil on the pharmacokinetics of ethinyl estradiol and triazolam in healthy volunteers. Clin Pharmcol Ther 2002; 71(1):46–56.
13. Dequardo JR. Modafinil-associated clozapine toxicity. Am J Psychiatry 2002; 7:1243.
14. Robinson RW, Zwillich CW. Medications, sleep, and breathing. In: Kryger MH, Roth T, Dement WC, eds. Principles of Sleep Medicine. 3rd ed, ch. 69. Philadelphia, PA: W.B. Saunders Co, 2000.
15. Sanders M. Medical therapy for obstructive sleep apnea-hypopnea syndrome. In: Kryger MH, Roth T, Dement WC, eds. Principles of Sleep Medicine. 3rd ed, Chapter 75. Philadelphia, PA: W.B. Saunders Co, 2000:879–892.
16. Inoue Y, Takata K, Sakamoto I, et al. Clinical efficacy and indication of acetazolamide treatment on sleep apnea syndrome. Psychiatry Clin Neurosci 1999; 53(2):321–322.
17. Kraiczi H, Hedner J, Dahlof P, et al. Effect of serotonin uptake inhibition on breathing during sleep and daytime symptoms in obstructive sleep apnea. Sleep 1999; 22(1):61–67.
18. Berry RB, Yamaura EM, Gill K, Reist C. Acute effects of paroxetine on geniogulossus activity in obstructive sleep apnea. Sleep 1999; 22(8):1087–1092.
19. Avidan AV. Sleep in the geriatric patient population. Semin Neurol 2005; 25(1):52–63.
20. Young T, Finn L, Austin D, et al. Menopausal status and sleep-disordered breathing in the Wisconsin Sleep Cohort Study. Am J Respir Crit Care Med 2003; 167:1181–1185.
21. Tun Ye, Hida W, Okabe S, et al. Can nasal continuous positive airway pressure decrease clinic blood pressure in patients with obstructive sleep apnea? Tohoku J Exp Med 2003; 201:181–190.
22. Bartel PR, Loock M, Becker P, et al. Short-term antihypertensive medication does not exacerbate sleep-disordered breathing in newly diagnosed hypertensive patients. Am J Hypertens 1997; 10:640–645.
23. Borgel J, Sanner BM, Keskin F, et al. Obstructive sleep apnea and blood pressure. Am J Hypertens 2004; 17:1081–1087.
24. Albarrak M, Banno K, Sabbagh AA, et al. Utilization of healthcare resources in OSA syndrome: a 5-year follow-up study in men using CPAP. Sleep 2005; 28(10):1306–1311.
25. Nozaki-Taguchi N, Isono S, Nishino T, et al. Upper airway obstruction during midazolam sedation: modification by nasal CPAP. Can J Anaesth 1995; 42(8):685–690.
26. Jain SS, Dhand R. Perioperative treatment of patients with obstructive sleep apnea. Curr Opin Pulm Med 2004; 10:482–488.
27. Wang D, Teichtahl H, Drummer O, et al. Central sleep apnea in stable methadone maintenance treatment patients. Chest 2005; 128:1348–1356.

28. White D. Central sleep apnea. In: Kryger MH, Roth T, Dement WC, eds. Principles of Sleep Medicine. 3rd ed, Chapter 71. Philadelphia, PA: WB Saunders Co, 2000:827–839.
29. Top 200 Prescription Drugs of 2005. Pharmacy Times, May 2006:26–30. www.pharmacytimes.com.
30. Camacho ME, Morin CM. The effect of temazepam on respiration in elderly insomniacs with mild sleep apnea. Sleep 1995; 18(8):644–645.
31. Benca R. Diagnosis and treatment of chronic insomnia: a review. Psychiatric Services. 2005; 56:332–343.
32. Lunesta, Package Insert. www.lunesta.com. (accessed 2-11-05).
33. Ambien CR Package Insert. www.ambiencr.com (accessed 1-12-06).
34. Terzano MG, Rossi M, Palomba V, et al. New drugs for insomnia: comparative tolerability of zopiclone, zolpidem and zaleplon. Drug Safety 2003; 26(4):261–282.
35. Girault C, Muir JF, Mihaltan F, et al. Effects of repeated administration of zolpidem on sleep, diurnal and nocturnal respiratory function, vigilance, and physical performance inpatients with COPD. Chest 1996; 110(5):1203–1211.
36. Bassiri AG, Guilleminault C. Clinical features and evaluation of OSA-HS. In: Kryger MH, Roth T, Dement WC, eds. Principles of Sleep Medicine. 3rd ed, Chapter 74. Philadelphia, PA: W.B. Saunders, 2000.

18 Snoring and Upper Airway Resistance Syndrome

Riccardo A. Stoohs
Somnolab Sleep Disorders Centers—Dortmund, Essen, Dortmund, Germany

Antoine Aschmann
Medica Surgical Private Clinics, Mülheim, Germany

INTRODUCTION

The term "upper airway resistance syndrome" (UARS) was first coined in 1992 (1) and 1993 (2). Prior to these reports, in the late 1980s, we conducted a series of studies at Stanford University aimed at the pathophysiologic mechanisms of subtle flow limitation associated with snoring during sleep. Using a pneumotachometer and esophageal pressure monitoring it became apparent that there existed a number of individuals with impaired respiration during sleep, who did not fit the typical diagnostic criteria of obstructive sleep apnea (OSA). This is to say that they presented with daytime sleepiness and snoring but without clear polysomnographic diagnostic criteria of apnea, hypopnea or oxygen desaturation. Despite the absence of these diagnostic criteria for OSA they still showed signs of abnormal breathing during sleep when investigated with pneumotachometers and esophageal pressure monitoring instead of oronasal thermistors. This led us to pose the question: "Obstructive sleep apnea or abnormal upper airway resistance during sleep?" (3). In 1991, we published the pathophysiologic phenomena of increased upper airway resistance leading to sleep fragmentation in the absence of apnea, hypopnea, and hypoxemia (4). For further reference into the historic development of UARS please refer to the article by Exar and Collop (5) for a more comprehensive review.

Fifteen years later, the majority of patients with UARS remain undiagnosed, although, a fair number of patients with OSA are being diagnosed with UARS. Others are diagnosed with "habitual" or primary snoring (PS). There are three reasons for this profound misunderstanding. First is the widespread use of the term "sleep-disordered breathing" (SDB) or "sleep-related breathing disorder" (SRBD). The fundamental problem in using these terms lies with the fact that they include any breathing abnormality during sleep, independent of type, pathogenetic background or clinical manifestation. The second reason is that many clinicians still do not have a clear understanding of the distinct diagnostic criteria and the differences in the clinical presentation of UARS and obstructive sleep apnea–hypopnea (OSAH) without daytime sleepiness and obstructive sleep apnea–hypopnea syndrome (OSAHS) (with daytime sleepiness). To make the issue even more complicated, in the second edition of *The International Classification of Sleep Disorders* (ICSD-2), the term "obstructive sleep apnea" (OSA) now incorporates the majority of these terms. UARS is also subsumed under this diagnosis because it was felt by the ICSD-2 SRBDs task force that pathophysiology does not significantly differ from that of OSA (6). And finally, many laboratories still do not use adequately sensitive methods to detect subtle flow limitation during sleep: they still use oronasal thermocouples.

The goal of this chapter is to review the current knowledge about snoring and UARS and to describe its typical clinical and diagnostic features.

PATHOPHYSIOLOGY

The pathophysiology of UARS has two components: a central component and a peripheral component. The central component is responsible for the adaptive mechanisms to the increase in upper airway resistance and ultimately its symptoms. The peripheral component is subdivided into the upper airway properties and functions during sleep. There is some considerable overlap of the behavior of these components in OSA and UARS. On the other hand, based on current knowledge there are also distinctive differences especially in the neural adaptive mechanisms between OSA and UARS. The interplay between overlap and difference is another reason for misdiagnosis of patients with UARS.

Peripheral Component

The extra-thoracic airways are comprised of the nasopharynx, oropharynx, and hypopharynx extending down to the supraglottic larynx. This anatomical system is highly compliant with a complex geometry. Its patency depends on muscular activity and is influenced by various factors such as sleep state, route of breathing, hypercapnia, hypoxia, and lung volume (7). In UARS and OSA, upper airway resistance during sleep can increase significantly so that ventilation becomes compromised triggering adaptive mechanisms. These adaptive mechanisms act to maintain the physiologic metabolic equilibrium as well as the behavioral state of sleep.

Adaptive Mechanisms

During conditions of upper airway collapse ventilation is compromised leading to a decrease in minute ventilation (V_I). Adaptive mechanisms counteracting the decrease in minute ventilation include an increase in mean inspiratory flow rate [tidal volume (V_T)/inspiratory time (T_I)] during the inspiratory phase of the respiratory cycle and prolongation of the inspiratory time of the respiratory cycle [also referred to as the duty cycle (T_I/T_{TOT})] (7–9). Under conditions of internal respiratory loading (increase of upper airway resistance) the V_T/T_I responds until it starts to decline. This is due to mechanical impediment increasing above levels where augmented neural drive reaches a ceiling where it cannot further increase inspiratory flow rate. At this point a second line of defense may be activated: the duty cycle, that is, prolongation of the inspiratory portion of the respiratory cycle. Previous and recent work has suggested that both compensatory mechanisms are distinct phenotypic traits and therefore genetically predetermined (7,10,11).

Respiratory Event Types

Why do patients exhibit apneas, others hypopneas or both and others (UARS) respiratory effort-related arousals (RERAs)? It could be related to either abnormal upper airway anatomical properties, the integrity of upper airway defense mechanisms, the chain of events at which arousal from sleep is the last resort, or a combination of all three factors. Upper airway anatomical factors include fat deposition, nasal resistance, tonsillar hypertrophy, and craniofacial abnormalities. Upper airway defense mechanisms translate into neuromuscular function whose net effect can be expressed as upper airway closing pressure (P_{CRIT}). In fact, Schwartz et al. (12) have shown that in normal individuals P_{CRIT} is markedly negative whereas in patients with predominantly apneas and hypopneas during sleep P_{CRIT} is relatively more positive. More recently, Gold et al. (13) have demonstrated that patients with UARS (P_{CRIT} −4.0 cm H_2O) present with P_{CRIT} levels, are intermediate between mild-to-moderate OSA (P_{CRIT} −1.6 cm H_2O) and normal controls (P_{CRIT} −15.4 cm H_2O). P_{CRIT} in patients with UARS is significantly different from asymptomatic primary snorers (PS) shown to have an average P_{CRIT} of −6.5 (14).

Electroencephalographic Arousal and Microstructure

As with OSA, respiratory abnormality in UARS is closely linked to its clinical presentation in terms of excessive daytime sleepiness (EDS). Other atypical signs of OSA (such as disorders of initiating and maintaining sleep) may be more frequent in UARS.

During inspiratory resistive loading, complex reflex mechanisms act to preserve upper airway patency (15) and metabolic demands. If this ultimate goal cannot be accomplished by respiratory compensation preserving sleep, only arousal from sleep will do so, at the cost of sleep integrity. The function of afferent upper airway receptors preserving metabolic demands during sleep in the face of flow limitation will likely depend on their status of impairment. Various studies in patients with OSA point to the fact that upper airway neurogenic pathology secondary to repetitive, prolonged stretching of pharyngeal tissue may be implicated in suboptimal load compensation. Data in support of this hypothesis of impaired sensory input come from two-point discrimination studies of the palatal mucosa (16,17) backed by biopsies from palatopharyngeal muscles (18), and histological studies in OSA patients (19,20). To further complicate the matters, there seems to be evidence that cortical processing of baroreceptor-mediated afferents may also be impaired in patients with OSA, while responses to auditory stimulation remain unaltered (21).

Taken together, these studies have produced evidence for the concept that in patients with OSA suboptimal load compensation and perhaps also impaired arousability could be interpreted on the basis of peripheral and central neurogenic alteration. The notion that patients with UARS present with abnormal upper airway closing pressures (P_{CRIT}) is not surprising and supports the clinical relevance of this sleep disorder. Gold et al. (13) have placed patients with UARS within the spectrum of severity between patients with OSA and normal individuals on the basis of P_{CRIT}. It would be inappropriate to infer from these studies that peripheral and central processing of a sleep-related inspiratory load can be placed equally on the scale of severity making UARS a less severe form of OSA. Gold et al. acknowledge this in their report. To the contrary, studies indicate that palatal two-point discrimination is preserved in patients with UARS, while it is obvious that such studies need to be controlled for the duration of respiratory abnormality (17). Further histologic studies in patients with UARS are needed.

Thus, while patients with OSA present with hyporeactivity to a respiratory load induced by increase of upper airway resistance during sleep, patients with UARS may actually respond in the opposite fashion. They may be hyper-reactive to inspiratory loading while the etiologic foundation for this abnormality is likely the same in OSA and UARS: increased P_{CRIT} leads to flow limitation, triggering load compensation.

Arousal from sleep under conditions of flow limitation due to increased upper airway resistance during sleep constitutes defeat. One of the objectives of load compensation apart from metabolic demands is sleep maintenance. Mean inspiratory flow and duty cycle act to protect it. However, their actions crucially depend on afferent sensory input from upper airway receptors, which seem to be impaired in patients with OSA. Thus, patients with OSA develop a second line of defense based on the time constants of biochemical feedback systems (hypoxia and hypercapnia). In patients with UARS the biochemical feedback system is not activated resulting in the absence of repetitive hypoxia in the chain of events. Based on these findings it appears that patients with UARS respond with a central activation to respiratory abnormality during sleep that is different from patients with OSA. Investigation of this response has been focused on macrostructural electroencephalographic (EEG) changes, that is, visible EEG arousal detected in recordings from central electrodes and microstructural analysis of EEG power spectrum changes (2). Early studies in patients with UARS have described the association between flow limitation/increase in respiratory effort and the termination of such events by α-EEG arousal using standard American Academy of Sleep Medicine (AASM) [formerly American Sleep Disorders Association (ASDA)] criteria (4,22). While the identification of EEG arousal according to AASM criteria (23) may be the most practical approach to identify associations between breathing abnormality and sleep disruption in patients with UARS, it may not be the most accurate one. As Carley et al. (24) have shown, respiratory adaptive mechanisms can act in the absence of EEG arousal, and we know that respiratory events in patients with OSA may not be terminated in association with a visible EEG arousal according to AASM criteria (25). More recently, using EEG spectral analysis, Guilleminault et al. (26) have demonstrated that patients with UARS compared to patients with predominant apneas or hypopneas during sleep present with a significantly higher power density in the slow α-EEG band (7–9 Hz). Differences for the 9 to 10 Hz band were not significant. Pooling of these two bands still showed significant differences between UARS and OSA, while there was no difference for the faster bands (10–12 Hz). Of note, there was no gradual decline in the α-EEG power density as sleep progressed. Similarly, UARS patients show a significantly higher EEG power density in the low Δ band (0.5–2 Hz) than OSA patients and normal controls with no significant decline throughout the night (26).

Guilleminault et al. interpreted these findings on the basis of a difference in the cortical response and cortical processing to respiratory load compensation between OSA and UARS patients. Blunted afferent upper airway reflex responses (25), and localized upper airway polyneuropathy in OSA (19) may contrast to hyperreactivity in patients with UARS as documented by the changes in the α-EEG band leading to a higher Δ pressure throughout the night. Similarly, to the incoherence between objective EEG findings and the clinical presentation of EDS in patients with OSA, little is known about this interplay in patients with UARS.

POLYSOMNOGRAPHIC DIAGNOSTIC CRITERIA AND MEASUREMENT TECHNIQUES
RERAs and RERA Index
By definition, the apnea–hypopnea index (AHI) in patients with UARS is smaller than five. The lowest oxygen desaturation in our initial report was greater than 92% (2).

However, based on the AHI criterion of < 5, it is conceivable that some patients with UARS may present with lowest SaO_2 values < 92%. AHI alone is not sufficient to diagnose UARS. It simply means that if the AHI criterion of OSA is met, UARS can be excluded and a diagnosis of OSA must be made with additional information from the clinical history (27). For the diagnosis of UARS, a clear presence of RERAs must be established. Oronasal thermistors lack the sensitivity to detect this respiratory abnormality (28). In some sleep clinics it has become common practice to use direct or indirect assessment of esophageal pressure or more sensitive respiratory flow measurement techniques such as a nasal cannula connected to a pressure transducer, calibrated thoracic/abdominal inductive plethysmography, or use of a pneumotachograph. While there is agreement regarding the type of sensors used to identify RERAs, there is little consensus in the definition of RERAs. Some investigators using nasal cannulas (28–30) and respiratory inductive plethysmography (31) require a "flattening" of the inspiratory flow curve in conjunction with an arousal according to AASM criteria to identify RERAs. While the term "flattening" is rarely defined, our own experience with the use of nasal cannulas suggests that the signal quality is often compromised especially in the presence of mouth breathing. Respiratory inductive plethysmography, however, is problematic because of position changes. Data from a 2005 study show that inspiratory flow limitation from nasal cannula recording was superior to esophageal pressure recording for the detection of RERAs (32). In this study of normal subjects, alcohol [which is known to depress arousal responses and ventilatory drive (33)] was given to induce a breathing abnormality. Taken together, it is fair to conclude that a nasal cannula flow signal and esophageal pressure signal are reliable methods to identify RERAs if waveform changes resulting in event detection are clearly defined.

Definition of RERA

Based on our initial investigations on RERAs (4), the development of a calibrated nasal pneumotachograph sensor with a small deadspace that could be comfortably worn throughout the polysomnographic study would be desirable. This sensor was developed by the Johns Hopkins sleep research group. Figure 1 shows the sensor with amplifier, and Figure 2 shows the correlation between values obtained with the sensor in comparison with a pneumotachograph. In Dortmund, we have used this sensor in 158 full-night sleep studies. This sensor allows quantitatively defining RERAs based on our initial investigations of peak inspiratory flow decrement (4).

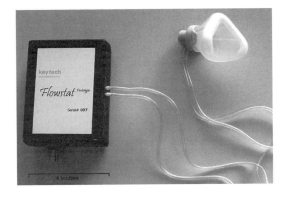

FIGURE 1 Novel flow sensor with amplifier.

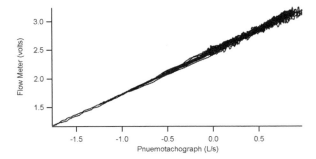

FIGURE 2 Relationship between a novel flow sensor and pneumotachograph.

This decrement was $43 \pm 14\%$ compared to silent unobstructed breathing. The decrement in V_T was 22% or 100 mL. These changes were often seen only within the last three breaths prior to arousal. In fact, during the early stages of periods with increased upper airway resistance (namely during slow wave sleep) we noted an increase in V_T and V_I suggesting a compensated state with higher metabolic demand that ultimately decompensates, leading to arousal from sleep. Based on the above mentioned studies, it seems appropriate to use cannula or pneumotachograph flow decrements of 30% (~ mean −1 SD as reported) (4) and/or esophageal pressure increments with P_{es} reversal (34) at arousal to determine RERAs when the arousal is taken as endpoint in the chain of events. In comparison to the definition of hypopnea, the distinct nature of RERA scoring lies in the fact that this event can be shorter than 10 seconds (one or two breaths) (4).

Guilleminault (26,35) and others (36) have suggested that an even subtler central endpoint may exist to increased upper airway resistance during sleep, which is not readily visible to the human eye in polysomnographic recordings. An article published in 2004, however, has challenged the arousal as endpoint for upper airway obstruction during sleep in OSA (37). More studies are needed to better define this endpoint and to develop simple methods for its assessment.

RERA Frequency
In addition to defining the event type (apnea, hypopnea, RERA), the frequency of these events occurring during sleep that defines the diagnosis has to be established. Based on data published in 1992, it was observed that patients with UARS who were subsequently treated with continuous positive airway pressure (CPAP) improved significantly in terms of daytime sleepiness when the RERA index (RERAs/hour of sleep) dropped below 10 (1). Therefore, the number of abnormal respiratory events (RERAs)/hour of sleep in UARS should be ≤ 10 in contrast with a cutoff point of ≥ 5 abnormal respiratory events (apneas and hypopneas) per hour of sleep for OSA. As these events are closely linked to transient events during sleep it is required that the definition of RERA should include a subsequent arousal from sleep. Until more specific measures of brain activation associated with these respiratory events have been identified, RERAs should be identified based on these criteria.

To this date no data are available on the occurrence of RERAs in PS.

Alternative, Noninvasive Measures of Respiratory Effort
The use of esophageal pressure sensors has disadvantages preventing its widespread use in polysomnographic diagnostic sleep studies. This is in part due to the

patient's fear of discomfort and the technician's hesitancy to apply the sensor. From our own experience in Dortmund, it is not uncommon that patients remove the esophageal balloon some time after successful application.

Several noninvasive measures have shown to correlate well with respiratory effort. Pulse transit time (PTT) has shown to detect inspiratory effort (38). This method is based on the time differential of the pulse wave between two points (39) within the arterial tree. PTT has also shown to detect arousals during sleep (40). More recently, noninvasive measurement of diaphragmatic electromyogram (EMG_{DI}) with surface electrodes (41) has shown to correlate with esophageal pressure in OSA (42) and partial upper airway obstruction as well (43). When snoring is present in patients with partial upper airway obstruction, sound pressure levels allow estimation of relative changes in esophageal pressure (44). Of course, this method will not work for complete upper airway obstruction where complete flow limitation will put an end to snoring. The forced oscillation technique (45) is based on the application of a high-frequency oscillation applied with a nasal mask to the upper airway (5–20 Hz). It continuously measures the relationship between pressure and flow. This technique has also shown to be useful in determining effective CPAP pressure (46). For further reference on the methods described above, a detailed review was published by Farré et al. (47) in 2004.

A summary of the diagnostic criteria for UARS versus OSA is given in Table 1.

EPIDEMIOLOGY

To date no study has been undertaken to determine the prevalence of UARS in the general population. A prerequisite for a study on this subject would be an unequivocal agreement on the diagnostic criteria for UARS (clinical and polysomnographic features), independent of whether researchers may or may not agree on the distinct nature of this diagnosis (48). In view of the lack of prevalence data we analyzed the Dortmund/Essen Sleep Disorders Center data from 1999 to 2006. From a total of 2768 diagnostic referrals for suspected OSA, 2174 (78%) were diagnosed with OSA. Fourteen percent ($n = 384$) of the patients were diagnosed with UARS and 210 (8%) with PS. The female to male ratio in patients with OSA was 1:8 while this ratio was 1:2 in patients with UARS and 1:5 in PS. While this data does not reflect true

TABLE 1 Polysomnographic Differential Features of Upper Airway Resistance Syndrome and Obstructive Sleep Apnea

Variable	UARS	OSA
AHI	< 5	≥ 5
Lowest oxyhemoglobin saturation	In most cases < 92%	In most cases > 92%
RERA (based on P_{ES}, cannula, or pneumotachograph)	≥ 10	< 10
EEG frequency analysis	α power increased REM Δ power increased	α power decreased REM Δ power decreased

Abbreviations: AHI, apnea-hypopnea index; EEG, electroencephalography; OSA, obstructive sleep apnea; P_{es}, esophageal pressure; REM, rapid eye movement; RERA, respiratory effort–related arousals; UARS, upper airway resistance syndrome.

prevalence in the general population, it shows that in a sleep clinic referral population, the female to male ratio for UARS is four-fold larger than for OSA, possibly suggesting a gender-specific genetic basis for inspiratory load compensation during sleep (49).

In children the female to male ratio of UARS appears to be closer to 1:1 (50). Similar gender ratios have been published for snoring in children (51). These data suggest that respiratory load compensation and/or upper airway properties are still similar in boys and girls at this developmental stage where the hormonal profile has not yet differentiated.

CLINICAL FEATURES
Insomnia Symptoms
Although diagnostic and polysomnographic signs of patients with UARS differ from patients with OSA, the clinical features between these two sleep disorders overlap. Differential clinical features are given in Table 2. Recently, it has been suggested that patients with UARS may present a link to functional somatic syndromes (52) and therefore differ from patients with OSA. However, this study included only 75 patients with 25 patients in each group (UARS with AHI < 10/hour, mild-to-moderate OSA and severe OSA). Among those functional somatic disorders, UARS patients presented significantly more often with headaches, irritable bowel syndrome, sleep-onset insomnia, and alpha-delta sleep. Also, the proportion of women in the UARS group was significantly higher than in the other two groups (52).

With respect to insomnia, data from Guilleminault et al. (53) show that sleep-onset insomnia as well as sleep maintenance insomnia are frequent complaints. The occurrence of insomniac problems being more frequent in UARS than OSA is also consistent with our own data. While sleep-maintenance problems are more frequent than sleep-onset problems, 25% of patients with UARS complain of sleep-onset insomnia, compared to 15% in OSA patients. As to sleep-maintenance insomnia 46% of patients with UARS as opposed to 43% of patients with OSA complain of this symptom (49).

Sleepiness
Without going into detail about the difficulties associated with the assessment of sleepiness, it should be mentioned that reports suggest that UARS is more commonly associated with a report of fatigue rather than sleepiness (52).

TABLE 2 Clinical Differential Features in Upper Airway Resistance Syndrome and Obstructive Sleep Apnea

Variable	UARS	OSA
Age	All ages, most < 50 at diagnosis	All ages
Male/female ratio	2:1	8:1
Sleep onset	Insomnia	Short
Body habitus	Normal	Overweight-obese
Functional somatic complaints	Often	Seldom
Blood pressure	Low to normal	Normal to high
Orthostatic symptoms	Often	Seldom

Abbreviations: OSA, obstructive sleep apnea; UARS, upper airway resistance syndrome.

Data on Epworth sleepiness scale (ESS) indexes (54) in patients with UARS have been reported (55), although this measure has been questioned in the past (56). Lofaso et al. (57) investigated nonapneic snorers with daytime sleepiness (who probably fit the diagnosis of UARS) and found that they had ESS scores > 10. For analysis of our dataset, we chose a combination of ESS ≥ 10 or a sleep-specialist's assessment of sleepiness from a comprehensive patient history indicating sleepiness on more than three days a week. ESS scores in UARS (9.4/24) were significantly lower than in OSA (10.4/24). The clinical usefulness of this absolute difference, however, should be questioned. As to a report of nonrefreshing sleep upon awakening, patients with UARS (77%) did not differ from patients with OSA (75%). Patients with PS presented the lowest frequency (28%) of nonrefreshing sleep being also significantly lower than in patients with OSA (41%) (49).

Physical Examination

Orthostatic hypotension has been reported in 25% of patients with UARS (58) contrasting with the frequent finding of arterial hypertension in patients with OSA (59). It has been hypothesized that nonhypoxic resistive respiration may alter parasympathetic control during sleep. Therefore, questions regarding this sign should be addressed in the history of the patients and blood pressure measurement should be included.

An oropharyngeal examination should be part of any clinical investigation in patients being evaluated for an SRBD. Allergy-related enlargement of the inferior nasal turbinates should be assessed (60). This finding is supported by our own data where patients with UARS presented with a higher frequency of seasonal allergies (40%) compared to all other groups (49).

At inspection, patients with OSA often tend to present with a crowded oral cavity primarily due to excess soft tissue, especially when patients are overweight or obese. A significant reason for this finding can also be attributed to a short intermolar distance, and overlapping teeth. Whether this holds true for patients with UARS still needs to be investigated. Questions about the effectiveness of nasal breathing are important since poor nasal ventilation precipitates mouth breathing. This is especially important in children where chronic mouth breathing may alter craniofacial growth.

Early reports about UARS have emphasized that patients with UARS are generally not considered obese (2). In our UARS population the mean body mass index (BMI) is 26.1 ± 4.1 kg/m^2 versus 29.3 ± 5.3 kg/m^2 in the OSA patients. Other investigations have reported a BMI ≤ 25 kg/m^2 for UARS patients (2,22). Of note, female UARS patients (25.2 kg/m^2) appear to be significantly less overweight than male UARS patients (26.4 kg/m^2). A similar gender-related BMI differential is seen in the OSA patients (49).

With respect to age, Gold et al. (52) reported that patients with UARS are younger than patients presenting with moderate and severe OSA. In their sample of 22 patients with UARS the mean age was 47.5 years. This is consistent with our data showing an age differential of −6.7 years for patients with UARS compared to OSA. Patients with UARS in our sample have a mean age of 44.9 ± 12.1 years compared to 51.7 ± 11.6 years in patients with OSA. Whether this finding may act in favor of the hypothesis that UARS may represent an early stage of OSA will have to be addressed by long-term, prospective studies. A 2006 study indicated that of 94 patients with untreated UARS only five progressed to OSA (55). The mean change in AHI between initial diagnosis and follow-up was nonsignificant. However, they did progress significantly in terms of their clinical symptoms (insomnia, fatigue, and depressive mood) (55) four years after the initial diagnosis.

TREATMENT
Nasal Continuous Positive Airway Pressure
Nasal CPAP treatment has been used in the initial description of UARS (2). It was demonstrated that CPAP was able to resolve inspiratory flow limitation by increasing the upstream pressure. Sleepiness as assessed by the multiple sleep latency test (MSLT) was also significantly improved. However, in this patient sample as well as in samples which followed (55,61,62) adherence with CPAP treatment continues to be a problem. Sleep-onset insomnia may be an important factor for this low adherence in that inspiratory load compensation at sleep onset may not be the only reason for the development of sleep instability at sleep onset. The addition of the therapeutic interface may add to sleep-onset disturbance and aggravate sleep-maintenance insomnia.

Despite the limited adherence with CPAP in the treatment of UARS, it still constitutes the first line of treatment. Side effects are limited and, unlike surgery, CPAP does not result in potential side effects that are nonreversible. The advantage of a CPAP trial is that in some patients it can yield additional diagnostic information by resolving daytime sleepiness.

Transnasal Insufflation
This novel technique is based on insufflation of high flow humidified air through a proprietary nasal cannula (63). While this new technique relieves inspiratory flow limitation especially in patients with UARS and patients with predominant hypopneas, its precise mechanism of action, efficacy, and adherence yet need to be determined.

Behavioral Treatment
For certain patients, especially those with symptoms of insomnia, cognitive behavioral treatment as an adjunct to CPAP may be beneficial (53,64). Avoidance of agents known to impair ventilation during sleep in patients with OSA including alcohol (65) and benzodiazepines (66) may have a positive effect.

Insufficient data exist on the potential effect of weight loss in UARS. However, weight loss, which has shown to reduce AHI in OSA (67,68), may also be a treatment option for UARS. Given the fact that the typical BMI in this patient group is well below 40 they are rarely candidates for surgical interventions for weight loss (69).

Oral Appliances
Considering the low adherence rates with CPAP and health insurance guidelines in patients with UARS (2,61,62) treatment with oral appliances is an important treatment alternative to surgical intervention. In this context an update of practice parameters for the treatment of snoring with oral appliances was published in 2006 (70). This American Academy of Sleep Medicine (AASM) practice recommendation defines the oral appliance treatment objective by separating patients with PS from patients with UARS and OSA. However, unlike for patients with OSA it does not

define the treatment outcome for patients with UARS. According to this guideline only patients with PS are excluded from the need of follow-up sleep studies to document treatment outcome. So far only three case studies have been published showing that oral appliances can successfully treat patients with UARS (71–73). Cohort studies are needed to confirm this finding in larger populations.

Surgery
In 1996, Pepin et al. (74) concluded that the studies on surgical intervention for UARS were descriptive rather than comparative. Recent studies on surgical intervention in UARS even include bariatric surgery (75) for UARS. According to the authors, the patients in this study included six women with UARS, who had a mean AHI of three events/hour and a mean low oxyhemoglobin saturation of 84%. They also considered an ESS of ≥ 8 as the sole criterion for daytime somnolence. It appears that the criteria for a diagnosis of UARS were inappropriate, aggravated by the fact that no BMI was mentioned for this subgroup. No follow-up outcomes were presented in this subgroup. Studies like this highlight the need for adherence to diagnostic criteria and randomized protocols; especially when treatment modalities are chosen, which are associated with surgical intervention where side effects and complications must be weighed against the potential gain.

Surgery and Site of Upper Airway Collapse
Different methods have been described to determine the site of collapse in the upper airway. These methods can be divided in those attempting to define the site of obstruction during wakefulness, normal sleep, and anesthesia-invoked sleep. Some of the techniques used include cephalometry, fluoroscopy, computed tomographic (CT)- and magnetic resonance (MR)-imaging, acoustic reflection, and nasopharyngoscopy.

Surgical success for uvulopalatopharyngoplasty (UPPP) in OSA is only 5% in patients with an obstruction at the base of the tongue (76). Since most patients present with multiple sites of upper airway obstruction during sleep (77), diagnostic techniques must be developed which can improve surgical outcome. However, this quest is hindered by the fact that upper airway obstruction during sleep is a dynamic process. Varying sites of obstruction have been documented within one individual (78,79).

As mentioned before, no systematic studies of surgical intervention for UARS have been conducted. UARS and upper airway obstruction in general share pathophysiologic mechanisms. Thus, it seems appropriate to hypothesize that similar surgical procedures used in the treatment of PS and OSA may have a positive effect on UARS. Among those specifically, the less intrusive surgical methods seem appropriate candidates, such as turbinectomy, septoplasty, UPPP, laser-assisted uvuloplasty, uvulopalatal-flap (80), radiofrequency-assisted uvulopalatoplasty, radiofrequency ablation of the palate and tongue, and more recently, distraction osteogenesis (81). As in surgical treatment for OSA these procedures may be combined in a stepwise approach, which has been referred to as multilevel surgery to improve surgical outcome (82).

Any surgical procedure should include follow-up polysomnographic investigations as it is required for surgical treatment of OSA (83). If multilevel surgery is performed, polysomnographic investigation should be conducted between each surgical intervention (83).

CONCLUSIONS

UARS is a clinically relevant SRBD. It shares some pathophysiologic features with other disorders associated with increased upper airway collapsibility during sleep such as OSA and PS. Other pathophysiologic features, however, appear to be different from OSA and PS. It differs particularly in its gender distribution, diagnostic criteria, and clinical presentation. At this time treatment outcome is poorly understood. Nasal CPAP treatment shows low adherence. Oral appliances may represent an important treatment modality. Surgical treatment should be focused on less invasive procedures with low side effects and lower potential for complications.

REFERENCES

1. Guilleminault C, Stoohs R, Clerk A, Simmons JL. From obstructive sleep apnea syndrome to upper airway resistance syndrome: consistency of daytime sleepiness. Sleep 1992; 15:S13–S16.
2. Guilleminault C, Stoohs R, Clerk A, Cetel M, Maistros P. A cause of excessive daytime sleepiness. The upper airway resistance syndrome. Chest 1993; 104:781–787.
3. Stoohs R, Guilleminault C. Obstructive sleep apnea syndrome or abnormal upper airway resistance during sleep? J Clin Neurophysiol 1990; 7:83–92.
4. Stoohs R, Guilleminault C. Snoring during NREM sleep: respiratory timing, esophageal pressure and EEG arousal. Respir Physiol 1991; 85:151–167.
5. Exar EN, Collop NA. The upper airway resistance syndrome. Chest 1999; 115:1127–1139.
6. American Academy of Sleep Medicine. International classification of sleep disorders, 2nd ed. Diagnostic and Coding Manual. Westchester, IL: American Academy of Sleep Medicine, 2005.
7. Schneider H, Patil SP, Canisius S, et al. Hypercapnic duty cycle is an intermediate physiological phenotype linked to mouse chromosome 5. J Appl Physiol 2003; 95:11–19.
8. Milic-Emili J, Grunstein MM. Drive and timing components of ventilation. Chest 1976; 70:131–133.
9. Clark FJ, von Euler C. On the regulation of depth and rate of breathing. J Physiol (London) 1972; 222:267–295.
10. Bendixen HH, Smith GR, Mead G. Pattern of ventilation in young adults. J Appl Physiol 1964; 19:195–198.
11. Tankersley C, Kleeberger S, Russ B, Schwartz A, Smith P. Modified control of breathing in genetically obese (ob/ob) mice. J Appl Physiol 1996; 81:716–723.
12. Schwartz AR, Smith PL, Wise RA, Gold AR, Permutt S. Induction of upper airway occlusion in sleeping individuals with subatmospheric nasal pressure. J Appl Physiol 1988; 64:535–542.
13. Gold AR, Marcus CL, Dipalo F, Gold MS. Upper airway collapsibility during sleep in upper airway resistance syndrome. Chest 2002; 121:1531–1540.
14. Gleadhill IC, Schwartz AR, Wise RA, Permutt S, Smith PL. Upper airway collapsibility in snorers and in patients with obstructive sleep apnea. Am Rev Respir Dis 1991; 143:1300–1303.
15. Eastwood PR, Curran AK, Smith CA, Demsey JA. Effect of upper airway negative pressure on inspiratory drive during sleep. J Appl Physiol 1998; 84:1063–1075.
16. Kimoff RJ, Sforza E, Champagne V, Ofiara L, Gendron D. Upper airway sensation in snoring and obstructive sleep apnea. Am J Respir Crit Care Med 2001; 64:250–255.
17. Guilleminault C, Li K, Chen NH, Poyares D. Two-point palatal discrimination in patients with upper airway resistance syndrome, obstructive sleep apnea syndrome, and normal control subjects. Chest 2002; 122:866–870.
18. Edstrom L, Larsson H, Larsson L. Neurogenic efforts on the palatopharyngeal muscle in patients with obstructive sleep apnea: a muscle biopsy study. J Neurol Neurosurg Psychiatry 1992; 55:916–920.
19. Friberg D, Ansved T, Borg K, Carlsson-Norlander B, Larsson H, Svanborg E. Histological indications of a progressive snorer's disease in an upper-airway muscle. Am J Resp Crit Care Med 1998; 157:586–593.

20. Friberg D, Gazelius B, Hokfelt T, Norlander B. Abnormal afferent nerve endings in the soft palatal mucosa of sleep apneics and habitual snorers. Regul Pept 1997; 71:29–36.
21. Afifi L, Guilleminault C, Colrain I. Sleep and respiratory stimulus specific dampening of cortical responsiveness in OSAS patients. Respir Physiol Neurobiol 2003; 136:221–234.
22. Guilleminault C, Stoohs R, Duncan S. Snoring (I). Daytime sleepiness in regular heavy snorers. Chest 1991; 99:40–48.
23. American Sleep Disorders Association Atlas Task Force EEG arousals: scoring rules and examples: a preliminary report from the Sleep Disorders Atlas Task Force of the American Sleep Disorders Association. Sleep 1992; 15:173–184.
24. Carley DW, Applebaum R, Basner RC, Onal E, Lopata M. Respiratory and arousal responses to acoustic stimulation. Chest 1997; 112:1567–1571.
25. Berry RB, Gleeson K. Respiratory arousal from sleep mechanisms and significance. Sleep 1997; 20:654–675.
26. Guilleminault C, Kim YD, Chowdhuri S, Horita M, Ohayon M, Kushida C. Sleep and daytime sleepiness in upper airway resistance syndrome compared to obstructive sleep apnea syndrome. Eur Respir J 2001; 17:1–10.
27. AASM taskforce report: sleep-related breathing disorders in adults: recommendations for syndrome definition and measurement techniques in clinical research. Sleep 1999; 22:667–689.
28. Norman RG, Ahmed MM, Walsleben JA, Rapoport DM. Detection of respiratory events during NPSG: nasal cannula/pressure sensor versus thermistor. Sleep 1997; 20: 1175–1184.
29. Hosselet JJ, Ayappa I, Norman RG, Krieger AC, Rapoport DM. Classification of sleep-disordered breathing. Am J Respir Crit Care Med 2001; 163:398–405.
30. Ayappa I, Norman RG, Krieger AC, Rosen A, O'Malley RL, Rapoport DM. Non-invasive detection of respiratory effort-related arousals (RERAs) by a nasal cannula/pressure transducer system. Sleep 2000; 23:763–771.
31. Loube DI, Andrada T, Howard RS. Accuracy of respiratory inductive plethysmography for the diagnosis of upper airway resistance syndrome. Chest 1999; 115:1333–1337.
32. Johnson PL, Edwards N, Burgess KR. Detection of increased upper airway resistance during overnight polysomnography. Sleep 2005; 28:85–90.
33. Berry RB, Bonnet MH, Light RW. Effect of ethanol on the arousal response to airway occlusion during sleep in normal subjects. Am Rev Respir Dis 1992; 145:445–452.
34. Guilleminault C, Poyares D, Palombini L, Koester U, Pelin Z, Black J. Variability of respiratory effort in relationship with sleep stages in normal controls and upper airway resistance syndrome patients. Sleep Med 2002; 2:397–406.
35. Guilleminault C, Lee JH, Chan A. Pediatric obstructive sleep apnea syndrome. Arch Pediatr Adolesc Med 2005; 159:775–785.
36. Chervin RD, Burns JW, Subotic NS, Roussi C, Thelen B, Ruzicka DL. Correlates of respiratory cycle-related EEG changes in children with sleep-disordered breathing. Sleep 2004; 27:116–121.
37. Younes M. Role of arousals in the pathogenesis of obstructive sleep apnea. Am J Respir Crit Care Med 2004; 169:623–633.
38. Argod J, Pepin JL, Levy P. Differentiating obstructive and central sleep respiratory events through pulse transit time. Am J Respir Crit Care Med 1998; 158:1778–1783.
39. Pitson D, Chhina N, Knijn S, van Herwaaden M, Stradling J. Changes in pulse transit time and pulse rate as markers of arousal from sleep in normal subjects. Clin Sci (Lond) 1994; 87:269–273.
40. Pitson DJ, Stradling JR. Autonomic markers of arousal during sleep in patients undergoing investigation for obstructive sleep apnoea, their relationship to EEG arousals, respiratory events and subjective sleepiness. J Sleep Res 1998; 7:53–59.
41. Stoohs RA, Blum HC, Knaack L, Guilleminault C. Non-invasive estimation of esophageal pressure based on intercostal EMG monitoring. Proceedings of the 26th Annual International Conference of the IEEE EMBS San Francisco, CA, USA September 1–5, 2004:3867–3869.
42. Stoohs RA, Blum HC, Knaack L, Butsch vd Heydt B, Guilleminault C. Comparison of pleural pressure and transcutaneous diaphragmatic electromyogram in obstructive sleep apnea syndrome. Sleep 2005; 28:321–329.

43. Knaack L, Blum H, Hohenhorst W, Ryba J, Guilleminault C, Stoohs RA. Comparison of diaphragmatic EMG and oesophageal pressure in obstructed and unobstructed breathing during sleep. Somnologie 2005; 9:159–165.
44. Stoohs R, Skrobal A, Guilleminault C. Does snoring intensity predict flow limitation or respiratory effort during sleep? Respir Physiol 1993; 92:27–38.
45. Rühle KH, Schlenker E, Randerath W. Upper airway resistance syndrome. Respiration 1997; 64(suppl 1):29–34.
46. Badia JR, Farre RO, Kimoff RJ, et al. Clinical application of the forced oscillation technique for CPAP titration in the sleep apnoea/hypopnoea syndrome. Am J Respir Crit Care Med 1999; 160:1550–1554.
47. Farré R, Montserrat JM, Navajas D. Noninvasive monitoring of respiratory mechanics during sleep. Eur Respir J 2004; 24:1052–1060.
48. Douglas NJ. Upper airway resistance syndrome is not a distinct syndrome. Am J Respir Crit Care Med 2000; 161:1413–1416.
49. Stoohs RA, Knaack L, Blum HC, Janicki J, Hohenhorst W. Differences in clinical features of primary snoring, upper airway resistance syndrome, and obstructive sleep apnea hypopnea syndrome. Sleep Med, 2006; submitted for publication.
50. Guilleminault C, Khramtsov A. Upper airway resistance syndrome in children: a clinical review. Semin Pediatr Neurol 2001; 8:207–215.
51. Zhang G, Spickett J, Rumchev K, Lee AH, Stick S. Snoring in primary school children and domestic environment: a Perth school based study. Respir Res 2004; 5:19.
52. Gold AR, Dipalo F, Gold MS, O'Hearn D. The symptoms and signs of upper airway resistance syndrome: a link to the functional somatic syndromes. Chest 2003; 123:87–95.
53. Guilleminault C, Palombini L, Poyares D, Chowdhury S. Chronic insomnia, post menopausal women, and SDB. Part 2: Comparison of non drug treatment trials in normal breathing and UARS post menopausal women complaining of insomnia. J Psychosom Res 2002; 53:617–623.
54. Johns MW. A new method of measuring daytime sleepiness: the Epworth Sleepiness Scale. Sleep 1991; 14:540–545.
55. Guilleminault C, Kirisoglu C, Poyares D, et al. Upper airway resistance syndrome: a long-term outcome study. J Psychiatr Res 2006; 40:273–279.
56. Chervin RD. Epworth sleepiness scale? Sleep Med 2003; 4:175–176.
57. Lofaso F, Goldenberg F, d'Ortho MP, Coste A, Harf A. Arterial blood pressure response to transient arousals from NREM sleep in nonapneic snorers with sleep fragmentation. Chest 1998; 113:985–991.
58. Guilleminault C, Faul JL, Stoohs R. Sleep-disordered breathing and hypotension. Am J Respir Crit Care Med 2001; 164:1242–1247.
59. Peppard PE, Young T, Palta M, Skatrud J. Prospective study of the association between sleep-disordered breathing and hypertension. N Engl J Med 2000; 342:1378–1384.
60. Chen W, Kushida CA. Nasal obstruction in sleep-disordered breathing. Otolaryngol Clin North Am 2003; 36:437–460.
61. Rauscher H, Formanek D, Zwick H. Nasal continuous positive airway pressure for nonapneic snoring? Chest 1995; 107:58–61.
62. Krieger J, Kurtz D, Petiau C, Sforza E, Trautmann D. Long-term compliance with CPAP therapy in obstructive sleep apnea and in snorers. Sleep 1996; 19:S136–S143.
63. McGinley BM, DeRosa P, Alan SR, et al. A novel strategy for treating upper airway obstruction (UAO) with transnasal insufflation (TNI). Sleep 2005; 28:A208.
64. Krakow B, Melendrez D, Lee SA, Warner TD, Clark JO, Sklar D. Refractory insomnia and sleep-disordered breathing: a pilot study. Sleep Breath 2004; 8:15–29.
65. Issa FG, Sullivan CE. Alcohol, snoring and sleep apnea. J Neurol Neurosurg Psychiatry 1982; 45:353–359.
66. Guilleminault C, Silvestri R, Mondini S, Coburn S. Aging and sleep apnea: action of benzodiazepine, acetazolamide, alcohol, and sleep deprivation in a healthy elderly group. J Gerontol 1984; 39:655–661.
67. Peppard PE, Young T, Palta M, Dempsey J, Skatrud J. Longitudinal study of moderate weight change and sleep-disordered breathing. JAMA 2000; 284:3015–3021.
68. Dixon JB, Schachter LM, O'Brien PE. Polysomnography before and after weight loss in obese patients with severe apnea. Int J Obes Relat Metab Disord 2005; 29: 1048–1054.

69. Kelly J, Tarnoff M, Shikora S, et al. Best practice recommendations for surgical care in weight loss surgery. Obes Res 2005; 13:227–233.
70. Kushida CA, Morgenthaler TI, Littner MR, et al. American Academy of Sleep. Practice parameters for the treatment of snoring and obstructive sleep apnea with oral appliances: an update for 2005. Sleep 2006; 29:240–243.
71. Loube DI, Andrada T, Shanmagum N, et al. Successful treatment of upper airway resistance syndrome with an oral appliance. Sleep Breath 1998; 2:98–101.
72. Rose E, Frucht S, Sobanski T, Barthlen G, Schmidt R. Improvement in daytime sleepiness by the use of an oral appliance in a patient with upper airway resistance syndrome. Sleep Breath 2000; 4:85–88.
73. Guerrero M, Lepler L, Kristo D. The upper airway resistance syndrome masquerading as nocturnal asthma and successfully treated with an oral appliance. Sleep Breath 2001; 5:93–96.
74. Pepin JL, Veale D, Mayer P, Bettega G, Wuyam B, Levy P. Critical analysis of the results of surgery in the treatment of snoring, upper airway resistance syndrome (UARS), and obstructive sleep apnea (OSA). Sleep 1996; 19:S90–S100.
75. Frey WC, Pilcher J. Obstructive sleep-related breathing disorders in patients evaluated for bariatric surgery. Obes Surg 2003; 13:676–683.
76. Sher AE, Schechtman KB, Piccirillo JF. The efficacy of surgical modifications for the upper airway in adults with obstructive sleep apnea syndrome. Sleep 1996; 19:156–177.
77. Rama AN, Tekwani SH, Kushida CA. Sites of obstruction in obstructive sleep apnea. Chest 2002; 122:1139–1147.
78. Katsantonis GP, Moss K, Miyazaki S, Walsh J. Determining the site of airway collapse in obstructive sleep apnea with airway pressure monitoring. Laryngoscope 1993; 103: 1126–1131.
79. Boudewyns AN, Van de Heyning PH, De Backer WA. Site of upper airway obstruction in obstructive sleep apnoea and influence of sleep stage. Eur Respir J 1997; 10:2566–2572.
80. Powell N, Riley R, Guilleminault C, Troell R. A reversible uvulopalatal flap for snoring and sleep apnea syndrome. Sleep 1996; 19:593–599.
81. Guilleminault C, Li KK. Maxillomandibular expansion for the treatment of sleep-disordered breathing: preliminary result. Laryngoscope 2004; 114:893–896.
82. Kao YH, Shnayder Y, Lee KC. The efficacy of anatomically based multilevel surgery for obstructive sleep apnea. Otolaryngol Head Neck Surg 2003; 129:327–335.
83. Thorpy M, Chesson A, Derderian S, et al. Practice parameters for the treatment of obstructive sleep apnea in adults: the efficacy of surgical modifications of the upper airway. Sleep 1996; 19: 152–155.

19 Central Sleep Apnea

M. Safwan Badr
Division of Pulmonary, Allergy, Critical Care, and Sleep Medicine, Wayne State University School of Medicine, Detroit, Michigan, U.S.A.

INTRODUCTION

Sleep apnea is a relatively common condition with significant adverse health consequences (1). Apneas are classified into three categories: obstructive, central, and mixed. Apnea is deemed to be of central etiology when it is caused by cessation of ventilatory motor output. Central sleep apnea (CSA) is a part of instability in a variety of conditions with diverse etiologies (2). In addition, central apnea is reported to occur at sleep onset. Thus, there is a significant overlap between obstructive and central apnea. This chapter will address the pathophysiology, clinical features, and management of normocapnic and hypercapnic CSA.

PATHOPHYSIOLOGIC CLASSIFICATION OF CENTRAL SLEEP APNEA

CSA is often classified according to the level of alveolar ventilation (Table 1) as hypercapnic or nonhypercapnic central apnea (3). The majority of central apnea noted in clinical practice is not associated with hypercapnia.

Hypercapnic Central Sleep Apnea

The loss of wakefulness stimulus to breathe is associated with decreased alveolar ventilation and increased arterial partial pressure of carbon dioxide (Pco_2). However, the manifestations depend on the underlying clinical condition. Therefore, removal of the wakefulness stimulus to breathe results in profound hypoventilation in patients afflicted with conditions associated with impaired diurnal ventilation, such as neuromuscular disease or abnormal respiratory mechanics. Hypoventilation manifests as a central apnea or hypopnea; the ensuing transient arousal partially restores alveolar ventilation until sleep resumes. Thus, central apnea under these circumstances represents nocturnal ventilatory failure in patients with marginal ventilatory status or worsening of existing chronic ventilatory failure.

Patients with this condition have blunted chemoreflex responsiveness, either due to weakness of the respiratory muscles or due to impaired pulmonary mechanics rather than diminished central chemoreflex responsiveness. The clinical picture contains features of the underlying medical condition as well as symptoms of obstructive sleep apnea. Thus, it is common for patients to present with underlying ventilatory insufficiency (e.g., morning headache, cor pulmonale, peripheral edema, polycythemia, and abnormal pulmonary function tests) and features of obstructive sleep apnea (e.g., poor nocturnal sleep, snoring, and daytime sleepiness).

Despite the common inclusion of this condition under the rubric of "central apnea," most such patients do not have frank central apnea or periodic breathing. Instead, polysomnography reveals periods of hypoventilation, hypopnea, poor nocturnal sleep, and sleep fragmentation without clear rhythmic instability akin to periodic breathing.

TABLE 1   Causes of Central Sleep Apnea

Hypercapnic central apnea	Nonhypercapnic central apnea
Central congenital hypoventilation	Central apnea of sleep onset
Arnold-Chiari malformation	Periodic breathing at high altitude
Muscular dystrophy	Congestive heart failure
Amyotrophic lateral sclerosis	Acromegaly
Postpolio syndrome	Hypothyroidism
Kyphoscoliosis	Chronic renal failure
	Idiopathic central sleep apnea

Nonhypercapnic Central Apnea

Nonhypercapnic central apnea is due to transient instability of the ventilatory control system, rather than a ventilatory control defect. Apnea occurs in cycles of apnea alternating with hyperpnea. Typically, patients with nonhypercapnic central apnea demonstrate increased chemoresponsiveness (4,5), in contradistinction to blunted chemoresponsiveness noted in hypercapnic central apnea. Nonhypercapnic central apnea occurs in a variety of clinical conditions including obstructive sleep apnea, congestive heart failure (CHF), and metabolic disorders. Male gender and older age are demographic risk factors for the development of central apnea.

PATHOGENESIS OF CENTRAL APNEA DURING SLEEP

Breathing during non-rapid eye movement (NREM) sleep is critically dependent on chemical stimuli, especially Pco_2 (6), owing to the removal of the wakefulness drive to breathe. NREM sleep unmasks a highly sensitive hypocapnic "apneic threshold." Thus, central apnea occurs if arterial Pco_2 is lowered below the apneic threshold (6). Hypocapnia during sleep is the most ubiquitous and potent influence leading to the development of central apnea. Experimental paradigms used to produce hypocapnic central apnea include nasal mechanical ventilation (Fig. 1) and brief (3–5 minutes) hypoxic exposure. Both methods increase minute ventilation and alveolar ventilation and decrease arterial Pco_2. Termination of hyperventilation would result in hypopnea or apnea depending on the degree of hypocapnia (7–10).

The effects of hypocapnia on ventilation are modulated by several mechanisms that mitigate the effect of hypocapnia on ventilatory motor output. For example, hypocapnic central apnea has not been shown conclusively during rapid eye movement (REM) sleep. Most, but not all studies suggest that breathing during REM sleep is impervious to chemical influences (8). Likewise, the duration of hyperpnea is another important determinant of central apnea following hyperventilation, as brief hyperventilation is rarely followed by central apnea in sleeping humans (11,12), perhaps due to the insufficient reduction in Pco_2 at the level of the chemoreceptors. Finally, intrinsic excitatory mechanisms may also mitigate the effects of hypocapnia. Specifically, brief hypoxic hyperventilation is associated with increased ventilatory motor output referred to as short-term potentiation (STP) (10,13,14). This results in persistent, but gradually diminishing hyperpnea upon cessation of the stimulus to breathe. The activation of STP may serve as a teleological purpose by mitigating the effects of transient hypoxia and hypocapnia, on subsequent ventilation during sleep (10).

Although hypocapnia is the most common influence leading to central apnea (3,6,11,15), other less common mechanisms include negative pressure-mediated upper airway reflexes (16,17) and normocapnic hyperpnea (18,19). However, the

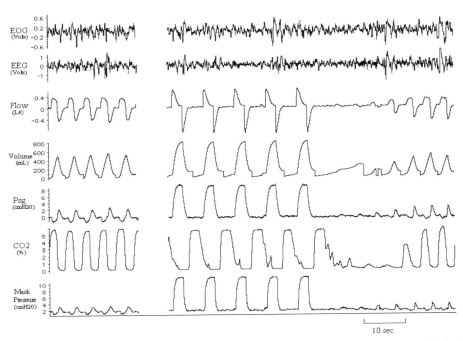

FIGURE 1   An example of hypocapnic central apnea induced by passive mechanical ventilation for three minutes. Note absence of flow and effort. Control represents room air breathing prior to initiation of mechanical ventilation; MV represents three minutes of mechanical ventilation, last five breaths are shown. Note the occurrence of central apnea upon termination of MV in the recovery period. *Abbreviations*: EOG, electro-oculogram; EEG, electroencephalogram; Flow, airflow; Volume, tidal volume (V_T); P_{sg}, supraglottic pressure, note positive pressure during nasal mechanical ventilation; CO_2, end-tidal Pco_2 ($P_{ET}CO_2$); Mask pressure (P_{mask}), note positive mask pressure during mechanical ventilation.

relevance of these mechanisms to the pathogenesis of central apnea in sleeping humans is yet to be determined.

Central apnea does not occur as an isolated event but as periodic breathing consisting of cycles of recurrent apnea or hypopnea alternating with hyperpnea. While hypocapnia can produce the initial event, additional factors are required to sustain breathing instability and periodic breathing. Upper airway narrowing or occlusion may occur during central apnea requiring additional effort to overcome craniofacial gravitational forces or tissue adhesion forces. In addition, breathing does not resume until arterial Pco_2 ($PaCO_2$) is elevated by 4 to 6 mmHg above eupnea owing to the inertia of the ventilatory control system (18,20). Consequently, the magnitude of hypoxia is enhanced and transient arousal may occur, leading to ventilatory overshoot, subsequent hypocapnia, and further apnea/hypopnea.

DETERMINANTS OF CENTRAL APNEA: RISK FACTORS

Several physiologic and pathologic conditions influence the vulnerability to develop central apnea for a given perturbation. These include age, gender, sleep state, CHF, thyroid disease and acromegaly.

Sleep State

Central apnea is reported to occur physiologically during sleep-wake transition at sleep onset. According to this theory, sleep state oscillates between wakefulness and light sleep (3,21), with reciprocal oscillation in $PaCO_2$ (partial pressure of alveolar carbon dioxide) around the apneic threshold. Hyperventilation produces central apnea during sleep (22), recovery from apnea is associated with transient wakefulness, hyperventilation and hence hypocapnia. The latter causes an apnea upon resumption of sleep. This cycle is broken once sleep is consolidated; sleep state and chemical stimuli are eventually aligned. The extent of sleep-onset central apnea has not been studied systematically. However, there is evidence that the phenomenon is present, at least on a physiological level. Transition from alpha (8–13 Hz) to theta (4–8 Hz) electroencephalographic frequencies in normal subjects is associated with prolongation of breath duration (23). Many authors believe that central apnea at sleep onset may be a normal phenomenon. Whether sleep-onset central apnea portends a benign natural history is an assumption pending experimental proof.

CSA is uncommon during REM sleep (15), possibly due to increased ventilatory motor output during REM sleep (24,25) relative to NREM sleep. However, it is unclear whether REM sleep is impervious to hypocapnic inhibition or whether the paucity of central apnea during REM sleep is due to sleep fragmentation preventing the progression to REM sleep. Furthermore, hypocapnia has been shown to decrease the amount of REM sleep in the cat (26). The clinical significance of this finding is unclear.

The loss of intercostal and accessory muscle activity during REM sleep leads to hypoventilation. If severe diaphragm dysfunction is present, nadir tidal volume may be negligible and the event may appear as central apnea. Thus, central apnea during REM sleep represents transient hypoventilation rather than posthyperventilation hypocapnia.

Aging

CSA occurs more frequently in older adults (27–29). Increased prevalence of sleep apnea and central apnea per se, may be due to increased prevalence of comorbid conditions such as CHF (30), atrial fibrillation (31), cerebrovascular disease (32), or thyroid disease (33). In addition, healthy older adults may also be at increased risk for developing CSA, attributed to sleep state (22). The clinical significance of aging-related central apnea in older adults is not certain.

Gender

Male gender is a risk factor for the development of central apnea. This assertion is supported by epidemiologic as well as empiric evidence. Epidemiologic studies demonstrate paucity of CSA in premenopausal women (34) and in patients with CHF and Cheyne-Stokes respiration (CSR) (35).

The hypocapnic apneic threshold during NREM sleep is higher in men relative to women. Using nasal mechanical ventilation, Zhou et al. (36) have shown that the apneic threshold was −3.5 mmHg versus −4.7 mmHg below eupneic breathing in men and women, respectively. In addition, no difference was noted in women in the luteal versus the follicular phase of the menstrual cycle. Thus, the gender difference was likely due to male sex hormones rather than progesterone.

The role of male sex hormones was confirmed in studies that manipulated the level of testosterone in men and women. Zhou et al. (27) have shown the administration of testosterone to healthy premenopausal women for 12 days resulted in an elevation of the apneic threshold and a diminution in the magnitude of hypocapnia required for induction of central apnea during NREM sleep. In fact, the apneic threshold in women after testosterone administration was identical to the apneic threshold in men (37). Conversely, suppression of testosterone with administration of long-acting gonadotropin-releasing hormone decreased the partial pressure of end-tidal carbon dioxide $P_{ET}CO_2$ that demarcates the apneic threshold (38). Thus, male sex hormones seem to play a critical role in the susceptibility to develop central apnea during NREM sleep.

Congestive Heart Failure

CHF is associated with CSR, characterized by a crescendo–decrescendo breathing pattern with central apnea or hypopnea occurring at the nadir of ventilatory drive. The prevalence of sleep apnea in patients with CHF is about 50% (30,39–41). In one prospective study, Javeheri et al. demonstrated that 51% of male patients with CHF had sleep-disordered breathing, 40% had CSA, and 11% had obstructive apnea. In another study, Sin et al. (35) identified CHF patients at high risk for the presence of sleep apnea in 450 consecutive patients with CHF who underwent polysomnography. Using an apnea–hypopnea index cutoff of 10 per hour of sleep, 302 patients had sleep-disordered breathing (66%). Risk factors for CSA were male gender, atrial fibrillation, age > 60 years, and daytime hypocapnia ($P_{CO_2} < 38$ mmHg). In contrast, risk factors for OSA differed by gender. Body mass index was the only independent determinant in men; age more than 60 years was the only independent determinant for women. Overall, there was a near-equal distribution between OSA and CSA. Thus, central apnea is common in patients with CHF; patients at high risk can be identified by history, electrocardiography, and arterial blood gases.

The precise mechanism(s) of central apnea in patients with CHF remain incompletely understood. The initial apnea is likely related to pulmonary congestion (30) leading to hyperventilation and hypocapnia. Thus, the initial central apnea may develop even after modest hyperpnea, owing to the precarious proximity of $PaCO_2$ to the apneic threshold. Xie et al. studied 19 stable patients with CHF with (12 patients) or without (7 patients) CSA during NREM sleep. Patients with central apnea showed no rise in $P_{ET}CO_2$ from wakefulness to sleep; eupneic $P_{ET}CO_2$ was closer to the apneic threshold than patients without central apnea as shown in Figure 2. The narrowed delta $P_{ET}CO_2$ predisposes the patient to the development of apnea and subsequent breathing instability.

The aforementioned mechanisms account for the occurrence of central apnea. However, the mechanism(s) of sustained breathing instability and periodic breathing is not clear. There is conflicting evidence regarding the role of prolonged circulatory delay in the genesis of periodic breathing in patients with heart failure (42–45).

Cerebrovascular Disease

Sleep apnea occurs frequently after a cerebrovascular accident (CVA) (32,46,47), and is an independent prognostic determinant of mortality following a first episode of stroke (48). CSA is the predominant type of sleep-disordered breathing in 40% of patients of sleep apnea after a CVA (47). The natural history of CSA with neurological recovery is yet to be determined.

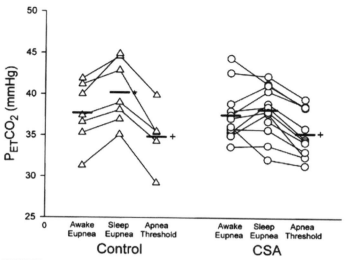

FIGURE 2 Awake and asleep eupneic $P_{ET}CO_2$ during stable breathing and apnea threshold during sleep. In the control group (*open circles*) there was a consistent and significant increase in eupneic Pco_2 during sleep ($p < 0.01$). In the central sleep apnea (CSA) group (*triangles*), there was no difference in eupneic Pco_2 between sleep and wakefulness ($p = 0.2$). In both groups, the apnea threshold was below both the sleep and awake eupneic $P_{ET}CO_2$. The threshold was closer to eupnea level in the CSA group compared with the control group. *$p < 0.05$ compared with awake $P_{ET}CO_2$; +$p < 0.05$ compared with sleep as well as awake $P_{ET}CO_2$. *Source*: Ref. 71.

Metabolic Disorders

Patients with hypothyroidism (49) and renal failure (50,51) have an unexpectedly high prevalence of sleep apnea. Nocturnal hemodialysis is associated with improvement in sleep apnea indices (50). Likewise, acromegaly (52,53) is associated with a high proportion of central apnea, which correlates with higher biochemical markers of disease activity and higher chemoresponsiveness.

Idiopathic Central Apnea

The prevalence of idiopathic CSA is unknown. Some patients may have occult cardiac or metabolic disease. For example, idiopathic CSA is more prevalent in patients with atrial fibrillation (31). Patients with idiopathic CSA demonstrate increased chemoresponsiveness and sleep state instability (54,55).

CLINICAL FEATURES AND DIAGNOSIS

The presenting symptoms for patients with hypercapnic CSA may include symptoms of the underlying disease and features of sleep apnea. These symptoms include daytime sleepiness, snoring, and poor nocturnal sleep, as well as morning headache, peripheral edema, and dyspnea.

Patients with nonhypercapnic central apnea can present with symptoms similar to obstructive sleep apnea including snoring and excessive daytime sleepiness. Alternatively, patients with CSA may present with insomnia and poor nocturnal sleep.

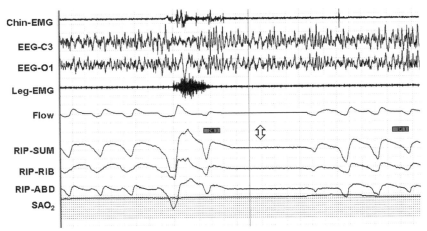

FIGURE 3 A polysomnographic segment showing central apnea in a patient with central apnea syndrome, electromyogram (EMG), electroencephalogram (EEG) leads are C3 (left central) and O1 (left occipital). *Abbreviations*: Flow, airflow; RIP, respiratory inductance plethysmograph, representing rib cage (RC) and abdominal (AB) effort signals, as well as a summed (SUM) signal; SAO_2, oxygen saturation. Note absence of flow and effort (*double arrow*) indicative of central apnea.

This may be due to frequent oscillation between wakefulness and stage 1 NREM sleep. Unfortunately, studies on the clinical features of patients with CSA are limited.

The diagnosis of CSA requires nocturnal polysomnography. Figure 3 shows a polygraphic example of a central apnea demonstrating absence of flow and effort.

MANAGEMENT

Management of CSA reflects the heterogeneity of the condition (2). Treatment decisions are based on the combination of clinical picture, findings on polysomnography, and clinical judgment. Comorbid conditions or concomitant obstructive sleep apnea influences the management strategy. For example, optimization of CHF treatment is essential to the successful treatment of central apnea in patients with CHF. Therapeutic options include positive pressure therapy, pharmacologic therapy, and supplemental oxygen therapy.

Hypercapnic Central Apnea

Noninvasive positive pressure ventilation (NIPPV) is the therapeutic intervention of choice (see also Chapter 10). Noninvasive ventilation using pressure support mode (bilevel nasal positive pressure) has virtually supplanted volume-preset ventilators. There is evidence that NIPPV exerts a salutary effect on survival in patients with ventilatory failure secondary to amyotrophic lateral sclerosis (56,57). Whether NIPPV exerts a similar effect in conditions associated with nocturnal ventilatory failure has yet to be determined.

Nonhypercapnic Central Apnea
Positive Pressure Therapy
Nasal continuous positive airway pressure (CPAP) therapy is the first-line therapy for obstructive sleep apnea (see also Chapter 6). CSA occurring in combination with

episodes of obstructive or mixed apnea may respond to nasal CPAP therapy. In addition, there is evidence that some patients with pure CSA may respond to nasal CPAP therapy (58), especially if central apnea is worse in the supine position. One possible explanation is that nasal CPAP increases lung volume and oxygen stores and alleviates hypoxia. Alternatively, nasal CPAP prevents the occurrence of upper airway narrowing or occlusion during central apnea (59). The net effect is to mitigate the ensuing ventilatory overshoot and perpetuation of ventilatory instability.

Nasal CPAP has been used to treat CSA in patients with CHF. It may be beneficial in these patients because of its direct effect as an upper airway pneumatic splint and the indirect effects on respiratory muscles and cardiac function. One study demonstrated increased left-ventricular ejection fraction and a reduction of combined mortality-cardiac transplantation risk by 81%. This effect did not manifest in patients without CSA (60).

Despite the promising early studies, a more recent randomized, controlled trial failed to demonstrate a survival benefit in patients with central apnea and heart failure receiving nasal CPAP. The Canadian Continuous Positive Airway Pressure (CANPAP) for patients with CSA and heart failure trial tested the hypothesis that CPAP would improve the survival rate of patients who have CSA and heart failure (61). The trial enrolled 258 patients who had heart failure and central apnea; these patients were randomly assigned to receive CPAP or no CPAP and were followed for a mean of two years. The CPAP group had greater reductions in the frequency of episodes of apnea and hypopnea and in norepinephrine levels and greater increase in the mean nocturnal oxygen saturation, ejection fraction and the distance walked in six minutes. However, there was no difference in the number of hospitalizations, quality of life, or atrial natriuretic peptide levels. More importantly, there was no difference in survival rate. The results of this study do not support the routine use of CPAP to extend life in patients who have CSA and heart failure.

Pharmacological Therapy
Pharmacological therapy for central apnea is of limited benefit. There are only two medications that have demonstrated promise in small clinical studies: acetazolamide and theophylline. Neither drug has been studied in large-scale clinical trials nor has been adopted widely (62).

Acetazolamide is a carbonic anhydrase inhibitor that causes mild metabolic acidosis; it is also a weak diuretic. Acetazolamide ameliorates CSA when administered as a single dose of 250 mg before bedtime in patients with idiopathic CSA and in patients with central apnea associated with heart failure (63,64). Nevertheless, the long-term effects of acetazolamide in patients with CSA are unknown. Likewise, theophylline ameliorates CSR in patients with CHF (65) without adversely affecting sleep quality or inducing cardiac arrhythmias. Nevertheless, the available findings are based on a small number of studies.

Supplemental O_2 and CO_2
Several studies have demonstrated a salutary effect of supplemental O_2 in patients with idiopathic CSA and patients with CHF-CSR (30,66). The postulated mechanism of benefit is ameliorating hypoxemia and minimizing the subsequent ventilatory overshoot. It is plausible that nocturnal oxygen therapy may improve outcome in patients with CHF and central apnea; however, long-term studies have yet to be conducted. Despite this limitation, it is prudent to evaluate the effect of supplemental O_2 in alleviating central apnea. Finally, elevation of $PaCO_2$ above the apneic threshold

is effective in eliminating central apnea. This can be accomplished by inhalation of supplemental CO_2 or added dead space (67–70). However, availability and a myriad of practical issues preclude widespread utilization of this therapy.

CONCLUSIONS

The heterogeneity of CSA mandates an individualized management approach. For example, treatment options for CSA associated with CHF begin with ensuring optimal CHF treatment with diuretics, beta-blockers, and reduction of afterload. Supplemental O_2 and nasal CPAP therapy are both valid options. Supplemental O_2 may be attempted during polysomnography in patients with significant hypoxia (oxyhemoglobin desaturation below 90%) following central events. For patients with idiopathic CSA, a trial of nasal CPAP or bilevel positive airway pressure is warranted, as many patients may respond to positive pressure therapy. However, nasal CPAP may aggravate central apnea in some patients. Finally, the development of effective, physiologically based pharmacological therapy for central apnea would be a major advance in the field.

REFERENCES

1. Young T, Palta M, Dempsey J, Skatrud J, Weber S, Badr S. The occurrence of sleep-disordered breathing among middle-aged adults. N Engl J Med 1993; 328:1230–1235.
2. Bradley TD, McNicholas WT, Rutherford R, Popkin J, Zamel N, Phillipson EA. Clinical and physiologic heterogeneity of the central sleep apnea syndrome. Am Rev Respir Dis 1986; 134:217–221.
3. Bradley TD, Phillipson EA. Central sleep apnea. Clin Chest Med 1992; 13:493–505.
4. Solin P, Roebuck T, Johns DP, Walters EH, Naughton MT. Peripheral and central ventilatory responses in central sleep apnea with and without congestive heart failure. Am J Respir Crit Care Med 2000; 162:2194–2200.
5. Javaheri S. A mechanism of central sleep apnea in patients with heart failure. N Engl J Med 1999; 341:949–954.
6. Skatrud JB, Dempsey JA. Interaction of sleep state and chemical stimuli in sustaining rhythmic ventilation. J Appl Physiol 1983; 55:813–822.
7. Berssenbrugge A, Dempsey J, Iber C, Skatrud J, Wilson P. Mechanisms of hypoxia-induced periodic breathing during sleep in humans. J Physiol 1983; 343:507–526.
8. Warner G, Skatrud JB, Dempsey JA. Effect of hypoxia-induced periodic breathing on upper airway obstruction during sleep. J Appl Physiol 1987; 62:2201–2211.
9. Tarbichi AG, Rowley JA, Shkoukani MA, Mahadevan K, Badr MS. Lack of gender difference in ventilatory chemoresponsiveness and post-hypoxic ventilatory decline. Respir Physiol Neurobiol 2003; 137(1):41–50.
10. Badr MS, Skatrud JB, Dempsey JA. Determinants of poststimulus potentiation in humans during NREM sleep. J Appl Physiol 1992; 73:1958–1971.
11. Badr MS, Kawak A. Post-hyperventilation hypopnea in humans during NREM sleep. Respir Physiol 1996; 103:137–145.
12. Badr MS, Kawak A, Skatrud JB, Morrell MJ, Zahn BR, Babcock MA. Effect of induced hypocapnic hypopnea on upper airway patency in humans during NREM sleep. Respir Physiol 1997; 110:33–45.
13. Georgopoulus D, Giannouli E, Tsara V, Argiropoulou P, Patakas D, Anthonisen NR. Respiratory short-term poststimulus potentiation (after-discharge) in patients with obstructive sleep apnea. Am Rev Respir Dis 1992; 146:1250–1255.
14. Eldridge FL. Central neural stimulation of respiration in unanesthetized decerebrate cats. J Appl Physiol 1976; 40:23–28.
15. Datta AK, Shea SA, Horner RL, Guz A. The influence of induced hypocapnia and sleep on the endogenous respiratory rhythm in humans. J Physiol 1991; 440:17–33.

16. Eastwood PR, Curran AK, Smith CA, Dempsey JA. Effect of upper airway negative pressure on inspiratory drive during sleep. J Appl Physiol 1998; 84:1063–1075.
17. Harms CA, Zeng YJ, Smith CA, Vidruk EH, Dempsey JA. Negative pressure-induced deformation of the upper airway causes central apnea in awake and sleeping dogs. J Appl Physiol 1996; 80:1528–1539.
18. Simon PM, Skatrud JB, Badr MS, Griffin DM, Iber C, Dempsey JA. Role of airway mechanoreceptors in the inhibition of inspiration during mechanical ventilation in humans. Am Rev Respir Dis 1991; 144:1033–1041.
19. Leevers AM, Simon PM, Dempsey JA. Apnea after normocapnic mechanical ventilation during NREM sleep. J Appl Physiol 1994; 77:2079–2085.
20. Leevers AM, Simon PM, Xi L, Dempsey JA. Apnoea following normocapnic mechanical ventilation in awake mammals: a demonstration of control system inertia. J Physiol 1993; 472:749–768.
21. Phillipson EA, Bowes G. Control of breathing during sleep. In: Cherniack NS, Widdicombe JG, eds. Vol. II. Control of Breathing, Part 2. Bethesda, MD: American Physiological Society, 1986. Ref Type: Generic.
22. Pack AI, Cola MF, Goldszmidt A, Ogilvie MD, Gottschalk A. Correlation between oscillations in ventilation and frequency content of the electroencephalogram. J Appl Physiol 1992; 72:985–992.
23. Thomson S, Morrell MJ, Cordingley JJ, Semple SJ. Ventilation is unstable during drowsiness before sleep onset. J Appl Physiol 2005; 99:2036–2044.
24. Orem J. Neuronal mechanisms of respiration in REM sleep. Sleep 1980; 3:251–267.
25. Orem J, Lovering AT, Dunin-Barkowski W, Vidruk EH. Tonic activity in the respiratory system in wakefulness, NREM and REM sleep. Sleep 2002; 25:488–496.
26. Lovering AT, Fraigne JJ, Dunin-Barkowski WL, Vidruk EH, Orem JM. Hypocapnia decreases the amount of rapid eye movement sleep in cats. Sleep 2003; 26:961–967.
27. Phillips B, Cook Y, Schmitt F, Berry D. Sleep apnea: prevalence of risk factors in a general population. South Med J 1989; 82:1090–1092.
28. Phillips BA, Berry DT, Schmitt FA, Magan LK, Gerhardstein DC, Cook YR. Sleep-disordered breathing in the healthy elderly. Clinically significant? Chest 1992; 101: 345–349.
29. Ancoli-Israel S, Kripke DF, Klauber MR, Mason WJ, Fell R, Kaplan O. Sleep-disordered breathing in community-dwelling elderly. Sleep 1991; 14:486–495.
30. Bradley TD, Floras JS. Sleep apnea and heart failure. Part II: central sleep apnea. Circulation 2003; 107:1822–1826.
31. Leung RS, Huber MA, Rogge T, Maimon N, Chiu KL, Bradley TD. Association between atrial fibrillation and central sleep apnea. Sleep 2005; 28:1543–1546.
32. Bassetti C, Aldrich MS. Sleep apnea in acute cerebrovascular diseases: final report on 128 patients. Sleep 1999; 22:217–223.
33. Kapur VK, Koepsell TD, deMaine J, Hert R, Sandblom RE, Psaty BM. Association of hypothyroidism and obstructive sleep apnea. Am J Respir Crit Care Med 1998; 158: 1379–1383.
34. Bixler EO, Vgontzas AN, Lin HM, et al. Prevalence of sleep-disordered breathing in women: effects of gender. Am J Respir Crit Care Med 2001; 163:608–613.
35. Sin DD, Fitzgerald F, Parker JD, Newton G, Floras JS, Bradley TD. Risk factors for central and obstructive sleep apnea in 450 men and women with congestive heart failure. Am J Respir Crit Care Med 1999; 160:1101–1106.
36. Zhou XS, Shahabuddin S, Zahn BK, Babcock MA, Badr MS. Effect of gender on the development of hypocapnic apnea/hypopnea during NREM sleep. J Appl Physiol 2000; 89:192–199.
37. Zhou XS, Rowley JA, Demirovic F, Diamond MP, Badr MS. Effect of testosterone on the apneic threshold in women during NREM sleep. J Appl Physiol 2003; 94:101–107.
38. Mateika JH, Omran Q, Rowley JA, Zhou XS, Diamond MP, Badr MS. Treatment with leuprolide acetate decreases the threshold of the ventilatory response to carbon dioxide in healthy males. J Physiol 2004; 561:637–646.
39. Javaheri S, Parker TJ, Liming JD, et al. Sleep apnea in 81 ambulatory male patients with stable heart failure. Types and their prevalences, consequences, and presentations. Circulation 1998; 97:2154–2159.

40. Javaheri S, Parker TJ, Wexler L, et al. Occult sleep-disordered breathing in stable congestive heart failure. Ann Intern Med 1995; 122:487–492.
41. Javaheri S. Central sleep apnea–hypopnea syndrome in heart failure: prevalence, impact, and treatment. Sleep 1996; 19:S229–S231.
42. Lange RL, Hecht HH. The mechanism of Cheyne-Stokes respiration. J Clin Invest 1962; 41:42–52.
43. Naughton M, Benard D, Tam A, Rutherford R, Bradley TD. Role of hyperventilation in the pathogenesis of central sleep apneas in patients with congestive heart failure. Am Rev Respir Dis 1993; 148:330–338.
44. Naughton MT. Pathophysiology and treatment of Cheyne-Stokes respiration. Thorax 1998; 53:514–518.
45. Khoo MC, Gottschalk A, Pack AI. Sleep-induced periodic breathing and apnea: a theoretical study. J Appl Physiol 1991; 70:2014–2024.
46. Bassetti C, Aldrich MS, Chervin RD, Quint D. Sleep apnea in patients with transient ischemic attack and stroke: a prospective study of 59 patients. Neurology 1996; 47:1167–1173.
47. Parra OLGA, Arboix ADRI, Bechich SIRA, et al. Time course of sleep-related breathing disorders in first-ever stroke or transient ischemic attack. Am J Respir Crit Care Med 2000; 161:375–380.
48. Parra O, Arboix A, Montserrat JM, Quinto L, Bechich S, Garcia-Eroles L. Sleep-related breathing disorders: impact on mortality of cerebrovascular disease. Eur Respir J 2004; 24:267–272.
49. Grunstein RR, Sullivan CE. Sleep apnea and hypothyroidism: mechanisms and management. Am J Med 1988; 85:775–779.
50. Hanly PJ, Pierratos A. Improvement of sleep apnea in patients with chronic renal failure who undergo nocturnal hemodialysis. N Engl J Med 2001; 344:102–107.
51. Venmans BJW, van Kralingen KW, Chandi DD, de Vries PMJM, ter Wee PM, Postmus PE. Sleep complaints and sleep disordered breathing in hemodialysis patients. Neth J Med 1999; 54:207–212.
52. Grunstein RR, Ho KY, Berthon-Jones M, Stewart D, Sullivan CE. Central sleep apnea is associated with increased ventilatory response to carbon dioxide and hypersecretion of growth hormone in patients with acromegaly. Am J Respir Crit Care Med 1994; 150:496–502.
53. Grunstein RR, Ho KY, Sullivan CE. Sleep apnea in acromegaly. Ann Intern Med 1991; 115:527–532.
54. Xie A, Rutherford R, Rankin F, Wong B, Bradley TD. Hypocapnia and increased ventilatory responsiveness in patients with idiopathic central sleep apnea. Am J Respir Crit Care Med 1995; 152:1950–1955.
55. Xie A, Wong B, Phillipson EA, Slutsky AS, Bradley TD. Interaction of hyperventilation and arousal in the pathogenesis of idiopathic central sleep apnea. Am J Respir Crit Care Med 1994; 150:489–495.
56. Aboussouan LS, Khan SU, Banerjee M, Arroliga AC, Mitsumoto H. Objective measures of the efficacy of noninvasive positive-pressure ventilation in amyotrophic lateral sclerosis. Muscle Nerve 2001; 24:403–409.
57. Aboussouan LS, Khan SU, Meeker DP, Stelmach K, Mitsumoto H. Effect of noninvasive positive-pressure ventilation on survival in amyotrophic lateral sclerosis. Ann Intern Med 1997; 127:450–453.
58. Issa FG, Sullivan CE. Reversal of central sleep apnea using nasal CPAP. Chest 1986; 90:165–171.
59. Badr MS, Toiber F, Skatrud JB, Dempsey J. Pharyngeal narrowing/occlusion during central sleep apnea. J Appl Physiol 1995; 78:1806–1815.
60. Sin DD, Logan AG, Fitzgerald FS, Liu PP, Bradley TD. Effects of continuous positive airway pressure on cardiovascular outcomes in heart failure patients with and without Cheyne-Stokes respiration. Circulation 2000; 102:61–66.
61. Bradley TD, Logan AG, Kimoff RJ, et al. Continuous positive airway pressure for central sleep apnea and heart failure. N Engl J Med 2005; 353:2025–2033.
62. Hudgel DW, Thanakitcharu S. Pharmacologic treatment of sleep-disordered breathing. Am J Respir Crit Care Med 1998; 158:691–699.

63. DeBacker WA, Verbraecken J, Willemen M, Wittesaele W, DeCock W, Van deHeyning P. Central apnea index decreases after prolonged treatment with acetazolamide. Am J Respir Crit Care Med 1995; 151:87–91.
64. Javaheri S. Acetazolamide improves central sleep apnea in heart failure: a double-blind, prospective study. Am J Respir Crit Care Med 2006; 173:234–237.
65. Javaheri S, Parker TJ, Wexler L, Liming JD, Lindower P, Roselle GA. Effect of theophylline on sleep-disordered breathing in heart failure. N Engl J Med 1996; 335:562–567.
66. Javaheri S, Ahmed M, Parker TJ, Brown CR. Effects of nasal O_2 on sleep-related disordered breathing in ambulatory patients with stable heart failure. Sleep 1999; 22:1101–1106.
67. Khayat RN, Xie A, Patel AK, Kaminski A, Skatrud JB. Cardiorespiratory effects of added dead space in patients with heart failure and central sleep apnea. Chest 2003; 123:1551–1560.
68. Lorenzi-Filho G, Rankin F, Bies I, Douglas BT. Effects of inhaled carbon dioxide and oxygen on Cheyne-Stokes respiration in patients with heart failure. Am J Respir Crit Care Med 1999; 159:1490–1498.
69. Xie A, Rankin F, Rutherford R, Bradley TD. Effects of inhaled CO_2 and added dead space on idiopathic central sleep apnea. J Appl Physiol 1997; 82:918–926.
70. Badr MS, Grossman JE, Weber SA. Treatment of refractory sleep apnea with supplemental carbon dioxide. Am J Respir Crit Care Med 1994; 150:561–564.
71. Xie A, Skatrud JB, Puleo DS, Rahko PS, Dempsey JA. Apnea-hypopnea threshold for CO_2 in patients with congestive heart failure. Am J Respir Crit Care Med 2002; 165:1245–1250.

20 Other Respiratory Conditions and Disorders

Francesco Fanfulla
Centro di Medicina del Sonno ad indirizzo cardio-respiratorio, Istituto Scientifico di Montescano IRCCS, Fondazione Salvatore Maugeri, Montescano (Pavia), Italy

INTRODUCTION

Sleep disturbance is a common problem in many medical disorders, including respiratory diseases, such as chronic obstructive pulmonary disease (COPD) and bronchial asthma. Impairment of sleep may worsen symptoms in these disorders and their prognosis. The diseases may also present particular clinical or functional patterns during sleep. Furthermore, since COPD, asthma, and sleep apnea are prevalent in the general population, associations between these disorders may often be found in the same patient, particularly in a hospital setting.

CHRONIC OBSTRUCTIVE PULMONARY DISEASE
Gas Exchange During Sleep

Recurrent episodes of nocturnal arterial oxyhemoglobin desaturation, especially during rapid eye movement (REM) sleep, have been extensively described in patients with COPD (1–3). Several definitions of nocturnal desaturations have been proposed:

1. 30% of sleep time with oxygen saturation < 90% (4,5).
2. ≥ 5 minute of sleep time spent with oxygen saturation below 90% and a nadir value < 85%, mostly during REM sleep (3).
3. Mean nocturnal SaO_2 < 90% or the time spent with an SaO_2 < 90% (6).

All patients with COPD are more hypoxemic during sleep than during a resting awake state. Generally, the patients who are most hypoxemic while awake are the ones most severely hypoxemic during sleep but the degree of nocturnal desaturation differs markedly among COPD patients (1,2,7–9). Results of pulmonary function tests correlate poorly with nocturnal hypoxemia, since this latter may be affected by comorbid conditions, such as heart failure and obstructive sleep apnea (OSA); however, the drop in oxygen saturation during sleep is higher than that observed during maximal exercise (10).

Sleep-related oxyhemoglobin desaturation generally occurs during REM sleep but is not specific to this sleep state. Indeed, desaturations may occur during non-REM (NREM) sleep, particularly during stages 1 and 2, but in this context their amplitude is generally less pronounced and their duration limited to a few minutes. There is a close relationship between the daytime and nocturnal level of PaO_2: patients who are most hypoxemic when awake became more hypoxemic when asleep (11,12). This relationship is mainly due to the shape of the oxygen dissociation curve: a drop in PaO_2 may have different consequences depending on the baseline level of SaO_2. The amplitude of desaturation is very large when the baseline SaO_2 is near or below the 90%.

Many of the physiological variables in COPD with nocturnal desaturation differ (13). A study published in 2005 showed that the variables that best identify patients with desaturation are the percentage of time spent with $SaO_2 < 90\%$ (T_{90}), mean pulmonary arterial pressure, and $PaCO_2$ values rather than the T_{90} alone (14).

Many studies were conducted to identify the best predictors of nocturnal SaO_2 dips, so that patients at risk may receive an appropriate diagnostic examination. In particular, the problem regards those patients with daytime $PaO_2 > 8$ kPa. Data obtained from different studies are summarized in Table 1 (3,6,13–15).

COPD was classified as a disease state characterized by airflow limitation that is not fully reversible. The airflow limitation is usually both progressive and associated with an abnormal inflammatory response of the lungs to noxious particles and gases (16). Declining lung function over time is an important component in the natural history of this disease. Different populations, such as susceptible smokers, nonsusceptible smokers, nonsmokers, have different trends in their lung function decline over time. Impaired lung function is a strong predictor of morbidity and mortality. However, COPD is a heterogeneous disease so that patients may present different phenotypes (17): for example, people who have frequent exacerbations or people who lose lung function at a faster rate than the rest of the population (18).

The role that nocturnal desaturations play in the natural history of COPD is not well known. More attention has been paid to patients, whose awake arterial oxygen tension is above 60 mmHg, in other words, patients with mild or absent daytime hypoxemia. It has been suggested that nocturnal desaturations occurring in patients without significant daytime hypoxemia could lead to permanent pulmonary hypertension, precipitating the development of cor pulmonale. Fletcher et al. (19) demonstrated that patients with nocturnal desaturation had a lower survival rate than those without; they also found that "desaturators" treated with nocturnal oxygen supplementation tended to survive longer than those who were not treated, although the difference was not statistically significant. However, Chaouat et al. (5) did not confirm that patients who had desaturations had higher pulmonary arterial pressures. Two different studies investigating the survival of COPD patients receiving long-term oxygen therapy for moderate hypoxemia found that long-term oxygen therapy treatment did not improve survival in this kind of patient (20,21). Furthermore, a two-year follow-up study by Chaouat et al. (22) suggested that the presence of isolated nocturnal hypoxemia or sleep-related worsening of moderate daytime hypoxemia in COPD patients neither favors the development of pulmonary hypertension nor leads to a worsening of daytime blood gases. However, more recently, a prospective study with a follow-up of 42 months indicated that nocturnal desaturation may represent an independent risk factor for the development of chronic respiratory failure in COPD patients with a daytime $PaO_2 > 60$ mmHg (23).

TABLE 1 Predictors of Nocturnal Hypoxemia in Patients with Chronic Obstructive Pulmonary Disease and Mild Daytime Hypoxemia

Predictors of nocturnal desaturation	
Fletcher et al. (3)	Lower PaO_2 and higher $PaCO_2$
Bradley et al. (13)	Daytime hypercapnia
Vos et al. (6)	Daytime PaO_2, hypercapnic ventilatory response and sleepiness
Little et al. (15)	Daytime $SaO_2 \leq 93\%$
Toraldo et al. (14)	Mean pulmonary artery pressure, daytime $PaCO_2$

This study, by Sergi et al., was conducted on 52 COPD patients with a stable day-time PaO_2 above 60 mmHg, absence of clinical or ECG signs of cor pulmonale and absence of OSA (apnea-hypopnea index < 5 events/hour). The patients were subdivided at enrollment in two groups on the basis of presence of nocturnal desaturations. The authors observed that the onset of chronic respiratory failure was much more common in desaturators than among those who did not (Fig. 1). Three independent factors were associated with the onset of chronic respiratory failure: $PaCO_2$, FEV_1 (forced expiratory volume in 1 second), and nocturnal desaturation.

Finally, many studies focus on one fundamental point: nocturnal desaturations that worsen over time are present in patients who have a more rapid derangement of their lung mechanics, as demonstrated by a more rapid decline of FEV_1, or a greater increase in $PaCO_2$ (13,14,23,24).

The development of nocturnal desaturations in COPD patients has been attributed to several causes including changes in respiratory mechanics, worsening in ventilation/perfusion ($\dot{V}/Q$) mismatch, increased airflow resistance, and progressive respiratory muscles weakness. Ballard et al. (25) found, in a group of COPD patients, that REM sleep caused a significant reduction in minute ventilation related to a decrease in tidal volume; increased resistances in the upper airway may contribute to this sleep-associated decrease in minute ventilation. During sleep there was a marked decrease in respiratory neuromuscular output, which fell by 39% during REM sleep. The authors concluded that sleep does not seem to alter lung volume or increase lower-airway resistance dramatically, but that a decrease in tidal volume and inspiratory flow are associated with increased upper airway resistance and reduced respiratory muscle activity. In another study, Becker et al. (26) investigated the mechanisms leading to hypoxemia during sleep in patients with various respiratory disorders including COPD. They found a more pronounced reduction in minute ventilation during REM sleep, irrespectively of the underlying disease, and concluded that reversal of hypoventilation during sleep should be a major therapeutic strategy for these patients. The work of breathing in COPD patients is already high while these patients are awake because of airways obstruction and

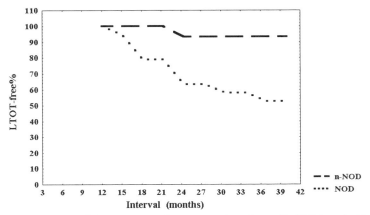

FIGURE 1 LTOT program enrollment curve in patient with (NOD) and without (n-NOD) nocturnal desaturations [see Ref. (23) for more details]. *Source*: S. Karger AG, Basel Editor.

lung hyperinflation. Respiratory muscles strength is reduced as a result of structural and functional abnormalities so that they are less able to support increased work of breathing (27). The diaphragm is the main respiratory muscle and plays the predominant role in inspiration. COPD challenges the diaphragm by increasing inspiratory muscle demands because of higher resistive, threshold, and elastic loads and by contributing to inspiratory muscle inefficiency or weakness. Like limb muscles, the diaphragm has been shown to respond to a work overload by cellular and functional adaptations (27–31). However, in contrast to models of limb muscle overload, in which periods of rest and recovery occur, diaphragmatic overload associated with COPD can be relentless and prolonged. The diaphragm's ability to adapt may be further impaired by factors that accentuate muscle weakness or limit regeneration. Such factors included impaired nutritional status, corticosteroids, and poor arterial blood gases (32). Thus, diaphragm dysfunction and injury may be due to the unremitting overload compounded by adverse clinical factors that exceed the diaphragm's capacity to adapt. Macgowan et al. (33) found that an increased severity of airflow obstruction is associated with an increased area of abnormal diaphragm muscle (and a decreased area of normal diaphragm muscle) in people with a large range of airflow obstruction undergoing thoracotomy surgery. The percentage of area of abnormal diaphragm ranged between 4% and 34% and included fibers with internally located nuclei, lipofuscin pigmentation, small angulated fibers, and some inflammation. The clinical significance of these findings is very important. Recovery of strength after injury is much slower than reversal of fatigue. For example, after eccentric loading of the elbow flexors, in otherwise healthy humans, the half-time of recovery was as long as five to six weeks. Finally, diaphragm contractility is reduced with hypercapnia and this can lead to muscle fatigue and further reduction in ventilatory responsiveness.

Respiratory muscle activity and chest wall motion differ markedly in the various stages of sleep. Normally, there is an increase in intercostal muscle activity during NREM sleep, thus increasing the rib cage's contribution to spontaneous ventilation over that provided during wakefulness (34,35). The changes in the electrical activity of the respiratory muscles are associated with a marked reduction in the rib cage's contribution to tidal volume and, consequently, a greater reliance on the diaphragm to maintain ventilation. In patients with a mechanically inefficient diaphragm or diaphragmatic weakness, the REM-induced loss of intercostal and accessory muscle activity causes a significant reduction in inspiratory pressure generation and impairs ventilation, contributing to the hypoventilation seen in such patients. It has been shown that accessory inspiratory muscles, such as the sternocleidomastoid and scalene muscles (36), as well as the abdominal muscles (37), play an important role in increasing ventilation during wakefulness and NREM sleep in patients with severe COPD and in those with generalized neuromuscular disorders. With loss of this activity during REM sleep, a significant degree of hypoventilation is expected to occur, which in turn is associated with deterioration in gas exchange. Sleep, especially the REM period, is also characterized by a major increase in upper airway resistance (34). In a group of patients with severe chronic airflow obstruction, O'Donoghue et al. (38) found that the development of nocturnal hypoventilation was related to baseline carbon dioxide, body mass index (BMI), severity of inspiratory flow limitation in REM sleep and the apnea–hypopnea index. Obesity and reduction in upper airway caliber in the absence of apnea or hypopnea episodes induce a further increase in inspiratory load.However, hypoventilation is not the only cause of hypoxemia. Oxygen desaturation during sleep in COPD may also be, in part, due to alterations in the distribution of $\dot{V}/Q$ relationships (39). Oxygen uptake is increased during REM sleep, and this may contribute to the desaturation. The dissociation between diaphragmatic and intercostal activity during REM sleep can also result in both hypoventilation and worsening of ventilation–perfusion disturbances. Indeed, a study published in 2003 found that patients with an FEV_1/FVC (forced vital capacity) ratio of less than 65% had an increased risk of sleep desaturation independent of their level of awake oxygen saturation and the presence of OSA (40). In the light of their findings, the authors proposed that overnight oximetry should be routinely considered in patients with an FEV_1/FVC of less than 65%. Mulloy and McNicholas (10) have found that transcutaneous PCO_2 level rose to a similar extent in patients who developed major nocturnal oxygen desaturation and in those who developed only a minor degree of desaturation, which suggests a similar degree of hypoventilation in both groups, despite the different degrees of nocturnal oxygen desaturation. The much larger fall in PaO_2 among the patients with major episodes of desaturation, in conjunction with the similar rise in transcutaneous $PaCO_2$ in both groups of patients, suggests that in addition to a degree of hypoventilation existing in all patients, other factors such as ventilation–perfusion mismatching must also play a part in the excess desaturation of some COPD patients.

Sleep-Disordered Breathing

A possible association between COPD and OSA was described in the mid-1980s by Flenley (41) who named this association the "overlap syndrome."

COPD is the most common chronic lung disease, since several epidemiological studies have shown that about 8% to 10% of the population above 30 years of age in developed countries is affected by this disorder (42–44). Morbidity from COPD results in a substantial use of secondary healthcare resources. Patients with severe COPD and other comorbid conditions absorb higher costs than patients with mild disease or no comorbidities (45). The prevalence of OSA is also very high (46), so that the presence of both diseases in the same subjects is not rare. An early report found a high prevalence of OSA in patients with COPD or, conversely, a high prevalence of chronic airways obstruction in OSA patients (46–50). However, a study conducted on 1132 participants using data of the Sleep Heart Health Study, found that OSA was not more prevalent in patients with mild COPD (40). The principal results of this study were: (*i*) prevalence of OSA is not greater in community patients with evidence of COPD; (*ii*) the proportion of participants with notable desaturation of oxyhemoglobin during sleep and the degree to which sleep is perturbed are greater in the presence of both disorders but are largely related to the contribution of OSA. The authors confirmed the hypothesis that when generally mild OSA and COPD coexist, it is on the basis of aggregation by chance rather than through a pathophysiological linkage. Participants with COPD had a significantly lower mean and median respiratory disturbance index (RDI) than those without COPD. In addition, the percentage of participants with a RDI greater than 10 or 15 was significantly lower in the group of subjects with COPD than in the group without COPD. Furthermore, RDI values were similar in subjects with and without COPD after stratification by quartiles of BMI. The RDI increased with higher BMI quartile independently of the presence of COPD. The authors examined the degree to which COPD and OSA independently and conjointly contributed to oxygen desaturation, assessing the risk of spending more than 5% of total sleep time with $SaO_2 < 90\%$ or 85%, in the presence of single disorders or their combination. The odds ratio for desaturation below the threshold levels considered was greatly increased in the presence of OSA, while that conferred by COPD in the absence of OSA was relatively lower (Table 2); the combination of OSA and COPD determined the highest risk of desaturation, being more or less double that observed in subjects with OSA alone.

The relatively low percentage of subjects with severe COPD in the study of Sanders et al. may limit the generalization of their results to more severely impaired individuals. The authors defined COPD subjects as those individuals with an FEV_1/FVC ratio less than 70%; however, given that normal aging may be accompanied by a decline in this ratio, it is possible that some normal subjects were misclassified as having COPD. Furthermore, the results can be biased by a survival effect. In other words, an association between COPD and OSA may not be detected because mortality causes and under-representation of participants with both disorders in the study population.

More recently, an epidemiological study performed in Poland on middle-aged and elderly subjects gave similar results to those of Sanders. Bednarek et al. (51) studied 676 subjects (age range 41–71 years), randomly selected from the general population. The prevalence of OSA was 11.3% while the prevalence of COPD was 10.7%. The overlap syndrome was found in only seven subjects (9.2% of OSAs population and 1% of total population). The authors concluded that the prevalence of COPD in OSA patients is similar to that in the general population, but that the severity of sleep-disordered breathing in subjects with coexisting COPD is high.

The overlap syndrome is said to predispose to daytime hypercapnia and hypoxemia independently of lung function (5). OSA appears to be an important cause of hypoxemia and hypercapnia in some groups of patients in whom these findings appear to be disproportionate to the level of lung function impairment (49,52,53). Chan et al. (52) showed that hypercapnic COPD patients had many more sleep-disordered breathing events, higher BMI, and smaller upper airway cross-sectional areas than did eucapnic controls matched for lung function.

Quality of Sleep

Sleep quality has been described to be different in patients with COPD and in age-matched healthy subjects. COPD patients seem to have a higher prevalence of insomnia, excessive daytime sleepiness, and nightmares than do the general population. The most frequent polysomnographic findings in COPD patients are a

TABLE 2 Adjusted Odds Ratio of Desaturation Based on Chronic Obstructive Pulmonary Disease and Obstructive Sleep Apnea Status

	OSA (+)		OSA (−)	
	COPD (+)	COPD (−)	COPD (+)	COPD (−)
> 5% TST with SaO_2 < 85%				
People %[a]	11.02	10.59	0.79	0.41
Odds ratio (CI)[b]	30.08 (13.21–73.18)	15.83 (7.23–34.67)	3.15 (1.07–9.26)	1 (reference)

[a]Overall χ^2 comparison significant at < 0.0001 level.
[b]Odds ratio (95% CI) adjusted for age, sex, height, weight, race, smoking status (former and current).
Abbreviations: CI, confidence interval; COPD, chronic obstructive pulmonary disease; OSA, obstructive sleep apnea; SaO_2, Oxyhaemoglobin saturation (%); TST, total sleep time.
Source: Modified from Ref. 40.

decreased sleep time, reduction in REM sleep and more changes in sleep stage (54). Poor sleep quality may represent a factor in the development of chronic fatigue and reduced quality of life usually reported by patients with severe COPD. The mechanisms of this disorganized sleep structure are debated. The disorganization may be related to alterations in gas exchange, medications or general debility associated with COPD (55). Although theophylline or β-agonists could be implicated in the insomnia, studies on these agents have failed to demonstrate any adverse effects on sleep stage or sleep efficiency. Maximization of drug therapy to prevent coughing and shortness of breath from disrupting sleep at night may help patients to cope with insomnia. Hypoxia stimulates the reticular activating system, and there is a strong association between hypoxemia and the incidence of arousals in COPD. The frequency of arousals does not, however, decrease after nocturnal oxygen therapy, suggesting it is not the hypoxemia but some related phenomenon, possibly hypercapnia, which is the principal stimulus to arousal (56).

Sandek et al. (57) showed that prolonged nocturnal hypoxemia and reduced whole night oxygenation are associated with increased superficial sleep. These authors found a correlation between the mean whole night SaO_2 and number of sleep stage changes during the night (Fig. 2), and as well as prolonged NREM sleep stage 1.

Diagnostic Approach and Management

The serious and potentially life-threatening disturbances in ventilation and gas exchange that may develop during sleep in patients with COPD raise the question of what investigations are appropriate in these patients (58). It is widely accepted that sleep studies are not routinely indicated in patients with COPD associated with respiratory failure. Although awake oxygen saturation is the best predictor of sleep desaturation in COPD, the degree of airflow obstruction also independently predicts sleep desaturation. Overnight oximetry should be considered in most COPD patients, irrespectively of whether they have symptoms of sleep disruption, to identify significant overnight desaturation that may be associated with reduced survival. Nocturnal oximetry is also mandatory in order to titrate the oxygen flow adequately

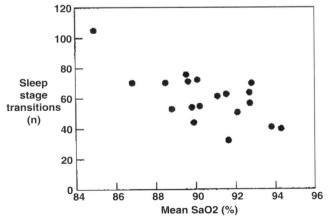

FIGURE 2 Correlation between mean SaO_2 and total numbers of sleep stage changes ($r = -0.54$; $p < 0.05$). *Source*: Modified from Ref. 57.

in patients who are eligible for long-term oxygen therapy (59). However, when performing overnight pulse oximetry, especially at home, it must be appreciated that patients with COPD considerable night-to-night variability in nocturnal desaturation so that only one recording may be insufficient for an accurate assessment (60).

Sleep studies are generally performed when there is a clinical suspicion of associated OSA or manifestations of hypoxemia not explained by the awake PaO_2 level or in the presence of daytime hypoxemia not adequately explained by the level of airflow obstruction.

The first step in the management of sleep-disordered breathing in COPD patients is optimal treatment of the underlying disease. Conventional O_2 therapy (both night-time and daytime) is the first-line treatment of nocturnal hypoxemia in COPD patients with stable respiratory failure ($PaO_2 < 55$–60 mmHg). However, COPD patients may have nocturnal desaturation even in the presence of only mild-to-moderate daytime hypoxemia ($PaO_2 > 60$ mmHg), thus not fulfilling the usual criteria for conventional oxygen therapy (40). According to the already mentioned results of Fletcher et al. (19) this group of patients usually receives oxygen therapy only during the night. However, the impact of nocturnal oxygen therapy in such patients is still debated since conflicting results are available both regarding the hypothesis that isolated sleep-related hypoxemia could favor the development of pulmonary hypertension or reduce the survival rate (61).

Noninvasive mechanical ventilation (NIMV) has been increasingly used as a treatment of chronic hypercapnic respiratory failure. Its use in patients affected by COPD is still controversial, while most of the studies performed in patients with restrictive thoracic disorders, and in particular in those with neuromuscular disorders, suggested that the symptoms of chronic hypoventilation were alleviated in the short-term, and in two small studies survival was prolonged (62–66). Indeed, a Cochrane review published in 2001 stated that "long-term mechanical ventilation should be offered as a therapeutic option to patients with chronic respiratory failure due to neuromuscular diseases" (67).

NIMV probably produces improvements in daytime blood gases through a number of mechanisms, including resting of the respiratory muscles, and a resetting of the respiratory drive. It was hypothesized that the nocturnal use of NIMV might prevent episodes of sleep-disordered breathing, reduce associated arousals, and improve the quality of sleep. In addition, NIMV during sleep would ameliorate nocturnal hypoventilation, leading to a downward resetting of the respiratory center's sensitivity to carbon dioxide. As a consequence, daytime gas exchange would improve, and the improved sleep quality would have a favorable impact on daytime function and quality of life. Elliot et al. (68) evaluated eight patients with severe COPD, six of whom had a reduction in daytime PaO_2 when treated with nocturnal nasal ventilation using a portable volume ventilator for six months. These patients had improved sleep quality and there was a significant correlation between the drop in $PaCO_2$ and the ventilatory response to CO_2, suggesting an increase in respiratory drive (69). In a controlled three-month crossover trial, Meecham-Jones (65) studied 18 patients receiving nasal bilevel positive airway pressure ventilation. Patients receiving NIMV had significant reductions in daytime $PaCO_2$, and the frequent oxygen desaturations and episodes of hypoventilation that occurred during control nights were ameliorated by NIMV. The authors concluded that NIMV improved sleep quality and nocturnal gas exchange, and that these benefits enhanced quality of life. Most of the papers published in the literature on the long-term efficacy of NIMV in patients with chronic hypercapnic respiratory failure do not have the effect of NIMV on sleep quality or the pattern of breathing during sleep (70). When the decision to initiate long-term NIMV is made, the ventilatory parameters to use during night-time are mainly decided according to the patient's tolerance when they are awake and records of diurnal arterial blood gases. However, the scenario during sleep may change considerably. Teschler et al. (71) studied the effect of mouth leak, very common on NIMV while asleep, on effectiveness of nasal bilevel ventilatory assistance and on sleep architecture. These investigators found that when the mouth was taped closed during nocturnal NIMV there was a significant reduction of transcutaneous carbon dioxide and a significant improvement of sleep quality as demonstrated by a reduction in arousal index and an increase in the amount of REM sleep. Finally, the effect of NIMV on sleep quality and improvement of gas exchange is also dependent on patient/ventilator interaction. Indeed, stable patients receiving nocturnal NIMV for chronic sleep hypoventilation or chronic hypercapnic respiratory failure may have a poor nocturnal gas exchange and disturbed sleep when the patient/ventilator interaction is not optimal, as was demonstrated by the presence of ineffective inspiratory efforts (72,73). Sleep quality and gas exchange improved after adjusting the ventilatory parameter according to a more physiological setting (Fig. 3).

At the moment, long-term oxygen therapy is the first-line treatment of COPD patients who are hypoxemic during the night but NIMV may become more important in the future. More studies are necessary to understand the true effect of NIMV on sleep quality and control of breathing during sleep. Until the mechanisms to explain the benefit of NIMV in COPD patients are better known, the indications, ideal ventilator settings, and expected response will remain unclear. The decision to start home NIMV during sleep should be individually defined on the basis of clinical and physiological response to a preliminary trial (74).

OBSTRUCTIVE SLEEP APNEA AND BRONCHIAL ASTHMA

OSA may represent a trigger for nocturnal acute asthma attacks. Indeed, in patients with concomitant OSA and bronchial asthma, CPAP therapy was demonstrated to be effective also in improving asthma control (75).

Bronchial asthma is a chronic inflammatory disease of the airways and is prevalent in the general population. Therapy usually results in a good control of symptoms and airway obstruction in the great majority of patients. However, some patients show frequent and severe exacerbations, with increased morbidity and

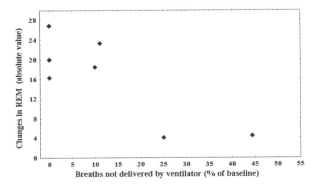

FIGURE 3 Correlation between changes in ineffective effort and changes in amount of REM sleep (expressed as % of total sleep time) observed during a more physiological setting of the ventilator ($r = -0.82$; $p = 0.02$). *Abbreviation*: REM, rapid eye movement. *Source*: From Ref. 72.

hospital admissions, frequently in emergency departments. Many factors have been identified or proposed to explain the instability of asthma control in these patients: a high-level of bronchial hyper-responsiveness, poor therapy compliance, inadequate use of inhalators, smoking, psychosocial factors as low income, inaccessibility of medical care, concomitant psychiatric disease, continuous exposure to allergens, and drugs such as β-blockers (76–80).

A study published in 2005, specifically designed to identify the main determinants of unstable severe asthma, was conducted on a group of patients with frequent severe exacerbation (81). As shown in Table 3, many factors were associated with the increasing number of exacerbations. All the patients included in the study had at least one of the identified risk factors, but three or more risk factors were present at the same time in more than half the patients. Sleep apnea was identified as an independent factor; the prevalence of OSA in this group of patients was higher than in the general population. These data suggest that the presence of sleep-disordered breathing should be adequately considered and investigated in patients with difficult-to-treat asthma.

Bronchial asthma and OSA are both associated with reduction in quality of life. Ekici et al. (82) investigated the impact of the association of both diseases on quality of life. They showed that there is a significant association between asthma symptoms, snoring, and complaints for apnea, also after adjusting data for sex, age, body weight, smoking, and socio-economic status. Subjects who experienced chronic symptoms of asthma and OSA had lower quality-of-life scores than did healthy or subjects with only one of the two diseases.

Finally, there is some experimental evidence suggesting that gastroesophageal reflux can worsen airway function, inducing cough, bronchospasm or asthma attacks. Gislason et al. (83) found that asthma attacks were more frequent in patients with nocturnal gastroesophageal reflux. The increase in bronchial tone may be caused directly by aspiration of gastric fluid into the trachea or indirectly by activity of afferent vagal fibers (84). The amplitude of the increase in respiratory resistance is correlated to the duration of the exposure to acid (85). OSA may worsen bronchial asthma indirectly, by increasing the episode of nocturnal gastroesophageal reflux. The relationship between gastroesophageal reflux and OSA is still unclear, but many studies reported that nocturnal gastroesophageal reflux is common in patients with OSA. Many patients with OSA experience a burning sensation or acid regurgitation during the night. The hypothesized explanation is that the pressure gradient between the esophagus and stomach increases due to augmented intrathoracic pressure with suction of gastric fluid into the esophagus. This produced a pharyngeal

TABLE 3 Odds Ratio for Factors Potentially Associated with Frequent Exacerbations in Difficult-to-Treat Asthma

	Odds ratio adjusted for age and asthma duration (95% CI)
Psychological dysfunctioning	10.8 (1.1–108.4)
Recurrent respiratory infections	6.9 (1.9–24.7)
Gastroesophageal reflux	4.9 (1.4–17.8)
Severe chronic sinus disease	3.7 (1.2–11.9)
OSA	3.4 (1.2–10.4)

Abbreviations: CI, Confidence interval; OSA, obstructive sleep apnea.
Source: From Ref. 81.

spasm in patients with sleep-related breathing disorders leading to bronchospasm or cough in asthmatic patients, by causing microaspiration (83,86).

CONCLUSIONS

Many patients with respiratory disorders experience worsening of their clinical and functional impairment during sleep. In chronic progressive disease, such as COPD, the onset of specific sleep-related phenomena is associated with worsening of daytime symptoms, poorer sleep quality and prognosis. Furthermore, the association of sleep apnea and concomitant chronic respiratory disorders increase the severity of each disease.

The evaluation of respiratory function during sleep should be performed routinely in patients with chronic progressive respiratory diseases, particularly in those with a more rapid worsening of symptoms or a more severe clinical status, not explained by the severity of functional impairment assessed during wakefulness.

REFERENCES

1. Trask CH, Cree EM. Oximeter studies on patients with chronic obstructive emphysema, awake and during sleep. N Engl J Med 1962; 266:639–642.
2. Douglas NJ, Claverly PMA, Leggett RJE, et al. Transient hypoxemia during sleep in chronic bronchitis and emphysema. Lancet 1979; i:1–4.
3. Fletcher EC, Miller J, Divine GW, et al. Nocturnal oxyhemoglobin desaturation in COPD patients with arterial oxygen tensions above 60 mmHg. Chest 1987; 92:604–608.
4. Levi-Valensi P, Weitzemblum E, Rida Z, et al. Sleep-related oxygen desaturation and daytime pulmonary haemodynamics in COPD patients. Eur Respir J 1992; 5:301–307.
5. Chaouat A, Weitzemblum E, Kessler R, et al. Sleep-related O2 desaturation and daytime pulmonary haemodynamics in COPD patients with mild hypoxaemia. Eur Respir J 1997; 10:1730–1735.
6. Vos PJE, Folgering HTM, Van Herwaarden CLA. Predictors for nocturnal hypoxaemia (mean SaO2 < 90%) in normoxic and mildly hypoxic patients with COPD. Eur Respir J 1995; 8:74–77.
7. Koo KW, Sax DS, Snider GL. Arterial blood gases and pH during sleep in chronic obstructive pulmonary disease. Am J Med 1975; 58:663–670.
8. Leitch AG, Clancy LJ, Leggett RJE, et al. Arterial blood gas tensions, hydrogen ion, and electroencephalogram during sleep in patients with chronic ventilatory failure. Thorax 1976; 31:730–735.
9. Flick MR, Bloch AJ. Continuous in vivo monitoring of arterial oxygenation in chronic obstructive lung disease. Am J Med 1979; 86:725–730.
10. Mulloy E, McNicholas WT. Ventilation and gas exchange during sleep and exercise in severe COPD. Chest 1996; 109:387–394.
11. Catterall HR, Douglas NJ, Calverly PMA, et al. Transient hypoxemia during sleep in chronic obstructive pulmonary disease is not a sleep apnea syndrome. Am Rev Respir Dis 1983; 128:24–29.
12. Connaughton JJ, Catterall JR, Elton RA, et al. Do sleep studies contribute to the management of patients with severe chronic obstructive pulmonary disease. Am Rev Respir Dis 1988; 138:341–344.
13. Bradley TD, Mateika J, Li D, et al. Daytime hypercapnia in the development of nocturnal hypoxemia in COPD. Chest 1990; 97:308–312.
14. Toraldo DM, Nicolardi G, De Nuccio F, et al. Pattern of variables describing desaturator COPD patients, as revealed by cluster analysis. Chest 2005; 128:3828–3837.
15. Little SA, Elkholy MM, Chalmers, et al. Predictors of nocturnal oxygen desaturation in patients with COPD. Respir Med 1999; 93:202–207.
16. World Health Organization. The GOLD global strategy for the management and prevention of CPOD, 2001. www.Goldcopd.org.

17. Mannino DM, Watt G, Hole D, et al. The natural history of chronic obstructive pulmonary disease. Eur Respir J 2006; 27:627–643.
18. Burrows B. Airways obstructive diseases: pathogenetic mechanisms and natural histories of the disorders. Med Clin North Am 1990; 74:547–559.
19. Fletcher EC, Donner CF, Midgren B, et al. Survival in COPD patients with a daytime PaO2 >60 mmHg with and without nocturnal oxyhemoglobin desaturation. Chest 1992; 101:649–655.
20. Gorecka D, Gorzelak K, Sliwinski P, et al. Effect of long term oxygen therapy on survival in patients with chronic obstructive pulmonary disease with moderate hypoxaemia. Thorax 1997; 52: 674–679.
21. Veale D, Chailleux E, Taytard A, et al. Characteristics and survival of patients prescribed long-term oxygen therapy outside prescription guidelines. Eur Respir J 1998; 12: 780–784.
22. Chaouat A, Weitzemblum E, Kessler R, et al. Outcome of COPD patients with mild daytime hypoxaemia with or without sleep-related oxygen desaturation. Eur Respir J 2001; 17:848–855.
23. Sergi M, Rizzi M, Andreoli A, et al. Are COPD patients with nocturnal REM sleep-related desaturations more prone to developing chronic respiratory failure requiring long-term oxygen therapy? Respiration 2002; 69:117–122.
24. Fletcher EC, Scott D, Qian W, et al. Evolution of nocturnal oxyhemoglobin desaturation in patients with chronic obstructive pulmonary disease and a daytime PaO2 above 60 mmHg. Am Rev Respir Dis 1991; 144:401–405.
25. Ballard RD, Clover W, Suh BY. Influence of sleep on respiratory function in emphysema. Am J Respir Crit Care Med 1995; 151:945–951.
26. Becker HF, Piper AJ, Flynn WE, et al. Breathing during sleep in patients with nocturnal desaturation. Am J Respir Crit Care Med 1999; 159:112–118.
27. Levine S, Kaiser L, Leferovich J, et al. Cellular adaptations in the diaphragm in chronic obstructive pulmonary disease. N Engl J Med 1997; 337(25):1799–1806.
28. Sliwinski P, Macklem PT. Inspiratory muscle dysfunction as a cause of death in COPD patients. Monaldi Arch Chest Dis 1997; 52:380–383.
29. Faulkner JA, Brooks SV, Opiteck JA. Injury to skeletal muscle fibers during contractions: conditions of occurrence and prevention. Phys Ther 1993; 73:911–921.
30. Poole DC, Sexton WL, Farkas GA, et al. Diaphragm structure and function in health and disease. Med Sci Sports Exerc 1997; 29:738–754.
31. Reid WD, Samrai B. Respiratory muscle training for patients with chronic obstructive pulmonary disease. Phys Ther 1995; 75:996–1005.
32. Reid WD, MacGowean NA. Respiratory muscle injury in animal models and humans. Mol Cell Biochem 1998; 179:63–80.
33. Macgowan NA, Evans KG, Road JD, et al. Diaphragm injury in individuals with airflow obstruction. Am J Respir Crit Care Med 2001; 163(7):1654–1659.
34. Tabacnick E, Muller NL, Bryan AC, et al. Changes in ventilation and chest wall mechanics during sleep in normal adolescents. J Appl Physiol 1981; 51:557–564.
35. Hudgel DW, Martin RJ, Johnson B, et al. Mechanics of the respiratory system and breathing pattern during sleep in normal humans. J Appl Physiol 1984; 56:133–137.
36. Johnson MW, Remmers JE. Accessory muscle activity during sleep in chronic obstructive pulmonary disease. J Appl Physiol 1984; 57:1011–1017.
37. White JES, Drinnan MJ, Smithson AJ, et al. Respiratory muscle activity and oxygenation during sleep in patients with muscle weakness. Eur Respir J 1995; 8:807–814.
38. O'Donoghue FJ, Catchside PG, Ellis EE, et al. Sleep hypoventilation in hypercapnic chronic obstructive pulmonary disease: prevalence and associated factors. Eur Respir J 2003; 21:977–984.
39. Stradling JR, Lane DJ. Nocturnal hypoxaemia in chronic obstructive pulmonary disease. Clin Sci 1983; 64:213–222.
40. Sanders MH, Newman AB, Haggerty CL, et al. Sleep and sleep-disordered breathing in adults with predominantly mild obstructive airway disease. Am J Respir Crit Care Med 2003; 167:7–14.
41. Flenley DC. Sleep in chronic obstructive pulmonary disease. Clin Chest Med 1985; 6:651–661.

42. Pena VS, Miravitlles M, Gabriel R, et al. Geographic variations in prevalence and under-diagnosis of COPD: results of the IPERPOC multicentre epidemiological study. Chest 2000; 118:981–989.
43. Viegi G, Pedreschi M, Pistelli F, et al. Prevalence of airways obstruction in a general population: European Respiratory Society vs. American Thoracic Society definition. Chest 2002; 117:S339–S345.
44. Pauwels RA, Buist AS, Calverly PM. Global strategy for the diagnosis, management, and prevention of chronic obstructive pulmonary disease: NHLBI/WHO Global Initiative for Chronic Obstructive Lung Disease (GOLD) Workshop summary. Am J Respir Crit Care Med 2001; 163:1256–1276.
45. Chapman KR, Mannino DM, Soriano JB, et al. Epidemiology and costs of chronic obstructive pulmonary disease. Eur Respir J 2006; 27:188–207.
46. Ferini-Strambi L, Zucconi M, Palazzi S, et al. Snoring and nocturnal oxygen desaturations in an Italian middle-aged male population. Epidemiological study with an ambulatory device. Chest 1994; 105(6):1759–1764.
47. Guilleminault C, Cummiskey J, Motta J. Chronic obstructive airflow disease and sleep studies. Am Rev Respir Dis 1980; 122:397–406.
48. Larsson LG, Lindberg A, Franklin KA, et al. Obstructive sleep apnoea syndrome is common in subjects with chronic bronchitis. Reports from the obstructive lung disease in northern Sweden studies. Respiration 2001; 68:250–255.
49. Chaouat A, Weitzemblum E, Krieger J, et al. Association of chronic obstructive pulmonary disease and sleep apnoea syndrome. Am Rev Respir Dis 1995; 151:82–86.
50. Bradley TD, Rutherford R, Lue F, et al. Role of diffuse airway obstruction in the hypercapnia of sleep apnea. Am Rev Respir Dis 1986; 134:920–924.
51. Bednarek M, Plywaczewki R, Jonczak L, et al. There is no relationship between chronic obstructive pulmonary disease and obstructive sleep apnea syndrome: a population study. Respiration 2005; 72:142–149.
52. Chan CS, Bye PT, Woolcock AJ, et al. Eucapnia and hypercapnia in patients with chronic airflow limitation. The role of the upper airway. Am Rev Respir Dis 1990; 141:861–865.
53. Berthon-Jones M, Sullivan CE. Time course of change in ventilatory response to CO2 with long-term CPAP therapy for obstructive sleep apnea. Am Rev Respir Dis 1987; 135:144–147.
54. Breslin E, Van der Schans C, Breubink S, et al. Perception of fatigue and quality of life in patients with COPD. Chest 1998; 114:958–964.
55. Mulloy E, McNicholas WT. Theophylline improves gas exchange during rest, exercise and sleep in severe chronic obstructive pulmonary disease. Am Rev Respir Dis 1993; 148:1030–1036.
56. Fleetham J, West P, Mezon B, et al. Sleep, arousals, and oxygen desaturation in chronic obstructive pulmonary disease. Am Rev Respir Dis 1982; 126:429–433.
57. Sandek K, Andersson T, Bratel T, et al. Sleep quality, carbon dioxide responsiveness and hypoxaemic patterns in nocturnal hypoxaemia due to chronic obstructive pulmonary disease (COPD) without daytime hypoxemia. Respir Med 1999; 93:79–87.
58. McNicholas WT. Impact of sleep in COPD. Chest 2000; 117:S48–S53.
59. Plywaczewski R, Sliwinski P, Nowinski A, et al. Incidence of nocturnal desaturation while breathing oxygen in COPD patients undergoing long-term oxygen therapy. Chest 2000; 117:679–683.
60. Lewis CA, Eaton TE, Ferfusson W, et al. Home overnight pulse oximetry in patients with COPD: more than one recording may be needed. Chest 2003; 123:1127–1133.
61. Chaouat A, Weitzemblum E, Kessler R, et al. A randomized trial of nocturnal oxygen therapy in chronic obstructive pulmonary disease patients. Eur Respir J 1999; 14:1002–1008.
62. Jones SE, Packham S, Hebden M, et al. Domiciliary nocturnal intermittent positive pressure ventilation in patients with respiratory failure due to severe COPD: long-term follow up and effect on survival. Thorax 1998; 53:495–498.
63. Gay PC, Hubmayr RD, Stroetz RW. Efficacy of nocturnal nasal ventilation in stable, severe chronic obstructive pulmonary disease during a 3-month controlled trial. Mayo Clin Proc 1996; 71:533–542.

64. Strumpf DA, Millman RP, Carlisle CC, et al. Nocturnal positive-pressure ventilation via nasal mask in patients with severe chronic obstructive pulmonary disease. Am Rev Respir Dis 1991; 144:1234–1239.
65. Meecham Jones DJ, Paul EA, Jones PW, et al. Nasal pressure support ventilation plus oxygen compared with oxygen therapy alone in hypercapnic COPD. Am J Respir Crit Care Med 1995; 152:538–544.
66. Clini E, Sturani C, Rossi A, et al. Rehabilitation and Chronic Care Study Group, Italian Association of Hospital Pulmonologists (AIPO). The Italian multicentre study on noninvasive ventilation in chronic obstructive pulmonary disease patients. Eur Respir J 2002; 20:529–538.
67. Annane D, Chevrolet JC, Chevret S, Raphael JC. Nocturnal mechanical ventilation for chronic hypoventilation in patients with neuromuscular and chest wall disorders. Cochrane Database Syst Rev 2000; (2).
68. Elliott MW, Steven MH, Phillips GD, et al. Non-invasive mechanical ventilation for acute respiratory failure. BMJ 1990; 300:358–360.
69. Elliott MW, Mulvey DA, Moxham J, et al. Domiciliary nocturnal nasal intermittent positive pressure ventilation in COPD: mechanisms underlying changes in arterial blood gas tensions. Eur Respir J 1991; 4:1044–1052.
70. Wijkstra PJ, Lacasse Y, Guyatt G, et al. A meta-analysis of nocturnal noninvasive positive pressure ventilation in patients with stable COPD. Chest 2003; 124:337–343.
71. Teschler H, Stampa J, Ragette R, et al. Effect of mouth leaks on effectiveness of nasal bi-level ventilatory assistance and sleep architecture. Eur Respir J 1999; 14:1251–1257.
72. Fanfulla F, Delmastro M, Berardinelli A, et al. Effects of different ventilator settings on sleep and inspiratory effort in neuromuscular patients. Am J Respir Crit Care Med 2005; 172:619–624.
73. Fanfulla F, Taurino E, D'Artavilla Lupo N, et al. Ineffective efforts during night-time non-invasive mechanical ventilation in COPD or RTD patients. Eur Respir J 2005; 26:S49.
74. Nava S, Fanfulla F, Frigerio P, et al. Physiologic evaluation of 4 weeks of nocturnal nasal positive pressure ventilation in stable hypercapnic patients with chronic obstructive pulmonary diseases. Respiration 2001; 68:573–583.
75. Chan CS, Woolcock AJ, Sullivan CE. Nocturnal asthma: role of snoring and obstructive sleep apnea. Am Rev Respir Dis 1988; 137:1502–1504.
76. Ulrik CS, Frederiksen J. Mortality and markers of risk of asthma death among 1075 outpatients with asthma. Chest 1995; 108:10–15.
77. Barnes PJ, Woolcock AJ. Difficult asthma. Eur Respir J 1998; 12:1209–1218.
78. Ten Brinke A, Zwinderman AH, Sterk PJ, et al. Factors associated with persistent airflow limitation in severe asthma. Am J Respir Crit Care Med 2001; 164:744–748.
79. Heaney LG, Conway E, Kelly C, et al. Predictors of therapy resistant asthma: outcome of a systematic evaluation protocol. Thorax 2003; 58:561–566.
80. Robinson DS, Campbell DA, Durham SR, et al. Systematic assessment of difficult-to-treat asthma. Eur Respir J 1998; 12:1209–1218.
81. Ten Brinke A, Sterk PJ, Masclee AAM, et al. Risk factors of frequent exacerbation in difficult-to-treat asthma. Eur Respir J 2005; 26:812–818.
82. Ekici A, Ekici M, Kurtipek E, et al. Association of asthma-related symptoms with snoring and apnea and effect on health-related quality of life. Chest 2005; 128:3358–3363.
83. Gislason T, Janson C, Vermeire P, et al. Respiratory symptoms and gastroesophageal reflux: a population based study of young adults in three European countries. Chest 2002; 120:158–163.
84. Berry RB, Harding SM. Sleep and medical disorders. Med Clin North Am 2004; 88:679–703.
85. Cuttitta G, Cibella G, Visconti A, et al. Spontaneous gastroesophageal reflux and airway patency during the night in adult asthmatics. Am J Respir Crit Care Med 2000; 161:177–181.
86. Demeter P, Pap A. The relationship between gastroesophageal reflux disease and obstructive sleep apnea. J Gastroenterol 2004; 39:815–820.

Other Sleep Disorders

Meeta H. Bhatt
*New York University School of Medicine and New York Sleep Institute,
New York, New York, U.S.A.*

Sudhansu Chokroverty
*Department of Neurology, NJ Neuroscience Institute at JFK Medical Center, Edison,
New Jersey and Seton Hall University, South Orange, New Jersey, U.S.A.*

INTRODUCTION

Sleep-related breathing disorders (SRBDs) are a group of disorders characterized by disordered respiration in sleep. Of these, obstructive sleep apnea (OSA), a form of sleep-disordered breathing (SDB), is the most commonly encountered condition. The syndrome of OSA is characterized by repetitive episodes of complete (apnea) or partial (hypopnea) upper airway obstruction during sleep, often resulting in snoring, arterial oxygen desaturation, and arousal from sleep. The upper airway resistance syndrome (UARS) is believed to be a milder version of OSA, although there is contradiction, and it is presumed to have the same risk factors as OSA (see also Chapter 18).

The prevalence of symptomatic OSA in adults aged 30 to 60 years has been reported as 4% in men and 2% in women, while asymptomatic OSA is reported in as many as 24% men and 9% women (1). The steepest prevalence increase is in the transition from middle-aged to older-aged adults. Prevalence of other sleep-related disorders, for example, insomnia, restless legs syndrome (RLS), periodic limb movement disorder (PLMD), and rapid eye movement (REM) sleep behavior disorder (RBD) also increase with age, likely contributing to the poor sleep quality of old age (2). Scharf et al. (3) reported concomitant sleep disorders in approximately one-third of 643 patients with OSA. The coexistence of sleep disorders may: (*i*) be incidental; (*ii*) originate from a shared pathophysiologic mechanism as seen in the increased prevalence of RBD in narcolepsy; (*iii*) stem from commonly shared risk factors, for example, obesity in major depressive disorder (MDD) and OSA; or (*iv*) provide a substrate for activation or exacerbation of another sleep disorder, as in the triggering of disorders of arousal secondary to sleep apnea-related arousals. The coexistence in turn may mask the symptoms or existence of a disorder preventing its adequate and timely treatment, for example, symptoms of OSA can mimic symptoms of depression. It can also potentially worsen sleep-related symptoms from a combined contributory effect, for example, excessive daytime sleepiness (EDS) from OSA can worsen the EDS from narcolepsy, when the two disorders coexist.

This chapter discusses the interaction between OSA and some of the most commonly occurring comorbid sleep disorders [e.g., epilepsy, insomnia, depression, narcolepsy, RLS, PLMD, and parasomnias].

SLEEP APNEA AND EPILEPSY

Prevalence and incidence of epilepsy are highest in later life with around 25% of new cases occurring in the elderly. OSA on the other hand may affect more than 50%

individuals over the age of 65 (4). Given the high prevalence of both conditions in the elderly population, coexistence is frequently likely. This section discusses the inter-relationship between epilepsy and sleep apnea (more information on sleep apnea and epilepsy can be found in Chapter 22).

Occurrence of epileptiform discharges is significantly influenced by the sleep-wake cycle and stages of sleep. Generalized epileptiform discharges are more frequent during non-rapid eye movement (NREM) sleep than during REM sleep or the awake state (5) and also increase gradually with deepening of NREM sleep (6). On the other hand, REM sleep is associated with a focalization of interictal discharges with restriction of the electrical field (7). Transitional sleep states, for example, sleep onset, sleep stage changes, and arousals may also be epileptogenic in susceptible individuals (8). More recently, the concept of cyclic alternating patterns (CAPs) further supports the observation that transitional CAPs activate epileptiform discharges (9).

During NREM sleep, virtually every cell in the brain discharges synchronously, which facilitates the spread of seizure discharges. In contrast, during wakefulness and REM sleep the brain cells discharge asynchronously and the divergent synaptic signals are less conducive for propagation of epileptic discharges. Also in REM sleep, there is tonic reduction in the interhemispheric transmission through the corpus callosum limiting the spread of epileptic discharges. REM deprivation may thus exacerbate epilepsy. It is well documented that sleep deprivation precipitates generalized epileptic seizures and particularly increases the epileptiform discharges in the sleep-wake transition state (10). Epileptic discharges may alter sleep regulation and cause sleep disruption, thus triggering seizures in turn.

Effect of Sleep Apnea on Epilepsy

OSA causes disruption and fragmentation of night sleep with intermittent hypoxemia. This provokes a state of chronic sleep deprivation that could decrease the seizure threshold in epileptic patients such that mild or even asymptomatic OSA might cause seizure exacerbation. Further, it is possible that epileptic patients have a low tolerance for intermittent hypoxemia thereby acting as a potential trigger for seizures in susceptible individuals. Also, disruption and fragmentation of the sleep architecture caused by the respiratory events provides a substrate for frequent transitional sleep states, for example, sleep stage changes, and arousals, which also activate epileptogenesis in susceptible individuals. Thus coexistent sleep apnea in patients with epilepsy can worsen seizure frequency, be responsible for poor response to conventional antiseizure medications and even lead to refractory seizures. Additionally, OSA can contribute further to impairment in daytime functions and quality of life.

Several investigators have reported the coexistence between sleep apnea and epilepsy in adults (11–16) and in neurodevelopmentally challenged children (17,18). Malow et al. (13) studied 39 candidates for epilepsy surgery without a history of OSA and diagnosed OSA by polysomnography (PSG) in one-third of the subjects, of which 13% had moderate-to-severe sleep apnea. Further, they suggested that OSA in patients with epilepsy was more common especially among men, older subjects, and those with seizures during sleep. In a larger study on 283 adult epilepsy patients, Manni et al. (19) reported a prevalence of polysomnographically proven OSA in 10.2% epilepsy patients, with mild sleep apnea in 66%, moderate in 22.2% and severe in 11.1% of the cases. They also suggested that "epilepsy + OSA" patients were older, heavier, more frequently male, and sleepier than those with "epilepsy only." de Almeida et al. (20) studied 39 patients with temporal lobe epilepsy and found OSA in 13% patients by PSG. Sonka et al. (21) did a retrospective survey of consecutive 480 adult patients with sleep apnea and reported a 4% incidence of new onset epilepsy (at least 2 seizures) in adults with 10 or more apneas per hour of sleep. The average age at first seizure was 48 years and notably, 79% had exclusively nocturnal seizures. The retrospective survey by Chokroverty et al. (16) of 478 adult patients with PSG diagnosis of OSA provided a figure of 6% with comorbid epilepsy and sleep apnea.

Effect of Treatment of Sleep Apnea on Epilepsy

Several researchers have demonstrated the effect of treating OSA on seizure frequency in patients with epilepsy. In one of the earlier studies, Devinsky et al. (11) showed a clear reduction in seizure frequency in four out of five patients with refractory partial epilepsy and sleep apnea, following treatment of sleep apnea with continuous positive airway pressure (CPAP). Vaughn et al. (22) evaluated response to treatment of sleep apnea in 10 patients with seizures and sleep apnea. Eight patients received CPAP and two patients were treated with positional therapy. Three patients became seizure free, and the others also showed a significant reduction in seizure frequency with treatment of sleep apnea. Malow et al. (23) selected 13 adults and five children from a clinic population based on seizure frequency and risk for OSA. Six out of 13 adults and three out of five children with epilepsy met PSG criteria for OSA. Of these, three adults and one child were treated with CPAP and all four reported at least a 45% reduction in seizure frequency during CPAP treatment.

Choice of anticonvulsant medication must also be taken into account as central nervous system (CNS) suppressants can aggravate breathing difficulty in sleep in a pre-existing or latent OSA. Antiepileptic drugs can promote weight gain (24) or affect upper respiratory airway tone (25). Vagal nerve stimulation (VNS) therapy for refractory epilepsy can cause dyspnoea, which is a well-recognized side effect. However, it is also documented to have an effect on respiration during sleep (26–28). Marzec et al. (28) did a baseline PSG followed by another PSG three months after VNS placement in 16 epilepsy patients. An apnea–hypopnea index (AHI) > 5 was reported in 1/16 at baseline and in 5/16 at three months following VNS treatment initiation. One patient with esophageal pressure monitoring showed crescendos in esophageal pressure during VNS activation, supporting an obstructive pattern. A patient with CPAP trial showed resolution in respiratory events with CPAP. Thus, anticonvulsant and VNS therapies can potentially worsen underlying sleep apnea in patients with epilepsy.

In cases selected for epilepsy surgery, it may be beneficial to evaluate for OSA preoperatively. It has been seen that the perioperative complication rate is higher in patients with coexistent OSA (29). With appropriate and adequate treatment of coexistent OSA, patients may either become seizure free or have significantly reduced seizure frequency. Thus all candidates for epilepsy surgery or refractory seizures should have a formal sleep evaluation and an overnight PSG performed. Also, seizures and interictal epileptiform discharges are generally suppressed during REM sleep while OSA has greatest respiratory disturbance during REM sleep. So, if a patient has a persistent tendency to REM-related seizures, a sleep evaluation may be helpful.

Conclusions

Thus, seizures, epilepsy and OSA have a very close relationship. It is suggested that a detailed sleep history should be obtained and PSG performed in: (*i*) epilepsy patients with risk factors for sleep apnea (e.g., obesity, craniofacial abnormalities) or markers for sleep apnea (e.g., loud, disruptive snoring, EDS); (*ii*) patients with refractory seizures and a change in seizure pattern to predominantly nocturnal seizures; and (*iii*) candidates for epilepsy surgery.

SLEEP APNEA AND INSOMNIA
Definition and Prevalence of Insomnia

Insomnia is defined as a repeated difficulty with initiating sleep, maintaining sleep, a final awakening that occurs much earlier than desired, sleep that is nonrestorative or of generally poor quality that occurs despite adequate time and opportunity for sleep and results in some form of daytime impairment (e.g., fatigue, daytime sleepiness, mood disturbance, cognitive difficulties, and social or occupational impairment) (30,31). It is well recognized that most of us have experienced insomnia at some time during our lives (31). In most cases, however, it is a transient problem in response to stress, illness or sudden change in life situations and resolves quickly when precipitating factors abate. Chronic insomnia that persists over time and contributes to various types of dysfunction remains a greater concern. Results of epidemiologic studies generally suggest that chronic or persistent forms of insomnia are relatively common but the prevalence estimates obtained in these studies have varied widely. In a review of these studies, Ohayon (32) observed that prevalence estimates for chronic insomnia ranged from a low of 4.4% to a high of 48% across numerous studies and he attributed this wide range to geographic and sociocultural characteristics of study samples but more importantly to the variation in insomnia definitions used. No matter how insomnia is defined, the pertinent research has clearly demonstrated that women are more prone to present with insomnia complaints than are men. Older adults are more prone to report these symptoms than are younger adults.

Relation Between Sleep Apnea and Insomnia

Insomnia and OSA are the two most common sleep disorders and yet peer-review publications based on state-of-the-art, evidence based literature are lacking in describing the interaction and implications emerging from the inter-relationship between the two. This has been well addressed in an editorial by Krakow (33). Insomnia is generally considered an infrequent presenting night-time complaint in patients with OSA. Yet review of limited literature shows a higher percentage than generally believed. In a retrospective study by Krakow et al. (34) 50% of patients with PSG-proven SDB, reported significantly problematic insomnia symptoms. More recently, Smith et al. (35) using a rigorous methodology reported a prevalence of significant insomnia in 39% of PSG-proven patients with OSA. Women with OSA are more likely to have insomnia than are men with the same degree of OSA (36).

Looking at the reverse picture, *what is the prevalence of SDB in insomnia patients?* Research shows that these numbers are similarly high. Guilleminault et al. (37) documented SDB in 83% of 394 postmenopausal women complaining of chronic insomnia using PSG studies with pressure transducer and esophageal manometry. The SDB was classified mainly in the low AHI range. Similarly, Lichstein et al. (38) reported sleep apnea in 29% to 43% of a recruited sample of older individuals with insomnia, depending upon whether an AHI of 15 or 5 was used for diagnosis. Thus, irrespective of whether it is SDB in insomnia patients or insomnia in patients with SDB, there is clear indication that a comorbid relationship exists between the two. This however, remains largely unrecognized as evidenced by a lack of established guidelines requiring routine use of PSG in the diagnosis of insomnia (39).

A few researchers have gone further to evaluate the relationship between SDB, the nature of insomnia and a possible mechanism of action to explain the interaction. Chung et al. (40) reported an interesting analysis of insomnia prevalence in 150 patients with suspected SDB, of which 119 were diagnosed to have an AHI $\geq$ 5 events per hour. It was noted that patients with difficulty going to sleep or returning to sleep after an awakening had significantly lower AHI than subjects with frequent awakenings and even those with no insomnia. He thus postulated that repeated apnea is not a single factor accounting for the insomnia symptoms in patients with SDB but that individual vulnerability must be considered. Krakow et al. (34) had observed similar findings of a statistically higher AHI in those without insomnia compared to those with insomnia. They suggested possibility of greater self-reported psychiatric distress and anxiety about sleep in contrast to SDB-induced respiratory compromise and sleep fragmentation. It may however be mentioned that the suggestion of increased prevalence of insomnia in patients with a lower AHI may need to be re-evaluated in the light of esophageal pressure monitoring and measurement of respiratory disturbance index (RDI) including respiratory effort-related arousals (RERAs) providing a more comprehensive picture of SDB. More recently, Chung (41) reported similar findings in another study in which 42% of 157 sleep apnea patients had at least one problematic insomnia symptom, with a prevalence of sleep onset insomnia of 6%, sleep maintenance insomnia of 26%, and early morning awakening in 19%. Patients with sleep onset insomnia had a significantly lower AHI and arousal index. There was a significant inverse relationship between sleep onset insomnia and measures of daytime sleepiness. On the contrary, subjects with repeated awakenings had more severe sleepiness. Results were similar in patients with AHI $\geq$ 5 or $\geq$ 15. Chung thus postulated that OSA with sleep onset insomnia may be a state of hyperarousal. This stresses the importance of evaluating insomnia subtypes in patients with SDB as it may help with treatment decisions.

There have been studies suggesting a higher than expected prevalence of SDB in patients with post-traumatic stress disorders (PTSDs). In one study Krakow et al. (42) reported the potential presence of SDB in 52% of female patients with PTSD, correlating positively with body mass index (BMI), increased arousal index, and PTSD severity. Improvement in insomnia and post-traumatic stress with successful treatment of SDB has also prompted the hypothesis of an arousal-based mechanism in trauma survivors and in patients with chronic insomnia (43). A greater than expected level of anxiety, depression, stress symptoms, and past history of psychiatric problems are also reported by Smith et al. (35) in patients with SDB and insomnia.

Effect of Insomnia on Sleep Apnea Treatment Outcomes

In addition to the role of insomnia in prevalence and diagnosis of sleep apnea, it must also be appreciated that it can have profound effect on treatment outcomes as well. For those practicing clinical sleep medicine, it is not difficult to understand that associated complaints of insomnia or depression, which are common in patients with SDB may contribute significantly not only to initial difficulty with acceptance and adjustment to CPAP therapy, but also contribute to suboptimal adherence for continued long-term use. This has been addressed to some extent by Engleman and Wild (44). Krakow et al. (45) demonstrated clinical cures or near-cures with combined cognitive behavioral therapy and CPAP treatment for SDB in 15 out of 17 subjects with SDB and chronic insomnia. It must also be noted that sedatives and hypnotics used for insomnia may have adverse effects on sleep apnea (46).

Conclusions

In summary, SDB and insomnia, two of the most prevalent sleep disorders, bear a comorbid relationship which needs future investigations for appropriate and timely diagnosis and management of each.

SLEEP APNEA AND DEPRESSION

OSA may affect more than 50% individuals over the age of 65 while depressive symptoms may be encountered in as much as 26% of a random community population of the elderly (4). As in adults apnea may have a profound effect on the pediatric age group as well (47,48) but may be difficult to recognize due to the subtle nature of the disorder, lack of daytime sleepiness, behavior problems including inattention, hyperactivity, and aggressiveness suggestive of attention-deficit hyperactivity disorder. In clinical practice the presence of depressive symptoms in patients with OSA are often noted and treated pharmacologically. On the other hand, the possibility of sleep apnea is not considered routinely in the evaluation of the depressed patient.

Relation Between Obstructive Sleep Apnea and Depression

OSA leads to EDS, fatigue, and impairment in daytime functioning in various neuropsychological, cognitive, behavioral, and social domains. Thus the symptoms of OSA can mimic symptoms of an MDD, leading to an erroneous diagnosis of depression, complicating the diagnosis, and management of both conditions. For over two decades clinical studies have suggested a relationship between OSA and depression. In recent years, a number of studies have confirmed an increasing prevalence and severity of depression in patients with OSA. Sharafkhaneh et al. (49) studied the prevalence of comorbid psychiatric conditions in 4,060,504 Veterans Health Administration beneficiaries with and without sleep apnea. They found a statistically significantly greater prevalence of depression (21.8%), anxiety (16.7%), PTSD (11.9%), psychosis (5.1%), and bipolar disorders (3.3%) in patients with sleep apnea as compared with patients without sleep apnea. While several investigators have reported an increasing prevalence of depression in OSA, very few have studied the prevalence and influence of OSA in patients with depression. Reynolds et al. (50) found that 15% of depressed inpatients had some evidence of SDB. Farney et al. (51) did a retrospective analysis using prevalence odds ratios and confidence intervals to show that the likelihood of having a diagnosis of OSA increases and must be considered when either antihypertensive or antidepressant medications have been prescribed. Ohayon (52) showed that 800 out of 100,000 individuals had both, a breathing-related sleep disorder and an MDD, with up to 20% of the subjects presenting with one of these disorders also having the other. The author suggested that identification of one of these two disorders should prompt the investigation of the other. It should however be noted that the study was conducted as a cross-sectional telephone survey in a randomly selected general population without PSG documentation of SDB. It must also be realized that other covariables, for example, obesity, hypertension, diabetes, medications, cardiovascular disease or other physical limitations in this patient population may also contribute to neuro-psychological dysfunction.

Studies have been conducted to study the effect and relationship of severity of SDB on depression. It is not known whether different clinical and PSG parameters, for example, BMI, RDI, and oxygen saturation contribute differentially to the occurrence and severity of depression in patients with OSA. It has yet to be established as to which factor of SDB has the greatest impact on mood and affect. The three parameters of greatest relevance include apnea/hypopnea associated hypoxia, sleep fragmentation related to arousal from respiratory events, and EDS resulting from the respiratory events. Sforza et al. (53) showed that depression was statistically significantly related to the Epworth sleepiness scale (ESS) reflecting daytime sleepiness, mean low SaO_2, and mean sleep latency of the maintenance of wakefulness test, but not to apnea density. Yue et al. (54) also found that severity of psychological symptoms in patients with OSA was positively related to ESS score. Aloia et al. (55) have suggested that OSA severity and obesity contribute differentially to symptoms of depression. Deldin et al. (56) evaluated 19 patients with MDD and 15 nondepressed controls using an unattended nasal pressure-based home sleep monitoring device. They reported that the respiratory variables distinguished between MDD patients and controls with an accuracy of 80%. The results are impressive, although electro-encephalographic (EEG) analysis was not included in the study, which invites further research into the interaction between depression and OSA.

In the general population, depression and anxiety are more prevalent in women and therefore gender differences in the psychological effects of OSA are likely expected. Pillar and Lavie (57) showed that in a large sample size of male subjects, neither the existence of nor the severity of OSA was associated with depression or anxiety. On the other hand, their smaller female population had significantly higher depression and anxiety scores than males and also revealed a positive relation between severity of OSA and depression scores.

Effect of Treatment of Sleep Apnea on Depression

The belief that depression is an actual phenomenon seen increasingly in patients with sleep apnea is well documented by numerous studies showing significant improvement in depression, daytime sleepiness, and quality of life following treatment of sleep apnea with CPAP (58–63). Schwartz et al. (62) demonstrated this effect in patients with RDI $\geq$ 15 and in patients with and without antidepressant pharmacotherapy. Hilleret et al. (64) reported an interesting case of a 50-year-old man with no previous history of bipolar disorder, diagnosed with severe depression and resistant to seven weeks of treatment with venlafaxine and trazodone. A diagnosis of OSA and use of CPAP was followed a few days later by a mood switch to first hypomania and then a mixed disorder. Thus OSA might not only be associated with a depressive syndrome but its presence may also be responsible for failure to respond to appropriate pharmacological treatment. Furthermore, undiagnosed OSA might be exacerbated by adjunct treatments to antidepressant medications, such as benzodiazepines. Also, high anxiety and/or depression scores can lead to CPAP nonadherence (65). Conversely, a few other studies have questioned the relation of mood improvement with sleep apnea treatment. Li et al. (66) reported moderate improvement in mood postoperatively after extended uvulopalatal flap surgery on 84 patients with sleep apnea. However, this improvement in mood was not significantly associated with changes in RDI, maximum arterial oxygen saturation, or the ESS scores. Yu et al. (67) conducted a randomized, placebo-controlled trial of CPAP treatment on patients with sleep apnea and compared mood improvement in the two groups seven days after starting CPAP. Both the CPAP treatment and placebo CPAP groups showed significant improvement in mood states, raising the possibility of placebo effect. A longer trial of CPAP versus placebo is suggested to truly evaluate and differentiate real differences from the placebo effect.

However, as suggested by O'Hara and Schröder (68), OSA and MDD do share some common pathophysiological mechanisms, for example, the serotonergic system central to depressive disorders is implicated in the regulation of mood as well as the sleep-wake cycle and upper airway muscle tone control during sleep. Further, the common risk factors and covariables (e.g., obesity, diabetes, hypertension, and cardiovascular disease) shared by OSA and MDD also suggest the presence of common pathophysiological mechanisms. This may be supported by imaging studies showing increased subcortical white matter hyperintensities in patients with severe compared to minimal OSA and also a trend for increased subcortical hyperintensities with an elevated level of depression (69).

Conclusions

Future research must continue to establish and explain the complex relationship between OSA and depression and to clarify which feature of OSA has the greatest impact on depression. In the interim, it may be important to convey that OSA must be excluded in depressed patients with risk factors for sleep apnea or in patients with chronic or resistant depression. Similarly, when OSA is diagnosed, it may be necessary to look for a possible depression. This would lead to appropriate and timely treatment of each condition.

SLEEP APNEA AND NARCOLEPSY

Narcolepsy is a CNS disorder of unknown etiology characterized by the classic pentad of EDS, cataplexy (muscle weakness precipitated by emotions), sleep paralysis (inability to move at sleep onset or upon awakening), hypnagogic or hypnopompic hallucinations (dream-like perceptions at sleep onset or upon awakening), and nocturnal sleep disturbance. Symptoms are believed to be physiologic correlates of intrusion of REM sleep or REM atonia into periods of wakefulness.

It is now believed that narcolepsy with and without cataplexy are two distinct clinicopathologic entities and they have been separated into two separate diagnostic categories (30). There are two main challenges in the diagnosis of narcolepsy, namely, identifying patients with clear-cut cataplexy and in the differentiation of narcolepsy without cataplexy from other conditions causing EDS, which are numerous and most commonly include SDB, chronic sleep deprivation and insufficient sleep syndrome, inadequate sleep hygiene, RLS, and PLMS with frequent nocturnal awakenings.

Relation Between Sleep Apnea and Narcolepsy

Narcolepsy may be associated with other comorbid sleep disorders such as RBD, OSA, PLMS, sleepwalking, and nightmares. It is often associated with an increased

BMI, which predisposes to the development of OSA. On average, narcoleptics have a BMI 10% to 20% higher than the normal population (70,71). A reduced metabolic rate, decreased motor activity or abnormal eating behavior have been suggested as possible explanations. SDB is found in 10% to 20% of patients (72). Chokroverty (73) documented repeated apneic episodes in 11 out of 16 narcoleptic subjects. Sleep apnea was predominantly central but obstructive and mixed apneas were also noted. In 1972, Guilleminault et al. (74) reported central sleep apnea in two patients with narcolepsy and later extended this observation and found central and OSA in a large number of patients with narcolepsy (75). Laffont et al. (76) noted sleep apnea (both central and obstructive) in five patients with narcolepsy.

In cases with possibilities for other coexistent sleep disorders liable to produce EDS, narcolepsy may be considered after appropriate and adequate treatment of associated comorbid sleep disorders, and can subsequently be confirmed by an overnight multiple sleep latency test (MSLT) (77). While the combination of EDS and cataplexy is highly sensitive and specific for narcolepsy, the diagnosis based on EDS requires further evaluation. Narcolepsy without cataplexy represents 10% to 50% of the narcoleptic population. A PSG will provide supportive evidence in terms of disturbed nocturnal sleep with frequent awakenings, decreased sleep latency, short nocturnal REM sleep latency, and fragmented night sleep. These are nonspecific and can be seen in other conditions, for example, prior sleep deprivation. A sleep-onset REM period (SOREMP) of less than eight minutes during a PSG is observed in 25% to 50% narcolepsy with cataplexy and is highly specific. A PSG will also help evaluate the presence of other or coexistent sleep disorders, for example, OSA or PLMS. The MSLT demonstrates a mean sleep latency of less than eight minutes, typically less than five minutes and two or more SOREMPs (78). A mean sleep latency of less than eight minutes can be found in up to 30% of the normal population but two or more SOREMPs are considered highly suggestive of narcolepsy in an appropriate clinical context. However, 15% of patients with narcolepsy with cataplexy especially older than 36 years of age may have a normal or more frequently borderline MSLT result (sleep latency of eight minutes or longer or only one SOREMP). Also population-based studies show that approximately 1% to 3% of adults may have multiple SOREMPs during random MSLTs. Up to 30% of patients presenting with EDS and both a mean sleep latency < 5 minutes + 2 SOREMPs have a condition other than narcolepsy (79). Bishop et al. (80) screened 139 healthy subjects and documented two or more SOREMPs in 17% of the subjects. These individuals were more likely to be male, younger, and sleepier than those with one or zero SOREMPs. In another study, Chervin and Aldrich (81) showed that 4.7% of 1145 patients suspected or confirmed to have OSA had two SOREMPs on the MSLT. Multiple SOREMPs can thus be seen in association with other sleep disorders, for example, SDB or behaviorally induced insufficient sleep syndrome. Measuring hypocretin-1 levels in CSF may be useful when the MSLT is difficult to interpret, in subjects already treated with psychoactive drugs, or in patients with other sleep disorders, for example, SDB, RBD, PLMD or insufficient nocturnal sleep (82,83).

Conclusions
In cases with possibilities for other coexistent sleep disorders liable to produce EDS, narcolepsy may be considered after appropriate and adequate treatment of associated comorbid sleep disorders, and can subsequently be confirmed by MSLT. Similarly, if a previously well-controlled narcoleptic patient relapses despite

adequate treatment, the presence of other comorbid disorders may be suspected particularly with increasing age, as prevalence of OSA increases in the elderly.

SLEEP APNEA AND RESTLESS LEGS SYNDROME—PERIODIC LIMB MOVEMENT DISORDER
Restless Legs Syndrome
RLS is a sensorimotor disorder, classified as a sleep-related movement disorder due to its close association with periodic limb movements in sleep (PLMS) (30). The diagnosis of RLS is subdivided into essential criteria, and supportive and associated features of RLS (84). The four essential criteria in adults are: an urge to move the legs usually accompanied or caused by uncomfortable and unpleasant sensations in the legs; the urge to move or unpleasant sensations begin or worsen during periods of rest or inactivity such as lying or sitting; the urge to move or unpleasant sensations are partially or totally relieved by movement, such as walking or stretching; and the urge to move or unpleasant sensations are worse in the evenings or night than during the day or only occur in the evening or night. The supportive clinical features of RLS include positive family history, presence of periodic limb movements during wakefulness (PLMW) or sleep (PLMS) and a positive response to dopaminergic therapy. The associated features of RLS include a variable clinical course, but typically chronic and often progressive, normal physical examination in idiopathic/familial forms, and sleep disturbance, a common complaint in more affected patients.

Effect of Restless Legs Syndrome on Sleep
Both the RLS sensory symptoms and PLMW occur at the transition between waking and sleep, disturbing sleep onset or the return to sleep. PLMS occur in at least 80% of patients with RLS. The PLMS of patients with RLS are frequently associated with arousal from sleep, which can then lead to long periods of wakefulness and cause sleep disruption. In a study of 133 patients with RLS, most of the patients (84.7%) frequently experienced difficulty falling asleep at night because of RLS, and 86% reported that symptoms woke them up frequently during the night. Several patients (46.2% of men and 22.2% of women) also reported excessive daytime fatigue or somnolence, probably as a consequence of disrupted nocturnal sleep (85).

PLMS are defined as repetitive and stereotyped limb movements in sleep typically characterized by rhythmic extensions of the big toe and dorsiflexion of the ankle with occasional flexion of knee and hip. The quantification of PLMS is routinely obtained by recording bilateral surface electromyographic (EMG) of the tibialis anterior muscles. It is defined as a brief increase in EMG amplitude lasting 0.5 seconds to 5 seconds and repeating every 4 seconds to 90 seconds in a sequence of at least four movements (86). PLMW are recorded similarly except the maximum duration is increased to 10 seconds. Occurrence of PLMS at a rate of five or more per hour of sleep and/or PLMW greater than 15 per hour of waking during the entire night sleep period support a diagnosis of RLS. Recording and scoring of PLMS must be an integral part of PSG evaluations to prevent misinterpretation of movements following EEG arousals from respiratory events (87). There are major controversies with regard to the functional significance of PLMS, and several authors have concluded that PLMS have little impact on nocturnal sleep or daytime vigilance. Recently, more attention has been paid to other signs of physiologic activation associated with PLMS. Regardless of the presence of EEG arousals, almost all PLMS are associated with a tachycardia (decreased R–R intervals for

5–10 beats) associated with a rise of blood pressure followed by a bradycardia and relative fall of blood pressure (88,89). Further, it has been shown that arousals often precede rather than follow the movements (90) and they are still present after suppression of leg movements with L-dopa, suggesting that leg movements are not a cause of the arousals but rather a phenomenon associated with an underlying disorder. These data show that EEG arousals are probably not the only parameter of activation to consider in the evaluation of sleep disruption secondary to PLMS (91). Although the functional significance of PLMS has been a matter of dispute their quantification is often used in sleep laboratory diagnostic procedures for RLS (92) and for monitoring treatment.

Relation Between Sleep Apnea and Restless Legs Syndrome
RLS and OSA are two common sleep disorders but there is not much in the peer-reviewed literature to define or evaluate a possible relationship between the two. In a study by Lakshminarayanan et al. (93) a prevalence of clinically significant RLS with symptoms at least two to three days per week in 8.3% was reported in 60 sequentially polysomnographically studied patients with clinically significant sleep apnea (RDI > 10). This figure is, however, not dissimilar to the prevalence figure for RLS, although age-matched spouses used as controls showed a prevalence of RLS at 2.5%. In a study Rodrigues et al. (94) observed improvement in sleep apnea and RLS symptoms in 17 patients with coexistent RLS and OSA following CPAP therapy. Coexistence of RLS symptoms can have significant impact on the adjustment, tolerance, and adherence to CPAP treatment of OSA. Similarly, arousals and sleep fragmentation from OSA can cumulatively worsen symptoms secondary to RLS.

Periodic Limb Movement Disorder
PLMD is a sleep-related movement disorder characterized by the presence of PLMS and by clinical sleep disturbance that cannot be accounted for by another primary sleep disorder (30). The PLMS are considered responsible for sleep fragmentation and a complaint of EDS. However, PLMS are present in 6% of the general population and in more than 45% of adults aged 65 years or older (95). Also, there are a number of conditions other than RLS where PLMS are also recorded, for example, in about 45% to 60% with narcolepsy (96), 70% with RBD (97,98), 27% to 38% with OSA (95,99–101) and also in insomnia, sleep-related eating disorder (SRED), fibromyalgia, and attention deficit-hyperactivity disorder. Medications, for example, selective serotonin reuptake inhibitors, tricyclic antidepressants, lithium, and dopamine receptor antagonists are also known to precipitate PLMS. Low brain iron, as reflected by serum ferritin may also play a role. Thus, persistence of PLMS and related clinical sleep disturbance after adequate treatment of associated sleep disorder would be required for a diagnosis of PLMD in such cases. In patients with suspected SDB, pressure transducer airflow monitoring or esophageal manometry should be used to monitor breathing during PSG to reasonably exclude SDB as the direct cause of the PLMS. When independent PLMS are present in patients with SDB, a separate diagnosis of PLMD may be considered if the PLMS persist despite adequate CPAP or other therapy and a clinical sleep disturbance remains that is not otherwise explained. Also, PSG must be performed after the biologic effect of a medication or substance, for example, antidepressant, known to aggravate PLMS has ended. Thus, although PLMS are quite common, the exact prevalence of PLMD is not known. Also, the extent to which PLMS contribute to daytime sleepiness is still controversial (96,102,103).

Relation Between Sleep Apnea and Periodic Limb Movement During Sleep
Chervin (104) studied 1124 patients with suspected or confirmed SDB. Surprisingly, increased leg movements were associated with decreased objective sleepiness (but explained less than 1% of the variance) and showed no association with subjective sleepiness or sleep propensity. These results are in accordance with those of Mendelson (102). It must, however, be realized that in both these studies, movements secondary to an arousal at the end of a respiratory event, could be misinterpreted as a PLMS. This absence of definitive correlation between PLMS and daytime sleepiness does not establish that PLMS are without significant clinical impact. Rather, it questions the sensitivity of ESS and MSLT as parameters for measurement of daytime sleepiness, as has been questioned by several researchers (105,106).

Researchers have tried to assess the role of PLMS in the development of EDS in patients with OSA before treatment and in residual sleepiness in successfully CPAP-treated patients. The appearance of PLMS or enhancement with CPAP has also been reported (101). Haba-Rubio et al. (95) compared PSG, MSLT, and ESS in 57 consecutively diagnosed patients with severe OSA, before and after one year of treatment with CPAP. A total of 38.5% had significant PLMS in absence of apneas with CPAP. They did not find any correlation in the PLMS patient group between PLM index, ESS score, and mean sleep latency by MSLT, before or after treatment with CPAP. It may be mentioned that in the absence of esophageal pressure monitoring during PSG, RERAs may not be entirely evaluated or eliminated with CPAP, and/or frank apneas or hypopneas may be converted to RERAs by CPAP resulting in persistence of respiratory-related leg movements that are misinterpreted as PLMS. Also, in the process of CPAP titration, respiratory events continue to occur till optimum CPAP pressure is reached, contributing to persistence of respiratory events and respiratory-related leg movements.

Conclusions
The precise mechanism of PLMS and its impact on sleep fragmentation, EDS, and cardiovascular morbidity may still be a matter of some controversy and future research. However, it appears that for RLS, PLMS, and OSA, these three common conditions may be more closely related than currently appreciated and their coexistence could greatly influence independent treatment outcomes.

SLEEP APNEA AND PARASOMNIAS

Parasomnias are undesirable physical events or experiences that occur during entry into sleep, within sleep, or during arousals from sleep (30). These events are manifestations of CNS activation transmitted into skeletal muscle and autonomic nervous system channels. Parasomnias encompass abnormal sleep-related movements, behaviors, emotions, perceptions, dreaming, and autonomic nervous system functioning. Furthermore, "basic drive states" can emerge in pathologic forms as seen with sleep-related aggression and locomotion, SRED, and abnormal sleep-related sexual behaviors. They often involve complex and seemingly purposeful behaviors over which there is no conscious control. Parasomnias are clinical disorders of importance because of the potential for sleep-related injuries.

The parasomnias frequently reported clinically in relation to sleep apnea are: disorders of arousal (107–109), RBD (110–112), and SRED (113–115).

Disorders of Arousal (From Non-rapid eye movement Sleep)
This category includes a group of parasomnias that typically occur in slow wave sleep (SWS, NREM stages 3 and 4) and include confusional arousals, sleepwalking, and sleep terrors. They typically occur during the first part of the night when SWS is most prevalent. Genetic factors have a strong influence on the occurrence of arousal disorders and both sexes are equally affected. No known specific mechanism for disorders of arousal is suggested but impaired arousal from sleep has been postulated as a cause for their occurrence. Conditions related to sleep, for example, sleep deprivation, CNS-depressant medications, medical conditions (e.g., metabolic, toxic, or other encephalopathies), idiopathic hypersomnia, symptomatic hypersomnias, and factors that disrupt SWS (e.g., pain, stress, distended bladder, OSA, PLMS) can trigger an attack. Experimentally induced forced arousals have been documented to induce episodes in chronic sleepwalkers.

Rapid Eye Movement Sleep Behavior Disorder
RBD is characterized by REM sleep-associated intense motor activity, REM-related oneirism (dream-enacting behavior) and absence of the normal atonia of REM (EMG finding of excessive amounts of sustained or intermittent elevation of submental EMG tone or excessive phasic submental or upper or lower limb EMG twitching) (30,110,111). Patients do not enact their customary dreams but rather they enact distinctly altered, unpleasant, action-filled, and violent dreams usually involving confrontation or aggression with unfamiliar people and animals. RBD behaviors are generally aggressive and never appetitive (feeding or sexual). The movements involved are often explosive or exploratory including kicking, punching, arm flailing, gesturing, shouting, crawling, running, diving from the bed, and rapid ambulatory collisions with walls or furniture. Complications include disruption of bed partner's sleep, sleep-related injury to self or to the bed partner, which can be life threatening. Episodes may recur cyclically every 90 minutes after sleep onset or may occur a few times a week. The duration of an attack is typically from 2 to 10 minutes. A quarter of patients have a prodrome of behavioral release during sleep (presumed REM), for example, talking, yelling, vigorous movements, which precede the full-blown episodes by a number of years. It usually affects middle-aged or older men but can affect either gender at any age. The estimated prevalence is 0.38% in the general population and 0.5% in the elderly population. A 2.1% prevalence of current sleep-related violence has been reported, of which 38% is associated with dream enactment.

Sleep-Related Eating Disorder
This condition consists of recurrent episodes of involuntary eating and drinking during arousals from sleep with adverse consequences (30,113,114). They typically occur during partial arousals from sleep with subsequent partial recall. The problematic features of SRED include one or more of the following: consumption of peculiar forms or combinations of food, and/or of inedible or toxic substances (e.g., frozen pizzas, raw bacon, cat food, ammonia cleaning solutions), insomnia from sleep disruption, sleep-related injury, morning anorexia, weight gain, and obesity.

SRED may be idiopathic but is most commonly associated with a primary sleep disorder (113,114,116) or other clinical condition, of which sleepwalking is the most common. Other sleep disorders that can be associated include RLS, PLMD, OSA, and circadian rhythm sleep disorders. Medication-induced SRED have also been reported with zolpidem, triazolam, and other psychotropic agents. Treatment includes treating the underlying primary sleep disorder (e.g., CPAP for OSA, dopaminergics/opiates/benzodiazepines for RLS/PLMD).

Relation Between Sleep Apnea and Parasomnias

Parasomnias can emerge in close association with OSA. The following associations have been noted between the two conditions (30).

1. OSA is becoming an increasingly recognized precipitant of sleepwalking (107,108). Guilleminault et al. (107) described 84 children (5 with sleep terrors and 79 with both sleep terrors and sleepwalking). Fifty-one (61%) of 84 children with parasomnia had a diagnosis of an additional sleep disorder: 49 with SDB and two with RLS. Forty-three of 49 children with SDB were treated with tonsillectomy, adenoidectomy, and/or turbinate revision. In all 43 children who received surgery, PSG performed three to four months later indicated the disappearance of SDB. The recordings also showed an absence of confusional arousals. In all surgically treated cases, parents also reported subsequent absence of the parasomnia. Parasomnias persisted in the six children who were untreated for SDB. Guilleminault et al. (109) studied CAP in 32 chronic sleepwalkers as well as age-matched normal controls and patients with mild SDB. More than 90% of these patients with mild SDB had UARS. Sleepwalkers on a nonsleepwalking night presented instability of NREM sleep, as demonstrated by CAP analysis of EEG activity. This instability was similar to the one noted in UARS patients. The authors suggest that subtle sleep disorders associated with chronic sleepwalking constitute the unstable NREM sleep background on which sleepwalking events occur. A subtle associated sleep disorder should be systematically searched for and treated in the presence of sleepwalking with abnormal CAP.
2. OSA-induced arousal from NREM sleep with complex or violent behaviors may be indistinguishable from primary disorders of arousal (confusional arousals, sleepwalking, and sleep terrors), nocturnal complex seizures, or nocturnal dissociative states. Time-synchronized video-PSG (VPSG) is essential for correct diagnosis. Espa et al. (117) studied 10 patients with sleepwalking, sleep terrors or both and 10 age- and sex-matched controls, who underwent PSG for three consecutive nights using esophageal pressure monitoring. Respiratory events occurred more frequently in parasomniacs than in controls. Respiratory effort seems to be responsible for the occurrence of a great number of arousal reactions in parasomniacs and is involved in triggering the parasomnia episodes.
3. Incidental association of RBD with OSA is sometimes noted and only VPSG can detect coexistence of both conditions. In a study by Olson et al. (110), PSGs of 93 subjects with RBD showed an AHI > 10 in 32 (34%) of the subjects.
4. OSA-induced arousals from REM sleep may mimic RBD ("pseudo-RBD"), with immediate post-arousal dream-related, complex or violent behaviors. Since OSA is a very common sleep disorder and OSA is most severe during REM sleep, this form of parasomnia may be more prevalent than currently believed. Iranzo and Santamaria (112) reported 16 patients presenting with dream-enacting behaviors and unpleasant dreams, in whom VPSG excluded RBD and was diagnostic of severe OSA, also demonstrating that the reported abnormal behaviors occurred only during apnea-induced arousals. Further, CPAP therapy eliminated the abnormal behaviors, unpleasant dreams as well as the snoring and daytime

sleepiness. There have been other prior anecdotal reports of OSA simulating the clinical features of RBD but this is the first study with formal clinical and VPSG documentation (111,118). It is important to distinguish the two conditions because they have different pathophysiological substrates, and separate clinical and therapeutic implications.

5. Nasal CPAP therapy of OSA may result in SWS rebound with emergent confusional arousals, sleepwalking, sleep terrors, or a combination thereof. Millman et al. (119) report two episodes of sleepwalking in an adult on nasal CPAP during SWS rebound.
6. OSA-induced arousals from NREM (or occasionally REM) sleep may trigger repeated episodes of SRED (113,114).
7. SRED causing excessive weight gain may eventually induce clinical OSA (115).
8. OSA-induced cerebral anoxia and nocturnal seizures may present with complex or violent parasomnia-like behaviors. Parasomnias are a major cause of sleep-related violence, the current prevalence of which is reported to be about 2.1%, with males having a significantly higher rate than females; 38% is associated with dream-enacting behaviors (111). The other most frequently reported parasomnias in association with sleep-related violence are RBD and sleep terrors/sleepwalking, nocturnal dissociative disorders, nocturnal seizures, and OSA.

Conclusions
Parasomnias and behaviors mimicking them are becoming increasingly recognized in association with OSA. The most common parasomnias thus reported are disorders of arousal, RBD, and SRED. Time-synchronized VPSG is essential for a correct diagnosis.

REFERENCES
1. Young T, Palta M, Dempsey J, et al. The occurrence of sleep-disordered breathing among middle-aged adults. N Engl J Med 1993; 328:1230–1235.
2. Avidan AY. Sleep disorders in the older patient. Prim Care 2005; 32(2):563–586.
3. Scharf SM, Tubman A, Smale P. Prevalence of concomitant sleep disorders in patients with obstructive sleep apnea. Sleep Breath 2005; 9(2):50–56.
4. Schroder CM, O'Hara R. Depression and obstructive sleep apnea (OSA). Ann Gen Psychiatry 2005; 4:13–20.
5. Gibbs EL, Gibbs FA. Diagnostic and localizing value of electroencephalographic studies in sleep. Res Publ Assoc Res Nerv Ment Dis 1947; 26:366–376.
6. Ross JJ, Johnson LC, Walter RD. Spike and wave discharges during stages of sleep. Ann Neurol 1966; 14:399–407.
7. Lieb J, Joseph JP, Engel J, et al. Sleep state and seizure foci related to depth spike activity in patients with temporal lobe epilepsy. Electroencephalogr Clin Neurophysiol 1980; 49:538–557.
8. Patry FL. The relation of time of day, sleep and other factors to the incidence of epileptic seizures. Am J Psychiatry 1931; 10:789–813.
9. Terzano MG, Parrino L, Anelli S, et al. Modulation of generalized spike-and-wave discharges during sleep by cyclic alternating pattern. Epilepsia 1989; 30:772–781.
10. Rowan AJ, Veldhuisen RJ, Nagelkerke NJ. Comparative evaluation of sleep deprivation and sedated sleep EEGs as a diagnostic aid in epilepsy. Electroencephalogr Clin Neurophysiol 1982; 54:357–364.
11. Devinsky O, Ehrenberg B, Barthlen GM, et al. Epilepsy and sleep apnea syndrome. Neurology 1994; 44(11):2060–2064.
12. Malow BA, Fromes GA, Aldrich MS. Usefulness of polysomnography in epilepsy patients. Neurology 1997; 48:1389–1394.

13. Malow BA, Levy K, Maturen K, et al. Obstructive sleep apnea is common in medically refractory epilepsy patients. Neurology 2000; 55(7):1002–1007.
14. Vaughn BV, D'Cruz OF. Obstructive sleep apnea in epilepsy. Clin Chest Med 2003; 24(2):239–248.
15. Chokroverty S, Sachdeo R, Goldhammer T, et al. Epilepsy and sleep apnea. Electroencephalogr Clin Neurophysiol 1985; 61:26 [Abstract].
16. Chokroverty S, Siddiqui F, Rafiq S, Walters A. Comorbid epilepsy and sleep apnea. J N J Neurosci Inst 2006; 1:12–15.
17. Tirosh E, Tal Y, Jaffe M. CPAP treatment of obstructive sleep apnoea and neurodevelopment deficits. Acta Paediatr 1995; 84:791–794.
18. Koh S, Ward SL, Lin M, et al. Sleep apnea treatment improves seizure control in children with neurodevelopmental disorders. Pediatr Neurol 2000; 22:36–39.
19. Manni R, Terzaghi M, Arbasino C, et al. Obstructive sleep apnea in a clinical series of adult epilepsy patients: frequency and features of the comorbidity. Epilepsia 2003; 44(6):836–840.
20. de Almeida CA, Lins OG, Lins SG, et al. Sleep disorders in temporal lobe epilepsy. Arq Neuropsiquiatr 2003; 61(4):979–987 [Article in Portuguese].
21. Sonka K, Juklickova M, Pretl M, et al. Seizures in sleep apnea patients: occurrence and time distribution. Sb Lek 2000; 101:229–232.
22. Vaughn BV, D'Cruz OF, Beach R, et al. Improvement of epileptic seizure control with treatment of obstructive sleep apnoea. Seizure 1996; 5:73–78.
23. Malow BA, Weatherwax KJ, Chervin RD, et al. Identification and treatment of obstructive sleep apnea in adults and children with epilepsy: a prospective pilot study. Sleep Med 2003; 4(6):509–515.
24. Dinesen H, Gram L, Anderson T, et al. Weight gain during treatment with valproate. Acta Neurol Scand 1984; 70:65–69.
25. Robinson R, Zwillich C. Drugs and sleep respiration. In: Kryger M, Roth T, Dement W, eds. Principles and Practice of Sleep Medicine. Philadelphia, PA: Saunders, 1994: 603–620.
26. Nagarajan L, Walsh P, Gregory P, et al. Respiratory pattern changes in sleep in children on vagal nerve stimulation for refractory epilepsy. Can J Neurol Sci 2003; 30(3): 224–227.
27. Holmes MD, Chang M, Kapur V. Sleep apnea and excessive daytime somnolence induced by vagal nerve stimulation. Neurology 2003; 61(8):1126–1129.
28. Marzec M, Edwards J, Sagher O, et al. Effects of vagus nerve stimulation on sleep-related breathing in epilepsy patients. Epilepsia 2003; 44(7):930–935.
29. Jarrell L. Preoperative diagnosis and postoperative management of adult patients with obstructive sleep apnea syndrome: a review of the literature. J Perianesth Nurs 1999; 14:193–200.
30. American Academy of Sleep Medicine: International Classification of Sleep Disorders: Diagnostic and Coding Manual, 2nd ed. Westchester, IL: American Academy of Sleep Medicine, 2005.
31. National Institutes of Health State of the Science Conference Statement on Manifestations and Management of Chronic Insomnia in adults. Sleep 2005; 28:1049–1057.
32. Ohayon MM. Epidemiology of insomnia: What we know and what we still need to learn. Sleep Med Rev 2002; 6:97–111.
33. Krakow B. An emerging interdisciplinary sleep medicine perspective on the high prevalence of co-morbid sleep-disordered breathing and insomnia. Sleep Med 2004; 5(5):431–433.
34. Krakow B, Melendrez D, Ferreira E, et al. Prevalence of insomnia symptoms in patients with sleep-disordered breathing. Chest 2001; 120(6):1923–1929.
35. Smith S, Sullivan K, Hopkins W, et al. Frequency of insomnia report in patients with obstructive sleep apnoea hypopnea syndrome (OSAHS). Sleep Med 2004; 5(5):449–456.
36. Shepertycky MR, Banno K, Kryger MH. Differences between men and women in the clinical presentation of patients diagnosed with obstructive sleep apnea syndrome. Sleep 2005; 28(3):309–314.

37. Guilleminault C, Palombini L, Poyares D, et al. Chronic insomnia, premenopausal women and sleep disordered breathing. Part 2: Comparison of nondrug treatment trials in normal breathing and UARS post menopausal women complaining of chronic insomnia. J Psychosom Res 2002; 53(1):525–527.
38. Lichstein K, Riedel B, Letere K, et al. Occult sleep apnea in a recruited sample of older adults with insomnia. J Consult Clin Psychol 1999; 67:405–410.
39. Littner M, Hirshkowitz M, Kramer M, et al. Standards of Practice Committee of the American Academy of Sleep Medicine. Practice parameters for using polysomnography to evaluate insomnia: an update for 2002. Sleep 2003; 26(6):754–760.
40. Chung KF, Krakow B, Melendez D, et al. Relationships between insomnia and sleep-disordered breathing. Chest 2003; 123(1):310–313.
41. Chung KF. Insomnia subtypes and their relationships to daytime sleepiness in patients with obstructive sleep apnea. Respiration 2005; 72(5):460–465.
42. Krakow B, Germain A, Tandberg D, et al. Sleep breathing and sleep movement disorders masquerading as insomnia in sexual-assault survivors. Compr Psychiatry 2000; 41(1):49–56.
43. Krakow B, Melendrez D, Warner TD, et al. To breathe, perchance to sleep: sleep-disordered breathing and chronic insomnia among trauma survivors. Sleep Breath 2002; 6(4):189–202.
44. Engleman HM, Wild MR. Improving CPAP use by patients with the sleep apnoea/hypopnoea syndrome (SAHS). Sleep Med Rev 2003; 7:81–99.
45. Krakow B, Melendrez D, Lee SA, et al. Refractory insomnia and sleep-disordered breathing: a pilot study. Sleep Breath 2004; 8(1):15–29.
46. Collop NA. Can't Sleep? You May Have Sleep Apnea! Chest 2001; 120:1768–1769.
47. Crabtree VM, Varni JW, Gozal D. Health-related quality of life and depressive symptoms in children with suspected sleep-disordered breathing. Sleep 2004; 27(6):1131–1138.
48. Brown WD. The psychosocial aspects of obstructive sleep apnea. Semin Respir Crit Care Med 2005; 26(1):33–43.
49. Sharafkhaneh A, Giray N, Richardson P, et al. Association of psychiatric disorders and sleep apnea in a large cohort. Sleep 2005; 28(11):1405–1411.
50. Reynolds CF III, Coble PA, Spiker DG, et al. Prevalence of sleep apnea and nocturnal myoclonus in major affective disorders: clinical and polysomnographic findings. J Nerv Ment Dis 1982; 170(9):565–567.
51. Farney RJ, Lugo A, Jensen RL, et al. Simultaneous use of antidepressant and antihypertensive medications increases likelihood of diagnosis of obstructive sleep apnea syndrome. Chest 2004; 125(4):1279–1285.
52. Ohayon MM. The effects of breathing-related sleep disorders on mood disturbances in the general population. J Clin Psychiatry 2003; 64(10):1195–1200.
53. Sforza E, de Saint Hilaire Z, Pelissolo A, et al. Personality, anxiety and mood traits in patients with sleep-related breathing disorders: effect of reduced daytime alertness. Sleep Med 2002; 3(2):139–145.
54. Yue W, Hao W, Liu P, et al. A case-control study on psychological symptoms in sleep apnea–hypopnea syndrome. Can J Psychiatry 2003; 48(5):318–323.
55. Aloia MS, Arnedt JT, Smith L, et al. Examining the construct of depression in obstructive sleep apnea syndrome. Sleep Med 2005; 6(2):115–121.
56. Deldin P, Phillips LK, Thomas RJ. A preliminary study of sleep-disordered breathing in major depressive disorder. Sleep Med 2006; 7(2):131–139.
57. Pillar G, Lavie P. Psychiatric symptoms in sleep apnea syndrome: effects of gender and respiratory disturbance index. Chest 1998; 114(3):697–703.
58. Millman RP, Fogel BS, McNamara ME, et al. Depression as a manifestation of obstructive sleep apnea: reversal with nasal continuous positive airway pressure. J Clin Psychiatry 1989; 50(9):348–351.
59. Sanchez AI, Buela-Casal G, Bermudez MP, et al. The effects of continuous positive air pressure treatment on anxiety and depression levels in apnea patients. Psychiatry Clin Neurosci 2001; 55(6):641–646.

60. McMahon JP, Foresman BH, Chisholm RC. The influence of CPAP on the neurobehavioral performance of patients with obstructive sleep apnea hypopnea syndrome: a systematic review. Wisconsin Med J 2003; 102:36–43.
61. Means MK, Lichstein KL, Edinger JD, et al. Changes in depressive symptoms after continuous positive airway pressure treatment for obstructive sleep apnea. Sleep Breath 2003; 7(1):31–42.
62. Schwartz DJ, Kohler WC, Karatinos G. Symptoms of depression in individuals with obstructive sleep apnea may be amenable to treatment with continuous positive airway pressure. Chest 2005; 128(3):1304–1309.
63. Kawahara S, Akashiba T, Akahoshi T, et al. Nasal CPAP improves the quality of life and lessens the depressive symptoms in patients with obstructive sleep apnea syndrome. Intern Med 2005; 44(5):422–427.
64. Hilleret H, Jeunet E, Osiek C, et al. Mania resulting from continuous positive airways pressure in a depressed man with sleep apnea syndrome. Neuropsychobiology 2001; 43(3):221–224.
65. Kjelsberg FN, Ruud EA, Stavem K. Predictors of symptoms of anxiety and depression in obstructive sleep apnea. Sleep Med 2005; 6(4):341–346.
66. Li HY, Huang YS, Chen NH, et al. Mood improvement after surgery for obstructive sleep apnea. Laryngoscope 2004; 114(6):1098–1102.
67. Yu BH, Ancoli-Israel S, Dimsdale JE. Effect of CPAP treatment on mood states in patients with sleep apnea. J Psychiatr Res 1999; 33(5):427–432.
68. O'Hara R, Schröder C. Unraveling the relationship of obstructive sleep-disordered breathing to major depressive disorder. Sleep Med 2006; 7(2):101–103.
69. Aloia MS, Arnedt JT, Davis JD, et al. Neuropsychological sequelae of obstructive sleep apnea–hypopnea syndrome: a critical review. J Int Neuropsychol Soc 2004; 10(5):772–785.
70. Schuld A, Hebebrand J, Geller F, et al. Increased body mass index in patients with narcolepsy. Lancet 2000; 355(9211):1274–1275.
71. Okun ML, Lin L, Pelin Z, et al. Clinical aspects of narcolepsy–cataplexy across ethnic groups. Sleep 2002; 25(1):27–35.
72. Harsh J, Peszka J, Hartwig G, et al. Night-time sleep and daytime sleepiness in narcolepsy. J Sleep Res 2000; 9(3):309–316.
73. Chokroverty S. Sleep apnea in narcolepsy. Sleep 1986; 9(1 Pt 2):250–253.
74. Guilleminault C, Eldrige F, Dement WC. Insomnia, narcolepsy and sleep apnea. Bell Eur Physiopathol Respir 1972; 8:1127–1138.
75. Guilleminault C, Van Den Hoed J, Mitler MM. Clinical overview of the sleep apnea syndrome. In: Guilleminault C, Dement WC, eds. Sleep apnea syndrome. New York: Alan R. Liss, Inc., 1978:1–12.
76. Laffont F, Autret A, Minz M, et al. Sleep respiratory arrythmia in control subjects, narcoleptics and non-cataplectic hypersomniacs. Electroencephalogr Clin Neurophysiol 1978; 44:697–705.
77. Carpio MV, Carmona BC, Garcia DE, Botebol BG, Cano GS, Capote GF. Association of obstructive apnea syndrome during sleep and narcolepsy. Arch Bronconeumol 1998; 34(6):310–311 [Article in Spanish].
78. Littner MR, Kushida C, Wise M, et al. Standards of Practice Committee of the American Academy of Sleep Medicine. Practice parameters for clinical use of the multiple sleep latency test and the maintenance of wakefulness test. Sleep 2005; 28(1):113–121.
79. Aldrich MS, Chervin RD, Malow BA. Value of the multiple sleep latency test (MSLT) for the diagnosis of narcolepsy. Sleep 1997; 20(8):620–629.
80. Bishop C, Rosenthal L, Helmus T, et al. The frequency of multiple sleep onset REM periods among subjects with no excessive daytime sleepiness. Sleep 1996; 19(9):727–730.
81. Chervin RD, Aldrich MS. Sleep onset REM periods during multiple sleep latency tests in patients evaluated for sleep apnea. Am J Respir Crit Care Med 2000; 161(2 Pt 1):426–431.
82. Mignot E, Lammers GJ, Ripley B, et al. The role of cerebrospinal fluid hypocretin measurement in the diagnosis of narcolepsy and other hypersomnias. Arch Neurol 2002; 59(10):1553–1562.

83. Kanbayashi T, Inoue Y, Kawanishi K, et al. CSF hypocretin measures in patients with obstructive sleep apnea. J Sleep Res 2003; 12(4):339–341.
84. Allen RP, Hening WA, Montplaisir J, et al. Restless legs syndrome: diagnostic criteria, special considerations, and epidemiology: a report from The RLS Diagnosis and Epidemiology Workshop at the National Institute of Health. Sleep Med 2003; 4(2):101–119.
85. Montplaisir J, Boucher S, Poirier G, et al. Clinical polysomnographic and genetic characteristics of restless legs syndrome: a study of 133 patients diagnosed with new standard criteria. Mov Disord 1996; 12:61–65.
86. American Sleep Disorders Association Task Force. Recording and scoring leg movements. Sleep 1993; 16:748–759.
87. Stoohs RA, Blum HC, Suh BY, et al. Misinterpretation of sleep-breathing disorder by periodic limb movement disorder. Sleep Breath 2001; 5(3):131–137.
88. Sforza E, Nicolas A, Lavigne G, et al. EEG and cardiac activation during periodic leg movements in sleep: Support for a hierarchy of arousal responses. Neurology 1999; 52:786–791.
89. Siddiqui F, Walters A, Ming X, Chokroverty S. Rise of blood pressure with periodic limb movements in sleep in patients with restless legs syndrome. Neurology 2005; 20:S65 [Abstract].
90. Karadenitz D, Ondze B, Besset A, et al. EEG arousals and awakenings in relation with periodic leg movements during sleep. J Sleep Res 2000; 9:273–277.
91. Martin SE, Wraith PK, Deary IJ, et al. The effect of nonvisible sleep fragmentation on daytime function. Am J Respir Crit Care Med 1997; 155:1596–1601.
92. Michaud M, Paquet J, Lavigne G, et al. Sleep laboratory diagnosis of restless legs syndrome. Eur Neurol 2002; 48:108–113.
93. Lakshminarayanan S, Paramasivan KD, Walters AS, et al. Clinically significant but unsuspected restless legs syndrome in patients with sleep apnea. Mov Disord 2005; 20(4):501–503.
94. Rodrigues RND, Rodrigues AAS, Pratesi R, et al. Outcome of restless legs severity after continuous positive air pressure (CPAP) treatment in patients affected by the association of RLS and obstructive sleep apneas. Sleep Med 2006; 7:235–239.
95. Haba-Rubio J, Staner L, Krieger J, et al. Periodic limb movements and sleepiness in obstructive sleep apnea patients. Sleep Med 2005; 6(3):225–229.
96. Montplaisir J, Michaud M, Denesle R, et al. Periodic leg movements are not more prevalent in insomnia or hypersomnia but are specifically associated with sleep disorders involving a dopaminergic impairment. Sleep 2000; 1:163–167.
97. Schenck CH, Hurwitz TD, Mahowald MW. Symposium: normal and abnormal REM sleep regulation: REM sleep behavior disorder: an update on a series of 96 patients and a review of the world literature. J Sleep Res 1993; 2:224–231.
98. Lapierre O, Montplaisir J. Polysomnographic features of REM sleep behavior disorder: Development of a scoring method. Neurology 1992; 42(7):1371–1374.
99. Warnes H, Dinner DS, Kotagal P. Periodic limb movements and sleep apnoea. J Sleep Res 1993; 2(1):38–44.
100. Briellmann RS, Mathis J, Bassetti C, et al. Patterns of muscle activity in legs in sleep apnea patients before and during nCPAP therapy. Eur Neurol 1997; 38(2):113–118.
101. Fry JM, DiPillipo MA, Pressman MR. Periodic leg movements in sleep following treatment of obstructive sleep apnea with nasal continuous positive airway pressure. Chest 1989; 96:89–91.
102. Mendelson WB. Are periodic leg movements associated with clinical sleep disturbance? Sleep 1996; **19:**219–223.
103. Mahowald MW. Assessment of periodic leg movements is not an essential component of overnight sleep study. Am J Respir Crit Care Med 2001; **167:**1340–1341.
104. Chervin RD. Periodic leg movements and sleepiness in patients evaluated for sleep-disordered breathing. Am J Respir Crit Care Med 2001; 164(8 Pt 1):1454–1458.
105. Johns M. Rethinking the assessment of sleepiness. Sleep Med Rev 1998; 2:3–15.
106. Cluydts R, De Valck E, Verstraeten E, et al. Daytime sleepiness and its evaluation. Sleep Med Rev 2002; 6:83–96.
107. Guilleminault C, Palombini L, Pelayo R, et al. Sleepwalking and sleep terrors in prepubertal children: what triggers them? Pediatrics 2003; 111(1):e17–25.

108. Guilleminault C, Kirisoglu C, Bao G, et al. Adult chronic sleepwalking and its treatment based on polysomnography. Brain 2005; 128(Pt 5):1062–1069.
109. Guilleminault C, Kirisoglu C, da Rosa AC, et al. Sleepwalking, a disorder of NREM sleep instability. Sleep Med 2006; 7(2):163–170.
110. Olson EJ, Boeve BF, Silber MH. Rapid eye movement sleep behaviour disorder: demographic, clinical and laboratory findings in 93 cases. Brain 2000; 123:331–339.
111. Schenck CH, Milner DM, Hurwitz TD, et al. A polysomnographic and clinical report on sleep-related injury in 100 adult patients. Am J Psychiatry 1989; 146:1166–1173.
112. Iranzo A, Santamaria J. Severe obstructive sleep apnea/hypopnea mimicking REM sleep behavior disorder. Sleep 2005; 28(2):203–206.
113. Schenck CH, Hurwitz TD, O'Connor KA, et al. Additional categories of sleep-related eating disorders and the current status of treatment. Sleep 1993; 16(5):457–466.
114. Schenck CH, Mahowald MW. Review of nocturnal sleep-related eating disorders. Int J Eat Disord 1994; 15(4):343–356.
115. Eveloff SE, Millman RP. Sleep-related eating disorder as a cause of obstructive sleep apnea. Chest 1993; 104(2):629–630.
116. Schenck C, Hurwitz T, Bundlie S, et al. Sleep-related eating disorders: polysomnographic correlates of a heterogeneous syndrome distinct from daytime eating disorders. Sleep 1991; 14:419–431.
117. Espa F, Dauvilliers Y, Ondze B, et al. Arousal reactions in sleepwalking and night terrors in adults: the role of respiratory events. Sleep 2002; 25(8):871–875.
118. Comella C, Tevens S, Stepanski E, et al. Sensitivity analysis of the clinical diagnostic criteria for REM behavior disorder (RBD) in Parkinson's disease. Neurology 2002; 58(suppl3):A434.
119. Millman RP, Kipp GJ, Carskadon MA. Sleepwalking precipitated by treatment of sleep apnea with nasal CPAP. Chest 1991; 99(3):750–751.

22 | Neurological Disorders

Maha Alattar and Bradley V. Vaughn
Department of Neurology, University of North Carolina, Chapel Hill, North Carolina, U.S.A.

INTRODUCTION

Sleep and breathing are both controlled by the brain. A wide range of neurological disorders has significant impact on sleep-related breathing. Features of hypoventilation, obstructive, and central apneas may all be manifestations of neurological disorders and these disorders may impact on the individual's neurological function. The dynamic relationship of the nervous system to sleep-related breathing is most striking in individuals who have lesions in their central nervous system (CNS) and sleep apnea. For some of these individuals, disruption of breathing in sleep results in worsening of their overall condition and improvement in breathing results in a global benefit. In others, however, the sleep-related breathing issue appears to parallel their neurological condition and treatment may result in little benefit. Unfortunately for the clinician, the distinction between these two groups is not always clear.

Although obstructive sleep apnea (OSA) may be one of the more common sleep-related breathing disorders (SRBDs), clinicians must also be aware that other respiratory issues may impact patients with neurological disorders. Treatment of any SRBD offers an opportunity to improve quality of life. In this chapter, we will explore the relationship of sleep and breathing to a variety of neurological conditions and describe some of the therapeutic approaches and pitfalls.

NEUROLOGICAL LOCALIZATION OF RESPIRATION

The organ of control over breathing, the brain, orchestrates respiration through many layers of neural circuitry. From the respiratory-related muscles, peripheral receptors and nerves to brainstem, midbrain and cortical feedback loops, a variety of inputs augment and regulate ventilation and respiration. This multilayered control system permits for a variety of ventilatory patterns that can give clues to the site of potential neurological dysfunction (1) (Table 1).

The ventilatory cycle relies upon sensory inputs to estimate the somatic requirements. This sensory input is derived primarily from three components: (*i*) the vagus nerve relaying information from the pulmonary stretch receptors in the lung and aorta, (*ii*) the intercostals nerves and spinal cord relaying positional sense from the chest wall, (*iii*) and the chemoception. Chemoception utilizes two sensory areas: central and peripheral. Central chemoceptors are predominantly on the ventral aspect of the medulla. These receptors sense acid and carbon dioxide. The peripheral chemoceptors are in the aorta and carotid body and their information are relayed via the glossopharyngeal nerve. The carotid chemoceptors detect the oxygen content of the arterial blood. These sensors increase their firing rates when oxygen levels fall. These sensory nerves are typically myelinated but also convey some input via partially myelinated and unmyelinated axons. Processes such as diabetes

TABLE 1   Central and Peripheral Nervous System Lesions and Their Associated Neurological Disorders, Ventilatory Patterns, and Potential Sleep-Related Breathing Disorders

Location	Non-state-dependent breathing issue	Disorders of the area	Potential sleep-related breathing disorder
Cerebral cortex	Cheyne-Stokes post-hyperventilation pause	Stroke, tumor, multiple sclerosis, trauma, encephalitis	Obstructive sleep apnea, central sleep apnea, Cheyne-Stokes breathing
Midbrain	Central hyperventilation	Progressive supranuclear palsy, Parkinson's disease, tumor	Central sleep apnea
Pons	Apneustic, biots	Multiple sclerosis, tumors, strokes	Central sleep apnea
Medulla	Ataxic breathing	Chiari malformations, multiple sclerosis, stroke, tumor	Central sleep apnea, obstructive sleep apnea
Spinal cord	At or above C3–5: no respiratory effort, C5–T8: potential impaired chest wall motion, difficulty with expiration and potential hypoventilation	Multiple sclerosis, trauma, myelitis, syringomyelia, tumor	Hypoventilation
Peripheral nerve	Respiratory cycle issues with severe sensory and motor neuropathies	Guillain-Barré syndrome, porphyria, diabetes mellitus	Central apnea, hypoventilation
Neuromuscular junction	Hypoventilation with fatigue	Myasthenia gravis, Lambert-Eaton syndrome	Obstructive sleep apnea, hypoventilation
Muscle	Hypoventilation with fatigue	Myotonic dystrophy, Duchenne muscular dystrophy, polymyositis	Hypoventilation

mellitus, Guillain-Barré syndrome or porphyria can damage these nerves. Although pure sensory loss of these nerves is exceedingly rare, damage of these nerves is typically accompanied with loss of motor function. If pure sensory nerve loss did occur the peripheral feedback of information to the medulla would be diminished, and patients would rely upon central chemoceptors for feedback regulation.

At the level of the medulla, we find the first layers of respiratory cycle generators. Neurons in the nucleus solitarius, ambiguous, and retroambigualis work in concert to initially match ventilation to respiratory demand. The ventilatory cycle is composed of three phases: inspiration, postinspiration, and expiration. Respiratory neurons in the medulla and pons discharge in a pattern correlating to one of these phases. Together these neurons form the central pattern generator that orchestrates the cyclic activation of the respiratory musculature.

This central pattern generator is composed of predominately three neuronal groups. Nogues categorized these as dorsal respiratory group, ventral respiratory group, and pontine respiratory group (2). The dorsal respiratory group is in the ventrolateral subnucleus of the nucleus tractus solitarius. This neuronal group is primarily active during inspiration receiving input from pulmonary vagal afferents. Many of these neurons excite lower motor cranial nerves that dilate the upper airway prior to excitation of the contralateral phrenic and intercostal neurons in the spinal cord. This coordinated output must occur in the correct timed sequence to permit the movement of air through a patent airway. Other neurons in this same group receive input from baroreceptors and cardiac receptors influencing several other respiratory-related reflexes (e.g., coughing, sneezing).

The ventral respiratory group is located in the ventral lateral medulla from the top of the cervical cord to the level of the facial nerve. This group contains the Bötzinger complex, the preBötzinger neurons, the rostral portion of nucleus ambiguous, and nucleus retroambigualis. The Bötzinger complex contains neurons that are active during expiration and inhibit inspiration. The preBötzinger complex contains propriobulbar neurons that participate in generating the rhythm of respiration. The caudal portion of this group is primarily composed of expiratory neurons that project to intercostal, abdominal, and external sphincter motor neurons. Although these primary drivers form a rudimentary cycle, neurons in the ventral and midline medulla appear to have plasticity in response to intermittent hypoxemia to augment respiratory responses (3). Lesions in the medulla may produce ataxic breathing, agonal respiration or an absence of respiration.

The pontine respiratory group adds another layer of control. This group is localized to the dorsal lateral pons and is important in stabilizing the respiratory pattern. These neurons are influenced by both inspiratory and expiratory inputs and help determine the length of inspiration and expiration (1). Typically, the destruction of these neurons lengthens the duration of inspiration. Lesions of the caudal pons may also produce apneustic respiration, and lesions in the midbrain or posterior hypothalamus may produce hyperventilatory responses. These types of respiratory abnormalities may result from strokes, tumors or demyelinating plaques.

The voluntary control over respiration primarily resides in the cerebral cortex and diencephalon. The cortex is responsible for initiating the intricate respiratory control involved in speech, eating, and singing. As an individual enters sleep, the cortical control over sleep is altered and may allow the emergence of SRBD. With cortical injury, patients may have prolonged posthyperventilatory apnea or Cheyne-Stokes respiration (CSR). The CSR may be more prominent or only present in sleep (4).

The output to the lower respiratory neurons requires transmission of the respiratory effort through the spinal cord to the peripheral nerves. The spinal cord respiratory motor output is divided into two components. The phrenic nerves emerge from the upper cervical cord region (C3–5) to maintain diaphragmatic function. The thoracic levels (T1–T12) innervate the intercostal muscles and the lower thoracic and upper lumbar levels (T6–L3) innervate the abdominal muscles. This division of labor adds a level of assurance of respiration despite the potential of spinal cord injury.

The peripheral nerves must deliver the sensory and motor signals. These peripheral nerves are generally well-myelinated, relatively protected from trauma by bone and have limited lengths. These characteristics assure these nerves are less vulnerable to damage compared to most nerves supplying the limbs. In general, nerves with longer courses have greater opportunity to incur injury from trauma, toxins or demyelination, and thus are more likely to demonstrate dysfunction. This may not be true for some etiologies such as porphyrias, or inflammatory polyradiculopathies, which can afflict more proximal nerves. Individuals with peripheral nerve disorders may demonstrate progressive nocturnal hypoventilation and respiratory failure requiring ventilatory assistance during the more severe portions of the disorder (5). In contrast, patients with multiple cranial neuropathies may also demonstrate features of upper airway obstruction.

The neuromuscular junction may also be associated with respiratory dysfunction. Respiratory muscles such as the diaphragm may require less depolarization to reach firing threshold and thus these muscles may not be the first affected by neuromuscular dysfunction. The range of SRBDs affected by neuromuscular dysfunction is exemplified in myasthenia gravis (MG), as noted subsequently.

At the level of the muscle, respiration depends upon adequate contraction of these muscles no matter the sleep–wake state. These lower respiratory muscles include slow-twitch muscle, which generally require the less amount of energy to contract and thus are generally more stable with fatigue (6). Some inherited muscle conditions such as Pompe's disease (acid maltase deficiency) may primarily affect respiratory muscles causing hypoventilation. This hypoventilation may be more obvious in sleep.

Overall, respiration during sleep offers a unique window to view the neurological control over breathing. The entrance into each sleep state creates a change in the regulation over breathing and may allow the emergence of disordered breathing. This window may aid in the localization of neurological disease as well as bring insight into the potential causes of SRBD. We have included a table of typical breathing patterns and localization of neurological dysfunction (Table 1). As the reader reviews the variety of neurological disorders, the table may provide additional clarity to the secondary respiratory issues.

SPECIFIC DISORDERS AND SLEEP APNEA
Central Nervous System Disorders
Alzheimer's Disease

Alzheimer's disease is the classical tauopathy characterized by diffuse neuronal loss primarily in the cortex associated with the formation of neurofibrillary tangles and neuritic plaques. The incidence of SRBD in patients with Alzheimer's disease is unclear. Some investigators have found an increase in SRBD, but in the more positive of studies, the degree of sleep apnea is relatively small. In a cohort of 139 patients, Hoch found that the average apnea–hypopnea index (AHI) for patients with Alzheimer's was 4.6 whereas the control group was 0.6 (7). This finding was in contrast to Smallwood's findings, which showed that apnea index was not greater in elderly men with Alzheimer's than healthy elderly men without sleep complaints (8). Despite the incidence, the question remains: *does the apnea drive the neuropathology or does the dementia cause the breathing disturbance?* Untreated sleep apnea has been linked to potential decline in neurocognitive function (9). Although this too has been under debate, some of this decline may be related to vascular issues (9). One component may be the potential link of genetic predisposition to cognitive decline. Apolipoprotein E (APOE) 4 alleles have been associated as a risk factor for the development of Alzheimer's disease (10). This gene has also been linked to SRBD but to date the resulting cognitive issues have not been linked to APOE 4. Sleep-related respiratory disorders may have a daytime effect in patients with Alzheimer's. Gehrman (11) found that institutionalized patients with OSA were more likely to have daytime agitation but not night-time agitation suggesting that the SRBD may have some influence on daytime behavior.

The diagnosis and treatment of SRBD in patients with Alzheimer's disease can create some challenges. Early in the course of the dementia, most patients can easily adapt to the testing environment with extra instructions. Technologists and healthcare providers must be attuned to the patient's limited ability to learn new skills and adapt to new settings. These same individuals must remain calm, take extra time to review the procedures, and incorporate multiple teaching aids to help the patient understand. Visual teaching aids along with verbal and written communication may decrease the likelihood of confusion. For many of these patients, the laboratory personnel will find advantageous in having a family member or familiar caregiver in the testing environment to reinforce the communication. In more severely impaired individuals, patients may present significant challenges for electrode application. Making the environment calm with few stimuli may help. Sleep studies may show the patient has typical OSA or mixed apnea. This population is also at risk for CSR more commonly in Stage 1 and 2 sleeps but this pattern is uncommon in slow-wave sleep and rapid eye movement (REM) sleep.

Patients with Alzheimer's disease and sleep apnea generally accept the continuous positive airway pressure (CPAP) therapy similar to the general population. Ayalon found that these patients used the device an average of 4.8 hours per night (12). The use of CPAP may improve daytime alertness and decrease irritable behavior. Some specific issues may arise in the treatment of this disorder. Individuals may not easily accept therapies such as CPAP or oral appliances thinking the therapy may harm them or that they are related to some other aspect of their health. Many of these individuals have memory difficulties and have periods of nocturnal confusion. In general, these individuals may have a better chance of adherence if a family member or caretaker is given the same information regarding the diagnosis and importance of therapy. The caretaker may also consider using some form of behavior modification to help the patient adjust to wearing the CPAP or oral appliance. These techniques may include notes or other messages in prominent and frequented areas, or serial verbal cues before bedtime reminding the patient to use the device. Many medications may influence the patient's behavior and cognition: thus caregivers should be alert to medications given in the evening that may further confuse the patient. This is also true when considering surgery. These patients have some inherent risk with anesthesia, and will require close supervision following surgery. Most patients with early disease are able to tolerate surgery; this postoperative period is a frequent time for greater confusion and behavior change.

Other Forms of Cognitive Impairment
Lewy body dementia is also associated with cognitive decline and particular impairment of visual spatial tasks. These disorders are noted to have high prevalence of sleep-related complaints based on survey questionnaires, but no study has shown the prevalence of polysomnographic abnormalities in these patients (13). A case report suggests that individuals with autonomic features may have SRBD (14). Cheyne-Stokes breathing and OSA are common findings, but there is no clear link between this form of dementia and sleep apnea.

In many of these individuals, treatment follows the same recommendations as those with Alzheimer's disease. A subgroup of these individuals will have loss of REM sleep atonia and have periods of dream enactment, consistent with a diagnosis of REM sleep behavior disorder. This can become quite dangerous if the patient has a CPAP machine and uncontrolled nocturnal events. For these patients, adequate control of the nocturnal events is paramount. This may take a combination of a benzodiazepine (such as temazepam or clonazepam), with melatonin or an acetyl-choline esterase inhibitor (such as donepezil or rivastigmine). If the patient is having significant nocturnal movements, the bed partner should be advised to avoid injury and/or to sleep in another bed or room.

Mentally Handicapped Individuals

Individuals with mental handicaps may have a variety of sleep issues. Although there are no large studies, these individuals are noted to have SRBD and frequently require treatment. Over half of children with Down's syndrome have obstructive or central sleep apnea (15). Although these patients frequently have anatomical features contributing to the obstruction, the brain dysfunction may also play a role in their SRBD. Patients with other etiologies for chronic encephalopathies such as Prader-Willi syndrome also appear to have a high prevalence of SRBD (16).

Many of these individuals can undergo evaluation and initiation of treatment requiring only few additional explanations, while others, may create significant challenges. Technologists and healthcare providers must be sensitive to the patient's limitations and strengths. Individuals may respond to positive rewards to reinforce the behaviors that allow the testing to occur and adherence with therapy. Healthcare providers should be willing to take extra time in reviewing the procedures and to utilize multiple teaching aids to help the patients and their families understand the diagnosis and therapy. Some patients will have cognitive strengths in specific areas. The healthcare provider can employ teaching aids directed toward these strengths to maximize the patient's understanding. Including a family member or familiar caregiver in the discussion in conjunction with placing familiar personal objects in the testing environment will improve the likelihood of the success. In some very problematic individuals, the technologist may need to wait until the patient is behaviorally asleep before applying the remaining sensors.

In our experience, CPAP can be used effectively in patients with mental handi-caps. Individuals usually have improved behavior and are less irritable following successful employment of therapy. Patients may respond well to positive reinforce-ment and incentive programs such as star charts rewarding adherence with therapy. The healthcare provider should insist upon the inclusion of the therapy into the daily routine. If possible, the patient should be involved in the general cleaning of the device and given a sense of ownership. Over time, these individuals adapt to and comply with the therapy. We have noticed that many of these patients will have improved behavior, less aggressive outbursts, and heightened engagement with others.

Stroke

Stroke is an acute neurovascular event characterized by interruption of blood flow resulting in neuronal cell death with temporary or permanent neurological deficit.

SRBD is common in stroke populations with a range of 45% to 79% (17). The mechanism of why patients with stroke have SRBD is unknown. Some of these patients have central apnea that clears with time. This may indicate that the neuro-logical deficit itself is causing the respiratory abnormality or a byproduct from the neuronal damage that influences respiratory control. OSA also appears to be more frequently seen in individuals with stroke. This may be related to a higher pre-existing prevalence of OSA, predisposing this group to have strokes.

Although the exact mechanisms of the relationship between OSA and vascular disease are not clear, intermittent hypoxemia and the mechanical effects on intrathoracic pressure may cause increased sympathetic activation and oxidative stress that lead to vascular endothelial dysfunction (18). Research of the association between OSA and hypertension is most convincing (19). Evidence shows that SRBD is an independent risk factor for hypertension (20). The causal association of apnea with stroke remains unclear, however. Young et al. (1996) (21) demonstrated a dose–response increase in daytime and nocturnal blood pressures with the severity of OSA. After adjustment for age, gender, race, smoking status, alcohol consumption status, body mass index (BMI), and the presence or absence of diabetes mellitus, hyperlipidemia, atrial fibrillation, and hypertension, OSA retains a statistically significant association with stroke and death (22). Patients with recurrent strokes have a greater OSA severity (defined by the AHI) than patients with first-ever stroke and OSA maybe an independent risk factor for stroke recurrence (23). Moreover, the severity of upper airway obstruction following an acute stroke is associated with a worse functional outcome and increased mortality at six months (24).

Polysomnography can be accomplished in patients with acute and subacute stroke. The technologists must pay extra attention to the patient who has sensory, motor or verbal deficits. Some patients may not sense the need to or have the ability to change positions and will require frequent repositioning. Others may not be able to communicate their needs or discomforts and therefore symptoms such as being awake with an increased heart rate may indicate discomfort. In the acute stroke period, the technologists should also be alert for cardiac arrhythmias or oxygen desaturations. Technologists should be instructed to intervene early in events of oxygen desaturation.

Treatment of OSA in stroke patients with CPAP therapy has been shown to prevent new cerebrovascular events. A prospective study by Martinez-Garcia (25) of 95 patients presenting with acute stroke in the prior two months demonstrated that CPAP treatment during 18 months in patients with significant sleep apnea afforded significant protection against new vascular events after ischemic stroke. CPAP therapy in this population raises some theoretical issues related to altering cerebral blood flow. CPAP increases intrathoracic pressure and thus intracranial pressure that might decrease cerebral perfusion pressure. Alternatively, CPAP may improve oxygenation and decrease the surges of sympathetic activity. Further studies are required to determine the impact of CPAP on the cerebral blood flow in these patients.

Patients with strokes may have CSR or periodic breathing superimposed on the obstructive component. In this case, low CPAP levels are more optimal than higher levels. Nocturnal oxygen supplementation might also relieve the central and/or periodic breathing noted in some patients. The acceptance rate of nasal CPAP in this population was found to be low and dropout was related to difficulties with CPAP usage, facial weakness, motor impairment and increased discomfort with a full-face mask (26). These patients should be assessed for assistive devices to aid in wearing CPAP. Education and special training for patients and caregivers are needed for optimal adherence.

Epilepsy (See Also Chapter 21)
Epilepsy is the chronic condition of recurrent unprovoked seizures, and can be caused by multiple etiologies that result in dysfunction of cortical neurons. SRBDs are common in individuals with epilepsy. Polysomnographic investigations by Malow (27) showed that nearly one-third of patients with medically refractory

epilepsy had a respiratory disturbance index of greater than five. Although the exact cause of this increased prevalence of OSA in this population is unknown, we have speculated that this may be in part related to the underlying CNS dysfunction similar to that seen in other neurological disorders such as stroke (28). Therapeutic intervention for epilepsy also may increase the risk of sleep apnea. Valproate, vigabatrin, and gabapentin are well known to promote weight gain thus increase the likelihood for sleep apnea (29–31).

Additionally, benzodiazepines and barbiturates may cause suppression in responsiveness to carbon dioxide and oxygen desaturation and increase upper airway musculature relaxation (30). Another form of therapy for epilepsy, vagus nerve stimulation, has been reported to potentially increase airway disturbance during sleep in some patients (31). This therapy may increase airway resistance from stimulation of the recurrent laryngeal nerve or by interfering with the respiratory sensory feedback. Seizures themselves can cause respiratory disturbance and apnea (Figs. 1 and 2). It is important for clinicians to differentiate the underlying etiology of the apnea for subsequent treatment.

OSA may also increase the recurrence of seizures. Mechanisms for the apparent increase in seizures may be two-fold. OSA may increase seizures based upon sleep fragmentation, or by the repetitive oxygen desaturation (32). Both of these mechanisms may lower the seizure threshold and may be active in patients with OSA. Several studies have shown that for some patients regardless of age, treatment

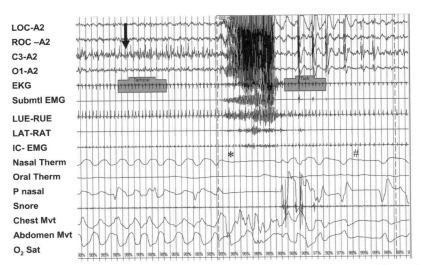

FIGURE 1 Focal onset seizure and obstructive sleep apnea. Polysomnographic epoch of a patient with history of epilepsy showing the onset of a focal seizure (*arrow*) with bi-frontal spread obscured by muscle activity then bilateral spike and wave activity. Following the onset of the seizure an ensuing obstructive apnea (*) is followed by a central respiratory pause (#). *Abbreviations*: A2, right auricular (reference) electrode; C3, left central electrode; EKG, electrocardiogram; IC-EMG, intercostal electromyogram; LAT, left anterior tibialis electromyogram; LOC, left outer canthi; LUE, left upper electro-oculogram; Mvt, movement; O1, left occipital electrode; O_2 Sat, oxygen saturation; P nasal, nasal pressure; RAT, right anterior tibialis electromyogram; ROC, right outer canthi; RUE, right upper electro-oculogram; Submtl EMG, submental electromyogram; Therm, thermocouple; Tachycar or Tach, tachycardia.

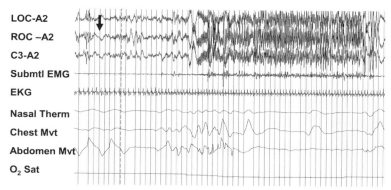

FIGURE 2 Focal onset seizure and central sleep apnea. Polysomnographic epoch of a patient showing the focal onset of seizure activity (*arrow*) with associated central apneas. *Abbreviations*: A2, right auricular (reference) electrode; C3, left central electrode; EKG, electrocardiogram; LOC, left outer canthi; Mvt, movement; O₂ Sat, oxygen saturation; ROC, right outer canthi; Submtl EMG, submental electromyogram; Therm, thermocouple.

of the OSA resulted in reduction of seizures in patients with focal onset seizures and generalized seizures (33–35).

Polysomnographic investigation of these patients does require additional precautions. The testing environment should be made safe for patients who may incur seizures during the testing procedure. These patients should be observed throughout the testing period and video recording should be time linked to the polysomnogram. Some patients may have events that cause them to fall out of bed. Therefore, the bed should not be near sharp edges and padding the bed rails may be helpful. Technologists should be familiar with recognizing the various types of seizures and the appropriate first aid. Physicians should also instruct the technologists on the appropriate emergency steps for prolonged seizures, status epilepticus, and airway management. Interpreting physicians should also consider expanding the number of electroencephalographic channels recorded. These channels should focus on the frontal and temporal regions, and the interpreting physician should review the electroencephalographic component with a 10-second per page window to aid in the identification of more subtle electroencephalographic features (36).

Treatment of sleep apnea in patients with epilepsy is similar to treatment of sleep apnea in the general population. Several case series have shown that treatment of OSA may improve seizure frequency (31–33). Our experience is that patients accept CPAP well. We have not had any significant patients become entangled in the tubing or injured with the device during a seizure. Patients who have postictal vomiting should not be considered candidates for oral appliances nor full-face masks because of the high potential risk of aspiration. Other investigators have promoted the use of respiratory stimulant medications such as protriptyline or acetazolamide (32,37).

Headaches
Migraines headaches are common neurovascular-based head pain that has both genetic and environmental etiologies. Patients with this disorder may develop OSA, but the prevalence of sleep apnea in these patients is unknown. Paiva (38) showed

that among individuals with frequent headache arising during the sleep period, 55% had an identifiable sleep disorder including sleep apnea. The mechanism of this relationship is unclear, but some of these individuals are vulnerable to headaches that are provoked by the sleep apnea.

These patients can be routinely studied and do not require any special monitoring. Some patients on opiates may demonstrate significant effect of the medication on respiration. For these individuals carbon dioxide monitoring may be helpful. However, patients otherwise tolerate the studies well and typically can handle CPAP intervention. Therapy for these patients is the same as therapy of the general population. In the general population, CPAP therapy appears to reduce the frequency of headache (39). Poceta (40) reported an individual who had a dramatic decrease in headaches following therapy for the OSA. To date there are no clinical trials demonstrating this effect, but these patients accept the therapy similarly to the general population.

Of note, some patients with trigeminal neuralgia may have difficulty tolerating the CPAP or oral appliance since this may trigger the pain. These patients may need trials with multiple delivery devices, more aggressive therapy for the trigeminal neuralgia or early consideration for neural ablative surgery.

Parkinson's Disease and Other Neurodegenerative Disorders

Parkinson's disease (PD) is characterized by a progressive loss of dopaminergic neurons, resulting in bradykinesia and a resting tremor. This disorder is reported to have a higher prevalence of sleep apnea ranging from 20% to 43% of the patients (41,42). The high prevalence of sleep apnea in this population occurs despite their lower average BMI that makes oxygen desaturation less prominent. Hogl (43) found snoring to be associated with daytime sleepiness. Yet, several investigators did not demonstrate a relationship of daytime sleepiness to AHI and the impact on the cardiovascular system is unknown (41).

Standard polysomnographic investigation of these patients should focus not only on respiration but also on other common issues including movements during sleep and sleep architecture. Because these individuals are less likely to have oxygen desaturations, more subtle forms of respiratory disturbance should be evaluated. Clinicians should be aware that patients with multiple system atrophy might present with nocturnal laryngeal stridor. This condition is an indication for tracheotomy.

Treatment for these individuals should include CPAP therapy. This requires the patient to have enough dexterity to manipulate the mask or have available assistance. Additionally, the medication therapy for the PD should be maximized to improve sleep and reduce rigidity that may be adding to the respiratory dysfunction (44). We have found patients note that they feel better with therapy; however, this may not reduce the daytime fatigue. Some patients may note that bedtime dosing of dopamine agonists may decrease rigidity and improve their ability to use the CPAP.

Multiple Sclerosis

Multiple sclerosis (MS) is a common neurological disorder affecting approximately 400,000 Americans. This autoimmune disorder targets the CNS causing demyelination and axonal loss. There is a high prevalence of sleep disturbance in MS patients and fatigue is especially a frequent and debilitating symptom.

Respiratory complications can occur in patients with advanced MS. However, sleep apnea in particular has only been presented in case reports. Of the 19 patients who presented with respiratory complications, only one was diagnosed with OSA (45). New onset sleep apnea syndromes were noted in cases of intractable hiccups (46). Of the six patients with definite MS and a complaint of insomnia, only one was diagnosed with central sleep apneas (47). Fatal sleep apnea (Ondine's curse) has also been reported in MS patients with medullary demyelination (48).

Respiratory complications and sleep apnea result from multiple factors relating to the disease state. Lesions located in areas dedicated to the regulation of respiration may significantly impair respiration. Additionally, bulbar and diaphragmatic weakness may result in airway obstruction or hypoventilation, respectively. MS lesions in the ventral medulla involving the chemoceptive areas may reduce sensitivity to CO_2 leading to fatal sleep apnea.

Patients with MS can be studied effectively in the sleep laboratory setting. Similar to other individuals with motor and sensory challenges, these patients may need handicap access and aid in transfer. Technologists should inquire if the patient needs assistance in turning during the night or has other special needs such as requirements for urinary catheterization or skin care needs. Since this disorder can result in hypoventilation and more subtle airway disturbance, these patients should be monitored for end tidal CO_2 and nasal pressure.

Treatment of the sleep apnea may improve the overall daytime sleepiness in some MS patients. No studies to date have been performed to evaluate the effect of treatment of sleep apnea on MS. CPAP is the standard treatment of sleep apnea in the general population. If sleep apnea is diagnosed in MS patients, CPAP use is advised. These patients must be evaluated for their dexterity and hand strength for application of CPAP or oral appliances. Motor and cognitive disability might make the use of CPAP a challenge. We have found that caregiver involvement in the fitting and education of CPAP use is very helpful. Many MS patients are using opiates for the relief of spasticity and pain. Physicians and patients must be aware of the risk of opiates on further respiratory compromise, especially during sleep.

Arnold Chiari Malformations
Arnold Chiari malformations are characterized by platybasia and decent of the cerebellar tonsils below the foramen magnum. Chiari malformations are associated with the production of central, obstructive, and mixed apneas (16). These respiratory events may be associated with wide swings in intracranial pressure and lead to the development of hydrocephalus and syringomyelia. Patients may have complex symptoms of headache, flushing, and autonomic instability. The respiratory events appear to be related to compression of the brainstem and upper cervical cord. This is probably in addition to the compromise of the vascular supply to those regions. These patients typically do not require any special assistive devices during the sleep study, but monitoring end tidal CO_2 may be helpful.

Treatment of patients with these malformations may involve the typical positive pressure support and device therapy. For many of these patients, surgical decompression of the posterior fossa may also relieve the central and potentially the obstructive events. Treatment series suggest that these patients feel better but no series to date show change in neurological state.

Spinal Cord Injury
Spinal cord lesions can cause sleep-related respiratory difficulties (49). SRBD can occur in more than 60% of individuals with tetraplegia after two weeks in acute spinal cord lesions (50). This finding persists and is evident even one

year after injury. There appears to be no relationship to pre-existing SRBD and the development of breathing issues after injury. Some of the SRBD may be related to loss of muscle strength or potentially increased abdominal girth but for others the use of respiratory suppressants such as opiates, muscle relaxants or benzodiazepines may contribute to the respiratory events. Partial damage of the spinal cord such as in transverse myelitis, trauma or compression may produce weakness of the chest wall and accessory muscles. This loss of strength may manifest as hypoventilation. Additionally, these individuals may fatigue to the level requiring nocturnal respiratory assistance. This assistance may be specifically evident in REM sleep for patients who have damage to the anterior horn cells of the phrenic nerves. These individuals may have limited to no respiratory motor output during REM sleep. Other lesions such as syringomyelia or other malformations such as Chiari Type 1 may compress proprioceptive sensory spinal pathways blocking the transmission of information for automatic breathing and result in central sleep apnea. Additionally, lesions in the high cervical cord and lower medulla may produce central apneas that typically occur in Ondine's curse.

Treatment of sleep apnea in patients with spinal cord lesions is generally well accepted. Burns found in his survey that 63% of patients diagnosed with OSA and spinal cord injury were continuing some form of therapy for sleep apnea. Most of these patients were treated with CPAP. Patients with spinal cord lesions generally tolerate the various treatments similarly to the general population. Patients who have hand co-ordination issues have a lower acceptance rate of CPAP masks but this would probably be similar to trouble with manipulating an oral appliance (51,52). Acceptance rate of the alternative therapies is not known. Yet, the physician needs to be cognizant of the individual's motor and co-ordination limitations as well as resources that may aid in overcoming these potential obstacles.

Amyotrophic Lateral Sclerosis

Amyotrophic lateral sclerosis (ALS), also known as Lou Gehrig's disease, affects approximately 30,000 individuals in the United States. This progressive and fatal illness results from degeneration of motor neurons in the brain, brainstem, and spinal cord. Skeletal muscle weakness such as that involving the extremities is observed first, but with time, bulbar, diaphragmatic and chest wall weakness cause respiratory compromise and eventual dependency upon mechanical ventilation. Although the exact prevalence of sleep apnea is not known in this population, respiratory insufficiency and failure are common. Most patients die from respiratory failure within five years from the onset of symptoms.

Respiratory insufficiency may occur during sleep despite normal daytime pulmonary function (53,54). One controlled study demonstrated a higher, though mild, AHI compared to controls. However, the subjects' sleep apnea predominated in REM sleep and consisted of periods of hypoventilation that accompanied significant oxygen desaturations (54). These nocturnal desaturations are related to hypoventilation rather than obstructive breathing (53). ALS patients with bulbar weakness or elderly with dyspnea are at higher risk for SRBD (55,56).

Respiratory symptoms and quality of life can be improved by intermittent mechanical ventilation (57). Orthopnea as well as daytime and nocturnal respiratory insufficiency improved after nocturnal nasal bilevel positive airway pressure (BPAP) therapy in one case (58). However, adherence to CPAP has been found to be poor in two other cases (59). Twenty-four-hour mechanical ventilation was associated with improved survival and quality of life especially in patients with orthopnea, daytime hypercapnea, and nocturnal desaturation (60). Polysomnographic investigation should focus on identifying features of hypoventilation and sleep apnea. ALS patients may frequently have difficulty turning, manipulating objects or even pushing a call button. Technologists should be aware of the patient's limitations and monitor the patient closely.

Clinicians should be aware that ALS patients have a progressive course and that their respiratory requirement will likely evolve as disease is worsened. Due to bulbar weakness, frequent leaks are encountered but may be reduced with the use of a full-face mask. Due to eventual upper extremity weakness, caregivers need to be involved in the placement of mechanical ventilation. Special attention to the effects of a sedative-hypnotic or pain medication is important to avoid further respiratory compromise.

Peripheral Nervous System Disorders
Peripheral Neuropathy
Peripheral neuropathy is ascribed when peripheral nerves are damaged. This condition is associated with impaired motor, sensory, and/or autonomic nerve dysfunction, and may be either inherited such as in Charcot-Marie-Tooth (CMT) disease or acquired. Acquired neuropathies are commonly caused by leprosy (most common world-wide), other diseases (diabetes mellitus, autoimmune disorders, toxins such as alcohol or heavy metals) or nutritional deficiencies (B_{12} or thiamine).

The prevalence of OSA in patients with peripheral neuropathy is unknown. This, in part, may be influenced by the underlying cause of disorder such as diabetes mellitus. In a group of nonobese diabetic patients, 30% demonstrated OSA (61). Patients with peripheral neuropathies such as CMT and familial dysautonomia are also predisposed to OSA (62,63). Sleep apnea may in itself pose a risk to the peripheral nervous system. Chronic hypoxemia is a known risk factor for polyneuropathy (64). OSA was shown to be associated with transient but severe peripheral vasoconstriction (65). Patients with OSA had clinical signs of polyneuropathy including axonal damage (66). Phrenic nerve dysfunction was documented in Guillain-Barre syndrome (GBS), CMT, ALS, and diabetes mellitus. Phrenic nerve dysfunction particularly avails the patient to hypoventilation and hypoxemia during REM sleep.

Polysomnographic investigation for most of these patients should be routine. Patients should be considered for hypoventilation syndromes and as such end tidal CO_2 measurements may be helpful. Patients must be observed in REM sleep for a complete evaluation. Esophageal reflux can also cause some of the apneic episodes in patients with autonomic nervous system dysfunction (67). Severe patients may require significant assistance with some activities of daily living.

Treatment of OSA in patients with peripheral neuropathy is similar to those in the general population and typically utilizes pressure support. Constant or bilevel pressure support can be used effectively. Patients need to be assessed for fine motor skills since distal extremities are typically involved with most peripheral neuropathies. Thus manipulation of these devices may require creative assistive devices such as large loops for quick-release straps or less intrusive delivery devices.

Guillain-Barré Syndrome
GBS is an acute inflammatory demyelinating polyradiculoneuropathy characterized by rapidly progressive muscle paresis and numbness of the extremities. Rapid respiratory deterioration is a short-term yet, serious complication that results from

bulbar, inspiratory, and expiratory muscle weakness. Bulbar dysfunction, autonomic instability, and early progression to disability predict development of respiratory paralysis in GBS (68). Although the prevalence of OSA or other respiratory disturbance during sleep has not been reported in GBS patients, respiratory compromise and failure may occur at anytime during the day or sleep. Continuous oxygen monitoring and frequent checks of vital capacity during the day and night in an intensive-care unit (ICU) setting are paramount to patient care during the acute phase of illness. The use of bilevel pressure support in two GBS patients with early deterioration of their respiratory systems was unsuccessful in preventing emergency intubation (69). Therefore, the use of CPAP or BPAP should not be a substitute for ICU admission and anticipation of emergency intubation. Whether patients develop OSA or other SRBD months or years later is unknown.

Neuromuscular Function Disorders
Myasthenia Gravis and Lambert-Eaton Syndrome
MG is the most common disorder of neuromuscular transmission that is usually due to acquired immunological dysfunction, but can rarely be caused by a genetic abnormality. There are approximately 36,000 cases in the United States. Patients complain of generalized skeletal muscle weakness that fluctuates throughout the day and is worse with sustained activity. Lambert-Eaton syndrome (LES) is another, yet rare disorder of neuromuscular transmission.

Sleep apnea has been reported in approximately 60% of patients with MG (70,71). The respiratory events occur predominantly in REM sleep and are associated with oxygen desaturations (70,72). Patients who are most vulnerable to the development of sleep apnea and oxygen desaturations are individuals with longer duration of the disease, older age, increased BMI, abnormal total lung capacity, and abnormal daytime blood gas concentrations (72,73). Patients with mild stable MG had infrequent respiratory abnormalities that were predominant in REM sleep (74). Our knowledge of patients with LES is limited. Other than one patient presented with rapidly progressive respiratory failure requiring ventilatory support, there are no reports of SRBD in these patients (75).

For these complex patients, the respiratory disturbance may be compounded by three potential issues. In addition to bulbar muscular weakness, inspiratory and expiratory muscle weakness with decreased chest wall compliance will worsen the severity of SRBD during REM sleep (72,76). Additionally, phrenic nerve conduction has been shown to be abnormal in patients during myasthenic crisis and some patients may have marked suppression of the intercostals muscle activity leading to central apneas (77,78).

Routine sleep studies can be performed in most of these patients. The clinician must be aware that the patient may demonstrate fatigue and changing respiratory status through the night. Significant differences in strength may occur in relationship to the timing of medication dosage, such as pyridostigmine. These patients are also at risk for hypoventilation and thus monitoring carbon dioxide levels may prove helpful. Although some patients may worsen through the night, others may have respiratory disturbance confined to REM sleep (72). Therefore, the study should include sufficient time in REM sleep to be considered an adequate evaluation.

Polysomnographic evaluation is needed in patients with MG or LES who develop signs of SRBD such as snoring, interrupted sleep, and/or daytime sleepiness. Optimization of the MG treatment with anticholinesterase agents may partially improve their ventilatory function, therefore leading to decreased respiratory disturbance during sleep (79). For some select patients thymectomy may resolve the sleep apnea, but CPAP therapy and/or nocturnal supplementation of oxygen continues to be the mainstay to improve their daytime function (73). Clinicians should be aware that patients with MG might have individual issues. Patients with MG may change through the course of their disease. During the period of recurring exacerbations, the clinicians should be attuned to changes in respiratory function and sleep-related symptoms, since these may change with change in muscle function. Patients may develop weakness of the bulbar musculature and require a full-face mask to limit air leakage. This may only be required during periods of exacerbation, and the patient may return to the pervious delivery device once bulbar strength has improved. The patients may also have significant hand weakness. For these patients the quick release headgear with pull loops may be helpful as well as ensuring that the patient understands that they may need assistance applying the headgear. Although these patients may require some creative problem solving, in general they do well with treatment.

Myopathies
Duchenne Muscular Dystrophy
Duchenne muscular dystrophy (DMD) is a degenerative disease of voluntary muscles that leads to generalized weakness and muscle wasting. It affects one in 3300 live male births. A less severe variant is known as Becker muscular dystrophy. Weakness of ventilatory muscles eventually develops in DMD patients, leading to eventual death typically in the third decade.

Respiratory insufficiency during sleep is the earliest sign of respiratory compromise in this patient population. REM-related hypoventilation and central apneas are common (80,81). Similarly to patients with MG, these patients are also at risk for isolated oxygen desaturation in REM sleep (Fig. 3). A bimodal presentation of SRBD was noted in 34 DMD patients, in which OSA was more prominent in the first decade and hypoventilation at the beginning of the second decade; lung function values did not accurately predict the severity of the SRBD (82). This study also recommends that each patient with SRBD be initiated on bilevel support at the start of treatment since transition from CPAP to bilevel was of short duration. Polysomnography should be considered when daytime $PaCO_2$ is ≥ 45 mmHg, and

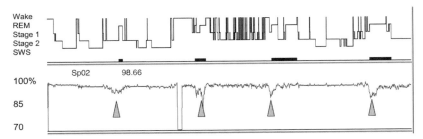

FIGURE 3 Muscular dystrophy and REM-related oxygen desaturations. Hypnogram of a young male with muscular dystrophy showing isolated oxygen desaturations occurring in association with each period of REM sleep (*arrow*). *Abbreviations*: REM, rapid eye movement; SWS, slow-wave sleep.

the study should include continuous end tidal CO_2 monitoring (82). Patients with DMD frequently require assistance to use CPAP/BPAP. They encounter similar issues as those seen in patients with MG or spinal cord disease.

Polymyositis and Dermatomyositis
Polymyositis and dermatomyositis (PM/DM) are chronic inflammatory myositis characterized by proximal muscle weakness. Respiratory complications due to pharyngeal and respiratory weakness are common.

Although SRBD has not been reported in these patients, alveolar hypoventilation is common (83). Patients with PM/DM, symptoms of snoring, hypersomnolence, and respiratory complications should undergo polysomnography to rule out sleep apnea or hypoventilation. CPAP or BPAP should be implemented if needed.

Myotonic Dystrophy
Myotonic dystrophy (MD) is a common type of muscular dystrophy and is a genetic disorder inherited with an autosomal dominant pattern. Myotonia, muscle weakness, and dystrophic changes in tissue are characteristic features of this disorder. Although this disorder is characterized by the muscle features, it is also associated with cognitive components, facial dysmorphic features, and sleep disturbance. Fatigue, tiredness, and excessive daytime sleepiness are very common in patients with MD.

Sleep apnea in MD patients is common and is more likely to be central than obstructive (84) (Fig. 4). In these patients, nocturnal hypoxemia and hypercapnea are often seen and may be more severe during REM sleep (85) (Fig. 5). Obese MD

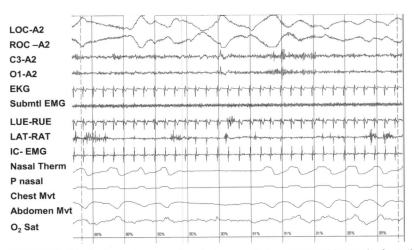

FIGURE 4 Myotonic dystrophy and central apnea. Polysomnographic epoch of a patient with myotonic dystrophy demonstrating central sleep apnea. Repetitive electromyographic activity is present in the limb (LAT–RAT) EMG channel. *Abbreviations*: A2, right auricular (reference) electrode; C3, left central electrode; EKG, electrocardiogram; EMG, submental electromyogram; IC-EMG, intercostal electromyogram; LAT, left anterior tibialis electromyogram; LOC, left outer canthi; LUE, left upper electro-oculogram; Mvt, movement; O1, left occipital electrode; O_2 Sat, oxygen saturation; P nasal, nasal pressure; RAT, right anterior tibialis electromyogram; ROC, right outer canthi; RUE, right upper electro-oculogram; Submtl EMG, submental electromyogram; Therm, thermocouple.

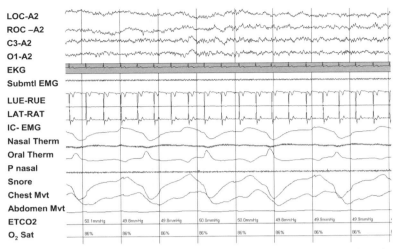

FIGURE 5 Myotonic dystrophy and hypoventilation. Polysomnographic epoch of a patient with myotonic dystrophy and hypoventilation. Note the presence of hypercapnea and oxygen desaturations in the absence of apneas or hypopneas. *Abbreviations*: A2, right auricular (reference) electrode; C3, left central electrode; EKG, electrocardiogram; ETCO2, end-tidal CO_2; IC-EMG, intercostal electromyogram; LAT, left anterior tibialis electromyogram; LOC, left outer canthi; LUE, left upper electro-oculogram; Mvt, movement; O1, left occipital electrode; O_2 Sat, oxygen saturation; P nasal, nasal pressure; RAT, right anterior tibialis electromyogram; ROC, right outer canthi; RUE, right upper electro-oculogram; Submtl EMG, submental electromyogram; Therm, thermocouple.

patients are at higher risk for nocturnal hypoxemia potentially due to the decreased functional reserve capacity (86). These respiratory disturbances appear to have consequences on general health. Guilleminault (85) discussed that MD patients with sleep apnea, are at risk of developing cardiopulmonary complications such as increased pulmonary and systemic arterial pressure and cardiac arrhythmias during sleep.

SRBD in MD patients may be secondary to a number of factors. Central apneas are probably a manifestation of the effects of the disorder on the CNS and maybe due to loss of catecholaminergic neurons in the medulla or dysfunction of the neurons involved in respiratory control during sleep (87). Reduced functional residual capacity may also result from respiratory muscle dysfunction, volume restriction, and supine position in sleep (84,88).

Technologists should be prepared for the cognitive, cardiac, and respiratory issues involved in patients with MD. Patients may require extra time for explanation and acclimatization to the study environment. Polysomnographic investigation of these patients should include measures of carbon dioxide and nasal pressure for subtle forms of breathing disorders. Technologists should also be attentive to cardiac rhythm and conduction abnormalities. Clinicians and technologists should also expect MD patients to frequently demonstrate sleep-onset REM periods during the overnight and the multiple sleep latency studies.

Treatment of these patients typically involves the use of medication or positive airway pressure support. Some patients respond to medication therapy such as protriptyline or acetazolamide (89). Studies show that patients have a subjective improvement with these medications with little improvement in the apnea index.

Others require pressure support. Due to the high prevalence of central apnea in this population, bilevel positive airway pressure with a timer may be necessary to restore nocturnal ventilation (90). Typically with effective therapy, patients feel better during the day and subjectively report better muscle usage.

Pompe's Disease

Pompe's disease is a glycogen storage disease due to acid maltase deficiency. It is an autosomal recessive disorder with a clinical course of progressive and severe muscle weakness. There is also involvement of respiratory muscles. Muscle replacement by fibro-fatty tissue was noted in the tongue and diaphragm in one autopsy case of a patient who developed severe OSA and respiratory failure (92). Nocturnal hypoventilation and REM-related hypopneas were noted (92). Patients with clinical symptoms of snoring, hypersomnolence, and respiratory problems should undergo polysomnography to rule out sleep apnea or hypoventilation. CPAP or bilevel pressure support should be used if needed.

CONCLUSIONS

Patients with neurological disease have an increased risk of a variety of sleep-related breathing disturbances that include OSA, periodic breathing, hypoventilation, and hypoxemia. These disturbances, in turn may have a negative impact on the patients' neurological state. Clinicians must therefore be cognizant of subtle sleep-related breathing issues that afflict each neurological disease and proceed with an appropriate evaluation and treatment tailored to the individual disease state.

Extremity weakness, decreased cognitive function, restricted movements during sleep and pain or spasticity are all issues that demand the physicians and polysomnographic technologists to come up with creative solutions for optimal use of CPAP/BPAP devices. Safety issues for patients with epilepsy, or those with limited sensory, motor or cognitive abilities should be outlined prior to patients' arrival to the sleep lab and considered in the choice of therapy. For all these patients, involvement of a caregiver is paramount to optimize adherence to the treatment plan. Yet, our real challenge is for clinicians to recognize SRBDs in these complex patients as opportunities to improve the quality of life and to have a potentially positive impact on their neurological state. Through this recognition, decisive investigation of the sleep related issues and customized effective therapies can make significant gains for these patients.

REFERENCES

1. Bianchi AL, Denavit-Saubie M, Champagnat J. Central control of breathing in mammals: neuronal circuitry, membrane properties and neurotransmitters. Physiol Rev 1995; 75:1–45.
2. Nogue MA, Roncoroni AJ, Benarroch E. Breathing control in neurological diseases. Clin Auton Res 2002; 12:440–449.
3. Morris KF, Baekey DM, Nuding SC, et al. Plasticity in the respiratory motor control, invited review: neural network plasticity in respiratory control. J Appl Physiol 2003; 94:1242–1252.
4. Janssens JP, Pautex S, Hilleret H, et al. Sleep disordered breathing in the elderly. Aging 2000; 12:417–429.
5. Chalmers RM, Howard RS, Wiles CM, et al. Respiratory insufficiency in neuronopathic and neuropathic disorders. QJM 1996; 89(6):469–476.

6. Coirault C, Chemla D, Pery-Man N, et al. Effects of fatigue on force–velocity relation of diaphragm. Energetic implications. Am J Respir Crit Care Med 1995; 151(1):123–128.

7. Hoch CC, Reynolds CF III, Kupfer DJ, et al. Sleep-disordered breathing in normal and pathologic aging. J Clin Psychiatry 1986; 47(10):499–503.

8. Smallwood RG, Vitiello MV, Giblin EC, et al. Sleep apnea: relationship to age, sex, and Alzheimer's dementia. Sleep 1983; 6(1):16–22.

9. Aloia MS, Arnedt JT, Davis JD, et al. Neuropsychological sequelae of obstructive sleep apnea–hypopnea syndrome: a critical review. J Int Neuropsychol Soc 2004; 10(5): 772–785.

10. Bliwise DL. Sleep apnea, APOE4 and Alzheimer's disease 20 years and counting? J Psychosom Res 2002; 53(1):539–546.

11. Gehrman PR, Martin JL, Shochat T, et al. Sleep-disordered breathing and agitation in institutionalized adults with Alzheimer disease. Am J Geriatr Psychiatry 2003; 11(4): 426–433.

12. Ayalon L, Ancoli-Israel S, Stepnowsky C, et al. Adherence to continuous positive airway pressure treatment in patients with Alzheimer's disease and obstructive sleep apnea. Am J Geriatr Psychiatry 2006; 14(2):176–180.

13. Grace JB, Walker MP, McKeith IG. A comparison of sleep profiles in patients with dementia with Lewy bodies and Alzheimer's disease. Int J Geriatr Psychiatry 2000; 15(11): 1028–1033.

14. Hishikawa N, Hashizume Y, Hirayama M, et al. Brainstem-type Lewy body disease presenting with progressive autonomic failure and lethargy. Clin Auton Res 2000; 10(3): 139–143.

15. de Miguel-Diez J, Villa-Asensi JR, Alvarez-Sala JL. Prevalence of sleep-disordered breathing in children with Down syndrome: polygraphic findings in 108 children. Sleep 2003; 26(8):1006–1009.

16. Kohrman MH, Carney PR. Sleep-related disorders in neurologic disease during childhood. Pediatr Neurol 2000; 23(2):107–113.

17. Turkington PM, Bamford J, Wanklyn P, et al. Prevalence and predictors of upper airway obstruction in the first 24 hours after acute stroke. Stroke 2002; 33(8):2037–2042.

18. Hayashi M, Fujimoto K, Urushibata K, et al. Hypoxia-sensitive molecules may modulate the development of atherosclerosis in sleep apnoea syndrome. Respirology 2006; 11(1): 24–31.

19. Brooks D, Horner RL, Kozar LF, et al. Obstructive sleep apnea as a cause of systemic hypertension. Evidence from a canine model. J Clin Invest 1997; 99(1):106–109.

20. Peppard PE, Young T, Palta M, et al. Prospective study of the association between sleep-disordered breathing and hypertension. N Engl J Med 2000; 342(19):1378–1384.

21. Young T, Finn L, Hla KM, et al. Snoring as part of a dose–response relationship between sleep-disordered breathing and blood pressure. Sleep 1996; 19(suppl 10):S202–S205.

22. Yaggi HK, Concato J, Kernan WN, et al. Obstructive sleep apnea as a risk factor for stroke and death. N Engl J Med 2005; 353(19):2034–2041.

23. Dziewas R, Humpert M, Hopmann B, et al. Increased prevalence of sleep apnea in patients with recurring ischemic stroke compared with first stroke victims. J Neurol 2005; 252(11):1394–1398.

24. Turkington PM, Allgar V, Bamford J, et al. Effect of upper airway obstruction in acute stroke on functional outcome at 6 months. Thorax 2004; 59(5):367–371.

25. Martinez-Garcia MA, Galiano-Blancart R, Roman-Sanchez P, et al. Continuous positive airway pressure treatment in sleep apnea prevents new vascular events after ischemic stroke. Chest 2005; 128(4):2123–2129.

26. Palombini L, Guilleminault C. Stroke and treatment with nasal CPAP. Eur J Neurol 2006; 13(2):198–200.

27. Malow BA, Fromes GA, Aldrich MS. Usefulness of polysomnography in epilepsy patients. Neurology 1997; 48(5):1389–1394.

28. Vaughn BV, D'Cruz OF. Obstructive sleep apnea in epilepsy. Clinics in Chest Medicine. Lee-Chiong T, Mohsenin V, eds. Philadelphia, PA: Elsevier Science, 2003; 24:239–248.

29. Lambert MV, Bird JM. Obstructive sleep apnea following rapid weight gain secondary to treatment with vigabatrin (Sabril). Seizure 1997; 6(3):233–235.

30. Takhar J, Bishop J. Influence of chronic barbiturate administration on sleep apnea after hypersomnia presentation: case study. J Psychiatry Neurosci 2000; 25(4):321–324.
31. Malow BA, Edwards J, Marzee M, et al. Effects of vagus nerve stimulation on respiration during sleep: a pilot study. Neurology 2000; 55(10):1450–1454.
32. Zgodzinski W, Rubaj A, Kleinrok Z, et al. Effect of adenosine A1 and A2 receptor stimulation on hypoxia induced convulsions in adult mice. Pol J Pharmacol 2001; 53:83–92.
33. Devinsky O, Ehrenberg B, Bathlen GM, et al. Epilepsy and sleep apnea syndrome. Neurology 1994; 44:2060–2064.
34. Vaughn BV, D'Cruz OF, Beach R, et al. Improvement of epileptic seizure control with treatment of obstructive sleep apnea. Seizure 1996; 5:73–78.
35. Koh S, Ward SL, Lin M, et al. Sleep apnea treatment improves seizure control in children with neurodevelopmental disorders. Pediatr Neurol 2000; 22:36–39.
36. Foldvary N, Caruso AC, Mascha E, et al. Identifying montages that best describe electrographic seizure activity during polysomnography. Sleep 2000; 23(2):221–229.
37. Ehrenberg B. Sleep apnea and epilepsy. In: Bazil CW, Malow BA, Sammaritano MR, eds. Sleep and Epilepsy: the Clinical Spectrum, Amsterdam: Elsevier 2002:373–382.
38. Paiva T, Farinha A, Martins A, et al. Chronic headaches and sleep disorders. Arch Intern Med 1997; 157:1701–1705.
39. Kiely JL, Murphy M, McNicholas WT. Subjective efficacy of nasal CPAP therapy in obstructive sleep apnoea syndrome: a prospective controlled study. Eur Respir J 1999; 13(5):1086–1090.
40. Poceta JS. Sleep-related headache syndromes. Curr Pain Headache Rep 2003; 7(4):281–287.
41. Arnulf I, Konofal E, Merino-Andreu M, et al. Parkinson's disease and sleepiness: an integral part of PD. Neurology 2002; 58:1019–1024.
42. Diederich NJ, Vaillant M, Leischen M, et al. Sleep apnea syndrome in Parkinson's disease. A case-control study in 49 patients. Mov Disord 2005; 20(11):1413–1418.
43. Hogl B, Seppi K, Brandauer E, et al. Increased daytime sleepiness in Parkinson's disease: a questionnaire survey. Mov Disord 2003; 18:319–323.
44. Yoshida T, Kono I, Yoshikawa K, et al. Improvement of sleep hypopnea by antiparkinsonian drugs in a patient with Parkinson's disease: a polysomnographic study. Intern Med 2003; 42(11):1135–1138.
45. Howard RS, Wiles CM, Hirsch NP, et al. Respiratory involvement in multiple sclerosis. Brain 1992; 115 (Pt 2):479–494.
46. Funakawa I, Yasuda T, Terao A. Intractable hiccups and sleep apnea syndrome in multiple sclerosis: report of two cases. Acta Neurol Scand 1993; 88(6):401–405.
47. Ferini-Strambi L, Filippi M, Martinelli V, et al. Nocturnal sleep study in multiple sclerosis: correlations with clinical and brain magnetic resonance imaging findings. J Neurol Sci 1994; 125(2):194–197.
48. Auer RN, Rowlands CG, Perry SF, et al. Multiple sclerosis with medullary plaques and fatal sleep apnea (Ondine's curse). Clin Neuropathol 1996; 15(2):101–105.
49. Burns SP, Rad MY, Bryant S, et al. Long-term treatment of sleep apnea in persons with spinal cord injury. Am J Phys Med Rehabil 2005; 84(8):620–626.
50. Berlowitz DJ, Brown DJ, Campbell DA, et al. A longitudinal evaluation of sleep and breathing in the first year after cervical spinal cord injury. Arch Phys Med Rehabil 2005; 86(6):1193–1199.
51. Burns SP, Little JW, Hussey JD, et al. Sleep apnea syndrome in chronic spinal cord injury associated factors and treatment. Arch Phys Med Rehabil 2000; 81:1334–1339.
52. Burns SP, Kapur V, Yin KS, et al. Factors associated with sleep apnea in men with spinal cord injury: a population-based case-control study. Spinal Cord 2001; 39:15–22.
53. Gay PC, Westbrook PR, Daube JR, et al. Effects of alterations in pulmonary function and sleep variables on survival in patients with amyotrophic lateral sclerosis. Mayo Clin Proc 1991; 66(7):686–694.
54. Ferguson KA, Strong MJ, Ahmad D, et al. Sleep-disordered breathing in amyotrophic lateral sclerosis. Chest 1996; 110(3):664–669.
55. Kimura K, Tachibana N, Kimura J, et al. Sleep-disordered breathing at an early stage of amyotrophic lateral sclerosis. J Neurol Sci 1999; 164(1):37–43.

56. Scelsa SN, Yakubov B, Salzman SH. Dyspnea-fasciculation syndrome: early respiratory failure in ALS with minimal motor signs. Amyotroph Lateral Scler Other Motor Neuron Disord 2002; 3(4):239–243.

57. Buhr-Schinner H, Laier-Groeneveld G, Criee CP. Amyotrophic lateral sclerosis and intermittent self ventilation therapy. Indications and follow-up. Med Klin (Munich) 1995; 90(1 suppl 1):49–51.

58. Takekawa H, Kubo J, Miyamoto T, et al. Amyotrophic lateral sclerosis associated with insomnia and the aggravation of sleep-disordered breathing. Psychiatry Clin Neurosci 2001; 55(3):263–264.

59. Barthlen GM, Lange DJ. Unexpectedly severe sleep and respiratory pathology in patients with amyotrophic lateral sclerosis. Eur J Neurol 2000; 7(3):299–302.

60. Bourke SC, Bullock RE, Williams TL, et al. Noninvasive ventilation in ALS: indications and effect on quality of life. Neurology 2003; 61(2):171–177.

61. Bottini P, Dottorini ML, Cristina Cordoni M, et al. Sleep-disordered breathing in non-obese diabetic subjects with autonomic neuropathy. Eur Respir J 2003; 22(4): 654–660.

62. Dematteis M, Pepin JL, Jeanmart M, et al. Charcot-Marie-Tooth disease and sleep apnoea syndrome: a family study. Lancet 2001; 357(9252):267–272.

63. Gadoth N, Sokol J, Lavie P. Sleep structure and nocturnal disordered breathing in familial dysautonomia. J Neurol Sci 1983; 60(1):117–125.

64. Mayer P, Dematteis M, Pepin JL, et al. Peripheral neuropathy in sleep apnea. A tissue marker of the severity of nocturnal desaturation. Am J Respir Crit Care Med 1999; 159(1):213–219.

65. Schnall RP, Shlitner A, Sheffy J, et al. Periodic, profound peripheral vasoconstriction—a new marker of obstructive sleep apnea. Sleep 1999; 22(7):939–946.

66. Ludemann P, Dziewas R, Soros P, et al. Axonal polyneuropathy in obstructive sleep apnoea. J Neurol Neurosurg Psychiatry 2001; 70(5):685–687.

67. Guilleminault C, Briskin JG, Greenfield MS, Silvestri R. The impact of autonomic nervous system dysfunction on breathing during sleep. Sleep 1981; 4(3):263–278.

68. Sundar U, Abraham E, Gharat A, et al. Neuromuscular respiratory failure in Guillain-Barre syndrome: evaluation of clinical and electrodiagnostic predictors. J Assoc Physicians India 2005; 53:764–768.

69. Wijdicks EF, Roy TK. BiPAP in early Guillain-Barre syndrome may fail. Can J Neurol Sci 2006; 33(1):105–106.

70. Stepansky R, Weber G, Zeitlhofer J. Sleep apnea in myasthenia gravis. Wien Med Wochenschr 1996; 146(9–10):209–210.

71. Shintani S, Shiozawa Z, Shindo K, et al. Sleep apnea in well-controlled myasthenia gravis. Rinsho Shinkeigaku 1989; 29(5):547–553.

72. Quera-Salva MA, Guilleminault C, Chevret S, et al. Breathing disorders during sleep in myasthenia gravis. Ann Neurol 1992; 31(1):86–92.

73. Amino A, Shiozawa Z, Nagasaka T, et al. Sleep apnoea in well-controlled myasthenia gravis and the effect of thymectomy. J Neurol 1998; 245(2):77–80.

74. Manni R, Piccolo G, Sartori I, et al. Breathing during sleep in myasthenia gravis. Ital J Neurol Sci 1995; 16(9):589–594.

75. Sugie M, Yanagimoto S, Mori K, et al. A case of combined paraneoplastic neurological syndrome, with Lambert-Eaton myasthenic syndrome manifesting as severe respiratory failure, and anti-Hu syndrome. Rinsho Shinkeigaku 2001; 41(7):418–422.

76. Mier-Jedrzejowicz AK, Brophy C, Green M. Respiratory muscle function in myasthenia gravis. Am Rev Respir Dis 1988; 138(4):867–873.

77. Lu Z, Tang X, Huang X. Phrenic nerve conduction and diaphragmatic motor evoked potentials: evaluation of respiratory dysfunction. Chin Med J (Engl) 1998; 111(6): 496–499.

78. White JE, Drinnan MJ, Smithson AJ, et al. Respiratory muscle activity and oxygenation during sleep in patients with muscle weakness. Eur Respir J 1995; 8(5):807–814.

79. Radwan L, Strugalska M, Koziorowski A. Changes in respiratory muscle function after neostigmine injection in patients with myasthenia gravis. Eur Respir J 1988; 1(2): 119–121.

80. Kirk VG, Flemons WW, Adams C, et al. Sleep-disordered breathing in Duchenne muscular dystrophy: a preliminary study of the role of portable monitoring. Pediatr Pulmonol 2000; 29(2):135–140.
81. Barbe F, Quera-Salva MA, McCann C, et al. Sleep-related respiratory disturbances in patients with Duchenne muscular dystrophy. Eur Respir J 1994; 7(8):1403–1408.
82. Suresh S, Wales P, Dakin C, et al. Sleep-related breathing disorder in Duchenne muscular dystrophy: disease spectrum in the paediatric population. J Paediatr Child Health 2005; 41(9–10):500–503.
83. Selva-O'Callaghan A, Sanchez-Sitjes L, Munoz-Gall X, et al. Respiratory failure due to muscle weakness in inflammatory myopathies: maintenance therapy with home mechanical ventilation. Rheumatology (Oxford) 2000; 39(8):914–916.
84. Matsumoto H, Osanai S, Onodera S, et al. Respiratory pathophysiology during sleep in patients with myotonic dystrophy. Nihon Kyobu Shikkan Gakkai Zasshi 1990; 28(7): 961–970.
85. Guilleminault C, Cummiskey J, Motta J, et al. Respiratory and hemodynamic study during wakefulness and sleep in myotonic dystrophy. Sleep 1978; 1(1):19–31.
86. Finnimore AJ, Jackson RV, Morton A, et al. Sleep hypoxia in myotonic dystrophy and its correlation with awake respiratory function. Thorax 1994; 49(1):66–70.
87. Ono S, Takahashi K, Jinnai K, et al. Loss of catecholaminergic neurons in the medullary reticular formation in myotonic dystrophy. Neurology 1998; 51(4):1121–1124.
88. Horikawa H, Takahashi K, Yoshinaka H, et al. Aggravation of hypoxemia in supine position in myotonic dystrophy. Rinsho Shinkeigaku 1992; 32(10):1057–1060.
89. Barthlen GM. Nocturnal respiratory failure as an indication of noninvasive ventilation in the patient with neuromuscular disease. Respiration 1997; 64 (suppl 1):35–38.
90. Guilleminault C, Philip P, Robinson A. Sleep and neuromuscular disease: bilevel positive airway pressure by nasal mask as a treatment for sleep disordered breathing in patients with neuromuscular disease. J Neurol Neurosurg Psychiatry 1998; 65(2):225–232.
91. Margolis ML, Howlett P, Goldberg R, et al. Obstructive sleep apnea syndrome in acid maltase deficiency. Chest 1994; 105(3):947–949.
92. Mellies U, Ragette R, Schwake C, et al. Sleep-disordered breathing and respiratory failure in acid maltase deficiency. Neurology 2001; 57(7):1290–1295.

23 Medical Disorders

Robert D. Ballard
*Advanced Center for Sleep Medicine, Presbyterian/St. Luke's Medical Center,
Denver, Colorado, U.S.A.*

INTRODUCTION

A multitude of medical disorders are commonly associated with sleep disturbances, including obstructive sleep apnea (OSA). Impaired sleep clearly worsens quality of life in affected patients, and may aggravate symptoms of the underlying disorder and possibly worsen the underlying disorder's prognosis. This chapter reviews the interactions of sleep and OSA with a variety of medical disorders, including asthma, chronic obstructive pulmonary disease (COPD), gastroesophageal reflux (GER), renal disease, acromegaly, hypothyroidism, and cardiovascular disease.

INFLAMMATION

Evidence has accumulated that OSA can be associated with upper airway inflammation. Olopade et al. (1) measured exhaled pentane (an indicator of oxidative stress) and nitric oxide as indicators of inflammation in 20 OSA patients and eight healthy controls. Exhaled nasal pentane and nitric oxide were increased after sleep only in OSA patients. Carpagnano et al. (2) reported elevated levels of both 8-isoprostane (another indicator of oxidative stress) and interleukin-6 (IL-6) in breath condensate from 18 OSA patients. These changes correlated with measured apnea–hypopnea index (AHI). Such findings present convincing evidence of increased nasal/upper airway inflammation in OSA patients.

Evidence is also accumulating that OSA is associated with changes in systemic indicators of inflammatory function. Schulz et al. (3) reported from 18 OSA patients that neutrophil superoxide generation was enhanced in comparison to controls, and this enhancement was immediately blunted by continuous positive airway pressure (CPAP) therapy. Dyugovskaya et al. (4) demonstrated increased reactive oxygen species production from monocytes and granulocytes in 18 OSA patients, an effect that was also blunted by subsequent CPAP therapy. These studies lend support to a role for cycling hypoxia/reoxygenation typical of OSA as a promoter of injury and inflammatory responses in OSA patients. This concept is further supported by two separate reports that OSA is associated with reduced circulating nitric oxide, and that this reduction can again be reversed by subsequent CPAP therapy (5,6).

There is now substantial evidence that OSA is associated with increased circulating levels of a variety of proinflammatory cytokines. Intercellular adhesion molecule-1 (ICAM-1), interleukin-8 (IL-8), and monocyte chemoattractant protein-1 (MCP-1) were all found to be elevated in OSA patients, and these changes were reversed by effective CPAP therapy (7). Serum interleukin-6 (IL-6) and tumor necrosis factor-alpha (TNF-alpha) were also found to be elevated in OSA patients, and this increase occurred independent of obesity but in correlation with OSA severity (8). Finally, Dyuogvskaya et al. (9) demonstrated evidence of cluster of differentiation 8 (CD8+) T-lymphocyte activation in OSA patients, which was reversed by CPAP therapy. It is tempting to speculate that the apparently pro-inflammatory effect of OSA could account for possible associations of this disorder with asthma severity and cardiovascular disease.

ASTHMA (SEE ALSO CHAPTER 20)

Nocturnal worsening of asthma symptoms has been an acknowledged feature of asthma since the fifth century A.D. when Aurelianus Caelius (10) described an increased nocturnal frequency of asthma attacks. Turner Warwick (11) observed that up to 64% of asthmatic patients were awakened with symptoms of asthma at least three nights per week. In a more recent questionnaire-based study, Bellia et al. (12) assessed the frequency of nocturnal asthma symptoms in 1100 patients randomly selected from general medical practices. Up to 24% of patients with the diagnosis of asthma experienced troublesome nocturnal symptoms "sometimes," while 15% of patients experienced such symptoms "often." Peak expiratory flow rate (PEFR) measurements are widely used to diagnose nocturnal worsening of asthma, which is typically indicated by at least a 15% decrement in PEFR from bedtime to morning awakening.

The etiology of the nocturnal worsening of asthma is controversial, and is likely multifactorial. Potential mechanisms include circadian changes in parasympathetic activity and circulating levels of corticosteroids and catecholamines. An early morning increase in airway inflammation associated with increased airflow obstruction and bronchial responsiveness has been reported by some investigators (13), although others have been unable to duplicate this finding (14).

There is evidence that sleep itself plays a role in this pattern of nocturnal worsening. Clark and Hetzel (15) studied asthmatic shift workers, observing that virtually all subjects immediately shifted their daily rhythm of PEFR in conjunction with changing their work shifts. These same investigators subsequently observed that sleep disruption had little effect on overnight worsening of PEFR, although total sleep deprivation eliminated overnight decrements in PEFR in about 50% of all asthmatic patients (16). Catterall et al. (17) evaluated the effect of complete overnight sleep deprivation in 12 asthmatic patients with regular nocturnal worsening. PEFR fell significantly overnight, regardless of whether patients were kept awake or allowed to sleep during the night. However, both absolute and percent overnight decreases in PEFR were greater when patients were allowed to sleep.

Nocturnal worsening of asthma is also apparently linked to snoring and sleep-disordered breathing. Chan et al. (18) evaluated nine patients with asthma and concurrent OSA, noting that all patients had frequent nocturnal exacerbations of their asthma. After initiating effective CPAP therapy, all patients demonstrated marked improvement in their asthma, with decreased symptoms, improved PEFR, reduced need for bronchodilator therapy, and resolution of their nocturnal worsening (Fig. 1). Guilleminault et al. (19) subsequently reported two separate populations of asthmatics, one group of middle-aged males with confirmed OSA, and a second group of younger males with recurrent snoring. Nocturnal worsening of asthma resolved in both groups after initiating CPAP therapy. Yigla et al. (20) studied 22 consecutive patients with severe, unstable asthma. Subsequent polysomnography detected OSA in 21 (95.5%) of these patients, although the patient group had a normal mean body mass index. These studies suggest strong relationships between snoring and/or sleep-disordered breathing and overall asthma severity

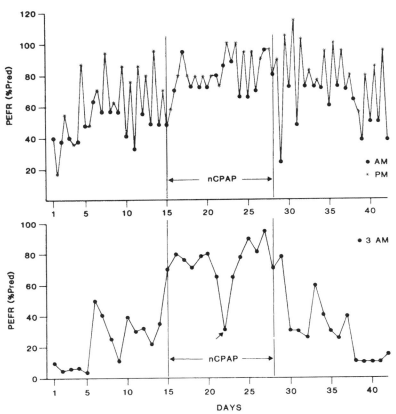

FIGURE 1 Overnight changes in peak expiratory flow rate (PEFR) in a single asthmatic patient. Top graph depicts bedtime (P.M.) to morning awakening (A.M.) changes in PEFR; bottom graph depicts three A.M. PEFR. Note how a two-week course of continuous positive airway pressure (CPAP) immediately improved early morning PEFR. Diagonal arrow on bottom graph indicates a single night without CPAP. *Source*: From Ref. 18.

and nocturnal worsening (Fig. 2). Effective CPAP therapy may improve asthma symptoms in affected patients.

Patients with nocturnal worsening of asthma are usually treated with the addition of, or an increase in the dose of, inhaled corticosteroid therapy. It is widely accepted that nocturnal worsening of asthma is a marker of overall asthma severity, and guidelines for asthma therapy emphasize the importance of inhaled corticosteroids in addressing nocturnal worsening. Patients who have persistent nocturnal worsening, despite adequate dosing of inhaled corticosteroids, may also be treated with long acting bronchodilators. Long acting inhaled beta-adrenergic agents, such as salmeterol and formoterol, are used widely to treat nocturnal worsening of asthma. Other investigators have suggested that sustained-release theophylline is effective for nocturnal worsening of asthma (21). Selby et al. (22) compared twice daily salmeterol with theophylline in 15 asthmatic patients with stable nocturnal worsening. The two agents had similar effects on overnight worsening of PEFR, but salmeterol use improved quality of life and was associated with fewer nocturnal awakenings and

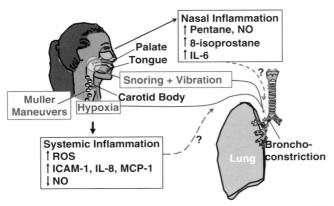

FIGURE 2   (See color insert.) Potential interactions between OSA, nasal inflammation, systemic inflammation, and their possible link to asthma severity. Abbreviations: NO, nitric oxide; IL-6, interleukin-6; ROS, reactive oxygen species; ICAM-1, intercellular adhesion molecule-1; IL-8, interleukin-8; MCP-1, monocyte chemoattractant protein-1; OSA, obstructive sleep apnea. Source: From Ref. 81.

arousals. In a similar study of asthmatic patients with nocturnal worsening, Weigand et al. (23) reported that salmeterol was superior to theophylline for improving nocturnal forced expiratory volume in the first second (FEV_1), reducing rescue therapy with albuterol, and improving perception of sleep. Shah et al. (24) reviewed the efficacy of long acting beta-adrenergic agents versus theophylline for maintenance treatment of asthma, and suggested that salmeterol is more effective than theophylline in reducing asthma symptoms (including nocturnal worsening), with fewer adverse side effects. Inhaled long acting beta-adrenergic agents should therefore routinely be considered before the addition of theophylline.

CHRONIC OBSTRUCTIVE PULMONARY DISEASE
(SEE ALSO CHAPTER 20)

COPD affects approximately 14 million adult Americans. COPD patients often report multiple problems with sleep, including insomnia and frequent awakenings. Sleep studies of COPD patients have revealed decreased total sleep time, frequent arousals and awakenings, and reduced amounts of slow-wave and rapid eye movement (REM) sleep. Impaired sleep quality likely results from a combination of factors, including chronic shortness of breath, nocturnal cough, and sleep-associated hypoxemia. In 1962, Trask and Cree (25) reported oximetry data from seven COPD patients, demonstrating oxygen desaturation to as low as 37% during subjective sleep. Pierce et al. (26) subsequently used electroencephalographic sleep staging and indwelling arterial catheters in 19 COPD patients to demonstrate a mean maximal fall in arterial partial pressure of oxygen (PaO_2) of 7.4 mmHg from wakefulness to sustained sleep. Douglas et al. (27) reported that 10 COPD patients all reduced their oxygen saturation by more than 10% during sleep, and eight of these patients demonstrated oxygen saturations that dipped below 50%. The lowest PaO_2s dropped into the range of 26 to 44 mmHg, which occurred predominantly during REM sleep. It has been widely observed that the most severe hypoxemia typically occurs during

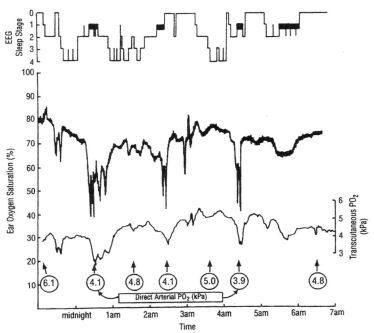

FIGURE 3 Overnight changes in sleep stage, oxygen saturation, and transcutaneous partial pressure of oxygen (PO_2), with intermittent measurement of arterial partial pressure of oxygen (PaO_2) in a chronically hypoxic chronic obstructive pulmonary disease patient. Note severe rapid eye movement (black bars on EEG Sleep Stage graph) associated hypoxemia. *Abbreviations*: EEG, electroencephalogram; kPa, kilopascals. *Source*: From Ref. 82.

REM sleep, when there is reduced inspiratory muscle activity and periods of hypoventilation characterized by small tidal volumes and variable respiratory effort. REM-associated hypoventilation can trigger severe hypoxemia even when the patient's waking PaO_2 is greater than 60 mmHg. However, COPD patients with lower levels of waking ventilation, manifested by higher arterial partial pressure of carbon dioxide ($PaCO_2$) with lower PaO_2, are likely to have the most severe nocturnal desaturation (Fig. 3).

Both episodic and relatively fixed pulmonary hypertension has been demonstrated in COPD patients with significant nocturnal oxygen desaturation, and nocturnal oxygen therapy can subsequently improve these abnormalities (28). Nocturnal supplemental oxygen can also improve sleep quality in COPD patients with nocturnal hypoxemia (29). The administration of low-flow supplemental oxygen by nasal cannula to COPD patients with a PaO_2 less than 55 mmHg was assessed in both the Nocturnal Oxygen Treatment Trial (30) and the Medical Research Council Working Party study (31). These studies demonstrated improved long-term survival in hypoxic COPD patients when supplemental oxygen was administered for at least 12 to 15 hours daily, which typically included the sleeping hours. It has therefore become standard care to administer 24-hour oxygen therapy in COPD patients with a waking resting PaO_2 of less than 55 mmHg, or in the range of 55 to 59 mmHg with evidence of end-organ damage (pedal edema, elevated hematocrit, or evidence of cor pulmonale). It has not been clearly established that nocturnal supplemental oxygen benefits COPD patients who have a waking PaO_2 of at least 60 mmHg with only isolated nocturnal arterial oxygen desaturation.

Although there is no evidence that COPD increases the risk for concurrent OSA, COPD can certainly be seen in association with OSA, which in combination has been termed the "overlap syndrome" (32). Treating such patients with nocturnal supplemental oxygen alone are unlikely to alleviate OSA-related symptoms of sleep disruption and nonrestorative sleep, and may actually increase apnea duration and contribute to greater sleep-associated increases in $PaCO_2$. These patients warrant therapy with CPAP, which reverses upper airway obstruction, improves gas exchange, and reduces inspiratory muscle work during sleep. There is some evidence that patients with "overlap syndrome" may be better candidates for bilevel positive airway pressure than standard CPAP (33).

Airflow obstruction in COPD frequently worsens in the early morning hours, in a fashion similar to asthmatic patients (34). Medical therapy for these worsening and associated symptoms usually consists of bronchodilator therapy, including long acting beta-adrenergic agents, anticholinergics, and theophylline. Berry et al. (35) observed in 12 normocapnic COPD patients that sustained-release theophylline improved morning FEV_1 and oxygen saturation plus $PaCO_2$ during non-REM (NREM) sleep, without adversely affecting sleep quality. Martin et al. (36) evaluated 36 patients with moderate-to-severe COPD during treatment with either four times daily nebulized ipratropium or placebo. Four weeks of treatment with ipratropium improved nocturnal oxygen saturation and perceived sleep quality, and increased time spent in REM sleep. McNicholas et al. (37) more recently assessed the utility of once daily inhaled tiotropium in 95 patients with moderate-to-severe COPD. Tiotropium improved FEV_1 and oxygen saturation during sleep, although there was no detected improvement in sleep quality. It appears that all of these bronchodilators may be useful for treatment of troublesome nocturnal symptoms in COPD patients. However, given the risks for potential side effects versus potential benefit from each medication, a reasonable approach is to initiate therapy at bedtime with tiotropium, to be followed by the administration of an inhaled long acting beta-adrenergic agent if warranted, with sustained-release theophylline reserved for those patients who continue to have troublesome night-time symptoms.

Nocturnal noninvasive positive pressure ventilatory support has been administered to many patients with COPD. Although this approach has been found quite useful in the treatment of acutely exacerbated COPD patients, those with severe but stable COPD have not as clearly benefited. Wijkstra et al. (38) conducted a meta-analysis of randomized controlled trials that assessed nocturnal noninvasive positive pressure ventilation in stable COPD patients. It was concluded that noninvasive ventilatory support did not improve lung function, gas exchange, or sleep efficiency. This therapy is therefore currently not widely advocated in patients with stable COPD, although it should be considered in patients with waking hypoventilation, especially in conjunction with the "overlap syndrome."

GASTROESOPHAGEAL REFLUX

Nocturnal GER is relatively common. One population survey reported that approximately 10% of all responders reported troublesome symptoms of night-time reflux (39). A Gallup poll reported that 79% of all people with heartburn had symptoms at night, and approximately 75% of these felt that heartburn impaired their sleep (40). Despite medical therapy, only half of all heartburn patients felt they had adequate control of night-time symptoms. Finally, in an analysis of 15,314 subjects surveyed as part of the Sleep Heart Health Study, 24.9% reported heartburn during sleep (41).

Sleep is associated with physiologic changes that can affect GER. The lower esophageal sphincter (LES) is the main barrier against GER. The LES appropriately relaxes during normal swallowing, but transient LES relaxation can also occur without swallowing, which accounts for the vast majority of GER episodes. Transient LES relaxations typically occur at night during wakefulness and after brief arousals from sleep. Sleep produces other physiologic changes that may enhance the impact of GER. For example, swallowed saliva neutralizes acid, but production of saliva normally ceases during sleep. Swallowing itself is also markedly reduced, if not absent, during continuous sleep, and swallowing episodes typically occur only after arousal from sleep. These physiologic changes impair esophageal acid clearance. More prolonged episodes of GER during the night also promote acid migration to more proximal regions of the esophagus.

Symptoms of nocturnal GER include disrupted sleep, chest discomfort, substernal burning, heartburn, and indigestion. With more proximal migration of esophageal acid, patients are more likely to awaken with a sour taste, coughing, and even choking. Nocturnal GER is best diagnosed via esophageal pH monitoring, with an esophageal pH probe positioned in the distal esophagus approximately 5 cm above the LES. Episodes of GER can thereby be defined by decreases in esophageal pH to less than four. Such studies are typically performed in the ambulatory setting, allowing 18 to 24 hours of continuous esophageal pH monitoring. Esophageal pH probes can also be utilized during standard polysomnography, allowing for the assessment of GER in relation to sleep disruption and obstructive apneas/hypopneas.

Nocturnal GER has been associated with other respiratory disorders at night, including OSA and asthma. OSA causes physiologic changes during sleep that promote GER, including frequent arousals and awakenings from sleep, plus increasingly negative intrathoracic pressure during discreet obstructive apneas/hypopneas. In addition, obesity is a common condition that is associated with both GER and OSA. Green et al. (42) prospectively evaluated 331 patients with diagnosed OSA. Significant nocturnal GER was detected in 62% of all patients at baseline. Subsequent CPAP therapy reduced nocturnal GER symptoms by 48% in CPAP adherent patients, but no change in GER symptoms occurred in CPAP nonadherent patients. This suggests that nocturnal GER is common in OSA patients, and that effective therapy with CPAP can reduce the frequency and severity of nocturnal GER episodes. The potential importance of diagnosing and treating GER in OSA patients is underscored by observations in 29 OSA patients that laryngeal inflammation correlated strongly with OSA severity (43).

There has also been extensive interest in the potential relationship between nocturnal GER and nocturnal worsening of asthma. Jack et al. (44) monitored both tracheal and esophageal pH in four asthmatic patients with a history of recurrent nocturnal worsening and GER symptoms. Thirty-seven episodes of GER were identified, of which five were also associated with a fall in tracheal pH, suggesting aspiration. The episodes of tracheal acidity were associated with more prolonged GER episodes, awakenings from sleep, and indications of bronchospasm.

Although aspiration of acidic reflux is clearly a potent trigger of bronchoconstriction, GER may not have to result in aspiration to trigger increased bronchomotor tone. Afferent vagal fibers are located in the distal esophagus, where they can be stimulated by exposure to acid reflux, leading to a reflex-induced increase in bronchomotor tone. Cuttitta et al. (45) monitored esophageal pH and lower respiratory resistance in seven asthmatics with a history of recurrent GER. They observed that GER episodes were associated with increased lower respiratory resistance, and that duration of esophageal acid exposure was an important predictor of an increase in lower respiratory resistance. However, Tan et al. (46) utilized virtually identical techniques, but were unable to demonstrate increases in lower respiratory resistance in response to either spontaneous episodes of GER or esophageal perfusion with acid.

In view of these discrepancies, there remains some uncertainty as to whether effective treatment of nocturnal GER can improve asthma severity. Several uncontrolled studies have demonstrated improvement in asthma after aggressive GER therapy. However, a systematic review of previous studies addressing this issue concluded that there is insufficient evidence that treatment of GER improves asthma in the general asthmatic population (47). It remains common practice to assess the clinical benefit from a three-month therapeutic trial with antireflux agents for individual patients with symptoms of both nocturnal GER and nocturnal worsening of asthma.

Both behavioral and pharmacologic interventions are typically employed to treat nocturnal GER. Patients should avoid eating at least two hours before bedtime, and should avoid high-fat content foods, caffeine, alcohol, chocolate, mint, citrus fruits, and caffeinated sodas, all of which may promote GER. Nicotine may decrease LES pressure, and patients should obviously be counseled to stop smoking. Obesity is associated with increased risk for GER, and obese patients should always be encouraged to lose weight via a combination of diet and exercise. Patients can be advised to sleep with the head of their bed elevated at least six inches, which can be achieved by placing blocks under the head of the bed. Evaluation of each patient's medical regimen is warranted, as many medications promote GER, including theophylline, calcium channel blockers, prostaglandins, and bisphosphonates.

Pharmacologic management of nocturnal GER typically includes antacids for immediate symptom relief, histamine H2 receptor antagonists, proton pump inhibitors, and esophageal motility agents. Once the mainstay of GER therapy, H2 receptor antagonists still provide symptomatic relief for 60% of treated patients, and can be dosed once daily at bedtime. However, proton pump inhibitors appear to provide superior suppression of gastric acid (48). GER therapy now commonly includes the bedtime administration of a proton pump inhibitor, such as omeprazole.

Esophageal motility agents, such as metoclopramide, may be considered in patients who remain refractory to H2 receptor antagonists and proton pump inhibitors. However, these agents have a high risk for side effects, limiting their utility. In those patients who remain refractory to all medical management, esophageal fundoplication surgery can be performed using laparoscopic methods. This procedure is often quite successful, yielding GER symptom control in 80% to 90% of treated patients.

RENAL DISEASE

Sleep complaints are common in patients with renal disease. Many studies have assessed end-stage renal disease (ESRD) patients treated with chronic dialysis. Strub et al. (49) evaluated 22 dialysis patients, finding that 14 (63%) of these patients reported sleep disturbances characterized by reduced, fragmented sleep, and increased wakefulness during the night. Holley et al. (50) subsequently assessed sleep quality in 48 hemodialysis patients and 22 continuous ambulatory peritoneal dialysis patients, comparing their perceptions of sleep with 41 healthy subjects. Approximately 50% of the dialysis patients complained of sleep problems, as opposed to only 12% of healthy control subjects. The most common sleep complaints were trouble falling asleep (67%), night-time awakening (80%), early morning awakening (72%), restless legs (83%), and jerking legs (28%). Many of these patients complained of daytime sleepiness, and dialysis patients reported napping an average of 1.1 ± 1.3 hours daily. Polysomnographic evaluations of such patients have confirmed disrupted sleep, with reduced total sleep times, low sleep efficiencies, frequent arousals, and increased periods of wakefulness throughout the night. Polysomnographic studies have also revealed that sleep architecture is usually "lighter," with increased amounts of NREM stage 1 and 2 sleep, and decreased amounts of NREM stage 3, 4, and REM sleep.

OSA also commonly occurs in patients with ESRD. Kimmel et al. (51) performed polysomnography on 30 ESRD patients, of whom 26 were on hemodialysis. Twenty-two of these 30 patients had symptoms suggestive of OSA, and 16 (73%) of these symptomatic patients were found to have clinically significant OSA. More recent studies have confirmed prevalence rates for OSA between 30% and 80% in the ESRD population, which is much greater than reported for the general population. The frequency and severity of OSA do not appear to vary substantially between patients treated with chronic hemodialysis and continuous ambulatory peritoneal dialysis.

This increased risk for OSA in the ESRD population is not well understood. It has been proposed that hypocapnia occurring as a respiratory response to metabolic acidosis and acidemia may predispose patients to an unstable respiratory pattern (52). Beecroft et al. (53) determined that ESRD patients with concurrent OSA have augmented responsiveness of both central and peripheral chemoreflexes, which could promote OSA by destabilizing respiratory control. Upper airway edema as a component of generalized volume overload could promote the development of OSA in this population. It has also been suggested that uremic toxins may depress the central nervous system, thereby reducing upper airway muscle tone during sleep. Both OSA and ESRD are more likely to present in older populations. In a possibly related fashion, dialysis for ESRD has been associated with hormonal changes that emulate the postmenopausal state in women. It has been established that the postmenopausal state substantially increases the risk for OSA in the female gender.

Therapy for OSA in the ESRD population usually includes CPAP therapy. It has also been reported that the use of bicarbonate-based versus acetate-based dialysate can decrease OSA severity. Hanly and Pierratos (54) reported that switching patients from the typical three times weekly daytime hemodialysis to more frequent, slower nocturnal hemodialysis sessions reduced the mean AHI from 25 to 8 events per hour in 14 ESRD patients. Tang et al. (55) reported that shifting from continuous ambulatory peritoneal dialysis to nocturnal peritoneal dialysis significantly reduced AHI in ESRD patients. The potential benefit from these changes in dialysis protocol clearly warrants further investigation.

Patients with ESRD frequently complain of daytime sleepiness, which has been confirmed by multiple sleep latency tests and maintenance of wakefulness tests. Potential contributors to daytime sleepiness could include underlying sleep disorders, such as OSA, restless legs syndrome (RLS), and periodic limb movement disorder (PLMD), all of which are more prevalent in the ESRD population. It has also been suggested that a subclinical uremic encephalopathy may be present in dialysis patients that may promote sleepiness (56). There is evidence that dialysis itself may predispose patients to somnolence, in that increased production of somnogenic cytokines, interleukin-1 and TNF-alpha, has been observed in association with both hemodialysis (57) and peritoneal dialysis (58). Therapy for problematic daytime sleepiness in this population remains focused upon treatable underlying causes, including OSA, RLS, PLMD, and insufficient sleep.

ACROMEGALY

Patients with acromegaly have well-described skeletal and soft tissue craniofacial changes that predispose them to the development of OSA. In one screening trial of 53 patients with acromegaly, 93% of patients with suspected OSA had the diagnosis confirmed, but 60% of patients not previously suspected of having OSA were also found to have this diagnosis (59). Weiss et al. (60) evaluated 55 patients with acromegaly, diagnosing OSA in 75% of their population. Surgical interventions and medical treatment (via somatostatin analogs) to reduce excess growth hormone (GH) in affected patients often improve OSA severity, although many patients have persistently severe disease (61). This implies that OSA in these patients likely results from a combination of pharyngeal soft tissue redundancy and skeletal craniofacial abnormalities, including vertical growth of the mandible (61). This also suggests that patients with residual OSA after successful treatment of their GH excess are even less likely to have successful outcomes from standard upper airway soft tissue surgery, such as uvulopalatopharyngoplasty.

HYPOTHYROIDISM

There are multiple case reports of OSA occurring in severely hypothyroid, myxedematous patients, and it has been commonly reported that effective thyroid supplementation subsequently normalized breathing during sleep in this population. This has lead to a common practice of screening for hypothyroidism via thyroid stimulating hormone (TSH) in all newly diagnosed OSA patients. However, multiple studies have now confirmed that the prevalence of undiagnosed hypothyroidism in the OSA population is similar to that of the general population, and the OSA population as a whole does not seem to be at higher risk for hypothyroidism. Kapur et al. (62) found hypothyroidism in only 1.41% of 336 adults referred for suspected OSA, and could find no significant association between OSA and hypothyroidism. Likewise, Mickelson et al. (63) found OSA in only 1.2% of 834 patients referred for suspected OSA, and that subsequent thyroid replacement therapy did not improve OSA in these patients. This latter finding was confirmed by Resta et al. (64). It is therefore now widely recommended that TSH levels be checked only in those OSA patients who present with other clinical signs and symptoms suggestive of hypothyroidism.

CARDIOVASCULAR DISEASE

Recent studies provide strong evidence that OSA is associated with several physiologic processes that could increase risk for cardiovascular disease. First, it has been well established that OSA is associated with sympathetic activation (65). This is most pronounced in association with obstructive apneas and hypopneas during

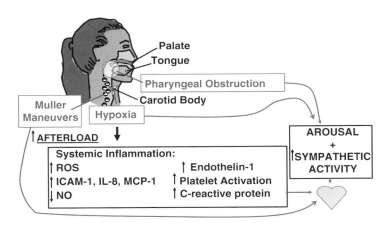

FIGURE 4 (*See color insert.*) Potential interactions between OSA, systemic inflammation, and their possible link to cardiovascular disease. *Abbreviations*: ROS, reactive oxygen species; ICAM-1, intercellular adhesion molecule-1; IL-8, interleukin-8; MCP-1, monocyte chemoattractant protein-1; NO, nitric oxide; OSA, obstructive sleep apnea.

sleep, but OSA patients also have evidence of increased sympathetic activity that persists during wakefulness (66). There is also evidence that therapy for OSA can reduce sympathetic activation, during both sleep and wakefulness (67). Obstructive apneas and hypopneas can thereby trigger significant surges in systemic blood pressure, and there is compelling evidence that OSA also increases risk for diurnal hypertension (68–70). An association between OSA and hypertension may at least partly explain the increased risk for heart disease reported in patients with OSA (71–73).

Evidence has also accumulated that OSA represents a state of oxidative stress, with increased levels of reactive oxygen species that could trigger a proinflammatory cytokine cascade (74). Proinflammatory cytokines, such as TNF-alpha, IL-6, and IL-8, as well as the adhesion molecules ICAM-1 and vascular cell adhesion molecule-1 (VCAM-1), are all increased in the presence of OSA (Fig. 4). It has been demonstrated that C-reactive protein, a strong marker of cardiovascular risk, is also elevated in patients with OSA (75). There is evidence that effective therapy for OSA can reduce these proinflammatory cytokines. Since cardiovascular disease is now widely thought to involve inflammatory processes, at least at the site of localized vascular lesions, the potential role of OSA as a promoter of inflammation also warrants consideration when assessing risk for cardiovascular disease.

Therapy for Obstructive Sleep Apnea—Effects upon Cardiovascular Disease

CPAP remains the most effective therapy for OSA. Although adherence with CPAP therapy can be challenging, it is widely accepted that adherence with this therapy will control OSA at least 90% of the time. Two studies have assessed the relative benefits of therapy with effective versus subtherapeutic, or sham, CPAP upon blood pressure (76,77). Both studies demonstrated that effective CPAP therapy significantly reduced nocturnal and diurnal blood pressures in comparison to sham CPAP therapy.

Two studies confirm that CPAP therapy in patients with OSA and concurrent congestive heart failure can also improve both cardiac function and quality of life. Kaneko et al. (78) treated 12 OSA patients with congestive heart failure for one month with CPAP. Treated patients demonstrated a 10 mmHg reduction in daytime systolic blood pressure in conjunction with an improvement in left ventricular ejection fraction from 25% to 34%. A control group of 12 similar patients demonstrated no significant changes. Mansfield et al. (79) evaluated the effects from three months of CPAP therapy upon quality of life and cardiac function in 19 OSA patients with congestive heart failure. Regular CPAP therapy improved left ventricular ejection fraction by 5% and improved quality of life indicators, whereas a control group of 21 untreated patients remained unchanged.

Marin et al. (80) monitored 1465 snorers referred for polysomnography over a mean of 10 years. During the 10 years after their diagnoses, patients with untreated severe OSA (AHI > 30) had a nearly three-fold increase in risk for fatal cardiovascular events when compared to healthy controls and other patients with severe OSA who were treated with CPAP. These studies suggest that OSA has adverse effects upon blood pressure, cardiovascular status, and probably cardiovascular mortality. There is evidence that effective therapy with CPAP can improve blood pressure and cardiac function in adult OSA patients.

CONCLUSIONS

It has now been clearly demonstrated that sleep and OSA commonly interact with a host of other medical conditions. Nocturnal worsening of asthma is a common manifestation of this disease, and is indicative of increased disease severity. Snoring and OSA may also contribute to such nocturnal worsening. Therapy focuses upon judicious use of long acting bronchodilators, but the presence of OSA should be evaluated and treated, if present. COPD is frequently associated with impaired sleep, likely as a result of chronic dyspnea and sleep-associated hypoxemia. Appropriate therapy again includes long acting bronchodilators and possibly nocturnal supplemental oxygen, but if concurrent OSA ("overlap syndrome") is present, therapy should include CPAP or bilevel positive airway pressure. GER during sleep may lead to prolonged episodes of esophageal acid exposure. This is a common sequela of OSA, and may trigger nocturnal worsening of asthma. ESRD and chronic dialysis are commonly associated with a host of troublesome sleep problems, including OSA, RLS, PLMD, and daytime sleepiness. Modification of dialysis schedules may improve OSA. A majority of acromegalic patients have OSA, which may respond to surgical and medical interventions to reduce excessive GH. The routine screening for hypothyroidism in the general OSA population is unwarranted, unless patients present with other clinical signs and symptoms of hypothyroidism. Extensive evidence links cardiovascular disease and OSA. OSA has adverse effects upon blood pressure, cardiovascular status, and mortality. Effective CPAP therapy can improve blood pressure and cardiac function in OSA patients.

REFERENCES

1. Olopade CO, Christon SA, Zakkar M, et al. Exhaled pentane and nitric oxide levels in patients with obstructive sleep apnea. Chest 1997; 111:1500–1504.
2. Carpagnano GE, Kharitonov SA, Resta O, et al. Increased 8-isoprostane and interleukin-6 in breath condensate of obstructive sleep apnea patients. Chest 2002; 122:1162–1167.

3. Schulz R, Mahmoudi S, Hattar K, et al. Enhanced release of superoxide from polymorphonuclear neutrophils in obstructive sleep apnea. Am J Respir Crit Care Med 2000; 162:566–570.
4. Dyugovskaya L, Lavie P, Lavie L. Increased adhesion molecules expression and production of reactive oxygen species in leukocytes of sleep apnea patients. Am J Respir Crit Care Med 2002; 165:934–939.
5. Ip MS, Lam B, Chan LY, et al. Circulating nitric oxide is suppressed in obstructive sleep apnea and is reversed by nasal continuous positive airway pressure. Am J Respir Crit Care Med 2000; 162:2166–2171.
6. Schulz R, Schmidt D, Blum A, et al. Decreased plasma levels of nitric oxide derivatives in obstructive sleep apnea: response to CPAP therapy. Thorax 2000; 55:1046–1051.
7. Ohga E, Tomita T, Wada H, et al. Effects of obstructive sleep apnea on circulating ICAM-1, IL-8, and MCP-1. J Appl Physiol 2003; 94:179–184.
8. Ciftci TU, Kokturk O, Bukam N, et al.The relationship between serum cytokine levels with obesity and obstructive sleep apnea syndrome. Cytokine 2004; 28(2):87–91.
9. Dyugovskaya L, Lavie P, Hirsh M, et al. Activated CD8+ T-lymphocytes in obstructive sleep apnea. Eur Respir J 2005; 25(5):820–828.
10. Caelius A. De Morbis Acutis et Chronicis. 1709, Amsterdam: Westeniand.
11. Turner-Warwick M. Epidemiology of nocturnal asthma. Am J Med 1988; 85(1B):6–8.
12. Bellia V, Pistelli R, Filippazzo G, et al. Prevalence of nocturnal asthma in a general population sample: determinants and effect of aging. J Asthma 2000; 37(7):595–602.
13. Martin RJ, Cicutto LC, Smith HR, et al. Airways inflammation in nocturnal asthma. Am Rev Respir Dis 1991; 143(2):351–357.
14. Oosterhoff Y, Timens W, Postma DS. The role of airway inflammation in the pathophysiology of nocturnal asthma. Clin Exp Allergy 1995; 25(10):915–921.
15. Clark TJ, Hetzel MR. Diurnal variation of asthma. Br J Dis Chest 1977; 71(2):87–92.
16. Hetzel MR, Clark TJ. Does sleep cause nocturnal asthma? Thorax 1979; 34(6):749–754.
17. Catterall JR, Rhind GB, Stewart IC, et al. Effect of sleep deprivation on overnight bronchoconstriction in nocturnal asthma. Thorax 1986; 41(9):676–680.
18. Chan CS, Woolcock AJ, Sullivan CE. Nocturnal asthma: role of snoring and obstructive sleep apnea. Am Rev Respir Dis 1988; 137(6):1502–1504.
19. Guilleminault C, Quera-Salva MA, Powell N, et al. Nocturnal asthma: snoring, small pharynx and nasal CPAP. Eur Respir J 1988; 1(10):902–907.
20. Yigla M, Tov N, Solomonov A, et al. Difficult-to-control asthma and obstructive sleep apnea. J Asthma 2003; 40(8):865–871.
21. Martin RJ, Cicutto LC, Ballard RD, et al. Circadian variations in theophylline concentrations and the treatment of nocturnal asthma. Am Rev Respir Dis 1989; 139(2):475–478.
22. Selby C, Engleman HM, Fitzpatrick MF, et al. Inhaled salmeterol or oral theophylline in nocturnal asthma? Am J Respir Crit Care Med 1997; 155(1):104–108.
23. Wiegand L, Mende CN, Zaidel G, et al. Salmeterol versus theophylline: sleep and efficacy outcomes in patients with nocturnal asthma. Chest 1999; 115(6):1525–1532.
24. Shah L, Wilson AJ, Gibson PJ, et al. Long acting beta-agonists versus theophylline for maintenance treatment of asthma. Cochrane Database Syst Rev 2003(3):CD001281.
25. Trask CH, Cree EM. Oximeter studies on patients with chronic obstructive emphysema, awake and during sleep. N Engl J Med 1962; 266:639–642.
26. Pierce AK, Jarrett CE, Werkle G Jr, et al. Respiratory function during sleep in patients with chronic obstructive lung disease. J Clin Invest 1966; 45(5):631–636.
27. Douglas NJ, Calverley PM, Leggett RJ, et al. Transient hypoxaemia during sleep in chronic bronchitis and emphysema. Lancet 1979; 1(8106):1–4.
28. Fletcher EC, Luckett RA, Miller T, et al. Exercise hemodynamics and gas exchange in patients with chronic obstruction pulmonary disease, sleep desaturation, and a daytime PaO_2 above 60 mmHg. Am Rev Respir Dis 1989; 140(5):1237–1245.
29. Calverley PM, Brezinova V, Douglas NJ, et al. The effect of oxygenation on sleep quality in chronic bronchitis and emphysema. Am Rev Respir Dis 1982; 126(2):206–210.
30. Nocturnal Oxygen Therapy Trial Group. Continuous or nocturnal oxygen therapy in hypoxemic chronic obstructive lung disease: a clinical trial. Ann Intern Med 1980; 93(3):391–398.

31. Medical Research Council Working Party. Long term domiciliary oxygen therapy in chronic hypoxic cor pulmonale complicating chronic bronchitis and emphysema. Lancet 1981; 28[1(8222)]:681–686.
32. Weitzenblum E, Krieger J, Oswald M, et al. Chronic obstructive pulmonary disease and sleep apnea syndrome. Sleep 1992; 15(suppl 6):S33–S35.
33. Resta O, Guido P, Picca V, et al. Prescription of nCPAP and nBIPAP in obstructive sleep apnoea syndrome: Italian experience in 105 subjects. A prospective two centre study. Respir Med 1998; 92(6):820–827.
34. Connolly CK. Diurnal rhythms in airway obstruction. Br J Dis Chest 1979; 73(4):357–366.
35. Berry RB, Desa MM, Branum JP, et al. Effect of theophylline on sleep and sleep-disordered breathing in patients with chronic obstructive pulmonary disease. Am Rev Respir Dis 1991; 143(2):245–250.
36. Martin RJ, Bartelson BL, Smith P, et al. Effect of ipratropium bromide treatment on oxygen saturation and sleep quality in COPD. Chest 1999; 115(5):1338–1345.
37. McNicholas WT, Calverley PM, Lee A, et al. Long-acting inhaled anticholinergic therapy improves sleeping oxygen saturation in COPD. Eur Respir J 2004; 23(6):825–831.
38. Wijkstra PJ, Lacasse Y, Guyatt GH, et al. A meta-analysis of nocturnal noninvasive positive pressure ventilation in patients with stable COPD. Chest 2003; 124(1):337–343.
39. Farup C, Kleinman L, Sloan S, et al. The impact of nocturnal symptoms associated with gastroesophageal reflux disease on health-related quality of life. Arch Intern Med 2001; 161:45–70.
40. Shaker R, Castell DO, Schoenfeld PS, et al. Nighttime heartburn is an under-appreciated clinical problem that impacts sleep and daytime function: the results of a Gallup survey conducted on behalf of the American Gastroenterological Association. Am J Gastroenterol 2003; 98(7):1487–1493.
41. Fass R, Quan SF, O'Connor GT, et al. Predictors of heartburn during sleep in a large prospective cohort study. Chest 2005; 127(5):1658–1666.
42. Green BT, Broughton WA, O'Connor JB. Marked improvement in nocturnal gastroesophageal reflux in a large cohort of patients with obstructive sleep apnea treated with continuous positive airway pressure. Arch Intern Med 2003; 163(1):41–45.
43. Payne RJ, Kost KM, Frenkiel S, et al. Laryngeal inflammation assessed using the reflux finding score in obstructive sleep apnea. Otolaryngol Head Neck Surg 2006; 134(5):836–842.
44. Jack CI, Calverley PM, Donnelly RJ, et al. Simultaneous tracheal and oesophageal pH measurements in asthmatic patients with gastro-oesophageal reflux. Thorax 1995; 50(2):201–204.
45. Cuttitta G, Cibella F, Visconti A. Spontaneous gastroesophageal reflux and airway patency during the night in adult asthmatics. Am J Respir Crit Care Med 2000; 151:177–181.
46. Tan WC, Martin RJ, Pandey R, et al. Effects of spontaneous and simulated gastroesophageal reflux on sleeping asthmatics. Am Rev Respir Dis 1990; 141(6):1394–1399.
47. Gibson PG, Henry RL, Coughlan JL. Gastro-oesophageal reflux treatment for asthma in adults and children. Cochrane Database Syst Rev 2003(2):CD001496.
48. Peghini PL, Katz PO, Bracy NA, et al. Nocturnal recovery of gastric acid secretion with twice-daily dosing of proton pump inhibitors. Am J Gastroenterol 1998; 93(5):763–767.
49. Strub B, Schneider-Helmart D, Gnirss F, et al. Sleep disorders in patients with chronic renal insufficiency in long-term hemodialysis treatment. Schweiz Med Wochenschr 1982; 112(23):824–828.
50. Holley JL, Nespor S, Rault R. Characterizing sleep disorders in chronic hemodialysis patients. ASAIO Trans 1991; 37(3):M456–M457.
51. Kimmel PL, Miller G, Mendelson WB. Sleep apnea syndrome in chronic renal disease. Am J Med 1989; 86(3):308–314.
52. Mendelson WB, Wadhwa NK, Greenberg HE, et al. Effects of hemodialysis on sleep apnea syndrome in end-stage renal disease. Clin Nephrol 1990; 33(5):247–251.
53. Beecroft J, Duffin J, Pierratos A, et al. Enhanced chemo-responsiveness in patients with sleep apnoea and end-stage renal disease. Eur Respir J 2006; 28(1):151–158.
54. Hanly PJ, Pierratos A. Improvement of sleep apnea in patients with chronic renal failure who undergo nocturnal hemodialysis. N Engl J Med 2001; 344(2):102–107.

55. Tang SC, Lam B, Ku PP, et al. Alleviation of sleep apnea in patients with chronic renal failure by nocturnal cyler-assisted peritoneal dialysis compared with conventional continuous ambulatory peritoneal dialysis. J Am Soc Nephrol 2006; 17(9): 2607–2616.

56. Parker KP. Sleep disturbances in dialysis patients. Sleep Med Rev 2003; 7(2):131–143.

57. Rousseau Y, Haeffner-Cavaillon N, Poignet JL, et al. In vivo intracellular cytokine production by leukocytes during haemodialysis. Cytokine 2000; 12(5):506–517.

58. Lai KN, Lai KB, Lam CW, et al. Changes of cytokine profiles during peritonitis in patients on continuous ambulatory peritoneal dialysis. Am J Kidney Dis 2000; 35(4):644–652.

59. Grunstein RR, Ho KY, Sullivan CE. Sleep apnea in acromegaly. Ann Intern Med 1991; 115(7):527–532.

60. Weiss V, Sonka K, Pretl M, et al. Prevalence of the sleep apnea syndrome in acromegaly population. J Endocrinol Invest 2000; 23(8):515–519.

61. Hochban W, et al. Obstructive sleep apnoea in acromegaly: the role of craniofacial changes. Eur Respir J 1999; 14:196–202.

62. Kapur VK, Koepsell TD, deMaine J, et al. Association of hypothyroidism and obstructive sleep apnea. Am J Respir Crit Care Med 1998; 158:1379–1383.

63. Mickelson SA, Lian T, Rosenthal L. Thyroid testing and thyroid hormone replacement in patients with sleep disordered breathing. ENT—Ear, Nose and Throat J 1999; 78(10):768–775.

64. Resta O, Carratu P, Carpagnano GE, et al. Influence of subclinical hypothyroidism and T4 treatment on the prevalence and severity of obstructive sleep apnea syndrome (OSAS). J Endocrinol Invest 2005; 28(10):893–898.

65. Somers VK, Anderson EA, Mark AL, et al. Sympathetic neural mechanisms in obstructive sleep apnea. J Clin Invest 1995; 96(4):1897–1904.

66. Narkiewicz K, Van deBorne PJ, Cooley RL, et al. Sympathetic activity in obese subjects with and without obstructive sleep apnea. Circulation 1998; 98(8):772–776.

67. Narkiewicz K, Kato M, Phillips BG, et al. Nocturnal continuous positive airway pressure decreases daytime sympathetic traffic in obstructive sleep apnea. Circulation 1999; 100(23):2332–2335.

68. Peppard PE, Young T, Palta M, et al. Prospective study of the association between sleep-disordered breathing and hypertension. N Engl J Med 2000; 342(19):1378–1384.

69. Nieto FJ, Young TB, Lind BK, et al. Association of sleep-disordered breathing, sleep apnea, and hypertension in a large community-based study. Sleep Heart Health Study. JAMA 2000; 283(14):1829–1836.

70. Lavie P, Herer P, Hoffstein V. Obstructive sleep apnoea syndrome as a risk factor for hypertension: population study. BMJ 2000; 320(7233):479–482.

71. Partinen M, Guilleminault C. Daytime sleepiness and vascular morbidity at seven-year follow-up in obstructive sleep apnea patients. Chest 1990; 97(1):27–32.

72. Shahar E, Whitney CW, Redline S, et al. Sleep-disordered breathing and cardiovascular disease: cross-sectional results of the Sleep Heart Health Study. Am J Respir Crit Care Med 2001; 163(1):19–25.

73. Lanfranchi PA, Somers VK. Sleep-disordered breathing in heart failure: characteristics and implications. Respir Physiol Neurobiol 2003; 136(2–3):153–165.

74. Lavie L, Vishnevsky A, Lavie P. Evidence for lipid peroxidation in obstructive sleep apnea. Sleep 2004; 27(1):123–128.

75. Shamsuzzaman AS, Winnicki M, Lanfranchi P, et al. Elevated C-reactive protein in patients with obstructive sleep apnea. Circulation 2002; 105(21):2462–2464.

76. Becker HF, Jerrentrup A, Ploch T, et al. Effect of nasal continuous positive airway pressure treatment on blood pressure in patients with obstructive sleep apnea. Circulation 2003; 107(1):68–73.

77. Pepperell JC, Ramdassingh-Dow S, Crosthwaite N, et al. Ambulatory blood pressure after therapeutic and subtherapeutic nasal continuous positive airway pressure for obstructive sleep apnoea: a randomised parallel trial. Lancet 2002; 359(9302):204–210.

78. Kaneko Y, Floras JS, Usui K, et al. Cardiovascular effects of continuous positive airway pressure in patients with heart failure and obstructive sleep apnea. N Engl J Med 2003; 348(13):1233–1241.

79. Mansfield DR, Gollogly NC, Kaye DM, et al. Controlled trial of continuous positive airway pressure in obstructive sleep apnea and heart failure. Am J Respir Crit Care Med 2004; 169(3):361–366.
80. Marin JM, Carrizo SJ, Vicente E, et al. Long-term cardiovascular outcomes in men with obstructive sleep apnoea–hypopnoea with our without treatment with continuous positive airway pressure: an observational study. Lancet 2005; 365:1046–1053.
81. Qureshi AR, Ballard RD. Obstructive sleep apnea: Current review. J Allergy Clin Immunol 2003; 112:643–651.
82. Douglas NJ. Sleep in patients with chronic obstructive pulmonary disease. Clin Chest Med 1998; 19:116.

24 Legal Implications of Obstructive Sleep Apnea

Daniel B. Brown
Greenberg Traurig, LLP, Atlanta, Georgia, U.S.A.

INTRODUCTION

The legal implications of obstructive sleep apnea (OSA) derive principally from the debilitating effects of the disease on a patient's general health and wakeful actions. Medical science concludes that OSA causes sleep fragmentation, nocturnal hypoxia, and hypersomnia, which impairs daytime functioning, including work and driving performance (1,2). Untreated, the disease is an independent risk factor for cardiovascular diseases (3) and, in certain situations, can lead to death (4).

American jurisprudence adopts these causal connections to impose an array of legal duties on the range of foreseeably affected persons. For example, the law expects patients to acknowledge that OSA, once diagnosed and properly explained, is likely to impair their driving or work performance if left untreated (5). Employers with knowledge of their employee's habitual drowsiness due to OSA have a duty to recognize the disease as an impairment and to accommodate the employee's activities in a manner that does not threaten the safety of the general public. Industries touching directly on public safety, such as transportation services and nuclear power plants, consider OSA to be a factor in their fitness for duty programs.

Upon a finding that a sleep doctor has entered into a physician-patient relationship with his or her OSA patient, the law imbues the physician with the duty to diagnose and treat the disease in a manner consistent with the community's standard of care (6). Because untreated OSA can impair a patient's driving or other daytime activity, a physician may have additional legal and ethical obligations to unknown third parties to warn the patient against driving in an untreated, drowsy state (6).

This chapter reviews the brief legal history of sleep apnea in American jurisprudence and discusses how existing principles of tort, employment, administrative, criminal, and healthcare law have adapted to the diagnosis and treatment of OSA.

SURVEY OF SLEEP APNEA IN THE LAW

Although medical science first described OSA in 1973 (7), the first reference to OSA in any reported legal decision appeared seven years later in 1980 in the social security benefits case of *Parks v. Harris* (8). Claimant Parks sued to overturn his benefits denial on the basis of his recently diagnosed sleep apnea. A vocational expert testified that if Parks suffered from uncontrolled somnolence due to a sleep disorder, then Parks was likely disabled for purpose of the Social Security Act (8). Because continuous positive airway pressure (CPAP) treatment for OSA appeared a year later in 1981 (9), it is not surprising that the case failed to consider disease treatment as a factor in determining disability status.

Legal recognition of OSA as a disease grew slowly after *Parks*. Only 12 reported cases followed in the entire decade of the 1980s. The law's notice of OSA has increased significantly since 1990, with over 753 additional reported and nonreported federal and state cases mentioning sleep apnea in any context through March 10, 2006 (10).

Most of these cases contain only a passing reference to the disease in unrelated contexts (11). Only 44 cases make any reference to malpractice. Certain cases described below touch upon the principles discussed here.

LEGAL OBLIGATIONS OF PERSONS WITH OBSTRUCTIVE SLEEP APNEA

Tort law presupposes some uniform standard of reasonable conduct for the protection of others against unreasonable risks (12). As such, persons generally have a duty to conform their conduct in light of the apparent risk (13). Applied to persons suffering from disease, general negligence principles recognize that it is reasonable conduct for such persons to refrain from seeking treatment (14). Nonetheless, the law requires persons with specific types of infections or mental or physical conditions to take reasonable precautions to protect the health and well-being of third parties (15). Thus, persons who are aware of their sleep apnea and its effects on their daytime performance have joined the class of individuals charged with a duty to take reasonable precautions in light of their disease.

Reasonable Care and the "Sudden Blackout" Doctrine

The driver of a car has the general duty to exercise ordinary and reasonable due care in controlling his vehicle so as to avoid colliding with other persons and property (16). Under general negligence principles, a driver's breach of that duty in a manner that proximately causes damages to person or property will be held liable to the injured party (5). However, the law has long recognized that damages caused by a driver's sudden and unforeseen onset of sleep while driving does not constitute negligence (17). The rationale for this "sudden blackout" rule derives, in part, on an examination in 1925 by the Connecticut Supreme Court of early 20th century medical understandings of sleep physiology (18).

The 1925 case of *Bushnell v. Bushnell* (18) involved an action brought by Mrs. Bushnell against her husband for injuries she sustained when Mr. Bushnell, then 61, fell asleep at the wheel and crashed their car into a tree. The couple was returning home to Connecticut after taking their son to school at Brown College in Providence, Rhode Island. The issue was whether Mr. Bushnell's momentary lapse into sleep constituted negligence on his part.

The Court reasoned that a person under the influence of sleep possess neither sense nor perception. Therefore, the issue of legal responsibility for his conduct could not be resolved by determining whether or not he exercised reasonable care during the period of his unconsciousness. The issue of the driver's legal responsibility instead turned on whether "he exercised such care in permitting himself to lose consciousness in the first instance" (18).

Granted this premise, Mr. Bushnell's lawyer argued that his client could not be charged with negligence because "no man can tell when sleep will fall upon him"

(18). The Court cited contemporary medical literature to dispute the implication that sleep comes about unheralded:

> Purves Stewart, in his "Diagnosis of Nervous Diseases," 3rd ed., page 423, thus describes the chief phenomena of ordinary, healthy sleep: "Firstly, there is diminution and then loss of conscious recognition of ordinary stimuli, such as would ordinarily attract our attention, whether these stimuli be derived from the outer world or from within the sleeper's own organism. There is also, as consciousness is becoming blunted, a characteristic and indescribable sense of well-being. Voluntary movements become languid and ultimately cease, and the muscles of the limbs relax. Meanwhile there develops double ptosis or drooping of the eyelids; the pupils contract; the respiratory movements become slower and deeper, the pulse is slowed, the cutaneous vessels dilate to a slight extent and the general temperature of the body falls, whilst many processes of metabolism, such as those of digestion and of certain secretions, are retarded.

Citing the *American Journal of Physiology*, the Court continued:

> Particularly would this be true where the onset of sleep is due to the prolonged action of a uniform excitant, associated with little voluntary movement and a large degree of muscular relaxation, acting upon one who has become more or less fatigued and is sitting down in a warm atmosphere." 66 American Journal of Physiology, pp. 83, 84 (19).

On the basis of this medical evidence, the Court determined that sleep does not ordinarily come about unawares and that a driver retains control either to stay awake or to stop driving (19). As such, the Court ruled that the jury had the right to hear Mr. Bushnell's testimony regarding the unexpected suddenness of his sleep episode.

The ultimate holding in *Bushnell* not only adopts the "sudden blackout" defense but also points to its limited scope. To benefit from the rule, the loss of consciousness must occur suddenly, without warning, and be unforeseeable (20). As pointed out by the Tennessee Supreme Court, "the key to establishing the physical capacity or loss of consciousness defense is foreseeability" (21).

Thus, depending on the jurisdiction, the defense fails if the driver knew he or she were becoming drowsy or if the driver ignores the treatment regimen prescribed to subdue the symptoms leading to loss of consciousness. Courts differ in the application of the foreseeable rule. Some courts hold that any driver suffering from a medical disorder capable of producing a seizure or unconsciousness is liable, as a matter of law, for driving at all (22). Other courts hold that the sudden blackout defense is inappropriate if the driver was aware of facts sufficient to cause a reasonably prudent person to anticipate that his driving would lead to an accident (21).

Under these principles, knowledge of one's sleep apnea and a propensity for drowsy driving alone will likely be insufficient to invoke the defense. An OSA driver who has been properly warned against sleepy driving and placed on a treatment regimen would very likely have knowledge sufficient to make a sleep episode foreseeable. Thus, much like the diabetic driver who crashed after he skipped lunch and felt hypoglycemic, but neglected to stop and eat (23), the sleepiness of a noncompliant CPAP driver with OSA is likely foreseeable, opening the recalcitrant OSA patient to liability for injuries caused by falling asleep at the wheel.

Criminal Responsibility for Recklessness

The political logic of exculpatory doctrines like the "sudden blackout" rule became apparent in the New Jersey case seeking criminal vehicular homicide penalties for the driver who killed college student Margaret "Maggie" McConnell in 1997. The driver admitted to police that he had smoked crack cocaine hours before his car crashed into Ms. McConnell and that he had not slept for 30 hours leading up to the crash (24). The New Jersey district Attorney intended to use evidence of the driver's fatigue to prove reckless behavior under the statute. The judge refused to admit evidence of the driver's sleep deprivation and the jury acquitted the driver (24).

In response to the token $200 penalty assessed against the driver, the New Jersey legislature introduced legislation in 2002 to establish driving while fatigued as recklessness under that state's vehicular homicide statute (25). Amended significantly in the 14 months leading up to its passage, the law, known as "Maggie's Law," is an evidentiary rule providing that proof of driving after 24 consecutive hours of sleeplessness "*may* give rise to an inference that the defendant was driving recklessly" (emphasis added) (26). Fatigue in the law should be contrasted with inebriation, which the New Jersey legislature determined in the Maggie's Law amendment to be a condition which "*shall* give rise to an inference that the defendant was driving recklessly" (26) (emphasis added). Interestingly, the law also provides that falling asleep while driving, whether due to sleep deprivation or not, may also infer recklessness (26).

Though less than advertised, the law does change the legal landscape regarding liability for drowsy driving, at least in New Jersey. First, it provides New Jersey prosecutors the opportunity to infer recklessness from sleep deprivation for purposes of convicting drivers of criminal homicide. Next, it sets a benchmark for employers who schedule employees for consecutive periods approaching 24 hours. Finally, and perhaps unintentionally, it chips away at any "sudden blackout" defense available in New Jersey because the inference of recklessness may arise anytime a driver falls asleep at the wheel, regardless of the foreseeability of the sleep episode.

LEGAL DUTIES OF PHYSICIANS WITH REGARD TO OBSTRUCTIVE SLEEP APNEA

As with the treatment of all disease states, physicians owe their OSA patients a duty to diagnose and treat the disease in a manner consistent with the standard of ordinary care in the community (6). Thus, upon establishment of the physician-patient relationship, a treating physician incurs legal duties to the patient to not only diagnose and treat the disease but also to inform the patient of the risks and possible outcomes of treatment modalities (27). Depending on the severity of the disease, a physician's legal duties may include the duty to warn the patient against driving (28) and, under certain state motor vehicle laws, to report the patient's condition to the state department of motor vehicles (29). Failure to warn against driving in light of a foreseeable risk of harm to others may extend the physician's legal liability beyond the patient to unknown third parties (30).

Physician's Duties to Their Obstructive Sleep Apnea Patients
Physician-Patient Relationship
An essential element of any medical malpractice action is the existence of a physician-patient relationship (31). Absence of a professional relationship between the physician and the patient, the physician owes no legal duty to the patient or others (31). Because polysomnographic data are easily digitized, instantly transmitted, and

clearly reproduced on a video monitor or a compact printer, the sleep specialist's interpretation of the test can occur anytime and at any place. Often the physician's diagnosis of OSA occurs without the physician examining or even speaking with the patient. Questions may arise whether the sleep study patient and the distant reading physician have established a physician-patient relationship for purposes of a malpractice action.

The trend in recent case law is for courts to imply the existence of a physician-patient relationship among physicians unknown to the patient if the physician affirmatively undertakes to diagnose and/or treat the patient (32). A Texas case, *Dougherty v. Gifford* (33), is instructive. There, the patient's specialist sent a biopsy to his contracted pathologist who practiced in the regional medical center in Paris, Texas. The pathologist diagnosed cancer and aggressive treatments ensued, only to be discontinued when the pathologist admitted to having misread the biopsy (34).

Like most distant readers of sleep tests, the pathologist in Paris never intended to create a professional relationship with the patient. The pathologist never met the patient, did not review the patient's records, and only reviewed the specimen provided. The pathologist communicated the results to the patient's treating physician, who retained primary responsibility for the patient's care (35).

Nonetheless, the court found on these facts that a physician-patient relationship was created by the acceptance of the pathology work, the conduction of the tests, the preparation of a lab report, and the acceptance of a fee for the services rendered. The court stated that there could be no doubt that the diagnostic services furnished on behalf of the patient constituted the practice of medicine (36). As stated by the Tennessee Supreme Court in a similar case:

> In light of the increasing complexity of the health care system, in which patients routinely are diagnosed by pathologists or radiologists or other consulting physicians who might not ever see the patient face-to-face, it is simply unrealistic to apply a narrow definition of the physician-patient relationship in determining whether such a relationship exists for purposes of a medical malpractice case. Based upon the foregoing authorities, we hold that a physician-patient relationship may be implied when a physician affirmatively undertakes to diagnose and/or treat a person, or affirmatively participates in such diagnosis and/or treatment (37).

Telemedicine Aspects of the Physician-Patient Relationship

The free flow of sleep data to physicians who are not only invisible to the patient but also reside in a state different from the patient challenges traditional notions of the physician's license to practice medicine. All states have adopted laws which define the types of activity constituting the practice of medicine within their borders. Such laws generally prohibit persons from engaging in the unlicensed practice of medicine, and further punish physicians for aiding and assisting others in the unlicensed practice of medicine.

The threshold question is whether the professional interpretation of a sleep study constitutes the practice of medicine. Although each state defines the practice of medicine somewhat differently, the recent trend is for states to include the interpretation of diagnostic tests within the practice of medicine definition. Colorado's practice of medicine definition, which specifically includes the interpretation of tests, is representative. In full, the Colorado law provides that:

> Practice of medicine In Colorado means holding out one's self to the public within this state as being able to diagnose, treat, prescribe for, palliate, or prevent any human

disease, ailment, pain, injury, deformity, or physical or mental condition, whether by the use of drugs, surgery, manipulation, electricity, telemedicine, *the interpretation of tests*, including primary diagnosis of pathology specimens, images, or photographs, or any physical, mechanical, or other means whatsoever (38) (emphasis added).

At least 14 states have passed legislation specifically restricting the practice of telemedicine across state lines. For example, the Missouri statute defines the "practice of medicine across state lines" to mean:

1. The rendering of a written or otherwise documented medical opinion concerning the diagnosis or treatment of a patient within this state by a physician located outside this state as a result of transmission of individual patient data by electronic or other means from within this state to such physician or physician's agent; or
2. The rendering of treatment to a patient within this state by a physician located outside this state as a result of transmission of individual patient data by electronic or other means from within this state to such physician or physician's agent, definition (39).

An Oregon law specifically issues a special purpose license to outside physicians to practice within Oregon by distant communications, but only after the physician has first personally examined the patient (40). Other states, such as Alabama, issue a three-year special purpose license (41).

If the interpretation of the sleep study constitutes the practice of medicine, the next question is "which licensing authority governs?" The general rule in malpractice actions is that the patient's location at the time of service determines the location where the treatment occurs (42). As stated by the Ninth Circuit Court of Appeals in *Wright v. Yackley* (43):

> In the case of personal services focus must be on the place where the services are rendered, since this is the place of the receiver's (here the patient's) need. This need is personal and the services rendered are in response to the dimensions of that personal need. They are directed to no place but to the needy person herself.

Although improper licensure may not, by itself, indicate negligence in all malpractice actions (44), proper licensure can be a condition to the presentation of a clean, nonfraudulent claim to a government healthcare program for reimbursement (45).

Physician's Duties to Diagnose and Treat Obstructive Sleep Apnea

Upon establishment of the physician-patient relationship, a physician owes his patient the duty of reasonable care present in the community when treating his patient (31). A 1993 Louisiana case found a hospital and its physicians liable for the death of patient William Cornett as a result of the defendants' failure to treat the decedent's OSA (6). Mr. Cornett suffered from acromegaly, a generally nonmalignant pituitary tumor causing excessive secretion of growth hormones and the resulting enlargement of facial features, limbs, and soft tissues of the body (46). The condition may cause OSA, from which Mr. Cornett also suffered (46).

In March 1986, a family practice resident at the defendant hospital examined Mr. Cornett, who complained of chest pains and sleep apnea. The resident referred the patient to the hospital's endocrinology clinic for acromegaly. The hospital failed to schedule the appointment (46).

Seven months later, Mr. Cornett presented at the hospital's emergency room believing he was in a diabetic coma. He again explained his four- to five-year history of sleep apnea, and Mr. Cornett fell asleep during his diabetes testing, which proved negative. Concerned about Mr. Cornett's somnolence, the emergency room physician ordered arterial blood gas testing, which indicated elevated carbon dioxide levels and low oxygen levels. The emergency room physician testified at trial that Mr. Cornett requested treatment for sleep apnea because he had fallen asleep while driving. The doctor diagnosed acromegaly and sleep apnea. To confirm the diagnosis of acromegaly, the physician ordered diagnostic tests at the hospital's endocrinology clinic. These tests confirmed the diagnosis of the pituitary condition (47).

Mr. Cornett presented at the endocrinology clinic two weeks later when a different hospital physician confirmed a diagnosis of acromegaly and central hypoxia. This physician ordered pulmonary function testing at the hospital's chest clinic, but Mr. Cornett died before his scheduled appointment date. The cause of death was documented as cardiopulmonary arrest as a consequence of pituitary tumor (47).

Expert testimony at trial indicated that Mr. Cornett's death was more likely caused by sleep apnea and, had the hospital and its physicians provided appropriate medical treatment for OSA, Mr. Cornett would have survived. The last two hospital physicians who examined Mr. Cornett acknowledged that OSA is a potentially fatal condition. Each also testified that they failed to inform Mr. Cornett of the risk of death presented by untreated sleep apnea. The hospital's own medical expert acknowledged that sleep apnea may lead to life-threatening cardio-respiratory events and that the disease is a recognized emergency. The appellate court affirmed the trial court's holding the hospital and the physicians liable for professional negligence (48).

Physician's Duty to Obtain Patient's Informed Consent for Obstructive Sleep Apnea Surgery

Physicians have a general duty to provide their patients with sufficient information concerning their diagnosis, the nature and reason for the proposed treatment, the risks or dangers involved, the prospects for success and alternatives methods of treatment and the risks and benefits of such treatment (49). An unpublished decision of the Tennessee Court of Appeals discusses a physician's duty to inform a sleep apnea patient of CPAP treatment before performing uvulopalatopharyngoplasty (UPPP) (50).

The case involved a board-certified otolaryngologist who scheduled a nonurgent tonsillectomy for his 49-year-old male patient. The patient asked whether the procedure would help his snoring. Examining the patient further, the physician diagnosed mild sleep apnea and recommended surgical treatment. The patient testified at trial that he heard the doctor say that the doctor would trim his uvula, but the physician's notes indicated "surgery discussed, risks, and complications, schedule tonsillectomy, septoplasty, UVPP (uvulopharyngoplasty)" (51). In fact, the defendant physician performed the UPPP procedure. At no time did the physician advise his patient as to any nonsurgical alternatives to remedy his snoring.

The patient suffered various neurological disorders following the surgery and brought a malpractice action against the physician. Plaintiff based his claim on the physician's failure to inform his patient of noninvasive alternatives and failure to inform him of the diagnosis of OSA so that the patient could be properly informed of risks that stemmed from that diagnosis. In support, Plaintiff's medical expert testified that the physician should have informed Plaintiff of noninvasive snoring treatments, such as CPAP and laser surgery. The expert further testified that the physician should have ordered a sleep study to determine the presence of sleep apnea and the severity of the condition. However, on cross-examination, the expert admitted that even he did not send all of his patients who presented with OSA symptoms for a sleep study and that a sleep study was not required to identify the location in the throat that caused the snoring (52).

The physician presented the medical testimony of two fellow otolaryngologists. These doctors testified that the treating physician informed the patient of the procedure and risks consistent with the standards of the community. The jury also considered the broad language of the written consent form signed by the patient. On the basis of the expert testimony and the patient's written consent, the jury determined that the physician properly informed his patient and found for the physician (53).

What is unknown is a physician's responsibility to recognize the documented link between sleep apnea and hypertension, cardiovascular disease, and other diseases (3) when performing routine examinations. The *Cornett* case discussed above indicates the risks attendant to physicians who fail to recognize the urgency of the disease. Increased awareness of sleep medicine and recognition by the American Board of Medical Specialties of sleep medicine as a subspecialty (54) may bring minimum sleep inquiries into the community standard of practice for cardiologists, pulmonologists or family practice physicians whose patients present with typical OSA markers.

Physician's Duties and Liabilities to Third Parties for the Acts of Their Obstructive Sleep Apnea Patients
Duty to Warn and Report Impaired Driving
Because hypersomnolence generally follows untreated OSA, a physician may have additional legal and ethical duties to the public to inform the patient of the risks of fatigued driving caused by the failure or refusal to treat the disease. In appropriate cases, the physician may be required by law to report the patient's condition to applicable state motor vehicle agencies.

Although no case found expressly discusses a physician's duty to third parties in the context of an OSA patient, under the proper facts, a physician owes a duty to use reasonable care to protect the driving public if the physician's negligence in diagnosis or treatment of his patient contributes to Plaintiff's injuries (55).

One principal case holds that a physician who "takes charge" of a patient whom the physician knew or should have known was likely to cause bodily harm to others adopts the duty of reasonable care to prevent the patient from causing harm to others (56). However, courts readily distinguish a physician's prescribing narcotic drugs or similar treatment plans from situations in which the physician "takes charge" of the patient. The courts reason "that whether the patient takes the medication and then drives is beyond the doctor's control. In fact, whether the patient consumes the medication at all is beyond the doctor's control" (57). This same result would logically follow upon an injury caused by an OSA patient's failure to comply with his or her CPAP treatment.

However, the law requires a physician to warn the patient of the risks flowing from the use or misuse of the treatment (58). In *Gooden v. Tips* (59), a physician prescribed Quaalude tablets for his patient but failed to warn her not to drive under its influence. The patient's drug-induced driving injured third parties, who brought suit against the physician. The court ruled that the physician was liable to the injured third parties not because the physician had a duty to prevent his patient from driving, but because the physician had the duty to warn the patient not to drive, which he failed to do (30). A treating physician may have a similar duty to warn an OSA patient that the disease may cause a risk of drowsy driving if left untreated or treated improperly.

In addition to legal duties under common law negligence, physicians may have a statutory obligation to report impaired driving to the department of motor vehicles. For example, Vermont, Oregon, New Jersey, California, Delaware, Pennsylvania, and Nevada require physicians to report specific disorders of their patients to appropriate state agencies, typically the state department of motor vehicles (60). Other states permit physicians to report their patients' impaired driving conditions, but do not require reporting. Still other state laws permit the report to be made anonymously, while some laws offer physicians complete immunity from liability if they have reported the patient's condition to the applicable agency prior to a patient's injury (61).

According to the American Medical Association's "Physician's Guide to Assessing and Counseling Older Drivers," patients with a diagnosis of narcolepsy should cease driving altogether (62). The Guide suggests that patients with sleep apnea may drive if they do not suffer excessive daytime drowsiness as a consequence of therapy or otherwise (63). Physicians in reporting states should check with the department of motor vehicles in their states to determine if a sleep disorder is a specified condition for which reporting is required.

Even if reporting is not required, physicians face legal and ethical dilemmas if they judge the patient unfit to drive but the patient refuses to comply. In 2000, the American Medical Association adopted Ethical Opinion E-2.24 to address physicians' ethical obligations in this regard (63). According to the Opinion, if clear evidence of substantial driving impairment implies a "strong threat" to patient and public safety, and if the patient ignores the advice to discontinue driving, then the AMA believes it is desirable and ethical for the physician to notify the applicable department of motor vehicles. However, the Opinion clarifies that the physician must follow state law if reporting is required. The Opinion also advises that physicians should disclose and explain their responsibility to report to their patients.

Reporting a patient's impaired driving condition impacts an array of legal issues, including patient confidentiality. If a state law requires or permits disclosure, patient authorization may be required prior to the disclosure. The Privacy Standards applicable to protected health information under the Health Insurance Portability and Accountability Act of 1996 (HIPAA) will not stand in the way if state law requires or permits disclosure without authorization. HIPAA permits healthcare providers to disclose protected health information without individual authorization as "required by law" (64) or to avert a serious threat to health or safety (65). However, HIPAAs provisions yield to more stringent state laws. Accordingly, prior patient authorization may still be required under state law even though HIPAA may permit an unauthorized disclosure.

LEGAL OBLIGATIONS OF PERSONS EMPLOYING OBSTRUCTIVE SLEEP APNEA PATIENTS

Because science and the law recognize OSA as an impairment which, if untreated, may adversely affect work performance and safety, the law imposes distinct legal duties on employers of OSA patients. These duties include taking reasonable accommodations to the extent required by federal and state disability laws, vicarious liability for the acts of drowsy employees, and, in certain industries, the adoption of fitness for duty standards that recognize the risks posed by employees with sleep apnea.

Disability Laws

The Americans with Disabilities Act (ADA) (66), along with the Rehabilitation Act of 1973 (67) and similar state civil rights laws (68), prohibits discrimination by certain employers against qualified individuals with a disability (69). A "qualified individual" is one who is capable of performing the essential function of a job with or without reasonable accommodations (70). For example, if driving is an essential function of one's job and if an employee cannot safely drive due to his combined conditions of severe OSA, narcolepsy and cataplexy, then the employee is not a "qualified individual" eligible for ADA protections (71). The same holds true if sleep apnea prevents an employee from working overtime in his job as a power company lineman when working overtime shifts is an essential function of being a lineman (72). If the employee is not a qualified individual, then the employer has no obligation under the ADA to make the employee's job easier or even to make the job available at all (73).

Qualified individuals have often claimed OSA is an ADA disability and that such persons therefore deserve redress for lost employee benefits, promotions or even their jobs due to their disability. However, the allegation of a particular diagnosis, standing alone, is insufficient to establish a disability under the ADA (74). The answer whether OSA is an ADA disability requires an individualized, case-by-case approach to evaluate whether the employee's impairment is severe enough to constitute a disability for ADA purposes (75). Thus, the proper legal inquiry in such matters is not whether sleep apnea is a disability for purposes of ADAs protections, but whether the individual's sleep apnea substantially limits his or her major life activities as those terms are defined by the ADA.[1]

To establish a *prima facie* case of discrimination under the ADA, the employee must show that: (*i*) he is disabled within the meaning of the ADA, (*ii*) he is qualified to perform the essential functions of his job either with or without reasonable accommodation, and (*iii*) he has suffered from an adverse employment decision because of his disability (76).

To prove the existence of a disability, the employee must show that (*i*) he suffers from an impairment; (*ii*) the impairment affects major life activities; and (*iii*) the impairment "substantially limits" such major life activities (77).

Although the ADA does not define "impairment," regulations promulgated under the ADA by the Employee Equal Opportunities Commission do (78). These regulations define a physical or mental impairment to include, in part, any physiological disorder or condition affecting a person's neurological, musculoskeletal, respiratory or cardiovascular systems (79).

---

[1]Under certain circumstances sleep apnea is considered a disability for some federal benefit programs, such as Veteran's Affairs, 38 CFR § 4.97. Persons seeking social security disability benefits must prove that they have a "disability," which is defined to mean the "inability to engage in any substantial gainful activity" due to a "physical or mental impairment" that could cause death or might reasonably be expected to last continuously for at least twelve months. *See* 42 U.S.C. § 423(d) (1) (A).

Courts discussing OSA in the context of these ADA regulations routinely find—and employers routinely concede—that OSA is a physical impairment in satisfaction of the first prong of the analysis (80). Sleep apnea affects one's ability to breathe during sleep. As a consequence, one may not achieve a sound sleep at night and may drop off to sleep uncontrollably during the work day. This condition could reasonably be considered a respiratory disorder within the definition of "physical impairment" (81).

The second prong of the test requires that the impairment affect a major life activity. The regulations make clear that "breathing" is included in the definition of a "major life activity" for purposes of meeting the ADA test (78). "Sleeping," however, is conspicuously absent from the regulatory list of major life activities. ADA claimants with OSA can finesse the point by claiming that their sleep apnea substantially limits their breathing during sleep, thus impacting both activities (82).

In fact, most courts interpret ADA regulations to find that "sleeping" is a major life activity for ADA purposes (83). "Sleeping is a basic activity that the average person in the general population can perform with little or no difficulty, similar to the major life activities" that do appear in the regulations: walking, seeing, hearing, speaking, breathing, learning, and working (84). Interestingly, courts have also ruled that staying awake, in and of itself, is not a major life activity (85), and that general sleeplessness is insufficient to show a significant impairment to one's activity of sleeping (86).

Having determined that sleep apnea is an "impairment" affecting a "major life activity," the determination whether sleep apnea is a disability under the ADA depends, in each case, whether the claimant can prove that sleep apnea substantially limits the claimant's sleep or breathing for purposes of ADA protection. Such proof must satisfy yet another three part evaluation relative to (*i*) the nature and severity of the impairment; (*ii*) the duration or expected duration of the impairment; and (*iii*) the permanent long-term impact, or the expected permanent or long-term impact of or resulting from the impairment (87). In addition, courts will consider the measures used by the claimant to mitigate or treat his condition (86), such as, in the case of sleep apnea, CPAP (82).

The courts recognize that a determination of ADA disability for persons with OSA depends on the severity of the impairment, which presents in a wide spectrum:

> In general terms sleep apnea can be so severe such that it does impact on the major life activity of sleep. [Citation omitted]. Sleep apnea, however, is also a condition that varies in severity from very mild asymptomatic snoring to severe snoring and extremely restless sleep with extreme daytime hypersomnolence or excessive sleepiness during the day (88).

The use of CPAP therapy to correct or mitigate OSA symptoms is a key factor in determining the severity of the employee's disease in the determination of ADA disability. Thus, in a situation where common OSA therapies such as CPAP and surgery failed to alleviate an employee's fatigue resulting from severe sleep apnea, the United States District Court of Eastern Pennsylvania permitted the jury to consider whether the employee's OSA constituted a severe impairment for ADA disability purposes (89).

Cases involving successful use of CPAP reach different conclusions (90). The case of an obese police officer, 46-year-old Ike Mont-Ros, is instructive (82). Officer Mont-Ros was diagnosed with sleep apnea in 1993. His employer paid for his CPAP machine to alleviate his symptoms and, when Officer Mont-Ros' knees became too brittle for regular police work, accommodated Mont-Ros' request for light-duty, daytime dispatch duties. Armed with a physician's opinion that Officer Mont-Ros was not qualified to perform police work due to his orthopedic problems, the police department fired Officer Mont-Ros on grounds that he was hired originally to perform police duties at police officer pay, not civilian dispatch duties compensated at lower rates. Mont-Ros sued the City of West Miami for intentional discrimination against him due to his sleep apnea disability.

Using the applicable three-part tests, the court held that Officer Mont-Ros failed to provide sufficient evidence to support his contention that his sleep apnea constituted a disability under the ADA. While expert testimony showed that OSA is a severe, potentially life-threatening disease, Mont-Ros failed to show the severity of the disease in his specific case. Finally, the court noted that because OSA is treatable and can be corrected with the use of CPAP at night, Officer Mont-Ros could not demonstrate that he is substantially limited in any major life activity. As Officer Mont-Ros' own medical expert point out, "much like the use of glasses to correct ones vision, the use of the nasal CPAP machine at night will alleviate Plaintiff's condition during sleeping hours and, thus, reduce the daytime drowsiness (91)." Thus, in the worker's compensation context, OSA patients using CPAP earn no impairment ratings because "treated OSA has no permanent disability" (92).

Employers' Liability for Employee's Negligence
The application of traditional vicarious liability rules renders employers vicariously liable for the acts of their employees when performed in the scope of their employment (93). Thus, when Norman Munnal killed a woman when he fell asleep at the wheel of a tractor-trailer while driving for his trucking company employer, it was W.L. Logan Trucking Company that faced liability for its driver's acts (94). The trucking company invoked Ohio's version of the "sudden blackout" doctrine to defend Munnal's conduct (95). The employer alleged that it was the driver's "sudden unconsciousness" that caused the truck to move left of center, and that Munnal cannot be liable for losing control under these circumstances (95).

As we have seen, the sudden blackout defense fails if defendant knew that consciousness loss was likely to occur or was otherwise foreseeable (95). Munnal testified that he had a propensity to fall asleep at unpredictable times and that he had fallen asleep at the wheel at least once before (96). A sleep test ordered after the accident revealed that he suffered from severe OSA (96). At trial, Munnal's sleep disorders specialist opined that many sleep apnea patients engage in automatic behavior, such as driving, while unknowingly unconscious (97). The expert distinguished automatic behavior from fainting following a sudden blackout, and opined that distance truck driving was not the right profession for someone with untreated sleep apnea (96).

Even though Munnal testified that he had no knowledge of his sleep apnea before the accident (96), the court ruled that the employee driver was aware of his excessive fatigue and propensity to falling asleep at inopportune times (98). Because of this prior knowledge, the court held Munnal negligent for failing to operate the truck in a safe manner, and further found Munnal's employer trucking company liable for the driver's acts while in the scope of his employment (98). Under the rule in this case, employers' risk management programs would likely benefit from an employee OSA screening and therapy compliance program for employees working at safety-sensitive tasks such as driving.

Employers are also exposed to allegations of direct liability if they negligently hire persons with OSA and entrust vehicles to them. To prevail on these direct liability allegations, the injured party must prove that the employee's fatigue was due to the disease, was known to the employer, and proximately caused the accident leading to damages (99).

Growing awareness of general sleep health and expressions of public policy against drowsy driving of the kind codified in New Jersey by Maggie's law and New York's Bell Regulations (limiting medical residents' work hours) (100) sets the stage for actions against employers brought by unknown third parties injured by overworked, and likely fatigued, employees.

The legal question in such circumstances is whether the employer owes a duty to control the off-duty conduct of its employee. Although the general rule is that employers owe no duty to third parties for the off-duty acts of their employees, (101) at least one court has re-fashioned tort principles to find an employer liable for accidents caused by employees presumably fatigued due to over-scheduling by their employer (102). The same result obtains on similar facts under workmen's compensation law (103).

Regulatory Screening for Obstructive Sleep Apnea in Safety-Sensitive Positions

Because sleep apnea is a relatively common medical condition which, if untreated, contributes to daytime sleepiness and impaired job performance (2), public policy suggests that certain industries directly affecting public safety screen employees in safety-sensitive positions for sleep apnea or other fatigue-enhancing sleep disorders. Thus, each of the air, rail, ferry, distance trucking, and nuclear power industries have or propose regulatory fitness for duty programs addressing OSA.

The National Transportation Safety Board (NTSB) has issued three investigation reports finding that the undiagnosed or untreated OSA of a train or ship operator contributed to the subject incident (104). The latest, in 2004, involved a 2001 collision of two trains arising from the crewmembers' fatigue caused primarily by the engineer's untreated and the conductor's insufficiently treated OSA (105). The 2004 NTSB Report recommended that the Federal Railroad Administration (FRA) take remedial steps regarding employee fatigue (106), and the FRA issued its Safety Advisory 2004-04 on September 21, 2004 in response. The Advisory suggests that railroads adopt procedures to recognize sleep disorders, screen employees, and permit impaired persons to perform safety-sensitive tasks only after proper treatment (107).

Federal regulations require that only physically fit persons are eligible to operate a commercial motor vehicle in interstate commerce (108). Persons are considered physically fit if they obtain medical certification from a physician certifying that the applicant does not have an established medical history or clinical diagnosis of, among other ailments, a respiratory dysfunction or other condition which is likely to cause loss of consciousness or any other loss of ability to control a commercial motor vehicle safely (109). The current Medical Examination Form, updated in 2000, makes specific inquiry whether the applicant suffers from "sleep disorders, pauses in breathing while asleep, daytime sleepiness, (or) loud snoring (110)."

In 1991, the Federal Motor Carrier Safety Administration published advisory criteria to assist medical examiners determine a driver's physical qualifications for commercial driving. The guidance regarding pulmonary/respiratory disorders identifies OSA as a condition which, if untreated, renders applicants unqualified to operate a commercial vehicle:

> Individuals with suspected or untreated sleep apnea (symptoms of snoring and hypersomnolence) should be considered medically unqualified to operate a commercial vehicle until the diagnosis has been dispelled or the condition has been treated successfully. In addition, as a condition of continuing qualification, commercial drivers who are being treated for sleep apnea should agree to continue uninterrupted therapy as long as they maintain their commercial driver's license. They should also undergo yearly multiple sleep latency testing (MSLT) (111).

Guidance respecting seizures, epilepsy and interstate commercial driving reaches a similar conclusion as to chronic sleep apnea:

> Patients with sleep apnea syndrome having symptoms of excessive daytime somnolence cannot take part in interstate driving, because they likely will be involved in hazardous driving and accidents resulting from sleepiness. Even if these patients do not have the sleep attacks, they suffer from daytime fatigue and tiredness. These symptoms will be compounded by the natural fatigue and monotony associated with the long hours of driving, thus causing increased vulnerability to accidents. Therefore, those patients who are not on any treatment and are suffering from symptoms related to EDS should not be allowed to participate in interstate driving. Those patients with sleep apnea syndrome whose symptoms (e.g., EDS, fatigue, etc.) can be controlled by surgical treatment, for example, permanent tracheostomy, may be permitted to drive after three-month period free of symptoms, provided there is constant medical supervision. Laboratory studies (e.g., polysomnographic and MSLTs) must be performed to document absence of EDS and sleep apnea (112).

As to pilots, the Federal Aviation Administration Guide for Aviation Medical Examiners provides that any degree of sleep apnea is disqualifying for medical certification for all classes of pilots (113). However, aviation medical examiners may reissue a pilot's medical certificate without administrative appeal if the pilot presents a current report of a treating physician that the pilot's OSA treatment therapy has eliminated symptoms of the disease along with specific comments regarding the pilot's daytime sleepiness (114).

In 1989, the Nuclear Regulatory Commission (NRC) adopted its first Fitness for Duty Program focusing on detection of drug and alcohol impairments on personnel with access to protected areas of nuclear power reactors licensed by the NRC (115). Congressmen and others petitioned the NRC to expand the regulations to expand the program to include screening for sleep apnea and other disorders. The NRC published proposed rules to that effect in August 2005 (116).

LAWS REGULATING DIAGNOSTIC TESTING AND TREATMENT OF OBSTRUCTIVE SLEEP APNEA
State Certificate of Need and Licensure Laws
The majority of states allocate healthcare resources within their borders through the Certificate of Need (CON) process. Most CON laws require healthcare facilities, such as hospitals, magnetic resonance imaging centers and other outpatient diagnostic centers, to apply for and receive a CON prior to obtaining a state license or otherwise operating. Penalties for operating a healthcare facility without a CON range from civil fines to criminal penalties.

CON laws routinely exempt a variety of healthcare activities from the lengthy and expensive CON process. These exemptions include the individual or group practice of physicians and, in many cases, facilities requiring equipment or capital expenditures below a certain dollar threshold. A review of applicable CON laws is necessary to determine the impact on sleep testing.

States will typically require healthcare facilities such as nursing homes, ambulatory surgical centers, and some outpatient diagnostic testing facilities to obtain a license prior to operating. Because polysomnograms have historically been categorized for reimbursement and other purposes as an extensive electroencephalographic (EEG)–electrocardiographic (EKG) modality, states do not usually require separate facility licenses for sleep testing. However, a license may be required for freestanding sleep testing facilities. Again, review of applicable state laws will be necessary.

Self-Referral Laws
Providers of healthcare must comply with applicable fraud and abuse laws. The risk most relevant to OSA is the so-called federal "Stark" law prohibition on patient self-referrals and related state laws (117). The Stark law prohibits a physician from making a referral for a designated health service to an entity in which the physician (or an immediate family member of such physician) has a financial relationship—including a compensation arrangement—if the service is reimbursed by a federal healthcare program (including Medicaid). Only referrals for designated health services are prohibited. Professional readings for pulmonary function testing, EKGs and EEGs are not designated health services, unless furnished in a hospital setting (118). For this reason, polysomnography is also not considered to be a designated health service. However, items of durable medical equipment, including CPAP and bilevel pressure and related supplies, are designated healthcare services under the Stark law (119). Consequently, a physician may not refer anyone to an entity owned, directly or indirectly, by the physician or his immediate family, for CPAP if the entity seeks reimbursement from a federal healthcare program for the CPAP.

Many states have their own laws restricting self-referrals. Many are modeled after the federal Stark law and prohibit referrals for durable medical equipment regardless of government reimbursement. Some are more restrictive, others are less. A review of the law applicable to the states in which the physician practices is necessary to determine compliance.

REFERENCES
1. Sassani A, Findley LJ, Kryger M, et al. Reducing motor-vehicle collisions, costs, and fatalities by treating obstructive sleep apnea. Sleep 2004; 27(d):453, 458.
2. Kryger MH, Roth T, Dement WC, eds. Principles and Practice of Sleep Medicine. Philadelphia, PA: W.B. Sanders, 1994.
3. Shahar E, Whitney CW, Redline S, et al. Sleep-disordered breathing and cardiovascular disease: cross-sectional results of the Sleep Heart Health Study. Am J Respir Crit Care Med 2001; 163:19–25.
4. Campos-Rodriguez F, Peña-Griñan N, Reyes-Nuñez N, et al. Mortality in obstructive sleep apnea–hypopnea patients treated with positive airway pressure. Chest 2005; 128(2):624-633.
5. See, e.g., McCall v. Wilder, *913 S.W.2d 150* (Tenn. 1995).
6. Cornett v. State, W.O. Moss Hospital, 614 So.2d 189 (La. App. 3rd Cir. 1993).
7. Guilleminault C, Eldridge FL, Dement WC. Insomnia with sleep apnea: A new syndrome, Science 1973; 181(102):856–858.
8. Parks v. Harris, 614 F.2d 83 (5th Cir. 1980).
9. Sullivan CE, Issa FG, Berthon-Jones M, Eves L. Reversal of obstructive sleep apnea by continuous positive airway pressure applied through the nares. Lancet 1981; 1(8225): 862–865.

10. Results of a March 10, 2006, Westlaw inquiry of all reported and unreported cases for the mention of "sleep apnea" in any context in any state or federal court.
11. See, e.g., Besaraba v. State, 656 So.2d 441 (Fla. 1995), Edwards v. Edwards, 140 Or. App. 409 (1996).
12. William L. Prosser, Law of Torts, 4th ed, St. Paul: West Publishing Co., 1980:143.
13. William L. Prosser, Law of Torts, 4th ed, St. Paul: West Publishing Co., 1980:324.
14. See, e.g., Cruzan v. Missouri Department of Health, 497 U.S. 261, 110 S.Ct. 2841, 111 L.Ed.2d 224 (1990).
15. Eric L. Schulman, Note, Sleeping with the Enemy: Combatting (sic) the Sexual Spread of HIV-AIDS Through A Heightened Legal Duty, 29 J. MARSHALL L. REV. 957, 971–976, 1996.
16. American Law Reports 3d, Liability for Automobile Accident Allegedly Caused by Driver's Blackout, Sudden Unconsciousness, or the Like, Section 2(a), 93 A.L.R. 326 (1979), (updated 2006).
17. American Law Reports 2d, Physical Defect, Illness, Drowsiness, or Falling Asleep of Motor Vehicle Operator as Affecting Liability for Injury, Section 3, 28 A.L.R.2d 12 (1953), (updated 2006).
18. Bushnell v. Bushnell, 103 Conn. 583, 131 A. 432 (1925).
19. Bushnell v. Bushnell, 103 Conn. 583, 591, 131 A. 432 (1925).
20. See, e.g., Estate of Embry v. GEO Transportation of Indiana, Inc., 395 F. Supp 2d 516 (E.D. Ky 2005), McCall v. Wilder, *913 S.W.2d 150* (Tenn. 1995).
21. McCall v. Wilder, *913 S.W.2d 150, 155* (Tenn. 1995).
22. See, Malcolm v. Patrick, 147 So.2d 188 (Fla.Ct.App. 1962); accord Eleason v. Western Cas. & Sur. Co., 254 Wis. 134, 35 N.W.2d 301 (1948).
23. Howle v. PYA/Monarch, Inc., 288 S.C. App. 586, 344 S.E. 2d 157 (1986).
24. Testimony of Darrell Drobnich before the House Subcommittee on Highways and Transit, Committee on Transportation and Infrastructure, 4, June 27, 2002, http://www.house.gov/transportation/highway/06-27-02/drobnich.html, (accessed March 2006).
25. Chapter 143, 2003 New Jersey Public Laws.
26. "Maggie's Law," N.J.S.2C:11-5(a).
27. See, e.g., Robinson v. Bleicher, 251 Neb. 752, 559 N.W.2d 473 (1997).
28. See, e.g., Gooden v. Tips, 651 S.W.2d 364 (Tex. App. 1983) (as to physician's failure to warn a patient not to drive while under the influence of a prescribed drug).
29. See, e.g., U.S. Department of Transportation, National Highway Traffic Safety Administration, "Strategies for Medical Advisory Boards and Licensing Review," DOT HS 809 874 (July 2005), available at http://www.nhtsa.dot.gov/people/injury/research/MedicalAdvisory/index.html, (accessed March 2006).
30. See, e.g., Gooden v. Tips, 651 S.W.2d 364 (Tex. App. 1983).
31. Kelly v. Middle Tennessee Emergency Physicians, P.C., 133 S.W.3d 587, 592 (Tenn. 2004).
32. Kelly v. Middle Tennessee Emergency Physicians, P.C., 133 S.W.3d 587, 593 (Tenn. 2004).
33. Dougherty v. Gifford, 826 S.W.2d 668 (Tex. App. 1992).
34. Dougherty v. Gifford, 826 S.W.2d 668, 672 (Tex. App. 1992).
35. Dougherty v. Gifford, 826 S.W.2d 668, 674 (Tex. App. 1992).
36. Dougherty v. Gifford, 826 S.W.2d 668, 674, 675 (Tex. App. 1992).
37. Kelly v. Middle Tennessee Emergency Physicians, P.C., 133 S.W.3d at 596 (Tenn. 2004).
38. CRS § 12-36-106(1) (a).
39. Missouri Revised Statutes Section 334.010.
40. ORS § 847.025.0010.
41. Ala. Code § *34-24-502*.
42. Wright v. Yackley, 459 F.2d 287 (9th Cir. 1972).
43. Wright v. Yackley, 459 F.2d 287, 289 (9th Cir. 1972).
44. Andrews v. Lofton, 57 S.E.2d 338, 342 (Ga. App. 1950); Irwin v. Arrendale, 159 S.E.2d 719, 725 (Ga. App. 1967).
45. See, e.g., 42 CFR 410.33(e) (requiring the supervising physician of an independent diagnostic testing facility to be licensed in each state in which the facility operates); 31 U.S.C. § 3729.

46. Cornett v. State, W.O. Moss Hospital, 614 So.2d 189, 193 (La. App. 3rd Cir. 1993).
47. Cornett v. State, W.O. Moss Hospital, 614 So.2d 189, 194 (La. App. 3rd Cir. 1993).
48. Cornett v. State, W.O. Moss Hospital, 614 So.2d 189,196 (La. App. 3rd Cir. 1993).
49. See, e.g. Shadrick v. Coker, 963 S.W.2d 726, 732 (Tenn. 1998).
50. Russell v. Brown, No. E2004-01855-COA-R3-CV, 2005 WL 1991609 (Tenn.Ct.App.) (August 18, 2005).
51. Russell v. Brown, No. E2004-01855-COA-R3-CV, 2005 WL 1991609 *2 (Tenn.Ct.App.) (August 18, 2005).
52. Russell v. Brown, No. E2004-01855-COA-R3-CV, 2005 WL 1991609 *5 (Tenn.Ct.App.) (August 18, 2005).
53. Russell v. Brown, No. E2004-01855-COA-R3-CV, 2005 WL 1991609 *13 (Tenn.Ct.App.) (August 18, 2005).
54. See, The American Board of Medical Specialties, 2005 Annual Report & Reference Handbook, available at http://www.abms.org/Downloads/Publications/AnnualReport2005.pdf, (accessed March 2006).
55. See, e.g., Wharton Transport Corp. v. Bridges, 606 S.W.2d 521 (Tenn. 1980); Gooden v. Tips, 651 S.W.2d 364, 396 (Tex. App. Tyler 1983).
56. Tarasoff v. Regents of University of California, 17 Cal 3d 425, 131 Cal. Rptr 14, 551 P.2d 334 (1976).
57. Taylor v. Smith, 892 So.2d 887, 895 (Ala. 2004).
58. See, e.g., McKenzie v. Hawai'i Permanente Med. Group, Inc., 98 Hawai'i 296, 309, 47 P.3d 1209, 1222 (2002) (physician "owes a duty to non-patient third parties" to warn patients of possible adverse effects of prescribed medication on patients' driving ability, "where the circumstances are such that the reasonable patient could not have been expected to be aware of the risk without the physician's warning"); Joy v. Eastern Maine Med. Ctr., 529 A.2d 1364 (Me. 1987) (physician who treated a patient by placing a patch over his eye owed a duty to motorists to warn the patient against driving while wearing the patch); Welke v. Kuzilla, 144 Mich.App. 245, 252, 375 N.W.2d 403, 406 (1985) (physician who injected a patient with an "unknown substance" owed a duty to motorists "within the scope of foreseeable risk, by virtue of his special relationship with [the patient]"); Wilschinsky v. Medina, 108 N.M. 511, 515, 775 P.2d 713, 717 (1989) (physicians owe a duty "to persons injured by patients driving automobiles from a doctor's office when the patient has just been injected with drugs known to affect judgment and driving ability"); Zavalas v. State Dep't of Corr.,124 Ore.App. 166, 171, 861 P.2d 1026, 1028 (1993) (rejecting the argument "that a physician has no duty to third parties… who claim that the physician's negligent treatment of a patient was the foreseeable cause of their harm"). But see Kirk v. Michael Reese Hosp. & Med. Ctr., 117 Ill.2d 507, 513 N.E.2d 387, 111 Ill.Dec. 944 (1987); Rebollal v. Payne, 145 A.D.2d 617, 536 N.Y.S.2d 147 (1988).
59. Gooden v. Tips, 651 S.W.2d 364, 370 (Tex. App. Tyler 1983).
60. See, generally, Massachusetts Medical Society, "Medical Perspectives on Impaired Driving" (July, 2003), available at http://www.massmed.org/AM/Template.cfm?Section=Home&CONTENTID=5027&TEMPLATE=/CM/HTMLDisplay.cfm, (accessed March 2006).
61. American Medical Association, "Physician's Guide to Assessing and Counseling Older Drivers," Chapter 8 (May 2003), providing a list of all 51 state laws regarding reporting of impaired drivers. The Guide is available at the American Medical Society Website, http://www.ama-assn.org/ama/pub/category/10791.html, (accessed March 2006).
62. See, American Medical Association, "Physician's Guide to Assessing and Counseling Older Drivers," Chapter 8 (May 2003).
63. See, American Medical Society, Ethics Opinion E-2.24, "Impaired Drivers and Their Physicians," (June 2004), available at http:// www.ama-assn.org (accessed March 2006).
64. See, 42 C.F.R. § 164.512(a).
65. See, 42 C.F. R. § 164.512(j).
66. 42 U.S.C. §1201, et seq.
67. 29 U.S.C. § 791, et. seq.
68. See, e.g., Minnesota Human Rights Act, Minn.Stat. § 363.01, Wisconsin Fair Employment Act, Wisc. Stats § 111.34, Maine Human Rights Act, 5 M.R.S.A. §§ 4551–4634.

69. See, e.g., Sutton V. United Air Lines, Inc., 527 U.S. 471, 477, 119 S.Ct. 2139 (1999).
70. See, e.g., EEOC v. Amego, Inc., 110 F.3d 135, 144 (1st Cir. 1997).
71. Matewski v. Orkin Exterminating Co., 2003 WL 21516577 *12 (D. Maine, July 1, 2003).
72. Sanders v. Firstenergy Corp., 157 Ohio App. 3d 826, 834 (2004).
73. Calef v. Gillette Co., 322 F.2d 75, 86 (1st Cir. 2003).
74. Tice v. Centre Area Transportation Authority, 247 F.3d 506, 513 (3rd Cir. 2001).
75. Albertson's, Inc. v. Kirkingburg, 527 U.S. 555, 566 (1999).
76. Dvorak v. Mostardi Platt Assoc., Inc., 289 F.3d 479, 483 (7th Cir. 2002); Bekker v. Humana Health Plan, Inc., 229 F3d 662, 669-70 (7th Cir. 2000).
77. Bragdon v. Abbott, 524 U.S. 624, 631 (1998).
78. 29 CFR § 1630.02(h).
79. 29 CFR § 1630.02(h)(1).
80. See, e.g., Kolecyck-Yap v. MCI Worldcom, Inc., No. 99 CV 8414, 2001 WL 245531 (N.D. Ill. 2001), Peter v. Lincoln Technical Institute, Inc., 255 F. Supp 417. 431 (N.D. Ill 2002).
81. Miller v. Centennial State Bank, 472 N.W.2d 349, 351 (Minn. Ct. App. 1991).
82. Mont-Ros v. City of West Miami, 111 F. Supp.2d 1338 (S.D. Fla. 2000).
83. See, Pack v. Kmart Corp., 166 F.3d 1300, 1305 (10th Cir. 1999); McAlindin v. County of San Diego, 192 F.3d 1226, 1234 (9th Cir. 1999), Bennett v. Unisys Corporation, No. 2:99CV0446, 2000 WL 33126583, at *5 (E.D.Pa. Dec.11, 2000); Reese v. American Food Service, No. CIV. A.99-1741, 2000 WL 1470212, at *6 (E.D.Pa. Sept.29, 2000), Tedeschi v. Sysco Foods of Philadelphia, No. CIV. A.99-3170, 2000 WL 1281266, at *5 (E.D.Pa. Sept.5, 2000); Enforcement Guidance on the Americans with Disabilities Act and Psychiatric Disabilities, Compliance Manual, COMPLIANCE MANUAL (CCH) P6906, at 5398 (1998) ("EEOC Compliance Manual"). But See, Sarko v. Penn-Del Directory Co., 968 F. Supp. 1026, 1034 n. 8 (E.D. Pa. 1997) (the ability to get a sound night's sleep and report to work on time and clear-minded was not a major life activity).
84. Sutton v. United Air Lines, 130 F.3d 893, 900 (10th Cir. 1997).
85. See Reberg, 2005 WL 3320780 at *5 (citing Katekovich v. TeamRent A Car of Pittsburgh, Inc., 36 Fed. Appx. 688 (3rd Cir.2002); Green v. Pace Suburban Bus, No. 02 C 3031, 2004 WL 1574246 (N.D. Ill. July 12, 2004)).
86. Pack v. Kmart Corp., 166 F.3d 1300, 1306 (10th Cir. 1999).
87. 29 C.F.R. § 1630.2(j)(2).
88. Mont-Ros v. City of West Miami, 111 F. Supp.2d 1338, 1355 (S.D. Fla. 2000).
89. Peter v. Lincoln Technical Institute, Inc., 255 F. Supp. 417, 434 (E.D. Pa. 2002) (ADA claim denied on other grounds).
90. See, e.g., Taylor v. Blue Cross Blue Shield of Texas, 1999 WL 451339 *4 (N.D. Tex. 1999), Pack v. Kmart Corp., 166 F.3d 1300, 1306 (10th Cir. 1999); Mont-Ros v. City of West Miami, 111 F. Supp.2d 1338 (S.D. Fla. 2000); Kolecyck-Yap v. MCI Worldcom, Inc., No. 99 CV 8414, 2001 WL 245531 (N.D. Ill. 2001); Wendt v. Village of Evergreen Park, No. 00 C 7730, 2003 WL 223443 (N.D. Ill. 2003).
91. Mont-Ros v. City of West Miami, 111 F. Supp.2d 1338, 1346 (S.D. Fla. 2000).
92. Long v. Mid-Tennessee Ford Truck Sales, 160 S.W.3d 504, 509 (Tenn. 2005).
93. Burlington Industries, Inc. v. Ellerth, 524 U.S. 742, 756 (1998).
94. Dunlap v. W.L. Logan Trucking Co., 161 Ohio App. 3d 51 (2005).
95. Dunlap v. W.L. Logan Trucking Co., 161 Ohio App. 3d 51, 66 (2005).
96. Dunlap v. W.L. Logan Trucking Co., 161 Ohio App. 3d 51, 67 (2005).
97. Dunlap v. W.L. Logan Trucking Co., 161 Ohio App. 3d 51, 68 (2005).
98. Dunlap v. W.L. Logan Trucking Co., 161 Ohio App. 3d 51, 69 (2005).
99. Martinez v. CO2 Services, Inc., No. 00-2218, slip op. at 7, (10th Cir. April 12, 2001).
100. 10 N.Y. Comp. Codes & Regs., tit. 10, § 405.4 (2002). First enacted in 1989, the regulations limit resident scheduling to no more than 80 hours per week, averaged over four weeks. Shifts are limited to 24 hours with flexibility for certain surgery residents. Violators face significant monetary fines.
101. Baggett v. Brumfield, 758 So.2d 332, 336 (La. App.3d Cir. 2000).
102. Faverty v. McDonald's Restaurants of Oregon, Inc., 133 Or. App. 514, 893 P.2d 703 (1995).
103. Snowbarger v. Tri-County Electric Coop., 793 S.W.2d 348 (Mo. 1990) (electric lineman worked 86 of 100 hour work period during snow emergency and fell asleep at the

wheel); Van Devander v. Heller Electric Co., 405 F.2d 1108 (D.C.Cir. 1968) (an electrical equipment installer worked twenty-six consecutive hours on the job and fell asleep from fatigue).

104. Maryland Transit Administration Light Rail Vehicle Accidents at the Baltimore-Washington International Airport Transit Station near Baltimore, Maryland, February 13 and August 15, 2000, Railroad Special Investigation Report NTSB/SIR- 01/02 (Washington, D.C: NTSB, 2001); and Grounding of the Liberian Passenger Ship STAR PRINCESS on Poundstone Rock, Lynn Canal, Alaska, June 23, 1995, Marine Accident Report NTSB/MAR-97/02 (Washington, D.C: NTSB, 1997).

105. National Safety Transportation Board Report No. RAR-02/04, 27, "Railroad Accident Report, Collision of Two Canadian National/Illinois Central Railway Trains Near Clarkston, Michigan, November 15, 2001," (November 19, 2002).

106. National Safety Transportation Board Report No. RAR-02/04, 28 (November 19, 2002).

107. Department of Transportation, Federal Railroad Administration, "Notice of Safety Advisory 2004-04; Effect of Sleep Disorders on Safety of Railroad Operations," 69 Fed. Reg. 190, 58995, 58996 (October 1, 2004).

108. 49 CFR § 391.41.

109. 49 CFR § 391.41(b)(5), (8).

110. 49 CFR § 391.43; Final Rule, Department of Transportation, Federal Motor Carrier Safety Administration, "Physical Qualification of Drivers; Medical Examination; Certificate," 65 Fed. Reg. 194, 59363-59380 (October 5, 2000).

111. Federal Motor Carrier Safety Administration, Advisory Criteria, The Conference on Pulmonary/Respiratory Disorders and Commercial Drivers, FHWA-MC-91-004, at 5 (1991), http://www.fmcsa.dot.gov/documents/pulmonary1.pdf, (accessed March 2006).

112. Federal Motor Carrier Safety Administration, Advisory Criteria; Conference on Neurological Disorders and Commercial Drivers at: http://www.fmcsa.dot.gov/rules-regs/medreports.html "Seizures, Epilepsy and Interstate Commercial Driving," http://www.fmcsa.dot.gov/documents/neuro2.pdf.

113. Electronic Guide for Aviation Medical Examiners, http://www.faa.gov/about/office_org/headquarters_offices/avs/offices/aam/ame/guide/media/sec3.pdf, 61, (July 31, 2005) (accessed March 2006).

114. Electronic Guide for Aviation Medical Examiners, "AASI For History of Sleep Apnea," (January 16, 2006), http://www.faa.gov/about/office_org/headquarters_offices/avs/offices/aam/ame/guide/media/aasisleep.pdf (accessed March 2006).

115. 10 CFR Part 26, 54 Fed. Reg. 24468.

116. Nuclear Regulatory Commission, Proposed Rule, "Fitness for Duty Programs," 70 Fed. Reg. 165 50442-50620 (August 26, 2005).

117. 42 U.S.C. § 1395nn.

118. 66 Fed. Reg. 3; 880 (January 4, 2001).

119. 42 U.S.C. § 1395nn(h)(6)(F).

25 · A Concluding Note and Future Directions

William C. Dement
Stanford Sleep Research Center, Palo Alto, California, U.S.A.

Obstructive sleep apnea (OSA) and other sleep-related breathing disorders are arguably the number one health problem in the United States if not the entire world. Given the high prevalence, it is amazing that this problem was completely unknown to the general public as well as health professionals as recently as 1965 and mostly unknown until the late 1970s. In addition to the actual obstructive sleep disorder itself, there are strong associations with cardiovascular disease, fatigue, mental impairment, diabetes, obesity, and probably a host of other less well-documented associations.

All of the above receives a detailed description in these two volumes. It is worth noting that early on, Stanford sleep specialists realized the high prevalence of OSA. We also realized that a standard model to deal with the condition should be established. Finally, we knew it would be necessary to start training other physicians to diagnose and treat OSA. This led directly to the establishment of the formal clinical practice specialty of sleep medicine, which deals exclusively with the diagnosis and treatment of sleep disorders.

As with anything else, there are those who insist on only the most high-tech approaches. This is no longer appropriate. I have always said probably 90% of victims can be identified by asking two questions: *(i)* Do you snore loudly or does the bed partner, if there is one, complain? and *(ii)* Are you unusually tired when you are awake throughout the daytime with no apparent cause? If the answers to both the foregoing questions are "yes," OSA is highly likely. Keep in mind that individuals often do not seem to be aware of their fatigue, and among other individuals there is often a misapprehension that the tiredness is caused by depression, anemia, or some other esoteric problem. Any time there is loud snoring, check it out. As I have indicated, checking it out could not be easier. In fact, an educated bed partner can easily assess the implications of the snoring.

One of the problems we have encountered is that this area of human behavior is strange and frightening to many people. Some years ago, we showed a film clip of patients being treated with continuous positive airway pressure (CPAP) to a group of burly, tough, long-haul truck drivers. They were visibly shaken by the strangeness of patients sleeping with CPAP machines. Therefore, bestowing the benefits of the diagnosis of OSA on most individuals will certainly require extra efforts of persuading and convincing.

All of this is very ambitious, but clearly, as the large-scale clinical trials such as the Apnea Positive Pressure Long-term Efficacy Study (APPLES) now being conducted demonstrate, there is a pressing need for additional research in the service of prevention and diagnostic methodologies for all potential patient populations, including infants and children. There is promise of meeting some of this need in the near future, as less expensive and more accessible diagnostic tools, such as portable monitoring, are now being evaluated as a reasonable alternative to the in-laboratory polysomnogram. Above all, there is an even greater need for research in the service of the development of new treatment modalities and conclusive testing of those currently available. Partnerships between academia and industry, once frowned upon but now viewed as almost a codependent relationship, can help to foster the development of these newer treatment technologies. It is important to realize that the field of apnea treatment has made significant advances since the development of CPAP a little over a quarter of a century ago, but much more needs to be accomplished in sleep apnea patient care and research to develop treatments that are more palatable and accessible to those with this debilitating condition.

I have taught "Sleep and Dreams," which is the largest undergraduate course at Stanford, for over 30 years. During this time, I have witnessed countless personal stories in which students have learned about sleep apnea through my course and then subsequently educated and encouraged their family and friends suspected of having sleep apnea to obtain professional help for their condition. Based on this experience, there is a need to promote more education about sleep apnea and other sleep disorders not only at the medical or graduate student, resident, and practicing physician levels, but also at the undergraduate student levels. Only in doing so can we increase the awareness of this condition within the general public as well as to encourage others to enter the field to find better diagnostic and treatment options for sleep apnea sufferers.

There have been strong efforts in the public awareness and advocacy sectors, notably the National Commission on Sleep Disorders Research which issued its final report "Wake Up America: A National Sleep Alert" in 1993 after its two-year study, and more recently, the Institute of Medicine's report, "Sleep Disorders and Sleep Deprivation: An Unmet Public Health Problem," which was released in 2006. Given the existence of the National Center on Sleep Disorders Research in the National Heart, Lung and Blood Institute and the scope of the problem, it is absolutely essential that this center be accorded a much higher priority and a much larger budget from its parent institute and/or the US Congress, or perhaps it should be a freestanding entity. At the moment, the will to strongly advocate such improvements does not seem to exist among patients and practitioners, but the professional organizations representing this field, to wit, the American Academy of Sleep Medicine, the Sleep Research Society, the American Association of Sleep Technologists, and the National Sleep Foundation must respond to the challenge. There are also patient organizations, in particular the American Sleep Apnea Association as well as smaller local organizations. The moral imperative, however, is that we can and therefore we must deplore the diminished health, quality of life, and shortened-life expectancy of human beings afflicted with OSA and because we can, we must work as hard as possible to change their lives for the better.

Index